Cardiovascular Surgery 1980

Proceedings of the 29th International Congress of the European Society of Cardiovascular Surgery

Edited by

W. Bircks, J. Ostermeyer, H.D. Schulte

With 300 Figures and 271 Tables

Springer-Verlag Berlin Heidelberg New York 1981

Professor Dr. W. Bircks
Chirurgische Universitätsklinik B
Moorenstraße 5, D-4000 Düsseldorf 1

Priv.-Doz. Dr. med. J. Ostermeyer
Chirurgische Universitätsklinik B
Moorenstraße 5, D- 4000 Düsseldorf 1

Professor Dr. H. D. Schulte
Chirurgische Universitätsklinik B
Moorenstraße 5, D-4000 Düsseldorf 1

ISBN -13 : 987-3-642-68174-5 e-ISBN -13 : 987-3-642-68172-1
DOI: 10.1007/987-3-642-68172-1

Softcover reprint of the hardcover 1st edition 1981

2127/3130-543210

Preface

This volume contains the revised texts of the presentations at the 29th International Congress of the European Society of Cardiovascular Surgery, held from July 2-5, 1980, in Düsseldorf under the presidency of Jan Nielobowicz (Warsaw).

We express our gratitude to all the authors who have been participating in the Congress, in particular to the invited speakers A.R. Castañeda (Boston), D.B. Effler (Syracuse), F. Fontan (Bordeaux), F. Robicsek (Charlotte), and D.N. Ross (London) for their cooperation.

We are grateful to our colleagues of the Surgical Department B at the University of Düsseldorf, J.A. Herzer, G. Irlich, R. Körfer, and A. Krian, for their help during preparation and organisation of the Congress.

Finally, we are indebted to Sanol Schwarz GmbH for its support of this publication.

Düsseldorf, June 1981

Wolfgang Bircks
Jörg Ostermeyer
Hagen D. Schulte

Contents

Session III Cardiac Surgery

Tachycardiac Rhythm Disorders Coronary Disease

Chairman: C. Hahn, Geneva; Co-Chairman: H.H. Bentall, London

Invited Lecture

Session IV Vascular Surgery

Combined Disease of the Aorto-iliac and Femoro-popliteal Arteries

Chairman: M. Vink, Leiden; Co-Chairman: J. Vollmar, Ulm

Vascular Forum II

Chairman: J. Sautot, Lyon; Co-Chairman: R. May, Innsbruck

Session IX Joint Session

Infections in Cardiovascular Surgery

Chairman: C. Hahn, Geneva; Co-Chairman: G. Poulias, Athens

Leriche Lecture

Session X Cardiac Surgery

Cardiac Forum II

Chairman: M.E.M. Macedo, Lisbon; Co-Chairman: P. Satter, Frankfurt

Author Index

Vascular Forum IV

Chairman: P. Balas, Athens; Co-Chairman: J. van der Stricht, Brusselles

Film Session Cardiovascular Surgery

Chairman: H. Dalichau, Cologne; Co-Chairman: J.C. Reidemeister, Essen

The Contribution of European Surgeons to the Development of Modern Vascular Surgery

J. Nielubowicz

Your excellencies Mr. Ministers, Rector Magnificus, Professor Hahn, Professor Bircks, Members and Guests of the Society.

It is a great honour and an extremely high distinction to be elected president of the European Society of Cardiovascular Surgery. I feel very grateful to you for that promotion the more so that I have been elected to that high post by the cardiovascular surgeons of Europe. Born and educated in the eastern part of our continent, I feel like other surgeons from that region strong ties and firm links with the spirit and culture of Europe. I feel strongly so and with this solemn opening address I want to pay tribute to the effort and success of European vascular surgeons for whom I have such a great admiration and who have contributed so much to the development of modern surgery (Fig. 1).

I have been always told that the Europeans, since the time of Descartes, have always excelled in their passion for analysis. Before doing anything that was really important, deciding something really valuable, discovering new rules, ideas or devising new constructions the European is used at first to divide every problem into separate parts. These parts are then developed, forming the basis for reevaluation of old ideas, new constructions or new concepts.

Following these I tried to divide into parts the modern vascular surgery looking for its most basic components. It was not easy but after many doubts and hesitations I came to the conclusion that contemporary vascular surgery is based on ten principal, crucial discoveries, statements or principles which might be considered as milestones. They are: 1) arterial suture, 2) sympathectomy, 3) heparin, 4) vascular grafts, 5) thromboendareterectomy, 6) synthetic grafts, 7) arteriography, 8) embolectomy catheter, 9) venous surgery, and 10) lymphography.

I gathered these milestones presenting them in form of symbols which might be understandable even to those who know nothing about our history and culture. Setting these symbols in the form of a message I tried to imitate those who launched in 1971 the Explorer providing it with well-know symbols which might be understandable to thinking beings (Fig. 2). Maybe somebody in Space would like to become a vascular surgeon.

Let me discuss these points more precisely (Fig. 1).

The Arterial Suture

With bad suture material and frequent infections the arterial sutures and arterial anastomoses of early times were usually bad. It comes from the nineteenth century writings that there were three principal things which surgeons of these times feared in respect to arterial suture: early thrombosis, a foreign body in form of a thread in the lumen of the artery and haemorrhage which was supposed to originate from the holes that were left by the suturing needle. Lambert, a surgeon at

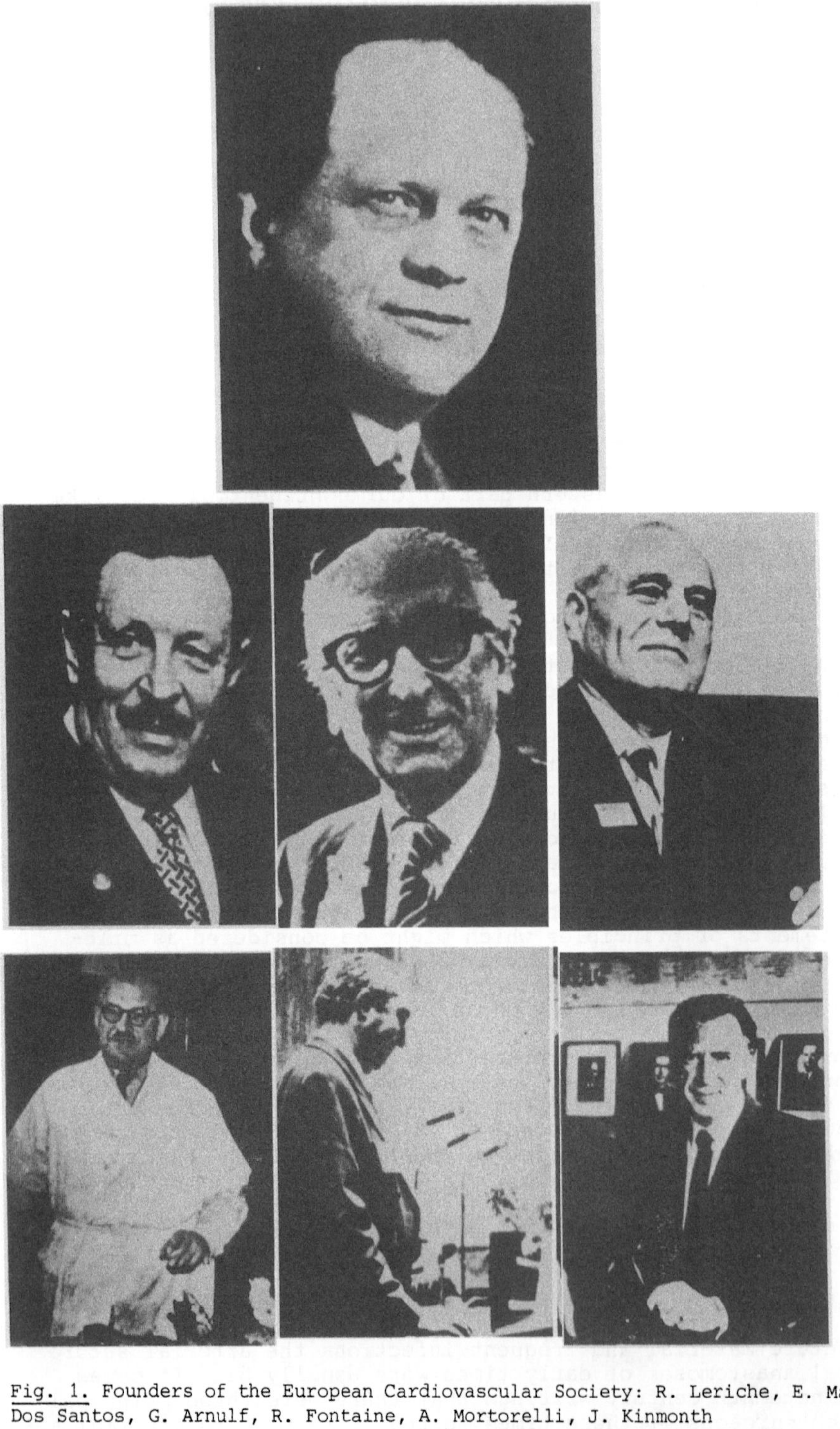

Fig. 1. Founders of the European Cardiovascular Society: R. Leriche, E. Malan, J. Cid Dos Santos, G. Arnulf, R. Fontaine, A. Mortorelli, J. Kinmonth

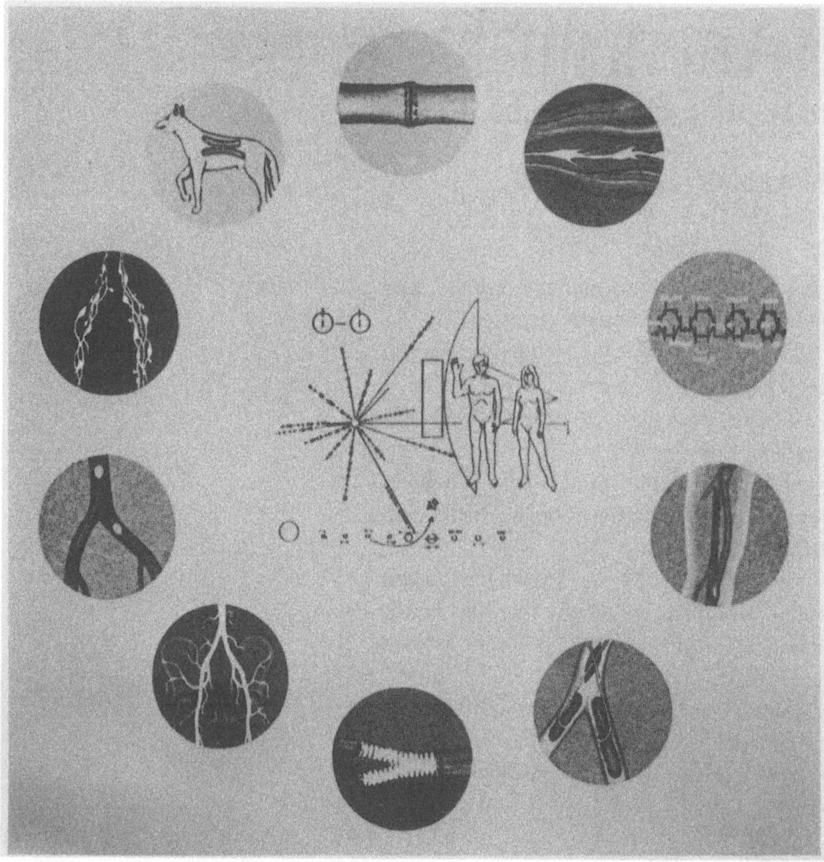

Fig. 2. Ten milestones of contemporary vascular surgery as imagined by the author: *1*, arterial suture; *2*, sympathectomy; *3*, heparin; *4*, vascular grafts; *5*, thromboendarterectomy; *6*, synthetic grafts; *7*, arteriography; *8*, embolectomy catheter; *9*, venous surgery; *10*, lymphography

Newcastle upon Tyne, was the first to make the suggestion in 1762 that an arterial suture should be done in the same way as sutures of other tissues. In 1759 Hallowell applied it clinically using a veterinary stitch which was usually applied to repair the cleft lips. A false aneurysm of the brachial artery was repaired in this way. The wound healed and the artery stayed patent but despite success nobody followed Hallowell at that time. It was Jassinowski from Vienna who is considered to be the next one to take over the problem again in 1889. Working on dogs, horses and lambs Jassinowski succeeded in obtaining in 10 out of 32 animals good healing of the severed artery without haemorrhag or thrombosis. To avoid the feared foreign body in the lumen of the sutured vessel Jassinowski sutured the arterial wall only partially. He passed with his needle only through the outer layer of the artery leaving the intima intact (Fig. 3).

Jassinowski's success stimulated others to continue the research in the field of arterial suture. In 1899 Dörfler proved that in arterial suture the thread which embraces the whole thickness of the artery does not provoke thrombosis (Fig. 4). With that statement ingenious techniques of arterial sutures were devised at that time by many European authors. Jaboulay and Briau signed in 1896 a circular anastomosis by means of interrupted mattress sutures. Other types of sutures were

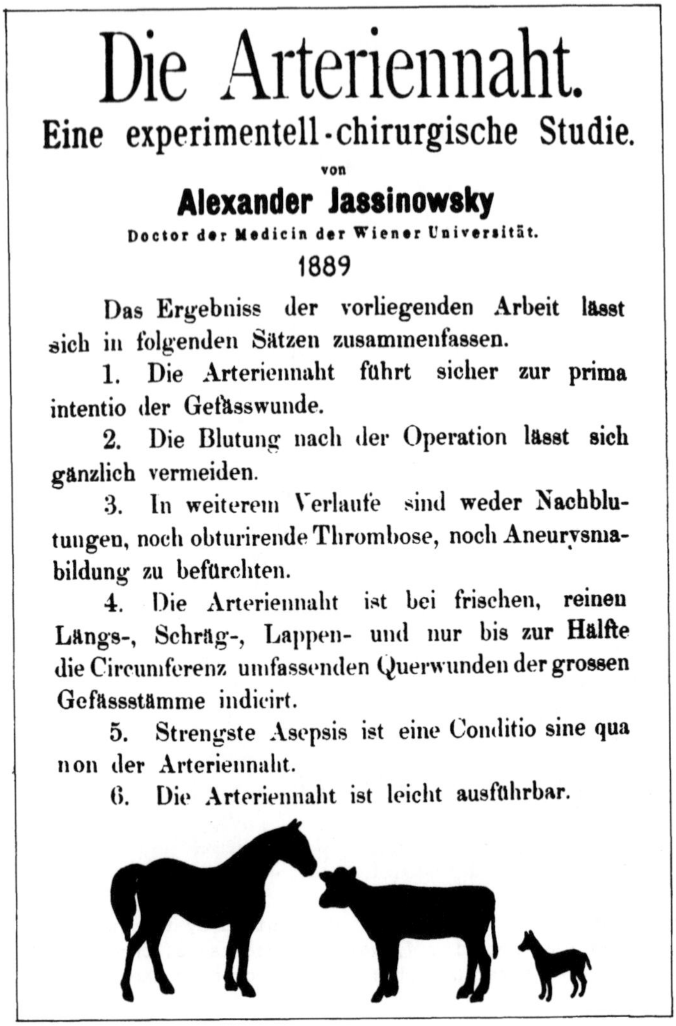

Die Arteriennaht.

Eine experimentell-chirurgische Studie.

von

Alexander Jassinowsky

Doctor der Medicin der Wiener Universität.

1889

Das Ergebniss der vorliegenden Arbeit lässt sich in folgenden Sätzen zusammenfassen.

1. Die Arteriennaht führt sicher zur prima intentio der Gefässwunde.

2. Die Blutung nach der Operation lässt sich gänzlich vermeiden.

3. In weiterem Verlaufe sind weder Nachblutungen, noch obturirende Thrombose, noch Aneurysmabildung zu befürchten.

4. Die Arteriennaht ist bei frischen, reinen Längs-, Schräg-, Lappen- und nur bis zur Hälfte die Circumferenz umfassenden Querwunden der grossen Gefässstämme indicirt.

5. Strengste Asepsis ist eine Conditio sine qua non der Arteriennaht.

6. Die Arteriennaht ist leicht ausführbar.

Fig. 3. Jassinowski's final conclusions. Photographed from his inaugural dissertation which was delivered in Dorpat in 1899

described by Gluck, Silberberger, Dorrance and others (Fig. 5). Soon after, the first successful circular arterial suture in man was performed in the USA by Murphy. In Europe according to what I found in the literature successful lateral arterial sutures were done in men in 1885 by Heidenhein, Zoege v. Manteuffell and Israel, in 1896 by Sabaniejeff and Marken and in 1896 by Dörfler, Lindner and Garre. In 1900 Payr fearing that a simple circular suture would not withstand the pressure within large arteries devised a method of uniting divided vessels by invaginating the ends of the arteries over absorbable magnesium rings (Fig. 6).

The modern methods of vascular anatomosis were elaborated by Alexis Carrel in 1902. The ends of the artery to be sutured were first united by three terminal stay sutures of fine silk positioned at equidistant points of the anastomotic line. With the difference that many surgeons use two stay sutures, the Carrel suture became the method of choice of many of us (Figs. 7 and 8).

BEITRÄGE

ZUR

KLINISCHEN CHIRURGIE

Von

Dr. Julius Dörfler,

approb. Arzt aus Weissenburg a/S.

TÜBINGEN 1899

VERLAG DER H. LAUPP'SCHEN BUCHHANDLUNG

Resumiere ich, so möchte ich die Frage, ob die Naht durch alle oder nur die beiden äussersten Schichten zu wählen sei, folgendermassen beantworten: Die Naht durch die ganze Wanddicke bietet dieselben günstigen Aussichten für ein Gelingen der Naht wie die Naht nur durch Adventitia und Media, kann also in allen Fällen, wo eine Arteriennaht in Frage kommt, unbedenklich angewendet werden. Auf jeden Fall lässt sie sich rascher ausführen und bietet grössere Sicherheit, als die Naht nur durch die beiden äussersten Schichten.

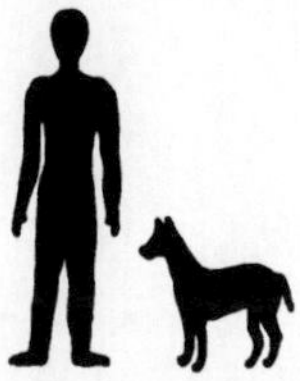

Fig. 4. Dörfler's statement: in arterial suture the thread can pass through all layers of the artery without provoking thrombosis

Considering the long-lasting history of arterial suture from 1759 to 1902 it is astonishing that something that seemed to be so simple took about 150 years to become generally accepted.

Sympathectomy

The first lumbar sympathectomy in a man was performed in 1924 by Julio Diaz. Although it was done in Argentina the idea of that operation was conceived in Europe. It was Claude Bernard who first observed that transsection of cervical sympathetic trunk of the rabbit is followed by warming of the ear (Fig. 9). The first clinical application of that rule was made by Leriche who started periarterial sympathectomies in 1920. In the previous generation of surgeons different types of sympathectomies had been repeatedly carried out all over the world. It was the operation of choice for all types of peripheral ischemia. It is still being performed in many vascular centers in the world.

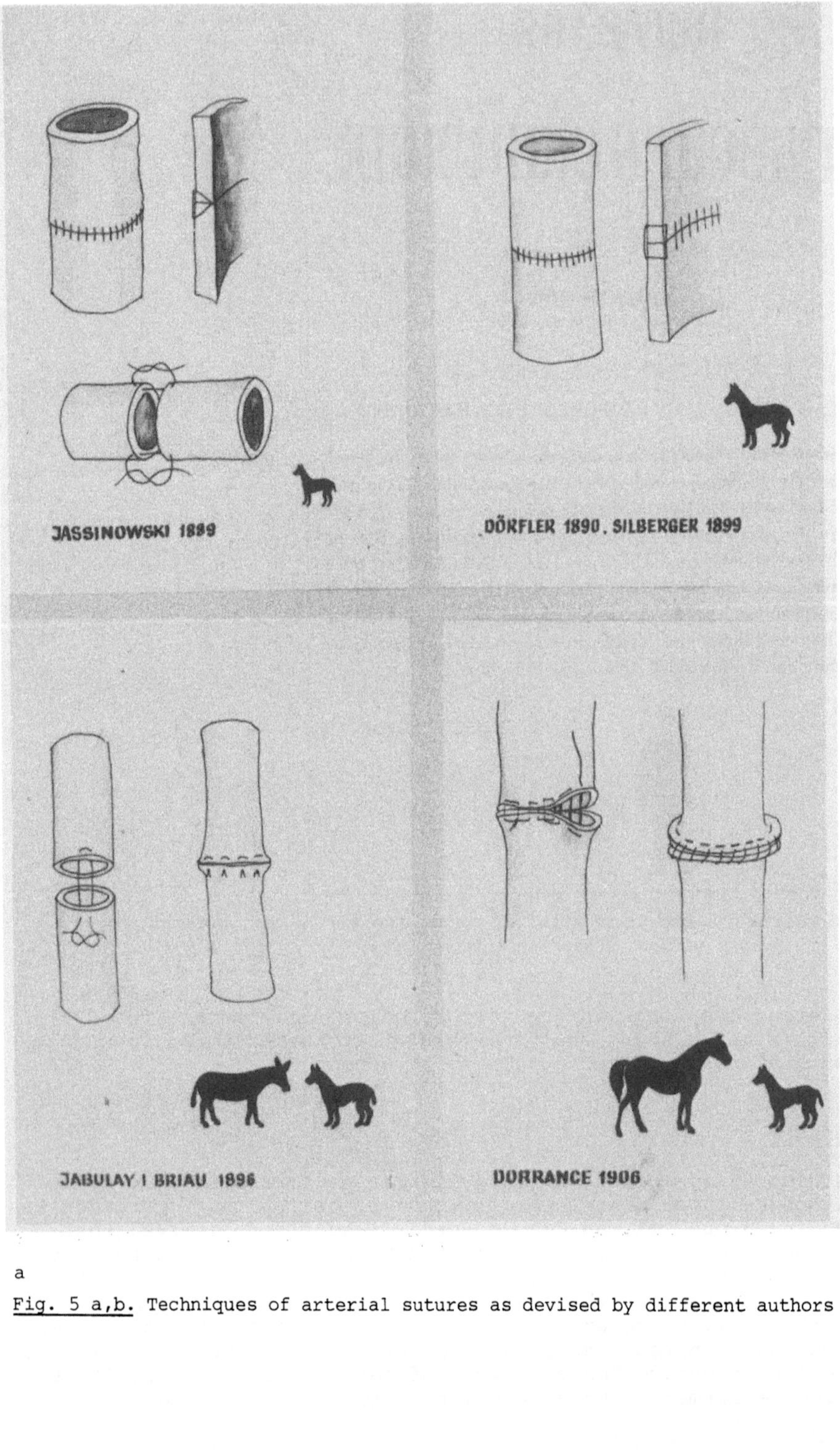

a

Fig. 5 a,b. Techniques of arterial sutures as devised by different authors

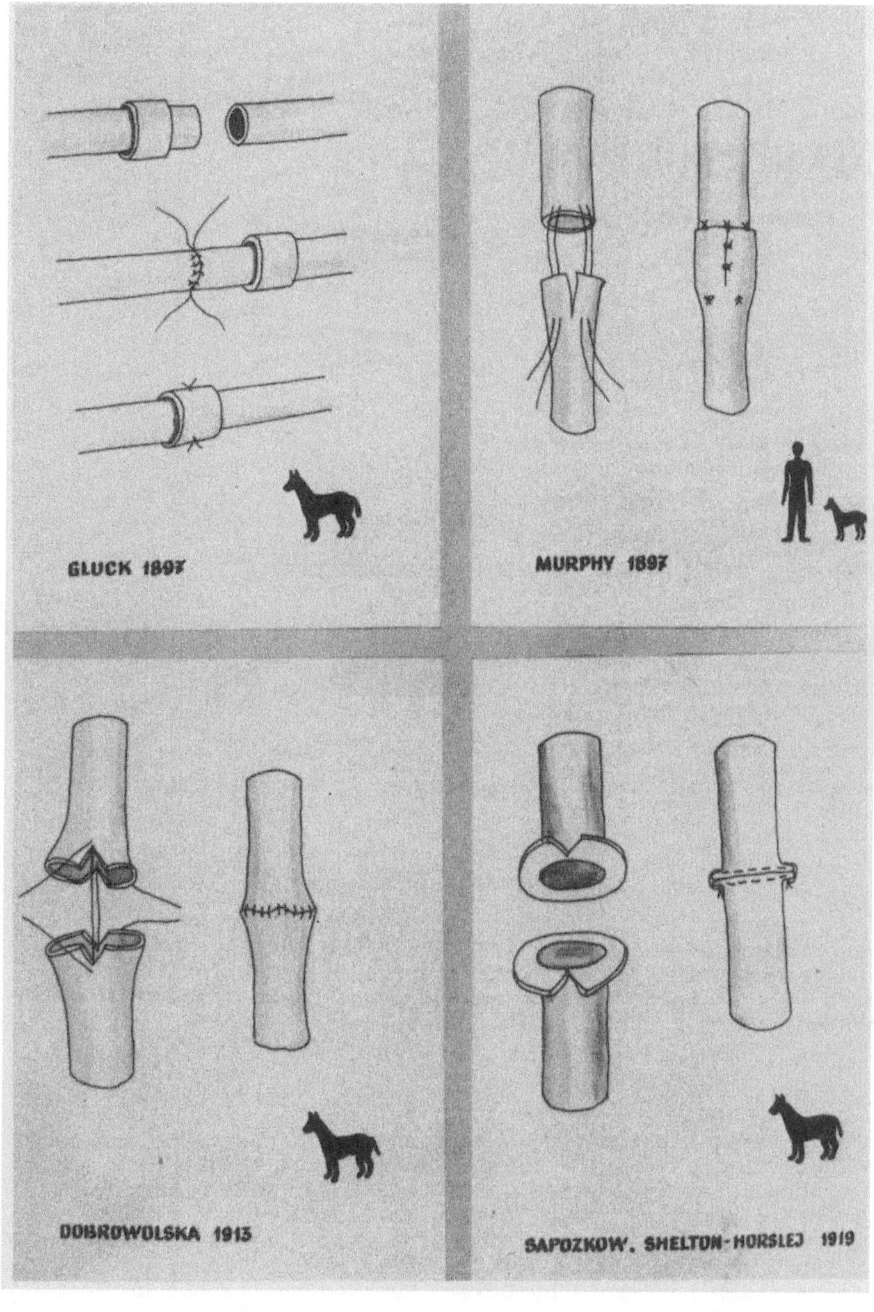
GLUCK 1897
MURPHY 1897
DOBROWOLSKA 1913
SAPOZKOW, SHELTON-HORSLEJ 1919

b

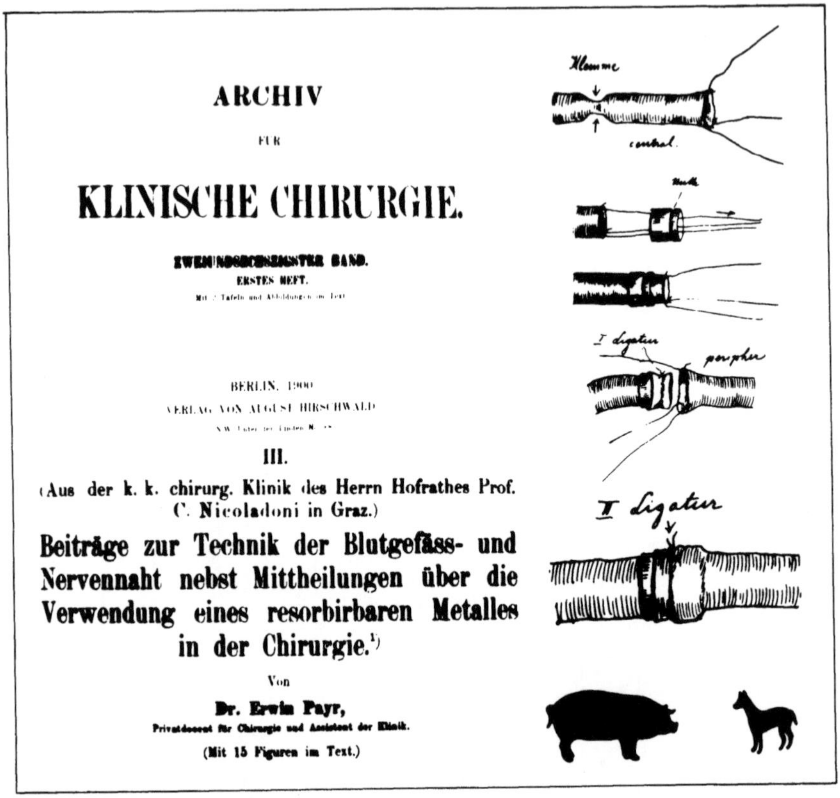

Fig. 6. Payr's method of uniting the ends of transsected artery over absorbable magnesium rings

Heparin

Heparin was discovered in the USA in 1911-1916 by Howell and McLean. The next phase began in 1933 with the preparation of purer heparin. A great part of that work was done in European laboratories by Charles and Scott Schmitz and Fisher and Jorpes.

Vascular Grafts

The first successful experimental venous autograft was performed by Carrel and Guthrie in 1906. The first clinical application of a vein graft was accomplished by Goyanes (1906) and Lexer (1907) (Fig. 10). Goayanes used the popliteal vein in situ to restore the continuity of the popliteal artery after excision of a luetic aneurysm. Eight days after the operation pedal pulses were palpable. The first free venous autograft was performed by Lexer. He used the saphenous vein in two cases to bridge a 3-cm-long defect in the axillary artery resected because of an aneurysm and in a similar way in a case of iliac artery aneurysm. These first vein grafts were followed by 13 cases which were published up to 1918 by Gorcke, Tuffier Pringle, Krause, Enderlen, Pizovano Mantelli Kaorn Omi. In six cases the results were excellent with peripheral pulses palpable 8-10 months postoperatively. During World War I good results of free saphenous vein autograft were reported by Sehert and Weglowski from Poland.

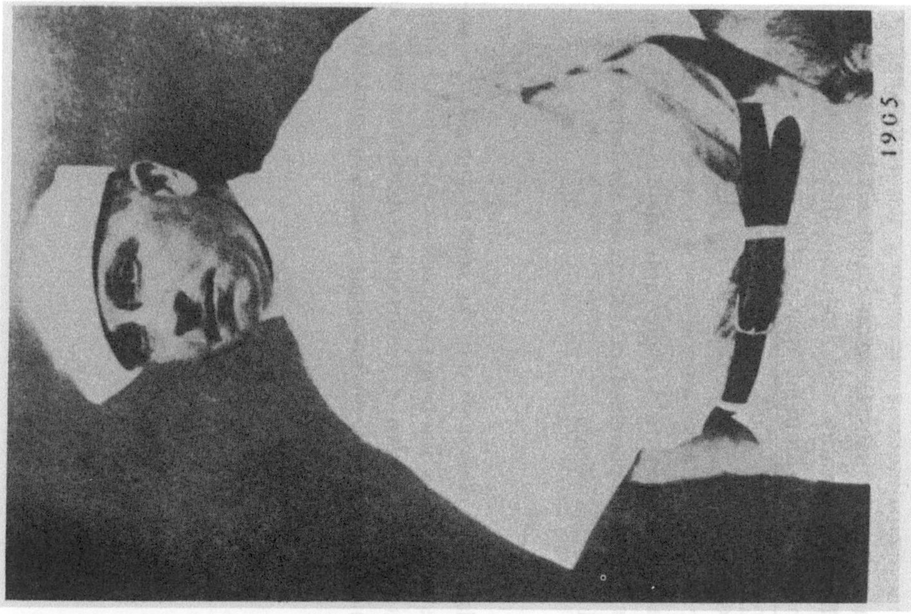
1905

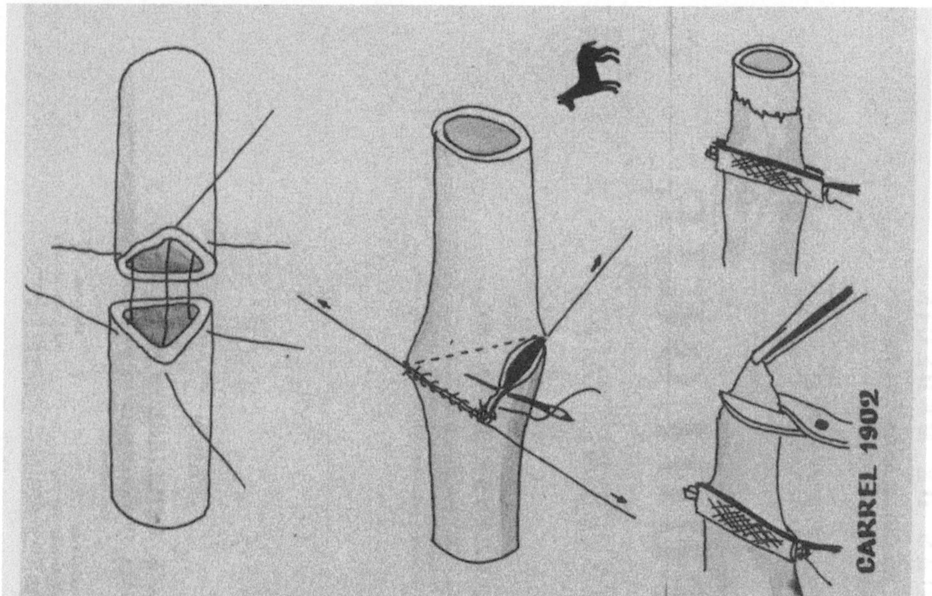
CARREL 1902

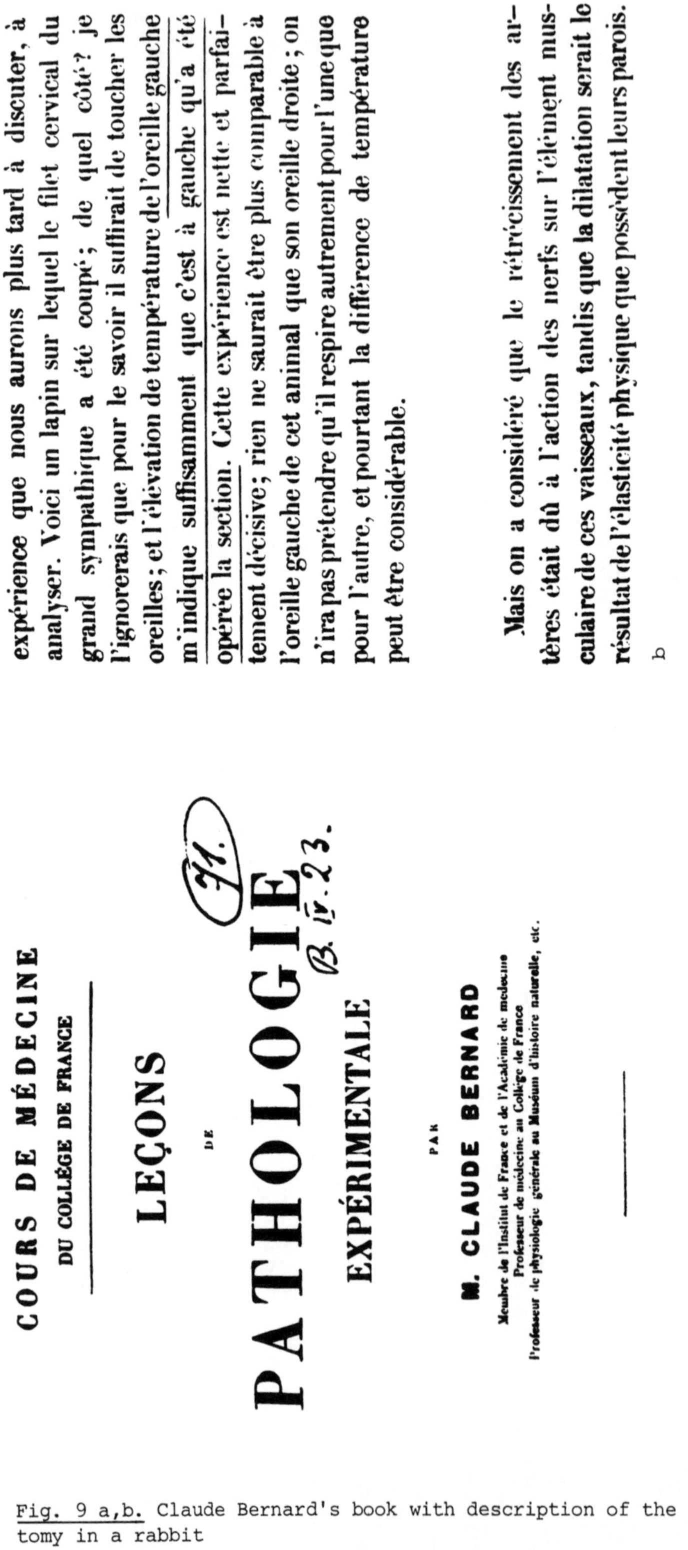
COURS DE MÉDECINE
DU COLLÈGE DE FRANCE

LEÇONS
DE
PATHOLOGIE
EXPÉRIMENTALE

PAR
M. CLAUDE BERNARD
Membre de l'Institut de France et de l'Académie de médecine
Professeur de médecine au Collège de France
Professeur de physiologie générale au Muséum d'histoire naturelle, etc.

PARIS
J. B. BAILLIÈRE ET FILS
LIBRAIRES DE L'ACADÉMIE DE MÉDECINE
Rue Hautefeuille, 19

Londres
Baillière, Tindall and Cox
20, King William street

Madrid
C. Bailly-Baillière
plaza de Topete, 8

1872

a

expérience que nous aurons plus tard à discuter, à analyser. Voici un lapin sur lequel le filet cervical du grand sympathique a été coupé; de quel côté? je l'ignorerais que pour le savoir il suffirait de toucher les oreilles; et l'élévation de température de l'oreille gauche m'indique suffisamment que c'est à gauche qu'a été opérée la section. Cette expérience est nette et parfaitement décisive; rien ne saurait être plus comparable à l'oreille gauche de cet animal que son oreille droite; on n'ira pas prétendre qu'il respire autrement pour l'une que pour l'autre, et pourtant la différence de température peut être considérable.

Mais on a considéré que le rétrécissement des artères était dû à l'action des nerfs sur l'élément musculaire de ces vaisseaux, tandis que la dilatation serait le résultat de l'élasticité physique que possèdent leurs parois.

b

Fig. 9 a,b. Claude Bernard's book with description of the first cervical sympathectomy in a rabbit

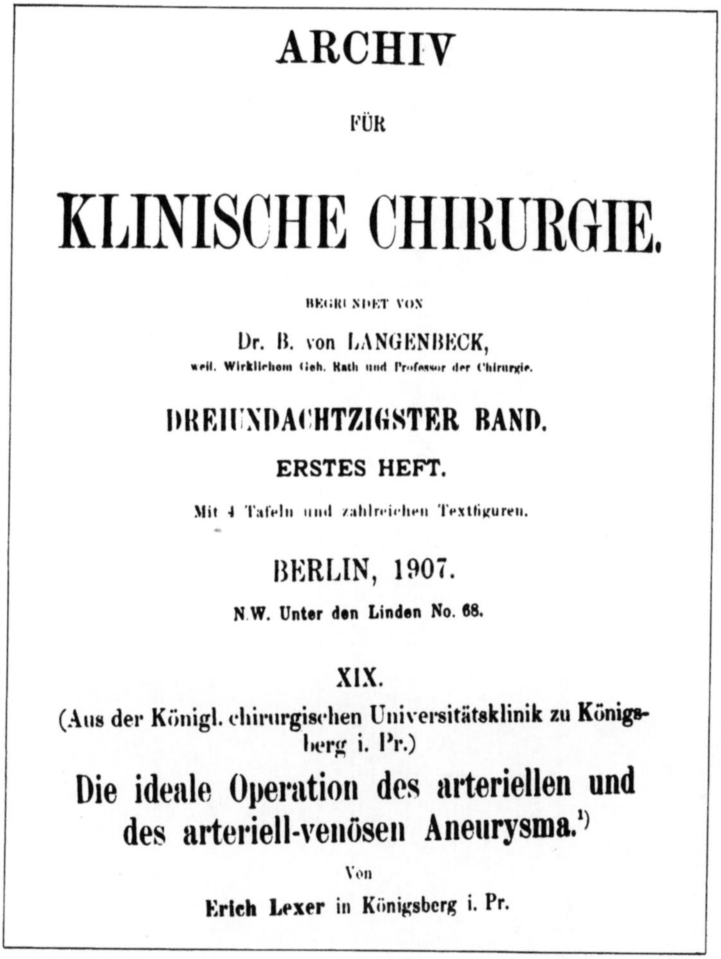

ARCHIV

FÜR

KLINISCHE CHIRURGIE.

BEGRÜNDET VON

Dr. B. von LANGENBECK,

weil. Wirklichem Geh. Rath und Professor der Chirurgie.

DREIUNDACHTZIGSTER BAND.

ERSTES HEFT.

Mit 4 Tafeln und zahlreichen Textfiguren.

BERLIN, 1907.

N.W. Unter den Linden No. 68.

XIX.

(Aus der Königl. chirurgischen Universitätsklinik zu Königsberg i. Pr.)

Die ideale Operation des arteriellen und des arteriell-venösen Aneurysma.[1])

Von

Erich Lexer in Königsberg i. Pr.

Fig. 10. The first free venous autograft performed by Lexer in 1907

In World War II several attempts at autogenous vein grafts were made but without success. Modern vascular grafting started with homografts which were used for congenital vascular abnormalities. This success inspired European surgeons to implant similar grafts in the aorta. In 1951 Oudot reported the first successful resection of aortic bifurcation followed by homograft replacement (Fig. 11). In the same year Dubost performed the successful resection of an aortic abdominal aneurysm with insertion of a formalin-preserved homograft (Fig. 12). These first successful reconstructions were followed in the USA by a great number of different aortic and aortic aneurysms operations with homograft replacements. A great contribution to vascular surgery in management of aortic aneurysm was the development of the graft inlay technique. At the same time that the first homograft was done in the USA, Kunlin of Paris introduced the bypass principle for surgical treatment of femoropopliteal obstruction. This very simple but very efficient method of restoring blood flow to the periphery had a lasting impact on the management of occlusive disease in different parts of the arterial tree (Fig. 13). Kunlin's idea was to perform a parallel shunt with the occluded artery using an end-to-side anastomosis.

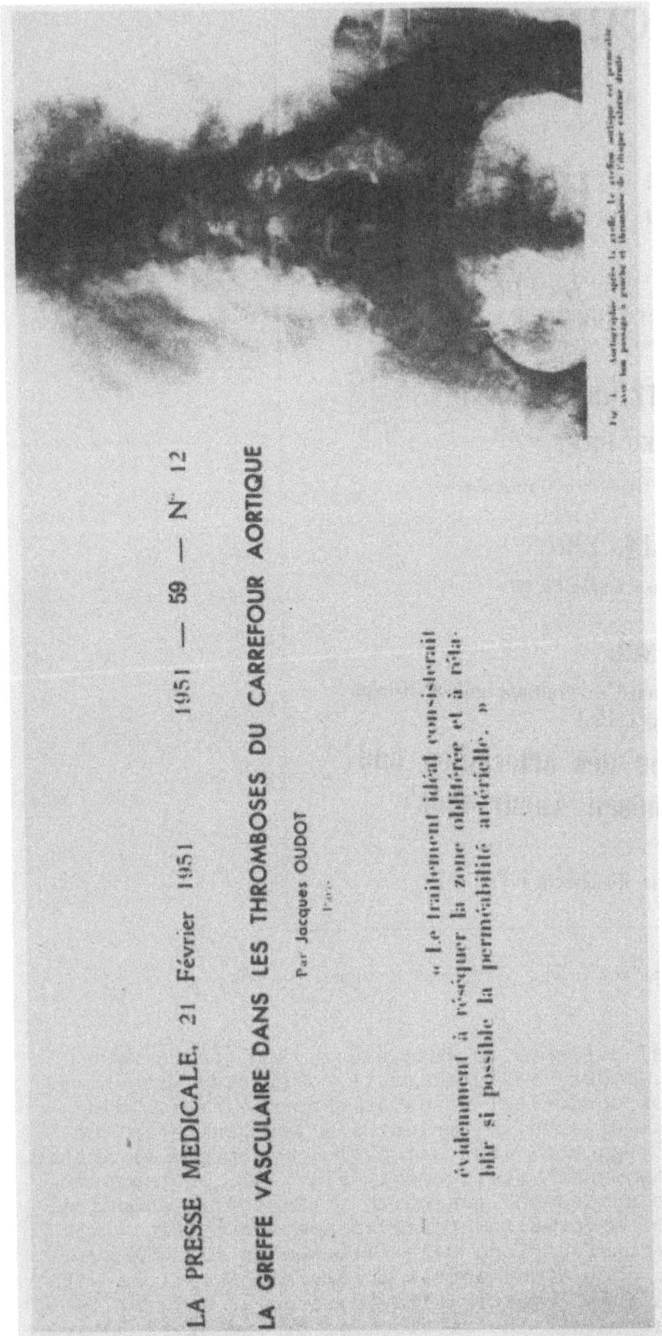

LA PRESSE MEDICALE, 21 Février 1951 — 1951 — 59 — N° 12

LA GREFFE VASCULAIRE DANS LES THROMBOSES DU CARREFOUR AORTIQUE

Par Jacques OUDOT

Paris

« Le traitement idéal consisterait évidemment à réséquer la zone oblitérée et à rétablir si possible la perméabilité artérielle. »

Fig. 11. First successful resection of aortic bifurcation followed by homograft replacement performed by Oudot in 1951

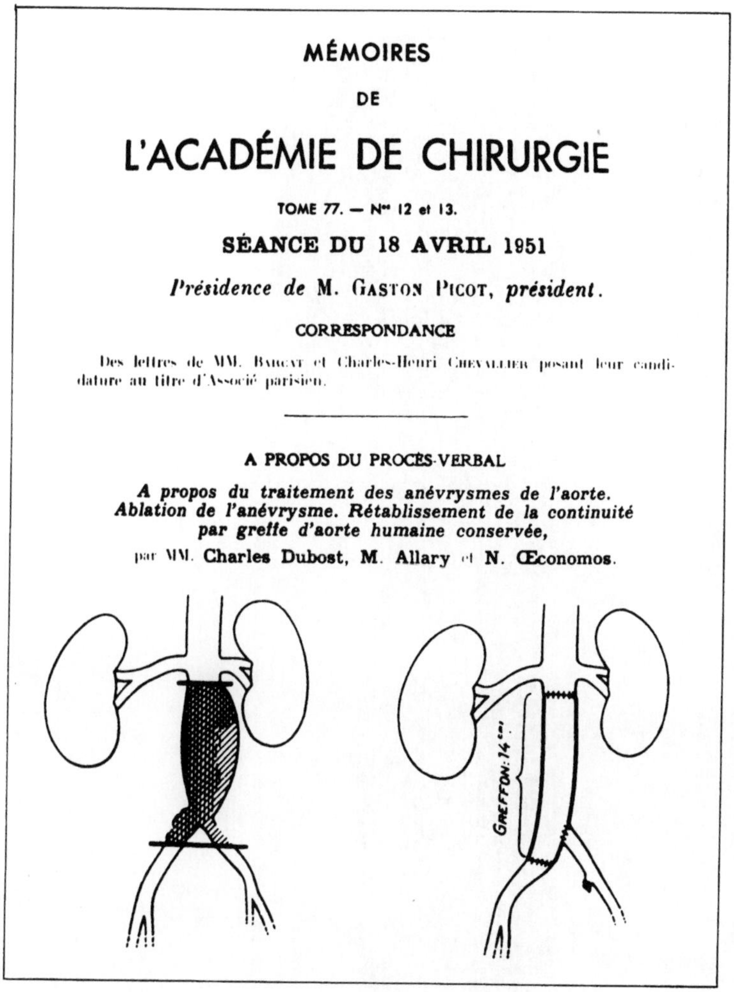

MÉMOIRES

DE

L'ACADÉMIE DE CHIRURGIE

TOME 77. — N°s 12 et 13.

SÉANCE DU 18 AVRIL 1951

Présidence de M. GASTON PICOT, *président*.

CORRESPONDANCE

Des lettres de MM. BAUCAT et Charles-Henri CHEVALLIER posant leur candidature au titre d'Associé parisien.

A PROPOS DU PROCÈS-VERBAL

A propos du traitement des anévrysmes de l'aorte. Ablation de l'anévrysme. Rétablissement de la continuité par greffe d'aorte humaine conservée,

par MM. **Charles Dubost, M. Allary** et **N. Œconomos**.

Fig. 12. First successful resection of aortic abdominal aneurysm performed by Dubost in 1951

Kunlin also devised his technique of end-to-side arteriovenous graft anastomosis, the technique which is used every day by almost all of us (Figs. 14 and 15).

Dr. Kunlin's operation has been rapidly and universally adopted all over the world. I remember Dr. R. Linton from Boston telling how much he was impressed with the original work of Dr. Kunlin when watching him in Paris doing a venous bypass graft in a patient with axillary artery obstruction. Dr. Linton on his return home became a great adherent of that method, using it routinely. Dr. Kunlin's technique was later applied to aortocoronary bypasses. It has been accepted all over the world.

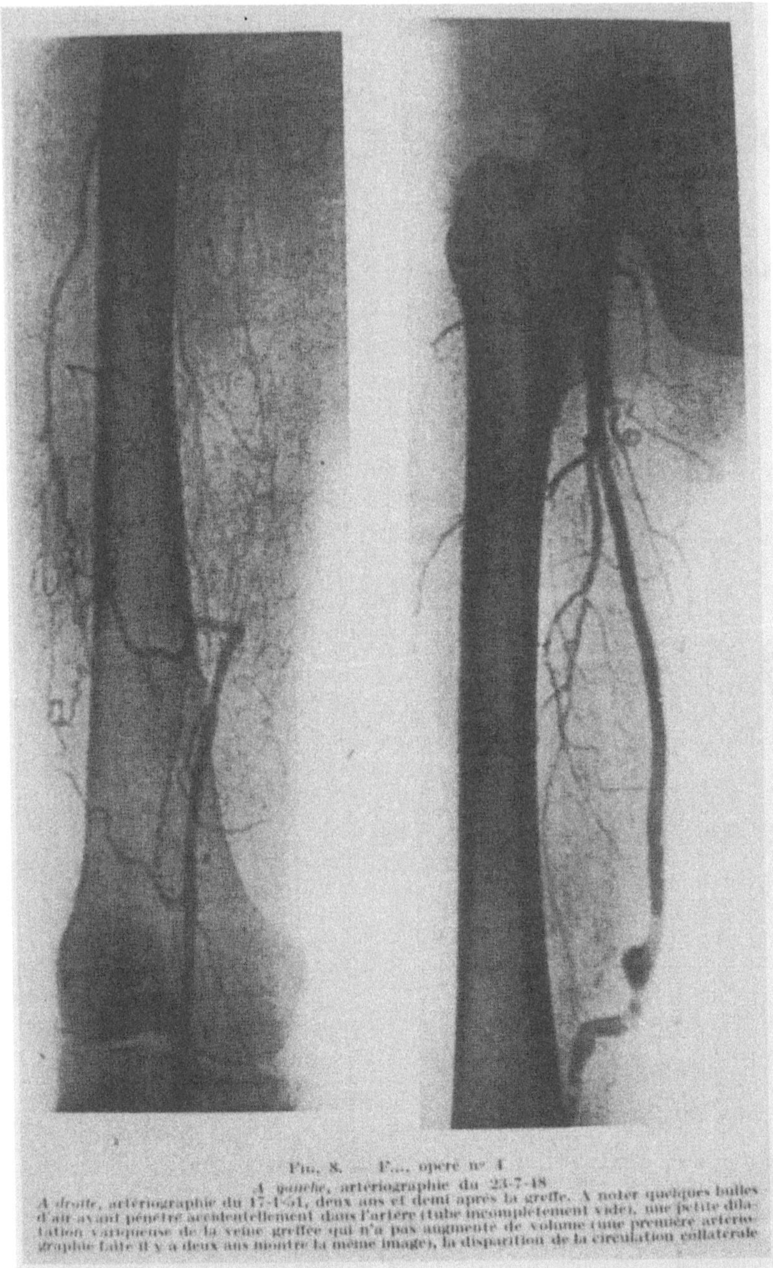

Fig. 13. Saphenous vein bypass graft devised by J. Kunlin in 1951. Arteriography 2 years after grafting

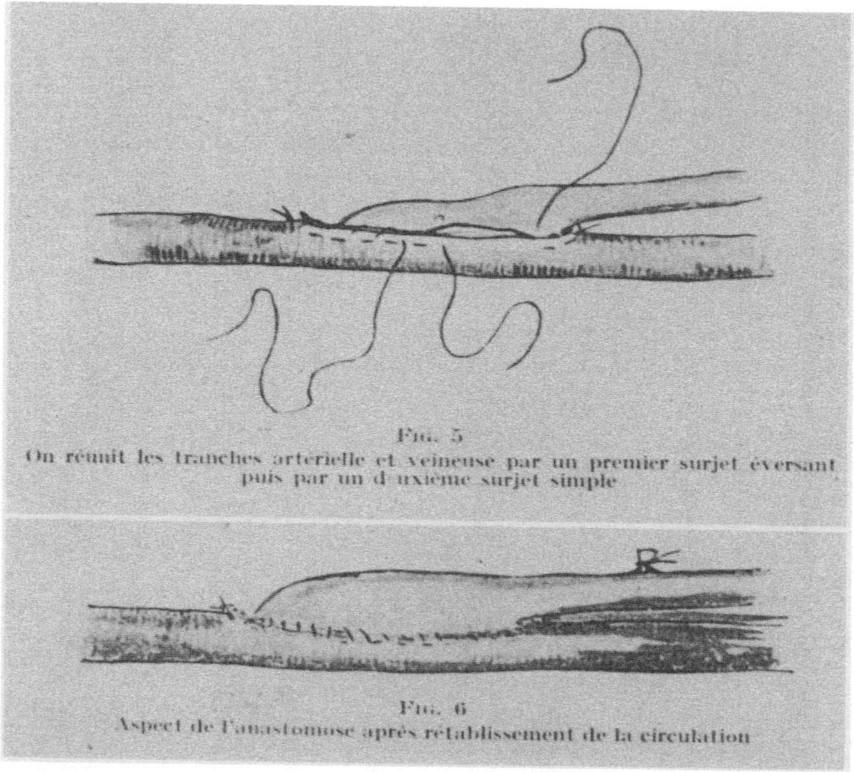

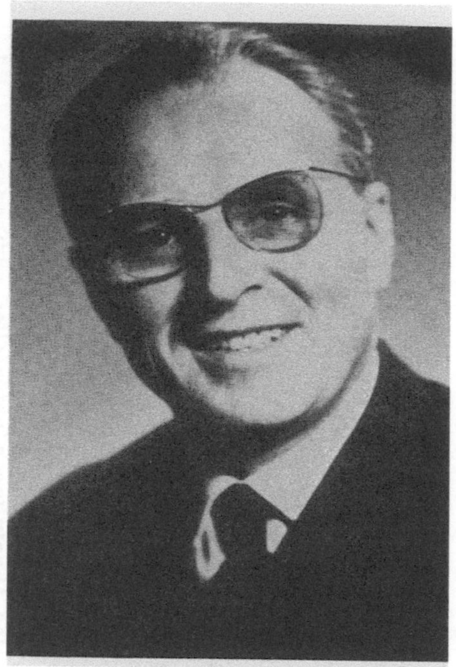

Fig. 14. Kunlin's technique of end-to-side bypassing vein anastomosis

MÉMOIRES DE L'ACADÉMIE DE CHIRURGIE

Séance du 28 Mai 1947.

Présidence de M. PIERRE BROCQ, *président.*

RAPPORT

Sur la désobstruction des thromboses artérielles anciennes,

par M. **Jean Cid dos Santos** (de Lisbonne).

Rapport de M. R. LERICHE.

mais il faut substituer à l'artériectomie la désobstruction à la façon de Santos. Probablement on aura là, avec l'héparine, une conservation de la fonction artérielle.

Fig. 16. J. Cid dos Santos' first thromboendarterectomies presented in 1947 by R. Leriche at the Academie de Chirurgie

Thromboendarterectomy

The credit of thromboendarterectomy goes to J. Cid dos Santos (Fig. 16) although Severeanu and Jianu in 1909 and Delbet in 1906 were probably the first to perform a thrombectomy on an occluded artery. Nevertheless, Cid dos Santos was the first to do what we all perform now as a routine operation, removing from the artery an organised thrombus with a part of media. Cid dos Santos' work is an excellent example of consequence and rational thinking. He tried to do an axillary embolectomy 4 days after its occurrence. Four days later the artery as proved at autopsy was patent. Cid dos Santos attributed his success to heparin which has been given to the patient at the time of the onset of symptoms. Later on, Cid dos Santos tried to do the same in his next patient with organised femoropopliteal arteriosclerotic thrombosis. His second case was as successful as the first one. Leriche when presenting Cid dos Santos' new method hoped that this operation would be superior to arteriectomy which was the operation of choice at that time. Cid dos Santos impressed me enormously in 1966 at the meeting in Brussels. Prominents in vascular surgery presented great statistics of thousands of cases operated upon because of arterial obstruction. Everybody waited with impatience for Cid dos Santos. He presented only about 30 cases. I realised then that in surgery not only figures are important. One can have smaller statistics but great ideas which pass into history.

L'encéphalographie artérielle, son importance dans la localisation des tumeurs cérébrales par Egas Moniz (de Lisbonne.)

(Travail de l'Institut d'Investigations scientifiques Rocha Cabral et de la Clinique neurologique de Lisbonne).

REVUE NEUROLOGIQUE
T. II. N° 1. Juillet 1927.

Communication Egas Moniz.
Société de Neurologie, séance du 7 juillet 1927.)

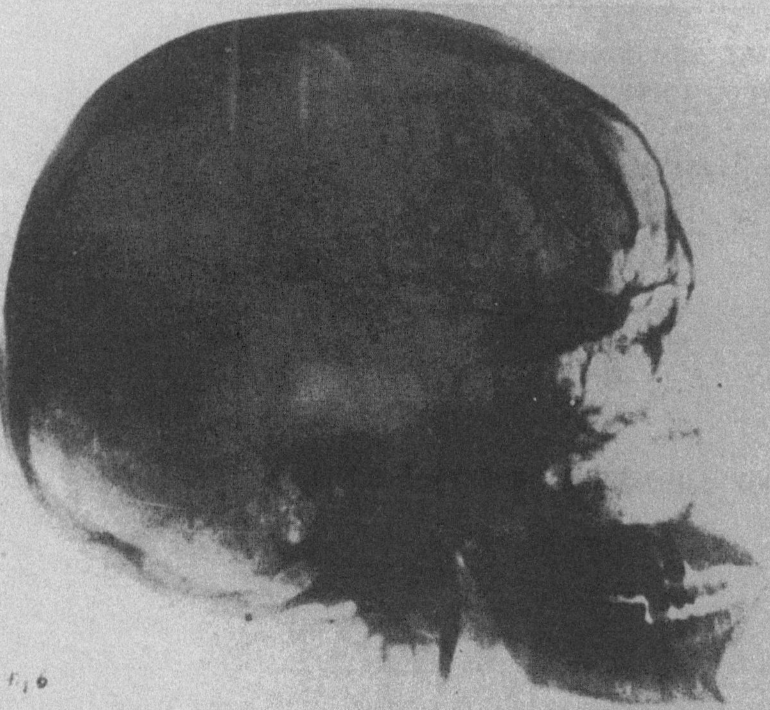

Fig 6. — L'encéphalographie artérielle du réseau cérébral carotidien chez l'homme vivant. Cas de grosse tumeur de l'hypophyse. La carotide est tirée en avant, bien que l'origine de la sylvienne soit plus haute. La cérébrale antérieure, très réduite de volume, est déformée dans sa direction.

Fig. 17. First arteriography in man performed by E. Moniz in 1927

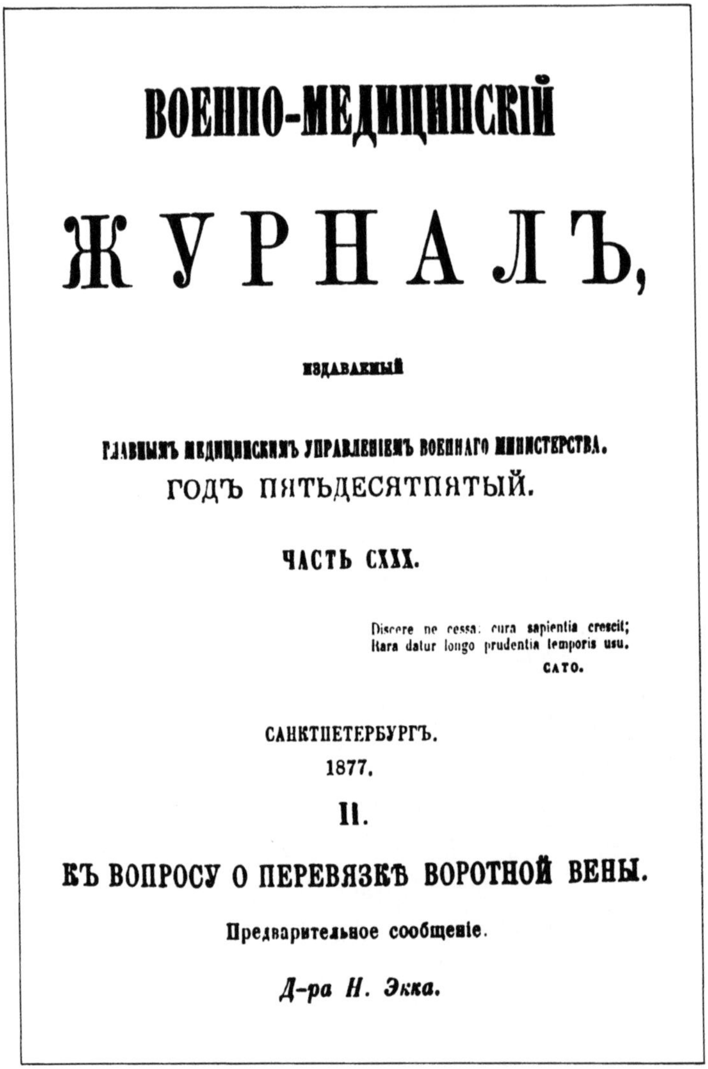

ВОЕННО-МЕДИЦИНСКІЙ

ЖУРНАЛЪ,

издаваемый

главнымъ медицинскимъ управленіемъ военнаго министерства.

ГОДЪ ПЯТЬДЕСЯТПЯТЫЙ.

ЧАСТЬ CXXX.

Discere ne cessa: cura sapientia crescit;
Rara datur longo prudentia temporis usu.
CATO.

САНКТПЕТЕРБУРГЪ.
1877.

II.

КЪ ВОПРОСУ О ПЕРЕВЯЗКѢ ВОРОТНОЙ ВЕНЫ.

Предварительное сообщеніе.

Д-ра Н. Экка.

Fig. 18. Front page and the title of the paper of N. Eck with the first description of an experimental venous side-to-side anastomosis. With that suture Eck performed a port-caval anastomosis known under the name of Eck's fistula

Synthetic Grafts

These were used for the first time clinically in 1953 by Voorhes, Jaretzki and Blakemore in the USA. This new ingenious substitute devised to replace the occluded arteries created enormous new possibilities. It was taken over and developed in Europe at almost the same time as in the USA. Successful aortic arch replacement was performed by Kremer in 1960.

CLINICAL SCIENCE

VOL. II.

LYMPHANGIOGRAPHY IN MAN.

A method of Outlining Lymphatic Trunks at Operation.

By J. B. KINMONTH.*

(*From the Surgical Professorial Unit, St. Bartholomew's Hospital.*)

Received May 9, 1951.

THE lack of a reliable method of studying the lymphatics in man has led to uncertainty about their function in many cases of œdema. In order to determine whether vital dyes could be used to delineate and test the function of main lymph trunks, two dyes were chosen for study. Table I describes their general features.

1952.

Fig. 19. Front page and the title of the paper on lymphography which was invented by J. Kinmonth in 1951

LERICHE R. Le syndrome de l' obliteration termino-aortique artérite. La Presse Médicale 1940. N. 54. 601.

MARTOREL F. in 1944 described the "Synchrome of supra-aortic trunks' obliteration in 1945 "Hypertension ulcers".

EASTCOTT H.H.G. PICKERING G.W. ROB C.G. Reconstruction of internal carotid artery in a patient with intermittent attacks of hemiplegia. Lancet 1954. II. 994.

MARTIN P. RENWICK S. STEPHENSON On the surgery of the profunda femoris artery. Brit. J. Surg. 1968. 55. 539.

Fig. 20. Important clinical descriptions of syndromes and special new indications for surgery which have been done by European surgeons, influencing the present status of vascular surgery

Arteriography

The first arteriography done in a living man for diagnostic purposes was a carotid arteriography. It was done in 1927 by Egaz Moniz (Fig. 17). Two years later Reynolds dos Santos developed the technique of translumbar arteriography. A further step was achieved in 1953 by Seldinger. His technique of transscutaneus arterial catheterisation allowed for more precise selective visualisation of particular arteries.

Embolectomy

Embolectomy, one of the earliest vascular operations, was successfully performed already in 1895 by Sabeniejeff and in 1907 by Moynihan. Nevertheless, the results despite heparin, earlier, better diagnosis and different technical refinements were not good. It was only in 1963 that the introduction by Fogarthy of the embolectomy balloon catheter improved the results in a spectacular way. It was immediately accepted in Europe.

Venous Surgery

Abundance of collatareal circulation lower pressure and slower blood flow in veins make venous surgery difficult. Grafting and thrombectomies are much more difficult than in arteries. The first venous suture was accomplished in 1877 in Petersburg by N. Eck (Fig. 18). Later on, direct lateral venous sutures were successful before arterial sutures. Payr united the divided ends of veins over magnesium rings in the same way as he did in arteries. The first experimental attempt at grafting in the venous system was reported by Exner. Successful clinical results of implanting synthetic grafts into the venous system have been achieved in superior vena cava and in portal vein. Palma from Montevideo obtained good results with crossover vein grafts in iliac and femoral vein thrombosis. Nevertheless, direct grafting of veins into the venous system is still far from definitely solved.

The great problem of chronic venous insufficiency of the leg with understanding of the communicating vein insufficiency has been clarified by Cockett and Dodd. Their contribution to the operation of subfascial leg vein ligation has solved the highly invaliding problem of postphlebitic syndrome and lower leg ulceration.

Lymphography

Direct lymphatic surgery is still more difficult if not impossible. For decades the origin and the mechanism of its formation remained unknown and the results of excisional operations were not good. It was John Kinmonth's great contribution to design in 1951 the lymphography which enabled us to understand the mechanism of lymphoedema formation (Fig. 19). J. Kinmonth is credited too with the generally accepted classification of lymphoedema. His work has stimulated others, creating new possibilities as, for example, the operation of Thompson.

This is the end of my list of milestones which we had to pass to come to the present state of vascular surgery. Besides the milestones which I considered crucial for the development of modern vascular surgery there are many other contributions which have been made in Europe.

Among the most important were the today historical descriptions of syndromes, special new indications and a multitude of technical improvements and refinements. This list is very long, so long that it would be impossible to repeat again what has been done in our part of the world in the last 100 years. May I list only some of them (Fig. 20).

It is time to draw conclusions. I have presented to you some fundamental principles and contributions which according to my understanding have created the modern vascular surgery. It appears from my survey that seven out of ten were conceived, started or discovered in Europe. That does not mean that they all were developed and improved in Europe. No, this happened in other parts of the world sometimes even on a much more spectacular scale. But the beginnings were in Europe. Why it happened so I do not know. May be because the European is more fond of thinking and deliberating than acting. It is a vice, a bad habit, as usually only action gives direct success. But thinking is so pleasant, and meditation may be so profitable, if not at once, if not directly for me then maybe for others, maybe in the future.

I think Europe was always a land of temptation. You see here Jupiter who captured Europe. I think he made a good choice.

Session I Cardiac Surgery

Valvular Surgery I

Chairman: V.O. Björk, Stockholm; Co-Chairman: A. Carpentier, Paris

Special Morphological Structures Along the Closing Zone of the Mitral Valve[1]

H. Heine and M. Laatz*

Introduction

The aim of these investigations was to study the functional morphology of the closing mechanism of the left atrioventricular valve (valva mitralis). The literature (cf. 1-4) describes only a strict closure during the systole of the valve edges thickened by connective tissue. The cordae tendineae prevent a tilt of the valve cusps into the atrium. It is still not known what morphological peculiarity causes the fitting of the valve edges.

Material and Methods

The valva mitralis together with the anulus fibrosus, chordae tendineae, and papillary muscles were taken out of 37 hearts of adults (female, male; different ages; preparatory session 1978/1979). The studies on the valve apparatus were performed by dissection under a magnifier or a light microscope after embedding in paraffin. The slices (10 μm) were stained after Romeis (1968) with H+E, trichrome, and resorcin-fuchsin (impregnation of elastic fibres).

Results

Under the magnifier the atrial area of the mitralis shows about 10-14 small balloon-like elevations in a row which are located at the very edge of the valves (Figs. 1,2). Towards the ventricular lumen these formations are in fact small tissular pockets with a diameter and depth of about 3-5 mm and an atrioventricular diameter of about 2.5 mm. Six to eight of these pockets can be found along the valve edge of the cuspis posterior of the valva mitralis; along the edge of the cuspis anterior there are four to six pockets (Figs. 1,2) which in the medial area are separated by a distance of 4-6 mm. This particular area directly covers the entrance to the conus aorticus of the

---

[1]Dedicated to Prof. Dr. J. Staubesand in honor of his 60th birthday

*The findings of this work are part of the doctoral thesis of M.L. (in preparation)
Anatomical Institute, University of Würzburg, Koellikerstr. 6, D-8700 Würzburg

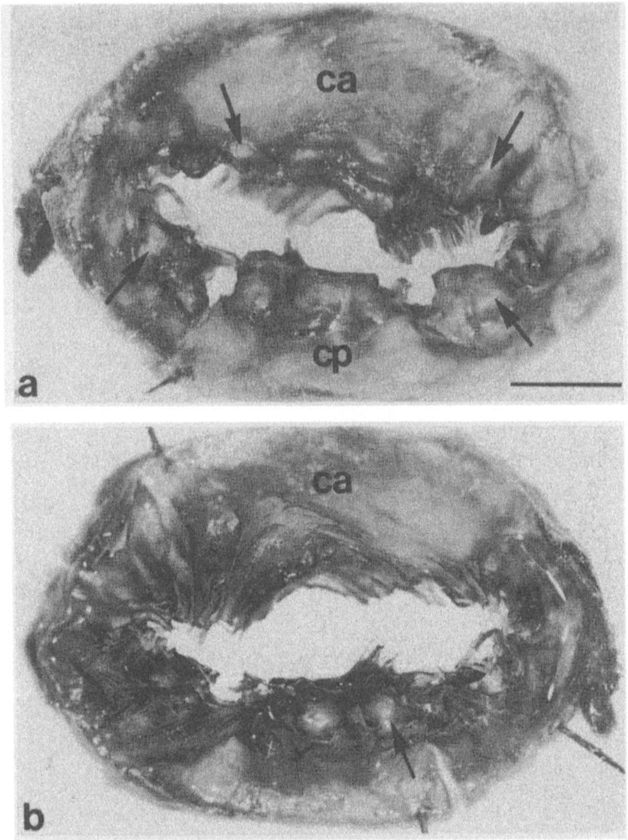

Fig. 1 a,b. Isolated human valva mitralis. a Atrial view, b ventricular view. Arrows point to the tissular pockets of the valve margin. *ca*, cuspis anterior; *cp*, cuspis posterior. Marker bar in all figures = 1 cm

left ventricle. Two to three of the tissular pockets follow on both sides.

The pockets are closely related to the chordae tendineae (Figs. 2,3). Tandler (1913) distinguished three orders of chordae: First-order chordae tendineae are directed towards the valve edge building up the frontal part of the pockets; they are the most numerous and their smallest diameter is about 0.65 mm. Second-order chordae tendineae are the strongest chordae (diameter approx. 1.0 mm) inserting in the ventricular area of the valve to the same distance as the depth of the pockets. First- and second-order chordae tendineae rise directly from the cupulae of the papillary muscles. Third-order chordae rise from the ventricular myocardium (sometimes from small accessory papillary muscles) and insert in front of the anulus fibrosus in the ventricular area of the valve. The structure of the mitral valve pockets consists exclusively of first- and second-order chordae tendineae.

The web-like spreading of delicate first-order chordae forms the frontal wall of the pockets acting as contact areas for the closure of the valve (Figs. 2,3). The second-order chordae tendineae also spread out close to the insertion, forming the rear wall of the pockets (Figs. 2,3). In this case, however, there are two additional fibre

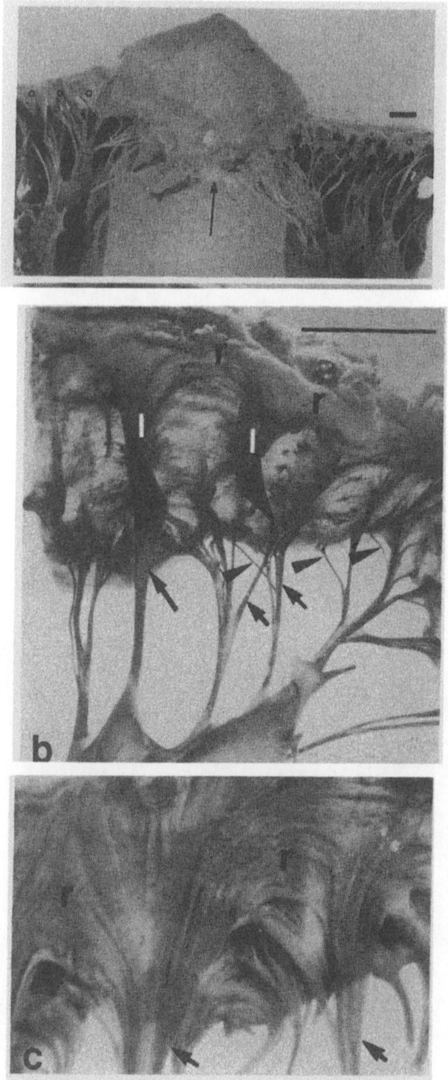

Fig. 2 a-c. Dissected valva mitralis with chordae tendineae and papillary muscles. a Anterior view of the closing zone of the valve with frontal walls of the tissular pockets (open rings). The arrow points to the pocket-free edge of the cuspis anterior. b Ventricular view of the mitral pockets. *Arrow heads:* First-order chordae tendineae to the frontal wall of the pockets. *Arrows:* Second-order chordae tendineae forming the lateral (*l*) and rear (*r*) wall of the pockets. c Higher magnification of the rear wall *r* of the pockets and ventricular area of the mitral valve. Arcade-like collagenous fibre systems of second-order chordae tendineae

systems involved coming from two neighbouring second-order chordae tendineae. As a result the rear wall consists of arcade-like overlapping collagenous fibre systems which continue to the ventricular side of the valves and are traceable up to the anulus fibrosus (Fig. 2). Because of the specific structure of the insertions of the second-order chordae the common lateral wall of two neighbouring pockets is also formed by second-order chordae. The first-order chordae tendineae are additionally involved by delicate intermediate chordae branching in the lateral pocket walls. The covering part of the pockets protruding towards the atrial lumen is constructed of crossing fibre systems from all the pocket walls. Histologically a collagenous fibre meshwork can be seen immediately in the subendocardial space reaching from the frontal wall of the pockets towards the valve insertion (Fig. 3). In the cross section a wedge-shaped dense connective tissue stripe is found in the transition area between the rear wall and the covering part of the pockets. In addition to a dense collagenous fibre meshwork

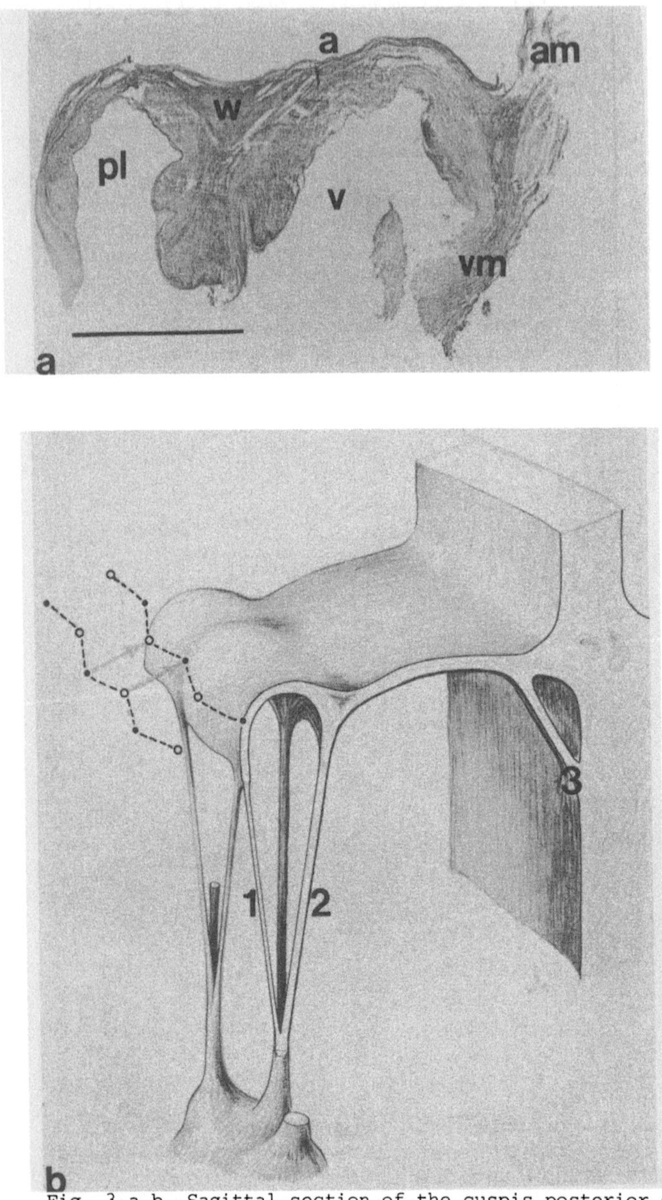

Fig. 3 a,b. Sagittal section of the cuspis posterior of the mitral valve. a Microanatomical structure of the valve. *a–v* atrial and ventricular side of the valve, *am–vm* atrial and ventricular myocardium, *pl* pocket lumen, *w* wedge of connective tissue in the back of the rear wall of a pocket. b Scheme of the closing zone of the mitral valve. *1, 2, 3* Insertion of first-, second-, and third-order chordae tendineae. The dashed line shows with an alternating row of circles and points along the frontal wall of the valvular pockets the zip fastener-like mechanism of the systolic closure of the valve

delicate elastic fibres exist in which a distinct frame about 10 µm thick forms in the lateral wall of the wedge. When the valves are closing a dense fitting of the contact zone of the valves takes place as the pockets alternatingly come together like a zip fastener.

Discussion

The results show that the closing edge of the mitral valve is morphologically characterized by small tissular pockets. When the mitral valve closes the opposite pockets of the edges of the cuspis anterior and posterior fit into each other like a zip fastener. During the systole the pockets are filled with blood, leading to a complete closure of the atrioventricular opening. The wedge-shaped stripe on the rear wall of the pockets may be interpreted as an important joint-like function during the systolic-diastolic rhythm.

Because the pockets are connected with the papillary muscles via the first- and second-order chordae tendineae any disturbance of this system (e.g. sclerosis of the mitral valve, endocarditis, damaged myocardial function) induces a disturbance of the function of the pockets and with it of the closing zone of the cuspis anterior and posterior of the left atrioventricular valve.

Summary

The margin of the valva mitralis shows a division in chambers unknown to the present which are mainly formed by inserting chordae tendineae. These tissular pockets have a decisive importance for the closing mechanism of the mitral valve.

References

1. Bargmann W (1963) Bau des Herzens. In: Bargmann W, Doerr W (eds) Das Herz des Menschen. Thieme, Stuttgart, pp 88-164
2. Burton AC (1969) Physiologie und Biophysik des Kreislaufes. Schattauer, Stuttgart, New York
3. Netter FH (1976) Farbatlanten der Medizin, vol 1: Herz. Thieme, Stuttgart (The Ciba collection of medical illustrations)
4. Rushmer RF (1970) Cardiovascular dynamics, 3rd edn. Saunders, Philadelphia, London
5. Tandler J (1913) Anatomie des Herzens. In: v. Bardeleben K (ed) Handbuch der Anatomie des Menschen, vol 3/1. Fischer, Jena

Conservative Surgery of the Mitral Valve. Annuloplasty on a new Adjustable Ring

M. Puig Massana, J. M. Calbet, and E. Castells*

Interest in conservative methods in mitral surgery has risen in accordance with the follow-up on operated patients demonstrating some difficulties after valve replacement and success in selective use of repair procedures. Mitral commissurotomy has always been accepted as a valid treatment of stenosis.

In treatment of mitral incompetence the efficiency of repair procedures is debatable, but there is no doubt that in selective groups, the quality of the correction obtained supported its use. Our actual policy in mitral surgery favours correcting, not substituting. This is based on experience acquired in 2536 operations on mitral valves performed between 1967 and 1980. Of these, 1135 have been valve replacements and 1401 conservative procedures. One hundred eighty-five mitral insufficiencies have been treated using repair methods, 79 by commissuroplasties or annuloplasties of the Wooler type and 106 by annuloplasties supported by a ring. In some cases, complementary techniques were used.

The Wooler annuloplasty for treatment of severe insufficiency demonstrated little reliability. Of 19 such operations performed before 1975, only 3 were free of systolic murmur, in 8 the systolic murmur was mild to moderate, and 5 presented severe regurgitation and had to be reoperated upon. There were two hospital deaths. This method was abandoned. Conversely, we consider commissuroplasties and little annuloplasties of the Wooler type suitable for the correction of less important insufficiencies, especially in residual postcommissurotomies.

Annuloplasties on a ring have shown better reliability in correcting severe regurgitation. In these, 53 rigid Carpentier rings and 53 flexible and adjustable rings were applied. The latter presented some advantages and permitted an increase in the number of reconstructive procedures in our group from 5% of the total mitral surgery to 15.7%. Now this is the preferred method.

The ring is totally flexible and is made of tubular braid 3 mm thick; its length can be reduced by traction threads passed through its interior. Once implanted, the ring can be reduced jointly with the organic valve annulus until the mitral leaflet becomes competent.

The ring has a nonretractable part, a segment of 33 mm. A different traction of the threads permits symmetrical or asymmetrical narrowing in order to give a more adequate correction of the deformed annulus with a minimal reduction in the mitral area. The size and distribution is secured by knotting the threads together.

*C. Sanitaria Principes de España, Feixa Llarga, s/n, Hospitalet, Barcelona, Spain

Clinical Material

Of 53 patients with an average age of 44.8 operated on, women were predominant. Functional affectation was severe in 44 cases (Table 1). The majority had a rheumatic cause; the aetiology was rheumatic (41), endocarditis (7), degenerative (3), and congenital (2). Most patients had double lesions, three showed eversion of the posterior leaflet due to ruptured chordae. Some of them had associated lesions, the most common was the association with other valve diseases (Table 2).

Table 1. Clinical material

Patients		53
Age: Average		44
Max.		67
Min.		11
Sex: Male		20
Female		33
NHYA Functional class:	IV	20
	III	24
	II	8
	I	1

Table 2. Anatomic diagnosis

Pure mitral insufficiency	16
Rupture of chordae	3
Stenosis and insufficiency	37
Associated lesions:	
Atrial myxoma	1
Coarctation of aorta	1
Atrial septal defect	1
Constrictive pericarditis	1
Ductus	1
Aortic valvular disease	6
Tricuspid insufficiency	6

Operative Procedure

The mitral annulus was presented by four cardinal points, two near the commissures and the others in the centre of anterior and posterior leaflet attachments. The nonretractile part should be sewed to the septal annulus (Fig. 1). The ring is sutured to the fibrous annulus of the valve. We prefer a continuous running suture but interrupted sutures are also satisfactory. The adjustment is made by pulling the retraction threads until the desired anatomical aspect of the valve is reached. Before final fixing of the size, the valve should be checked and modified until the desired result is obtained.

It is very important to check the function correctly. Different complementary methods may be used:

1) Visual inspection with the ventricle full and beating. If there is a significant aortic insufficiency it is enough to take off the aortic clamp. If not, the filling can be completed by a perfussion catheter passing through the apex.

2) By finger, with the left atrium closed and normal systolic pressure. The degree and characteristics of the regurgitation jet are tested. This is the method we prefer.

3) Checking by pressure graph, adjusting until disappearance of the V wave (Fig. 2). Sometimes traction of the threads has been effected from outside passing them through the atrial wall and knotting them to a Rummel tourniquet.

To avoid residual stenosis, once the critical area is approached, adjustment is done on a sizer. Diameters employed are 25, 23, 21.5, and 20. It is not advisable to go over this area, corresponding to the 27 Björk-Shiley or 20 Lillehei prostheses.

Finally, the size is secured by knotting the two threads together, but only after having ascertained that the result is functionally satisfactory. Sometimes associated procedures have been performed (Table 3).

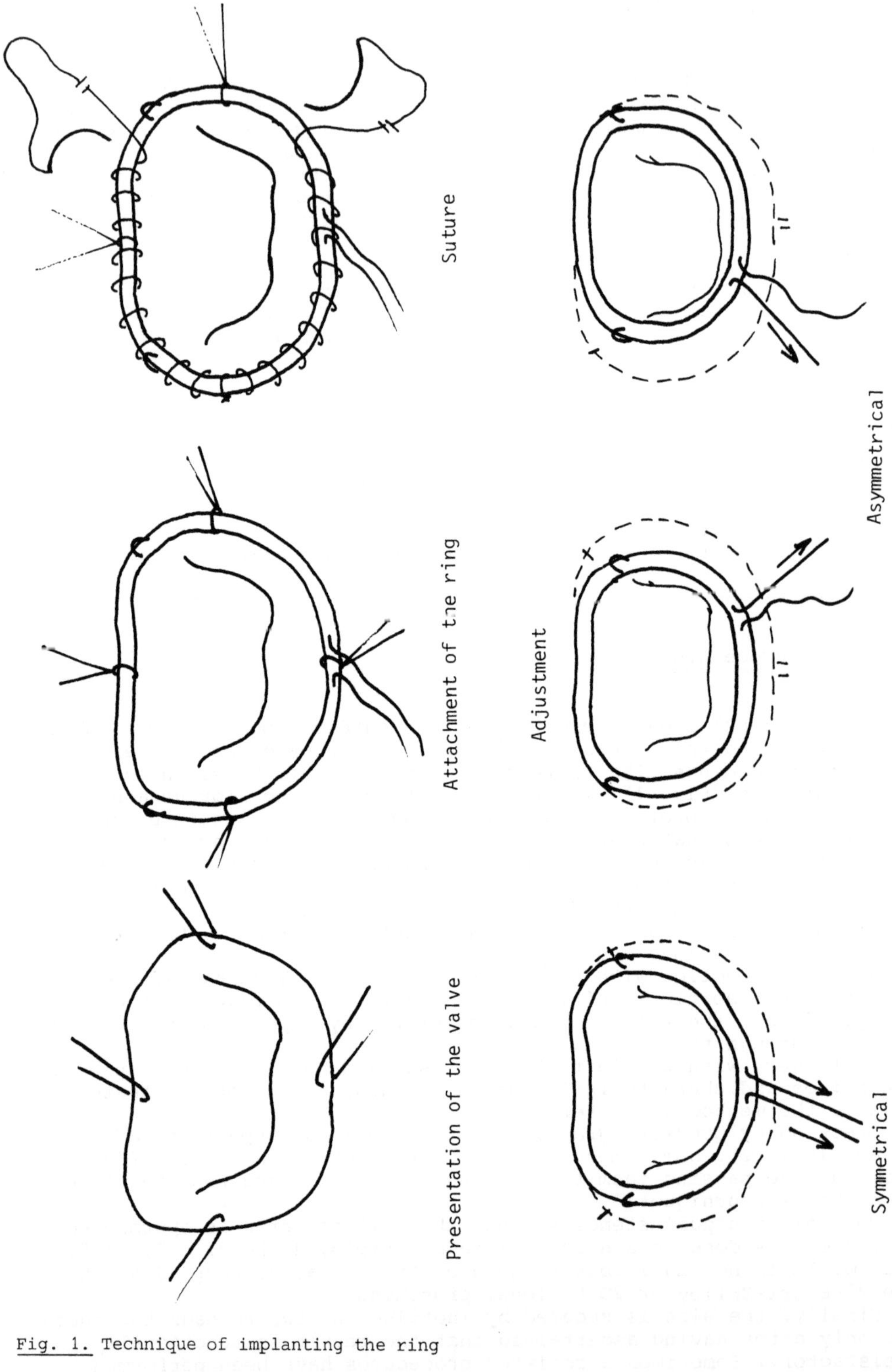

Fig. 1. Technique of implanting the ring

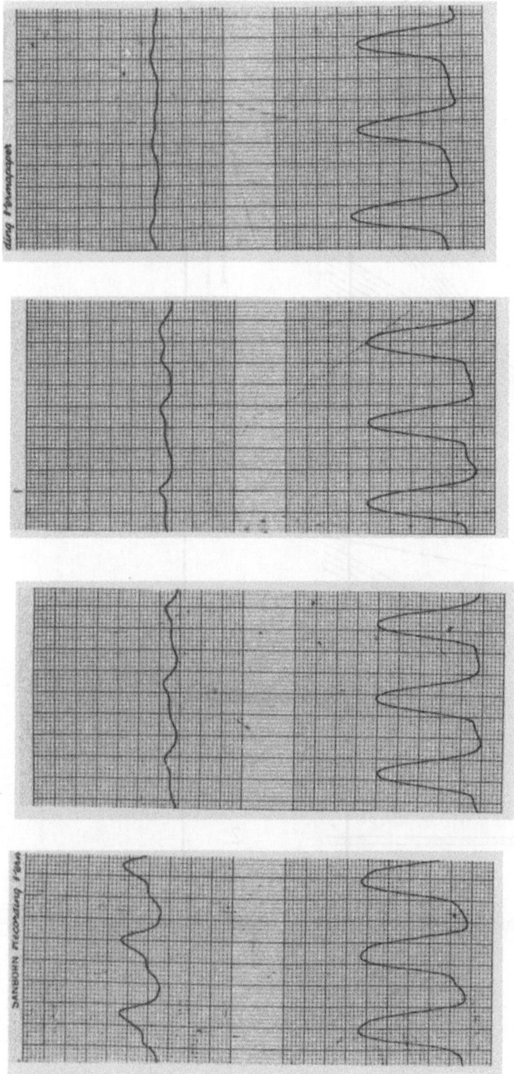

Fig. 2. Pressure graph, disappearance of the V wave according to the adjustment of the ring

Table 3. Associated procedures

Mitral commissurotomy	37
Resection of calcification	3
Repair of valvular perforations	3
Removal of mitral Carpentier ring	1
Partial resection of the posterior leaflet	1
Plication of the posterior leaflet	1
Removal of myxoma	1
Closure of atrial septal defect	1
Correction of coarctation of aorta	1
Closure of ductus	1
De Vega's tricuspid annuloplasty	6
Aortic valve replacement	6

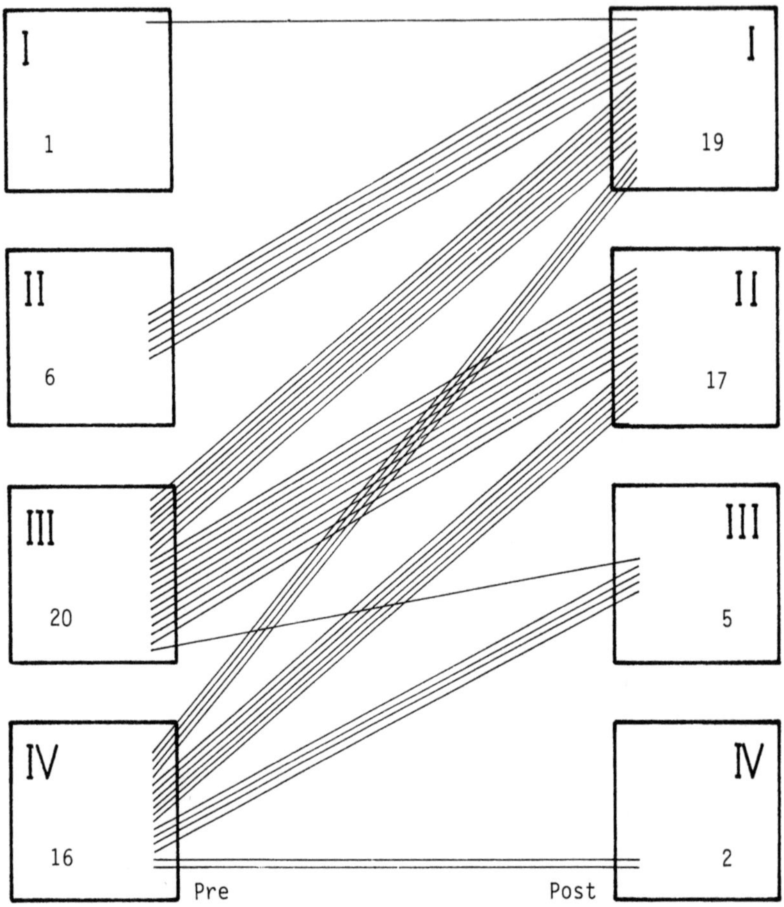

Fig. 3. NYHA functional class before and after annuloplasty on the adjustable ring

Results

Aortic patients are not included in the postoperative study. Total disappearance of regurgitation was frequently achieved after adjustment of the ring. Results were no regurgitation (33), grade 1/6 (9), grade 2/6 (7), grade 3/6 (1), and nonrecorded (4). There have been no hospital deaths. Forty-three patients have been followed up during a period of between 6 months and 3 years. Clinical evolution, treatments, and activity were evaluated according to the NYHA functional classification and showed a significant improvement with an average drop of 2 degrees (Fig. 3). The systolic murmur found in the long-term postoperative was no systolic murmur (19), grade <3/6 (21), and grade >3/6 (3).

Anticoagulant drugs were not used in any cases. There was one microembolic episode in late postoperative. Fifteen hemodynamic controls were done. The low number and a discriminate selection reduced the statistical value, but demonstrate the movement of the marked rings, changes of the atrial V wave, and the disappearance of the regurgitation which have been parallel to the surgical control and the clinical result. On the contrary, the area, gradient, and cardiac index sometimes have given paradoxical results to the ring diameter, being influenced by the pathologic condition of the corrected valve. Four patients were reoperated on for bacterial endocarditis (1), dehiscence of the ring (2), and progression of mitral incompetence (1). A patient was readmitted into hospital with endocarditis. On reoperation, destruction and extended vegetations were found in the septal leaflet; the prosthetic ring was not affected. Two cases of dehiscences were of special interest. In one patient, symptoms reappeared suddenly after 12 months. One stitch sewed parallely when changing direction of the suture became detached in the middle of the anterior leaflet attachment; in the second instance the annulus fibrosus was not enclosed by the suture. One progression of mitral incompetence after operation was due to elongated chordae which had not been properly corrected. The results in the three ruptured chordae have been very good, with a hemodynamic check-up in two of them.

Discussion

The disproportion between the mitral opening and the covering area of the leaflets is an important cause of mitral incompetence. The regurgitation contributes to the enlargement of the annulus and so increases the insufficiency, producing a vicious circle.

Different annuloplasty procedures offer good surgical results interrupting this progressive evolution by adapting the mitral ring to the surface area of the diseased leaflets. The annuloplasties supported by a ring, according to the Carpentier studies, provided a more confident solution. Flexible rings offer some advantages to the rigid ones in respect to better adaptation to the particular anatomy of each heart, producing fewer changes in cardiac movements. The flexible and adjustable ring also adds the advantages of the constrictive annuloplasties such as De Vega's in tricuspid valves or Parneth's mitral plication suture, but with more reliability because the suture stitches cross the fibres of the mitral annulus instead of being parallel to them.

Our results with the flexible and adjustable ring as compared with the nonflexible one have been encouraging (44.1% versus 37.7% without systolic murmur, and 48.8% versus 33.3% mild systolic murmur). Average area of the mitral opening measured by sizers at the end of the operation (Table 4) has been 5.5 cm^2, that is to say, higher than with other techniques including prosthetic replacement.

Table 4. Areas after adjustment of the ring

Sizer	Area	Number of patients
Two fingers	7.5 cm	18
S 25	4.8 cm	16
S 23	4.1 cm	13
S 21.5	3.6 cm	1
S 20	3.1 cm	1
Nonrecorded		4

One microembolic episode in the 43 controlled patients not taking anticoagulants is acceptable as far as the method is concerned, but it is a matter of discussion whether the anticoagulant therapy need be discontinued in patients maintaining after operation emboligenous factors such as atrial fibrillation, aneurysmatic dilatation, or endothelial changes.

The two ring dehiscences can be related to an incorrect technique of implantation as we pointed out before. A relapse of mitral incompetence caused by failure of one stitch of the septal ring attachment demonstrates that a complete ring is perhaps more reliable than the partial C-shaped ring.

Frequently, complementary techniques must be performed to correct associated lesions as well as to achieve a perfect valve repair and can result in difficulty in recognizing when it is justifiable to utilize high complexity techniques to prevent valve replacement, which in some instances continues to be the procedure of choice. Mitral reconstructive procedures do not alter the progression or the development of all subsequent pathological changes in the valve, so prudence is advisable in choosing reconstructive complex methods, especially when the long-term results cause doubt. Therefore, a simple method that prevents a valve replacement must be preferred at all times.

The adjustable ring simplifies the remodelling of the valve and increases the reliability of the method by securing the ring characteristics, size, and distribution after the result has been tested.

Acknowledgement. We would like to thank Miss Pili Perez for solving the problems encountered in making the ring in a simple and competent way.

References

1. Björk VO, Malers E (1964) Annuloplastic procedures for mitral insufficiency: late results. J Thorac Cardiovasc Surg 48:251
2. Burr HL, Krayenbuhl C, Sutton MSJ, Paneth M (1977) The mitral plication suture. J Thorac Cardiovasc Surg 73:589
3. Carpentier A (1969) La valvuloplastie reconstitutive. Une nouvelle technique de valvuloplastie mitrale. Presse Med 77:251
4. Carpentier A, Deloche A, Dauptain J, et al. (1971) A new reconstructive operation for correction of mitral and tricuspid insufficiency. J Thorac Cardivasc Surg 61:1
5. Carpentier A, Chauvaud S, Fabiani JN, et al. (1980) Reconstructive surgery of mitral valve incompetence. J Thorac Cardiovasc Surg 79:338
6. Cooley DA, Frazier OH, Norman JC (1976) Mitral leaflet prolapse: surgical treatment using a posterior annular collar prosthesis. Cardiovasc Dis Bull Texas Heart Inst 3:438
7. De Vega NG (1972) La anuloplastia selectiva regulable y permanente. Rev Esp Cardiol 25:6
8. Duran CG, Ubago JLM (1976) Conservative mitral valve surgery and developments in the technique of prosthetic ring annuloplasty. In: Kalmanson D (ed) The mitral valve. Acton, London
9. Duran CG, Pomar JL, Revuelta JM, et al. (1980) Conservative operation for mitral insufficiency. J Thorac Cardiovasc Surg 79:326
10. Ellis FJ Jr, Frye RL, McGoon DC (1966) Results of reconstructive operations for mitral insufficiency due to ruptured chordae tendinae. Surgery 59:165
11. McGoon DC (1960) Repair of mitral insufficiency due to ruptured chordae tendinae. J Thorac Cardiovasc Surg 39:357

12. Oury JH, Peterson Kl, Folkerth TL, et al. (1977) Mitral valve replacement versus reconstruction. An analysis of indications and results of mitral valve procedures in a consecutive series of 80 patients. J Thorac Cardiovasc Surg 73:825
13. Puig Massana M, Castells E, Calbet JM, et al. (1979) Prótesis anular regulable para anuloplastia mitral. Ann Med Soc Catalana Cir Cardíaca 9:1361
14. Reed GE, Pooley RW, Moggio RA (1980) Durability of measured mitral annuloplasty. J Thorac Cardiovasc Surg 79:321
15. Shore DF, Wong P, Paneth M (1980) Results of mitral valvuloplasty with a suture plication technique. J Thorac Cardiovasc Surg 79:349
16. Tandon AP, Lukacs LI, Smith DR, Ionescu MI (1977) Mitral annuloplasty – A long term clinical and haemodynamic study. Thorac Cardiovasc Surg 27:3944
17. Wooler GH, Nixon PGF, Grimshaw VA, et al. (1962) Experiences with the repair of the mitral valve in mitral incompetence. Thorax 17:49

Ruptured Mitral Chordae Tendineae: Surgical Experience in 102 Cases and Observations on the Valve Ultrastructure in this condition[1]

L. Zacharopoulos, J. K. Ross, J. L. Monro, and P. J. Gallagher*

Introduction

The functional anatomy of the mitral valve apparatus has been well documented in recent years (2, 3, 13). Normal function of the mitral valve requires delicately co-ordinated movement of its components – the leaflets, chordae, papillary muscles, and the supporting annulus and left ventricular myocardium. The chordae tendineae serve an essential role in the mechanics of mitral valve closure during ventricular systole. Rupture of one or more leads to mitral regurgitation. The pathological description of ruptured chordae probably begins with Corvisart in 1812. Older publications have stressed bacterial endocarditis (often with pre-existing rheumatic heart disease), rheumatic heart disaease alone, trauma, myocardial infarction, and connective tissue disorders as the common causes (16, 20, 21, 24). Recently, much attention has been directed towards the "floppy" mitral valve as the cause of innocent clicks or murmurs, and for its association with chest pain, atrial and ventricular arrhythmias and/or sudden death in elderly people (5, 6).

Material and Methods

Patients: Clinical Status

Between January 1974 and November 1979, 102 patients with chordal rupture were operated on at the Wessex Cardiac & Thoracic Centre in Southampton. Our experience from this series, drawn from a regional population of just under 3 million is that (Fig. 1) the rupture of chordae tendineae affects older patients (mean age 60 years), mostly males (72%) despite clinical, echocardiographic and necropsy studies which suggest that the incidence is higher in women (5, 18, 19, 26), while those presenting with chordal rupture after bacterial endocarditis tend to be younger with a shorter history. In the majority of our cases (73%) no obvious cause for the chordal rupture was present. Rheumatic valvulitis, with or without evidence of active healed bacterial endocarditis, was present in only 27% (with three cases of iatrogenic chordal rupture after closed valvotomy). Of the cases with "spontaneous" chordal rupture, there was reason to believe that 40

[1] Supported by Smith & Nephew Fellowship Grant

*Wessex Cardiac & Thoracic Centre, Western Hospital, Oakley Road, Southampton, SO9 4WQ, Great Britain

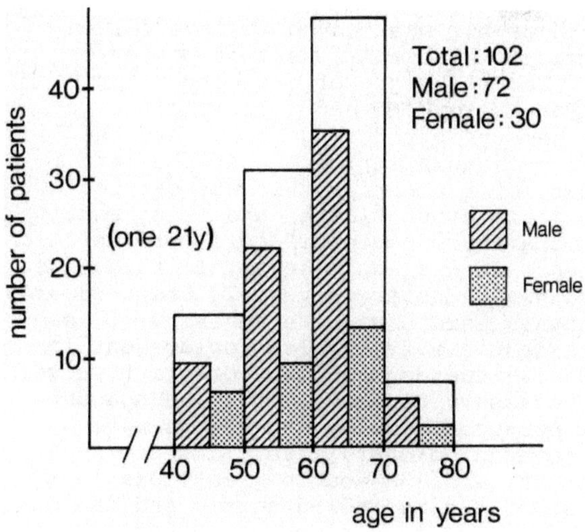

Fig. 1. Nomogram showing the age and sex incidence of patients undergoing operation for ruptured chordae tendineae

out of 74 were uncomplicated "floppy" valves before the rupture, but in none was there identifiable generalised connective tissue disorder. There was a significant incidence of associated systemic hypertension (14) and of aortic valve disease (18%). There were two cases with "floppy" aortic cusps, both in patients with "floppy" mitral valves. These figures suggest that important systemic hypertension and the volume overload of aortic regurgitation affect the functional state of the left ventricle and may play a significant part in some cases of ruptured chordae. An atrial septal defect of the secundum variety was found once with mitral regurgitation due to ruptured chordae (14, 15, 17). Reid (23) and Barlow (1) both showed that late systolic murmurs and clicks at the apex can originate from the mitral valve and 45% of our patients had a late systolic or pansystolic murmur, diagnosed many years before the onset of any symptoms. (As an aside, it is interesting that one of our patients was an Olympic runner in Berlin in 1936, presumably with a "floppy" valve.) These figures and the clinical course followed by the affected patients in our series suggest that such murmurs cannot be regarded as innocent, and demand full investigation (initially non-invasive) to clarify their cause. Our experience also confirms that the sudden onset of cardiac symptoms or an abrupt worsening of previous symptoms, with a pansystolic murmur radiating to apex or axilla, often with a third heart sound, should suggest a diagnosis of ruptured chordae in a middle-aged or elderly person in sinus rhythm with a normal-sized left atrium.

Operative Findings and Procedure

All our patients were selected for surgery on the basis of severe mitral regurgitation and 8 out of 102 were treated as emergencies because of intractable left ventricular failure. At operation the posterior leaflet was affected in 69 patients, the anterior in 29, and both leaflets in 4. Significant annular dilatation was noted in 75 patients and in all with "floppy" valves, without this being a constant finding in the other groups described. Eighty-seven patients had their valves replaced and 15 were reconstructed. Reconstruction of the valve was attempted in a further five instances but was judged to have failed when the valve was tested. This was so with four cases of posterior chordal rupture and one anterior. The technique of reconstruction of the valve was that described by Carpentier (4) and following the reconstruction, the valves were tested by introducing blood into the left ventricular cavity by way of a cannula introduced at the left ventricular apex. In the early part of the series this was carried out with the heart beating, with the aorta cross-clamped and using aortic root perfusion. Later, following the introduction of cold cardioplegic arrest, this was done with the heart in a flaccid state. In the valve replacement group, 9 received Braunwald-Cutter valves, 20 Starr-Edwards, 37 Björk-Shiley, and 21 bioprostheses were used. The severity of associated aortic valve disease necessitated aortic valve replacement in 13 patients: 8 Björk-Shiley, 4 Starr-Edwards, and one homograft valve being used. In two cases it was necessary to carry out a De Vega annuloplasty of the tricuspid valve. Aortocoronary bypass grafts were carried out for incidentally discovered coronary artery disease in 9 patients, 8 receiving a single graft, and 1 a double graft. One left ventricular aneurysm, one aneurysm of the ascending aorta, and one of the descending aorta were resected at the same time in 3 other patients, and in 1 associated atrial septal defect was closed.

Results

There were 3 peri-operative deaths (3% hospital mortality). The average follow-up for the surviving 99 patients was 35 months (6-76 months) [see Fig. 2]. Eighty-five of these showed a remarkable improvement in clinical status. There were 19 late deaths, 7 non-cardiac (cancer 4, lupus erythematosos 1, bronchopneumonia 2, all at least 2 years after operation). Of 13 emboli, 7 were fatal, all in patients with mechanical valves. Two patients died from myocardial infarction (3 and 4 years later), one from cerebral haemorrhage (on anticoagulants), and 3 from poor left ventricular function.

Pathology

Twenty mitral valves with spontaneous chordal rupture were examind by light, scanning, and transmission electron microscopy. Changes identified at rupture sites included oedema and necrosis of collagen, endothelial loss and, in some cases, partial or complete re-endothelialisation of the disrupted ends. With a solitary exception these abnormalities were confined to chordae which had actually ruptured. Some non-ruptured chordae were irregularly thinned and stretched, but were normal by light and electron microscopy. Mucoid degeneration was almost invariable in mitral valve leaflets.

Discussion

Since 1960, when McGoon (18) published a method for surgical repair of the valve affected by ruptured chordae, a number of reports describing various methods for dealing with this condition have been published. One author (J.K. Ross) after some years of experience with the technique advocated by Gerbode et al. (1968) continued a conservative approach wherever possible, using the technique described by Carpentier (4). The criteria adopted for attempted valve conservation by the

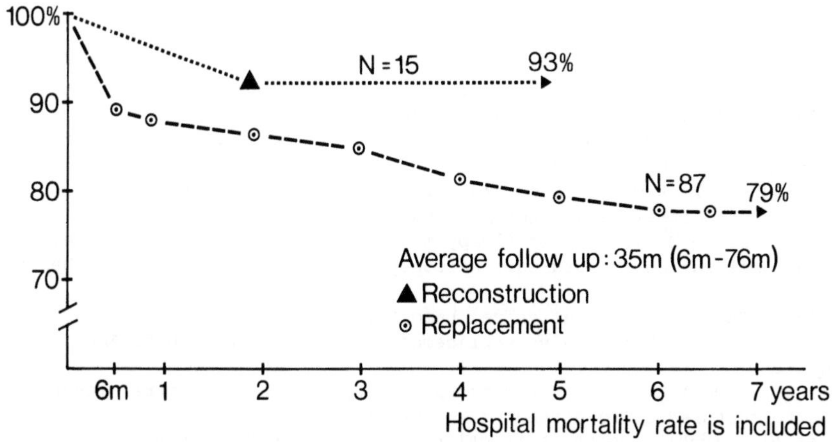

Fig. 2. Graph showing the survival of patients undergoing valve replacement and repair for ruptured chordae tendineae

Carpentier method include 1) chordal rupture confined to the posterior leaflet, 2) the flail segment being less than half the total length of the posterior leaflet, and 3) macroscopically unaffected anterior leaflet chordae. No attempt was made in the group treated by valve reconstruction to shorten chordae or carry out any other associated procedure on the subvalve mechanism. All received an annuloplasty using the Carpentier ring. The method of valve testing has already been referred to, and is probably less than ideal in the cold cardioplegic heart; however, to date, no discrepancy has been discovered between the assessment made of the valve using this method and the subsequent clinical course of the patient. The results to date in the conservatively treated group show less morbidity than in the group with valve replacement described below, with no evidence of declining valve function during a follow-up period extending to 60 months. There has been no incidence of late chordal rupture or disrupted repair as a result of late death. These facts, together with the original observations made on the ultrastructure of the mitral valve in spontaneous chordal rupture (25), suggest that the changes predisposing to rupture are not necessarily present in un-ruptured chordae in the same valve. This gives support to the policy of valve reconstruction whenever possible and justifies the continuation of this policy. One author (J.L. Monro) applies valve replacement in all cases of chordal rupture, and owing to the nature of the condition, and the strict criteria for reconstruction, the valve replacement group naturally represents the majority in this series. In this group there have been 13 embolic incidents, 7 of which were fatal, and none of which occurred in patients with bioprostheses. There was an 8% incidence of perivalvar leak, which we believe refects the technical problems associated with valve replacement in these patients who often have very poor connective tissue, combined with annular dilatation. As with all patients presenting with valve disease, part of the pre-operative investigation includes selective coronary arteriography and this is particularly important in the patients in the older age group who present with chordal rupture.

In conclusion, although the majority of patients suffering from chordal rupture require valve replacement, it is maintained that there is a place for reconstruction, specifically in those with posterior chordal rupture and a flail segment of manageable size, and that the results to date showing decreased mortality in the group with valve reconstruction compared with those with valve replacement justifies the continuation of this policy.

References

1. Barlow JB, et al. (1968) Br Heart J 30:203
2. Becker AE, De Wit (1979) Mitral valve apparatus. Br Heart J 42:680
3. Bulkley BH, Roberts WC (1975) Dilatation of the mitral annulus. A cause of mitral regurgitation. Am J Med 59:457
4. Carpentier A (1976) Plastic and reconstructive mitral valve surgery. In: Kalmanson D (ed) The mitral valve. Acton, London
5. Davies MJ, Braimbridge MV (1978) The floppy mitral valve. Study of incidence, pathology and complication in surgical, necropsy and forensic material. Br Heart J 40:468
6. Editorial (1979) The floppy mitral valve. Lancet 1:138
7. Effler DB, et al. (1965) Heart valve replacement, clinical experience. Ann Thorac Surg 1:4
8. Ellis HE, et al. (1966) Results of reconstructive operations for mitral insufficiency due to ruptured chordae tendineae. Surgery 59:165
9. Gerbode F, et al. (1968) Surgical correction of mitral insufficiency due to ruptured chordae tendineae. Circulation [Suppl II] 37-38:119
10. Guthrie RB, Edwards JE (1976) Pathology of the myxomatous mitral valve. Nature, secondary changes and complication. Minn Med 59:637
11. Hammer D, et al. (1979) Altered collagen composition in a prolapsing mitral valve with ruptured chordae tendineae. Am J Med 67:863
12. Higgins CB, et al. (1976) The significance of mitral valve prolapse in middle-aged and elderly men. Am Heart J 91:292
13. Kalmanson D (ed) (1976) The mitral valve. Acton, London
14. Lachman AS, et al. (1976) Association of ostium secundum atrial septal defects with mitral prolapse. Am J Cardiol 38:167
15. Littler WA, et al. (1973) Acute mitral regurgitation resulting from ruptured or elongated chordae tendineae. Q J Med 42:87
16. Manhas, et al. (1971) Ruptured chordae tendineae. Circulation 43:688
17. McDonald, et al. (1971) Association of prolapse of posterior cusp of mitral valve and atrial septal defect. Br Heart J 33:383
18. McGoon CD (1960) Repair of mitral insufficiency due to ruptured chordae tendineae. J Thorac Cardiovasc Surg 39:357
19. McKay, Yacoub M (1973) Clinical and pathological findings in patients with "floppy" valves treated surgically. Circulation [Suppl III] 47-48:63
20. Menges HJ, et al. (1964) Clinical diagnosis and surgical management of ruptured mitral chordae tendineae. Circulation 30:8
21. Osmudson PJ, et al. (1961) Ruptured mitral chordae tendineae. Circulation 23:8
22. Procacci PM, et al. (1976) Prevalence of clinical mitral valve prolapse in 1169 young women. N Engl J Med 294:1086
23. Reid JV (1961) S Afr J 35:353
24. Sanders AC, et al. (1967) Diagnosis and surgical treatment of mitral regurgitation secondary to ruptured chordae tendineae. N Engl J Med 276:943
25. Scott-Jupp, et al. (to be published) Ultrastructural changes in spontaneous rupture of mitral chordae tendineae. J Pathol
26. Silver M (1976) Recent advances in the knowledge of pathology of normal and artificial valves. In: Kalmanson D (ed) The mitral valve. Acton, London, p 53

Long Term and Sequential Hemodynamic Investigations in Patients With Ionescu-Shiley Pericardial Xenografts

D. R. Smith, A. P. Tandon, S. S. Hassan, and M. I. Ionescu*

The glutaraldehyde stabilized pericardial xenograft[1] has been in clinical use since 1971 and has gained much wider usage since 1976 when it was released for general use. The clinical experience has been gratifying (6, 7, 10). We present herewith the reults of hemodynamic investigations undertaken in 75 patients with pericardial xenograft heart valve replacement.

Material and Methods

Hemodynamic studies were undertaken in 68 patients with single and 7 patients with multiple heart valve replacement. The criteria for selection were the informed consent of the patient and the availability of preoperative investigations. Long-term hemodynamic studies were undertaken in 36 patients with aortic, 29 with mitral, 3 with tricuspid and in 7 patients with multiple valve replacement at mean duration of 41.2 (range 22 to 59), 40.2 (range 24 to 59), 47.7 (range 24 to 66), and 12 (range 9 to 21) months postoperatively, respectively.

Sequential hemodynamic investigations were undertaken in 13 patients with aortic and 6 patients with mitral valve replacement. The 13 patients with aortic pericardial xenografts had one preoperative and three separate postoperative studies at 9.9 ± 0.8, 42.2 ± 0.8, and 68.3 ± 1.0 months after valve replacement. The six patients with mitral valve replacement had, in addition to the preoperative, three cardiac catheterisations at 11.2 ± 1.6, 42.8 ± 3.3, and 68.7 ± 1.3 months postoperatively. The methodology of hemodynamic investigations has been described previously (6).

Results

Mitral Valve Replacement

Long-Term Study. A significant increase in cardiac index and oxygen uptake was noticed both at rest and during exercise, but the cardiac output response to exercise was impaired (Table 1). A highly signifi-

---

*Departments of Cardiology and Cardiothoracic Surgery, Royal Halifax Infirmary and Leeds General Infirmary, Great Britain

[1]Shiley Laboratories Inc., Irvine, California, USA

Table 1. Pre- and postoperative hemodynamic data (mean values ± SEM and statistical significance) of 29 patients having mitral valve replacement with pericardial xenografts

	Cardiac index ($l/min/m^2$)		PWP (mm Hg)		MDG (mm Hg)		XSA (cm^2)	
	R	E	R	E	R	E	R	E
Preoperative	1.9 ±0.1	3.0 ±0.3	23.0 ±1.9	40.4 ±2.7	- -	- -	- -	- -
Postoperative	2.6 ±0.2	4.1 ±0.2	13.8 ±0.8	29.4 ±1.5	6.4 ±0.5	15.3 ±0.9	2.0 ±0.1	2.3 ±0.1
p value	<0.001	<0.01	<0.001	<0.01	-	-	-	-

SEM, standard error of the mean; *PWP*, mean pulmonary wedge pressure; *MDG*, mean diastolic gradient; *XSA*, calculated xenograft surface area; *R*, rest; *E*, exercise

cant reduction was noted in the postop study both at rest and during exercise in the mean pulmonary wedge and pulmonary artery pressures and pulmonary vascular restistance. However, the pressures were abnormally elevated during exercise. The mean diastolic gradient was 6.4 ± 0.5 and 15.3 ± 0.9 mm Hg at rest and during exercise respectively at the postop study. The calculated xenograft surface areas were 2.0 ± 0.1 and 2.3 ± 0.1 cm^2 respectively.

Sequential Hemodynamic Studies. The results are summarized in Table 2. The data obtained at the first postoperative study were similar to those described above. No significant change was noted in the parameters recorded between the three postoperative studies.

Aortic Valve Replacement

Long-Term Study. The long-term study undertaken in 36 patients showed significant increase in cardiac index and stroke volume, both at rest and during exercise, as compared to preoperative values (Table 3). The mean pulmonary wedge and left ventricular end-diastolic pressures showed significant reduction when compared with the preoperative levels, both at rest and during exercise. The peak systolic gradient was 6.4 ± 1.0 at rest and 9.6 ± 1.6 mm Hg during exercise at the postop study. The mean peak systolic gradient was 8.3 mm Hg in patients with xenograft size 19 and it decreased with the corresponding increase in valve size, so that with the 27 mm pericardial xenograft it was hardly measurable. Similarly, the calculated surface area was lowest with the smallest xenograft implanted and rose with increasing xenograft size ($r = 0.996$ at rest and $r = 0.951$ during exercise).

Sequential Hemodynamic Studies. The data are detailed in Table 4. The cardiac catheterisation results at the first postoperative investigation were similar to those obtained in the long-term study. No significant change was noted between the three postop investigations, although there was a marginal reduction in systolic gradients and an increase in xenograft surface area.

Table 2. Sequential hemodynamic data of six patients with mitral valve replacement (mean values ± SEM)

Study number	CI ($l/min/m^2$)		PWP (mm Hg)		MDG (mm Hg)		XSA (cm^2)	
	R	E	R	E	R	E	R	E
Preop	1.8 ±0.2	3.4 ±0.3	23.2 ±2.1	44.0 ±3.0	- -	- -	- -	- -
Postop I	2.7 ±0.3	4.2 ±0.6	13.8 ±1.6	27.2 ±3.1	7.1 ±1.2	20.1 ±2.1	2.2 ±0.19	2.6 ±0.16
Postop II	2.8 ±0.3	4.6 ±0.5	13.6 ±2.2	25.0 ±2.4	6.6 ±1.5	19.1 ±2.3	2.3 ±0.27	2.7 ±0.15
Postop III	2.7 ±0.4	4.7 ±0.7	14.4 ±1.4	27.8 ±2.1	6.8 ±1.4	19.6 ±1.8	2.2 ±0.2	2.7 ±0.2
Statistical significance								
Pre- and postop I	<0.05	NS	<0.01	<0.001	-	-	-	-
Postop I and II	NS	NS	NS	NS	NS	NS	NS	NS
Postop II and III	NS	NS	NS	NS	NS	NS	NS	NS

SEM, standard error of the mean; *CI*, cardiac index; *PWP*, mean pulmonary wedge pressure; *MDG*, mean diastolic gradient; *XSA*, xenograft surface area; *NS*, not significant

Table 3. Pre- and postoperative hemodynamic data (mean values ± SEM and statistical significance) of 36 patients having aortic valve replacement with pericardial xenograft

	Cardiac index ($l/min/m^2$)		LVEDP (mm Hg)		PSG (mm Hg)		XSA (cm^2)	
	R	E	R	E	R	E	R	E
Preoperative	2.4 ±0.2	4.2 ±0.3	19.1 ±2.8	32.7 ±5.8	83.3 ±10.0	- -	- -	- -
Postoperative	2.7 ±0.1	4.6 ±0.2	9.9 ±0.7	18.3 ±1.6	6.4 ±1.0	9.6 ±1.6	1.6 ±0.07	2.0 ±0.1
p value	<0.05	<0.05	<0.01	<0.01	<0.001	-	-	-

SEM, standard error of the mean; *LVEDP*, left ventricular end-diastolic pressure; *PSG*, peak systolic gradient; *XSA*, calculated xenograft surface area; *R*, rest; *E*, exercise

Table 4. Sequential hemodynamic data in 13 patients with aortic valve replacement (mean values ± SEM)

Study number	CI ($l/min/m^2$)		LVEDP (mm Hg)		PSG (mm Hg)		XSA (cm^2)	
	R	E	R	E	R	E	R	E
Preop	2.4 ±0.2	4.1 ±0.3	19.0 ±2.4	33.0 ±6.0	49.0 ±17.7	-	-	-
Postop I	2.7 ±0.2	4.7 ±0.3	8.0 ±0.5	17.0 ±2.1	6.0 ±1.6	11.0 ±1.9	1.6 ±0.06	2.0 ±0.1
Postop II	2.6 ±0.6	4.5 ±0.2	9.0 ±0.5	16.0 ±1.7	6.0 ±1.2	9.0 ±1.7	1.6 ±0.07	2.1 ±0.1
Postop III	2.8 ±0.1	5.1 ±0.2	9.0 ±0.7	19.0 ±1.8	7.0 ±1.2	10.0 ±1.6	1.6 ±0.06	2.1 ±0.2
Statistical significance								
Pre- and postop I	<0.05	<0.05	<0.01	<0.01	<0.05	-	-	-
Postop I and II	NS	NS	NS	NS	NS	NS	NS	NS
Postop II and III	NS	NS	NS	NS	NS	NS	NS	NS

SEM, standard error of the mean; *CI*, cardiac index; *LVEDP*, left ventricular end-diastolic pressure; *PSG*, peak systolic gradient; *XSA*, xenograft surface area; *NS*, not significant

Tricuspid Valve Replacement

The hemodynamic studies in three patients with isolated tricuspid replacement showed significant reduction in right-sided pressures with marginal increase in cardiac index (Table 5). The diastolic gradients across the tricuspid xenografts were minimal ranging from 2 to 4 mm Hg.

Multiple Valve Replacement

The postoperative hemodynamic data of 7 patients with multiple valve replacement are summarized in Table 5. The transvalvular gradients were similar to those observed with single valve replacement.

Angiography

Ventricular or aortic root angiography performed at the end of each study confirmed the competence of the pericardial xenografts in all the patients.

In Vitro Studies

In vitro studies have been performed both at pulsatile and continuous flow (6, 17, 18). These studies have demonstrated that the pericardial xenograft has superior hydraulic characteristics when compared with currently available tissue valves.

Table 5. Postoperative hemodynamic data of patients with tricuspid and multiple valve replacement

Valves replaced	No. of patients	CI ($l/min/m^2$)	Transvalvular gradient (mm Hg) Mitral	Aortic	Tricuspid	Cal. Xen. Surface Area (cm^2) Mitral	Aortic	Tricuspid
Tricuspid	3	2.7 ±0.2	-	-	3.4 ±0.7	-	-	2.4 ±0.1
Mitral and tricuspid	3	2.6 ±0.6	6.6 ±0.6	-	2.8 ±0.5	1.9 ±0.1	-	2.2 ±0.1
Mitral and aortic	1	2.7	6.4	6.0	-	2.0	1.4	-
Mitral, aortic and tricuspid	3	2.4 ±0.2	6.2 ±1.4	7.0 ±1.0	3.0 ±0.6	1.9 ±0.2	1.3 ±0.2	2.1 ±0.1

CI, cardiac index

Discussion

The clinical experience with the Ionescu-Shiley pericardial xenograft over a period of more than 10 years has shown very favourable results (6, 7, 10). The results of the hemodynamic studies presented here from 75 patients have shown significant overall circulatory improvement.

In patients with mitral valve replacement, a significant increase in cardiac output and oxygen uptake was noted at the postoperative study as compared to the preoperative data. Postoperatively the mean pulmonary artery and wedge pressures approached normal figures at rest but rose to abnormal levels with exercises. Thus the hemodynamic response to exercise was still impaired. This seems to be the common finding with all types of mitral valve substitutes currently used (2, 5, 8, 11, 13-15). The mean diastolic gradient across the pericardial xenograft of 6.4 mm Hg compares favourably with gradients obtained with other mitral valve substitutes (2, 8, 11, 14).

In patients with aortic valve replacement, both the cardiac output and the oxygen utilisation increased marginally but significantly and their response to exercise was normal. Both the left ventricular end-diastolic and pulmonary wedge pressures showed normalisation at rest and diminished significantly during exercise at the postoperative study. The raised left ventricular end-diastolic pressure on exercise after successful aortic valve replacement has been previously reported (1, 3, 12, 16). A probable explanation for this phenomenon could be the presence of a certain degree of irreversible left ventricular dysfunction from long-standing valvular disease or myocardial injury sustained at the time of valve replacement.

The pericardial xenograft offers the least resistance to forward flow when compared with other valve substitutes (7, 10, 15-18). In practical terms the most important hemodynamic determinant of a valve substitute is the effective surface area available to flow as measured in vivo. None of the patients investigated in the present series had a calculated surface area of less than 1 cm^2. Further, Walker et al. (17) have recently demonstrated that the use of the Gorlin formula underestimates the calculated pericardial xenograft areas. Effective orifice areas less than 1 cm^2 are common findings in patients with the smaller sizes of porcine valves in the aortic position (4, 9).

The results of the sequential studies in 13 patients with aortic and 6 with mitral valve replacement are of considerable significance. The investigations have demonstrated that the initial circulatory improvement is maintained and that there is no alteration in the essential hemodynamic parameters up to 73 months following the operation.

Conclusions

The hydrodynamic characteristics of this valve, as demonstrated in in vitro studies are superior to all other tissue valves currently available.

The hemodynamic investigations on a large number of patients have shown very good performance of the pericardial xenograft in the aortic and atrioventricular positions. The transvalvular gradients are insignificant, even with small-size aortic valves.

The maximum hemodynamic improvement was achieved within 12 months postoperatively and sequential studies have shown that the improvement was maintained up to 73 months following valve replacement.

References

1. Björk VO, Holmgren A, Olin C, Ovenfors C (1971) Clinical and haemodynamic results of aortic valve replacement with the Björk-Shiley tilting disc valve prosthesis Scand J Thorac Cardiovasc Surg 5:177
2. Book K (1974) Mitral valve replacement with Björk-Shiley tilting disc valve – A clinical and haemodynamic study in patients with isolated mitral valve lesions. Scand J Thorac Cardiovasc Surg [Suppl 2] 12
3. Bristow JD, Kremkau EL (1975) Hemodynamic changes after valve replacement with Starr-Edwards prostheses. Am J Cardiol 35:716
4. Cohn LH, Sanders JH, Collins JJ (1976) Aortic valve replacement with the Hancock porcine xenograft. Ann Thorac Surg 22:221
5. Hulgren H, Hubis H, Shumway NE (1968) Cardiac functions following mitral valve replacement. Am Heart J 75:302
6. Ionescu MI, Tandon AP (1979) The Ionescu-Shiley pericardial xenograft heart valve. In: Ionescu MI (ed) Tissue heart valves. Butterworths, London, p 201
7. Ionescu MI, Tandon AP, Mary DAS, Abid A (1977) Heart valve replacement with the Ionescu-Shiley pericardial xenograft. J Thorac Cardiovasc Surg 73:31
8. Johnson AD, Daily PO, Peterson KL, Le Winter M, Di Donna GJ, Blaire G, Niwayama G (1975) Functional evaluation of the porcine heterograft in the mitral position. Circulation [Suppl 1] 52:40
9. Jones EL, Craver JM, Morris DC, King SB III, Douglas JS Jr, Franck RH, Hatcher CR Jr, Morgan EA (1978) Hemodynamic and clinical evaluation of the Hancock xenograft bioprosthesis for aortic valve replacement (with emphasis on management of the small aortic root). J Thorac Cardiovasc Surg 75:300
10. Ott DA, Coelho AT, Cooley DA, Reul GJ Jr (1980) Ionescu-Shiley pericardial xenograft valve: Hemodynamic evaluation and early clinical follow-up of 326 patients. Cardiovasc Dis Bull Texas Heart Inst 7:137
11. Pietras RJ, Long DM, Rosen KM (1974) Late postoperative clinical and hemodynamic assessment of the early cloth-covered Starr-Edwards mitral valve prosthesis. J Thorac Cardiovasc Surg 67:450
12. Rodriguez L (1970) Haemodynamic and angiographic findings in patients with isolated aortic valvular disease before and after insertion of a Starr-Edwards ball-valve prosthesis. Scand J Thorac Cardiovasc Surg [Suppl 1] 5

13. Russell T II, Kremkau EL, Kloster P, Starr A (1972) Late haemodynamic function of cloth-covered Starr-Edwards valve prostheses. Circulation [Suppl 1] 45-46:8
14. Sigwart U, Schmidt H, Gleichmann U, Borst HG (1976) In vivo evaluation of the Lillehei-Kaster heart valve prosthesis. Ann Thorac Surg 22:213
15. Tandon AP, Smith DR, Ionescu MI (1978) Hemodynamic evaluation of the Ionescu-Shiley pericardial xenograft in the mitral position. Am heart J 95:595
16. Tandon AP, Smith DR, Whitaker W, Ionescu MI (1978) Long-term haemodynamic evaluation of the aortic pericardial xenograft. Br Heart J 40:602
17. Walker DK, Scotten LN, Modi VJ, Brownlee RT (1980) In vitro assessment of mitral valve prostheses. J Thorac Cardiovasc Surg 79:680
18. Wright JTM (1979) Hydrodynamic evaluation of tissue valves. In: Ionescu MI (ed) Tissue heart valves. Butterworths, London, p 29

Pros and Cons of the Ionescu-Shiley Bioprosthesis

J.M. Revuelta, J.L. Pomar, J.L. Ubago, A. Figueroa, A. Ochoteco, and C.M.G. Duran*

Since the beginning of our unit, its geographic characteristics determined our valve replacement policy which favours the use of bioprosthesis. From May 1974 until May 1980, 836 Hancock valves were used in 755 patients with very satisfactory clinical results (1). The hemodynamic data obtained postoperatively in 305 valves recatheterized (2) showed significant residual gradients in the smaller size valves in both the aortic and mitral positions. Encouraged by the reported hemodynamic characteristics of the Ionescu-Shiley xenografts (3), a small series was started in August 1977, particularly in the cases with small annulus, while continuing with the routine use of the porcine xenografts. We report here our initial experience with the Ionescu-Shiley pericardial xenografts.

Material and Methods

Between August 1977 and May 1980, 104 Ionescu-Shiley pericardial valves were placed in 97 patients. Thirty-nine were male and 58 female. The average age was of 48.2 years (range 19 to 78 years). Eighty-two percent of the lesions were rheumatic in origin. Among the remaining patients the cause of the valve lesion was: congenital (3), degenerative (2), ischaemic (5), secondary to bacterial endocarditis (6), and prosthesic valve failure (1). Twenty patients were preoperatively in functional Class I-II and 77 in Class III-IV (Table 4).

Seventy-eight patients had their aortic valve, 11 their mitral, 7 their aortic and mitral, and 1 the pulmonary valve replaced with the Ionescu-Shiley bioprosthesis.

All patients were operated upon through a midline sternotomy. Standard cardiopulmonary bypass with a bubble oxygenator, hemodylution, and general body hypothermia to approximately 30-32^{0}C were employed. In all cases, topical hypothermia through a continuous perfusion system and intermittent lavage of the left ventricular cavity with cold saline at 4^{0}C were used. The whole intracardiac surgery except procedures on the right side of the heart was performed with a single uninterrupted period of aortic cross clamping. A 500 ml bolus of crystalloid cold cardioplegia was pressure infused in all cases. An apical left ventricular vent was routinely placed. The bioprosthesis was sutured with interrupted inverted "U" stitches in the aortic or pulmonary position. In the mitral, interrupted "figure 8" stitches in 12 cases and continuous suture in the remaining six patients were also used. The valve sizes employed in each position are listed in Table 1. Table 2 shows the associated surgery performed in this group of patients.

*Centro Medico Nacional Valdecilla. Universidad de Santander. Santander, Spain

Table 1. Ionescu-Shiley pericardial xenograft. Valve sizes used

Position	(N)	19	21	23	25	27	29	31
Aortic	85	7	38	26	11	1	2	
Mitral	18				1	11	5	1
Pulmonary	1			1				
	104	7	38	27	12	12	7	1

Table 2. Surgery performed

		Isolated	Associated	
Aortic group	n: 85	30	Replacement	Conservative
Mitral			40	15
Tricuspid			3	32
Mitral group	n: 18	7		
Aortic			7	-
Tricuspid			-	4

The anticoagulation policy was similar to that used for all our valvular surgery. All aortic patients received antiaggregants for 3 months, similar to the mitral patients in sinus rhythm. The latter, when in atrial fibrillation, were anticoagulated for 3 months and permanently if a giant left atrium or intraatrial thrombi were present.

Results

Aortic Valve Replacement

Among the 85 patients with aortic pericardial valves 30 had an isolated replacement (Table 3). There was one early death (3.3%) due to low cardiac output. There were 8 early deaths among the remaining 55 patients with concomittant surgery. The causes of death were low cardiac output (1), dysrhythmias (2), sepsis (2), neurological damage (1), and hemorrhage (2), one of them due to a left ventricular rupture in a patient with a simultaneous mitral replacement. The overall hospital mortality rate was 9.4%. There was one late death 2 months after surgery, due to acute bacterial endocarditis on a patient admitted to hospital and dying before emergency surgery could be attempted. Two other patients suffered bacterial endocarditis on the bioprosthesis (one by proteus and the other by staphylococcus epidermidis) both successfully reoperated upon. No valve structural failures have been detected in this group of patients. No thromboembolic episode occurred among the 76 surviving patients. Currently no case is in functional Class III-IV. Sixty-one are in Class I and the remaining 15 in Class II (Table 4).

Table 3. Ionescu-Shiley pericardial xenograft

Mortality	Aortic group	Mitral group	Overall
Early	8	4	12
Late	1	-	1
			9.4%

Table 4. Ionescu-Shiley pericardial xenograft
Functional class and cardiothoracic index

FC	I	II	III	IV
Preop	4	16	52	25
Postop	70	15	-	-
CTI	Preop	$\bar{x}$ =	61 ± 8	
	Postop	$\bar{x}$ =	52 ± 6	

Twelve Ionescu-Shiley aortic valves have been recatheterized between 1 and 6 months postoperatively. The results are presented in Table 5b. The average peak systolic gradient at rest was 5.2 ± 5 mm Hg. In four patients, including one with a 21-mm valve size, no resting gradients were detected.

The mean effective orifice area was 1.77 ± 0.48 cm^2 although it could not be calculated in those cases without gradients and therefore the effective area for this group of patients must be larger.

Mitral Valve Replacement

Eighteen patients had their mitral valve replaced with an Ionescu-Shiley bioprosthesis. Seven of them were isolated mitral replacements. The remaining 11 had simultaneously 7 valves replaced by other bioprosthesis and 4 conservative procedures on the tricuspid valve (Table 2). The operative mortality was four cases, one due to low cardiac output and three due to massive hemorrhage secondary to a left ventricular rupture. Their clinical and surgical characteristics are presented in Table 6.

Among the 14 surviving patients, one had a massive thrombosis of the atrial aspect of the valve 7 months after its implantation. Bacteriological examination was negative and the patient survived the reoperation. No thromboembolic phenomena have been detected and all patients are in functional Class I.

Six patients were recatheterized. One of them, with the thrombosed bioprosthesis, had a mean diastolic gradient of 16 mm Hg at rest. The remaining five patients had an average mean diastolic gradient of 6.0 ± 1.6 mm Hg at rest and 10.5 ± 3 mm Hg after volume overload. The effective orifice area was 2.16 ± 0.41 cm^2. The remaining data are presented in Table 5a.

The pulmonary valve replacement was on a patient with tetralogy of Fallot and pulmonary valve agenesia. The follow-up was uneventful.

Table 5a. Pre- and postoperative haemodynamic data (mean values ± SD) of 5 patients having mitral valve replacement with pericardial bioprosthesis

	CI ($l/min/m^2$)		PWP (mm Hg)		PAP (mm Hg)		PVR ($dynes.s.cm^{-5}$)		MDG (mm Hg)		MVA (cm^2)	
	R	VO	R	VO	R	VO	R	VO	R	VO	R	VO
Preoperative	2.36	2.82	18.4	28.0	29	37	561	-	17.5	22.6	-	-
	±0.52	±0.76	±5.9	±4.3	±7	±5	±211	-	±4.9	±0.6	-	-
Postoperative	2.89	3.29	8.6	15.0	19	25	308	-	6.0	10.5	2.16	-
	±0.22	±0.55	±3.4	±4.9	±4	±3	±101	-	±1.6	±3.5	±0.41	-
P value	NS	NS	<0.02	<0.005	<0.05	<0.005	<0.05	-	<0.02	<0.005	-	-

CI, cardiac index; *PWP*, mean pulmonary wedge pressure; *PAP*, mean pulmonary artery pressure; *PVR*, pulmonary vascular resistance; *MDG*, mean diastolic gradient; *MVA*, mitral valve area; *R*, rest; *VO*, volume overload; *SD*, standard deviation; *NS*, not significant

Table 5b. Pre- and postoperative haemodynamic data (mean values ± SD) of 12 patients having aortic valve replacement with pericardial bioprosthesis

	CI ($l/min/m^2$)		PWP (mm Hg)		LVEDP (mm Hg)		PSG (mm Hg)		AVA (cm^2)	
	R	VO	R	VO	R	VO	R	VO	R	VO
Preoperative	2.76	2.74	15.9	25.4	16.7	19.4	54.6	60.8	-	-
	±0.72	±0.58	±6.7	±10.4	±3.0	±7.7	±28.3	±34.0	-	-
Postoperative	2.98	2.94	8.6	14.7	6.0	10.1	5.2	5.4	1.77	-
	±0.5	±0.37	±3.9	±6.2	±2.0	±3.9	±5.0	±5.8	±0.48	-
P value	NS	NS	<0.005	<0.02	<0.001	<0.005	<0.001	<0.001	-	-

CI, cardiac index; *PWP*, mean pulmonary wedge pressure; *LVEDP*, left ventricular end-diastolic pressure; *PSG*, peak systolic gradient; *AVA*, aortic valve area; *R*, rest; *VO*, volume overload; *SD*, standard deviation; *NS*, not significant

Table 6. Left ventricular ruptures

Case	Age	Sex	Diag	FC	CTI	LVEDVI	Surgery[a]
1	65	F	MML	III	75	180	MVR - IO 31
			MAL				AVR - IO 25
			MTL				T Com - Flx
2	60	F	MML	III	64	105	MVR - IO 29
3	49	F	MML	IV	65	125	MVR - IO 27
			TI				T Flx

[a]Cold cardioplegia and apical vent in all cases

MML, mixed mitral lesion; *MAL*, mixed aortic lesion; *MTL*, mixed tricuspid lesion; *TI*, tricuspid insufficiency; *CTI*, cardiothoracic index; *LVEDVI*, left ventricular end-diastolic volume index.
Surgery: *MVR*, mitral valve replacement; *AVR*, aortic valve replacement; *T Com*, tricuspid commissurotomy; *Flx*, Duran flexible ring annuloplasty

Discussion

The inability to control adequate levels of anticoagulation in a large number of our patients together with the inherent danger of hemorrhage determined our selection of valve prosthesis. Since the beginning of our unit 836 Hancock valves were used with very satisfactory clinical results both in terms of thromboembolism and valve durability. Our hemodynamic data obtained from 305 recatheterized valves showed that the flow-related effective orifice of the Hancock valve is always stenotic particularly significant in the small sizes (2). The lower valvular gradients of the Ionescu-Shiley, as reported both in vitro by Gabbay et al. (4) and in vivo by Tandon et al. (3), encouraged us to initiate a short series of aortic replacements in patients with annuli smaller than 25 mm while continuing with the routine use of porcine xenografts.

Our initial surgical experience in the aortic position showed that the design of the Ionescu-Shiley valve with its prominent struts makes its placement technically more difficult than our standard porcine xenograft insertion. This is particularly so when tying the sutures and closing the aortotomy. It has, however, to be considered that experience with a particular prosthesis necessarily makes its surgical handling easier.

The operative mortality of 3.3% for the isolated aortic replacement and 9.4% overall mortality compares favourably with our experience with the porcine valve which is 4.6% and 8.7% respectively.

Medium-term results show a very satisfactory evolution with only one death due to bacterial endocarditis and no incidence of thromboembolism or valve failures. Two patients needed reoperation for endocarditis. This figure of three patients with infective valve endocarditis is, however, slightly worrisome although it is a constant feature of all types of valve surgery. Ott et al. (5) reports one instance of pericardial valve dehiscence contaminated with mycobacterium chelonei, a problem also present in the glutaraldehyde-preserved porcine valves.

A better sterilization should be expected in those valves preserved with formaldehyde.

The postoperative hemodynamic data show a net superiority of the pericardial valve over the porcine xenograft. The residual gradients were always inferior to those found with the Hancock valve in every size and at similar average flow. Unpublished data from our laboratory indicate that this is also true for the Carpentier-Edwards xenograft.

Encouraged by the early results of the pericardial valve in the aortic position we started using it in the mitral area, particularly in patients with annuli below 29 mm. Our experience is too limited to make any significant statement. However, again its design characteristics, with longer prongs than the porcine valves, makes it, at least initially, more difficult to place. Furthermore, the presence of three ventricular ruptures, not necessarily due to this only factor, cooled our initial enthusiasm. Cobbs et al. (6) have characterized the possible causes of midventricular disruption after mitral valve replacement with Hancock valves. It is not apparent which is the cause for our ruptures although it has to be pointed out that all were subjected to cold cardioplegia and a left apical vent (Table 6). On the other hand, our experience with the Hancock valve, using a similar surgical technique, does not show – to our knowledge – a single case of rupture.

Those patients who survived had a remarkably problem-free follow-up with the exception of one case of valve thrombosis. However, it is too short a period to conform the durability reported by other authors (3).

Our hemodynamic data show very similar results to those presented by Tandom et al. (3). Again the transvalvular gradients are lower in the pericardial than in the Hancock valves for any given size. The Ionescu-Shiley valves, by achieving lower gradients at flows similar to those of the porcine valves, must offer less resistance to their

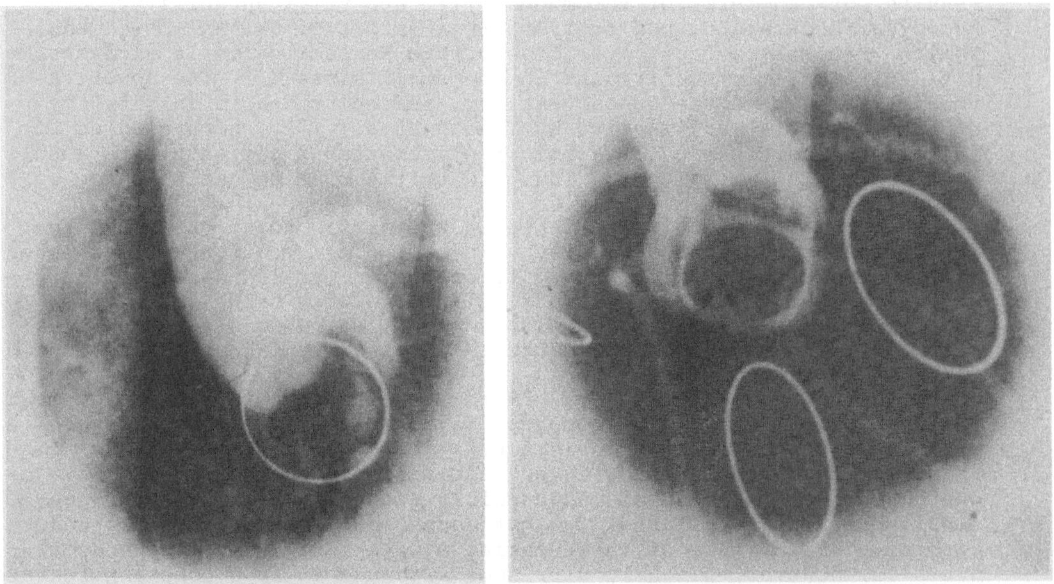

a b

Fig. 1a,b. Angiographic views of a Hancock valve a and an Ionescu-Shiley xenograft b in the aortic position. Note the triangular opening of the porcine valve compared with the circular orifice of the pericardial valve opening and larger physical orifices for the same patient's annulus. Figure 1 clearly shows this difference in vivo.

It is therefore felt that the Ionescu-Shiley pericardial xenograft, because of its design, represents, from a hemodynamic point of view, an advance with subsequent lower gradients and thromboembolic rate. But simultaneously, this geometry entails some negative surgical implications.

Addendum. Since writing the manuscript two transient embolic accidents, occurring in one patient with an Ionescu aortic and Hancock mitral replacement, have been brought to our attention.

References

1. Carrion MF, Gallo JI, Berrazueta JR, Duran CMG (1979) Valvular replacement with Hancock prosthesis. 14th World Congress of the International Cardiovascular Surgery Society, San Francisco, September 2-8, 1979
2. Ubago JL, Figueroa A, Colman T, Ochoteco A, Duran CMG (1980) Hemodynamic factors that affect calculated orifice areas in the mitral Hancock xenograft valve. Circulation 61:388
3. Tandom AP, Smith DR, Ionescu MI (1978) Hemodynamic evaluation of the Ionescu-Shiley pericardial xenograft in the mitral position. Am Heart J 95:595
4. Gabbay S, McQueen D, Yellin EL, Baker RM, Frater RWM (1978) In vitro hydrodynamic performance of mitral valve prosthesis in high flow rates. 48th Annual Meeting of the AATS, New Orleans, Louisiana, May 8-10, 1978
5. Ott D, Norman J, Cooley D (to be published) Experience with the Ionescu-Shiley xenograft. Cardiovasc Dis Texas Heart Inst
6. Cobbs BW, Hatcher CR, Craver JM, Jones EL, Sewel CW (1980) Transverse midventricular disruption after mitral valve replacement. Am Heart J 99:33

Criteria for Evaluation of Material for Porcine Heterograft Valves

L. Anisimowicz, M. Trenkner, S. Raczyński, A. Gorczyński, R. Gutkowski, and A. Drapella*

Preface

During the initial period of the study of aortic valves (1) in 1974 it was found that a number of porcine valves was incompetent at pressures as low as 50-60 mm Hg while others remained fully competent at pressures over 300 mm Hg. On some days almost all harvested valves were incompetent, while on others the reverse was true. A correlation with the method of feeding was suggested but not investigated at that time because the study dealt with the valves competent at high pressures only.

This hypothesis, if validated, seems to be of importance both from the theoretical point of view and for the process of obtaining material for valvular heterografts. No data on this subject, as well as on the criteria of selection of valves or the details of the manufacturing process, are available in the literature. The heterograft manufacturing companies must have undoubtedly done a lot of research on this problem but refuse any comment, considering it a "know-how" secret

An assumption was made that the valve which is a candidate for heterograft should in an unstented state sustain pressures of at least 160 mm Hg for AVR and 300 mm Hg for MVR. The reasons for using such criteria will be discussed.

In the first part of the study we tried to find simple criteria making it possible to eliminate the groups of donors with a small proportion of valves which may be used as heterografts. In the second part we tried to find the correlation between the shape of the aortic root at low pressures and the competence of the valve at maximal pressures.

Material and Methods

Material consisted of 100 porcine hearts harvested 20 min after slaughtering. All animals were of the Wielka Biala Polska (Big White Polish) breed. Pigs were raised using three types of feeding:

1) Natural feeding with human leftovers (small farms, army barracks),
2) Mixed type feeding – natural feeding plus approximately 50% special pig food,
3) "Industrial" raising of pigs in large farms – in artificial conditions, feeding exclusively with special food with added vitamins, antibiotics, and mineral salts.

*Institute of Surgery, Medical Academy Gdańsk, Poland, and Institute of Electronic Technology, Gdańsk Polytechnic, Gdańsk, Poland

Sex, weight, and heart weight were known in every case examined. Hearts were stored in a refrigerator and studied 3-7 h after slaughtering. Hearts were suspended on a stative, both coronary arteries ligated at the origin, left ventricle cut off transversally approximately 2-3 cm below aortic valve level, and atrial walls removed. A Y cannula was introduced into the ascending aorta and the aorta filled with normal saline. The filling branch of the cannula was clamped and intraaortic pressure increased using sphygmomanometer measurements at 40 mm Hg intervals. The study was terminated at the moment of appearance of aortic valve incompetence, manifested as transvalvular leak. The pressure at wich this occurred was labeled "incompetence pressure" (P_n). Aortic dimensions were measured at two levels. Direct measurement with the use of a tape was made at the lower level, i.e., at the level of the lowest point of leaflet attachments, and indirectly at the upper level, i.e., at the level of leaflet commissures. The latter method consisted of measuring the sides of the triangle formed by the three commissures. Aortic circumference and diameter were calculated from the formula for the dimensions of a circle circumscribed on a triangle. The rationale for use of this method and details were described in another paper (2). These measurements also made possible the evaluation of the valve symmetry, which seems to be an important criterion for the usefulness of the valve as a heterograft. Specimens for microscopy were obtained from the ascending aorta of every heart. Thickness of the aortic wall was measured using a MNP-1 microscopic projector. Routine hematoxylin-eosin stain and Fränkl stain for elastic fibers were applied.

Statistical analysis consisted of an x^2 test and correlation factor calculation using a Hewlett-Packard HP-9830 computer. Only valves competent at pressures over 160 mm Hg were used for studies of correlation between the value of incompetence pressure (P_n) and the behavior of the two aortic diameters in the increasing pressures. An index:

$$\frac{\text{upper diameter} - \text{lower diameter}}{\text{lower diameter}}$$

was introduced. At 120 mm Hg there was distinct negative correlation between the incompetence pressure value's logarithm and the value of the index mentioned. Use of log P_n instead of the P_n value proved to be essential because it made it possible to "comprise" values having naturally large dispersion, and the correlation between P_n and index values was less significant.

Results and Discussion

The dependence between such single factors as donor's sex and weight and the percentage of valves competent at given pressures is shown in Figs. 1 and 2. The histogram in Fig. 1 shows that there is almost equal distribution of the sexes of donors of valves competent at pressures up to 160 mm Hg, but a distinct prevalence of males in the group of extremely "strong" valves (competent up to 300 mm Hg) was present. Analysis of Fig. 2 reveals that there is a significant increase in the percentage of "strong" valves from pigs weighing from 95 to 105 kg.

The experimental distribution of natural logarithms of incompetence pressure values (L_nP_n) was studied. The highest average L_nP_n values were found in groups fed naturally and with mixed food.

In order to find which group is most suitable for large-scale production, the probability of finding a valve of a given incompetence pressure was calculated. The results are shown in Fig. 3. It may be

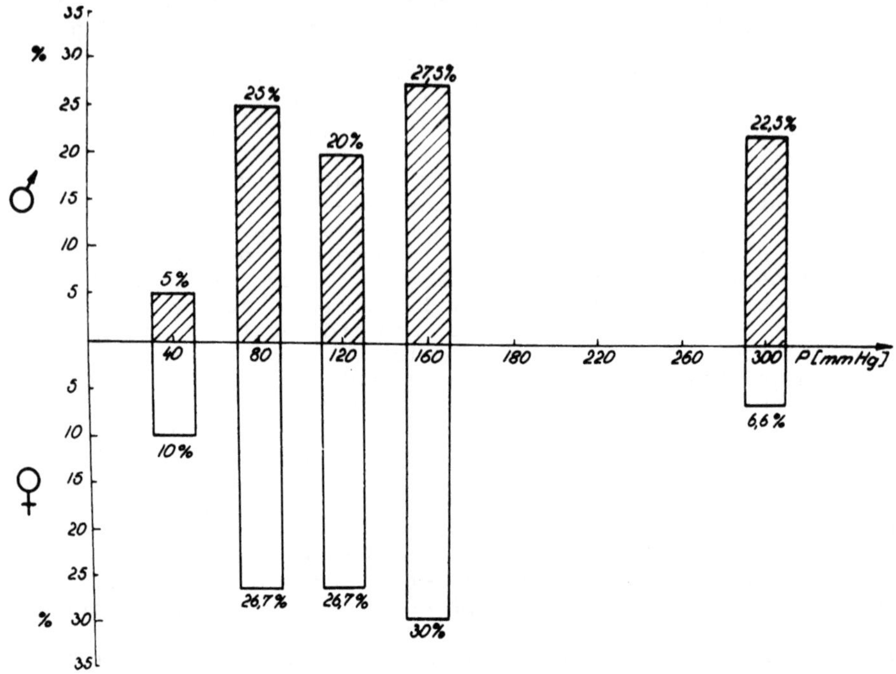

Fig. 1. Percentage of valves of a given P_n in male and female donors

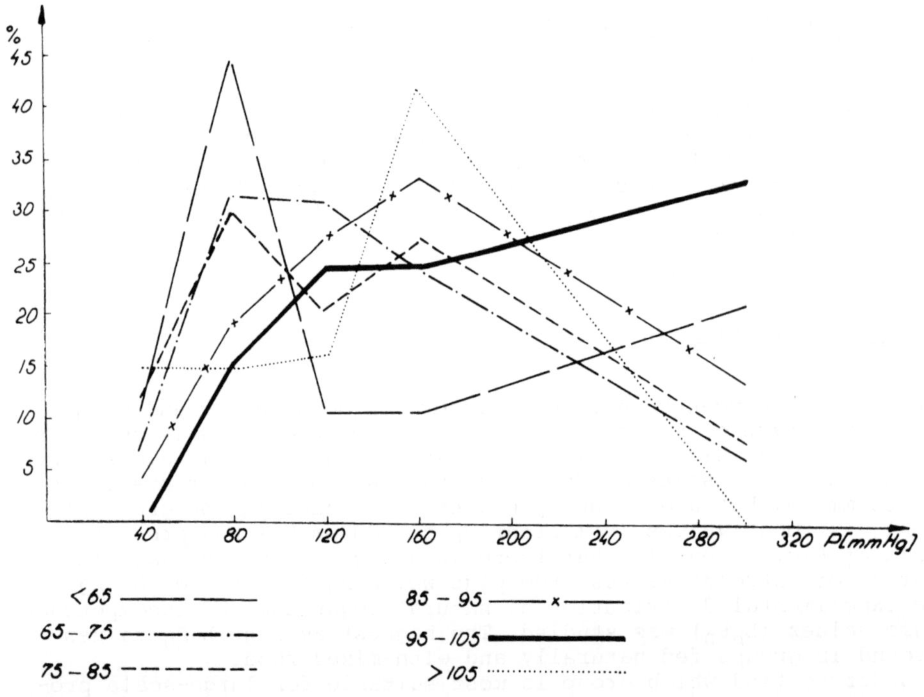

Fig. 2. Percentage of valves of a given P_n in six weight groups

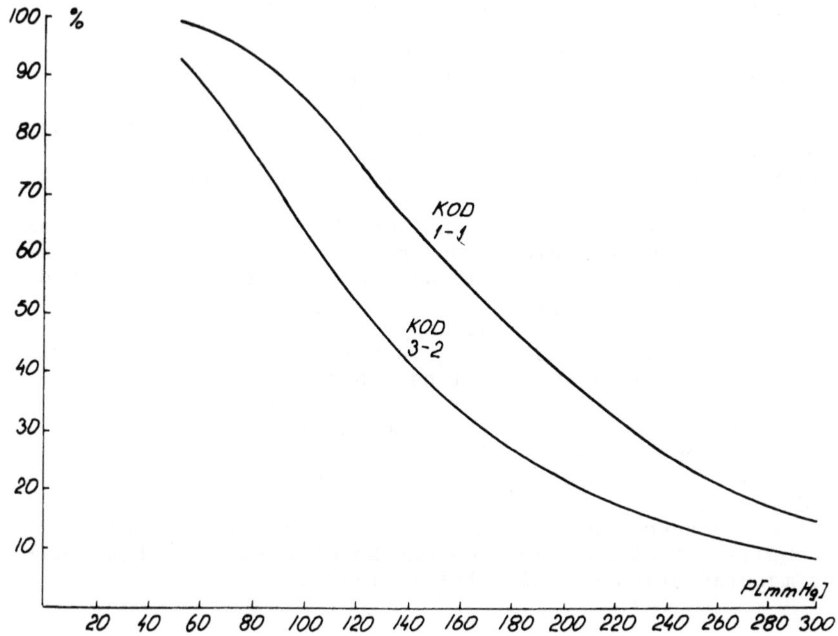

Fig. 3. Probability of finding a valve of given P_n. Code 1-1: females fed naturally, code 3-2: males fed artificially

seen that in animals fed naturally there is a 55% probability of finding a valve competent at a pressure of 160 mm Hg, while in group fed artificially it is only 30%. Respective values are in the same relation for pressures of 300 mm Hg.

No correlation was found between the P_n values and heart weight and single aortic diameters, but there was correlation between the product of the upper and lower diameter values.

As indicated previously the indirect measurement of the upper aortic diameter made possible the evaluation of the symmetry of the valve. Valves showing differences of 2 mm and more between the dimensions of the sides of the triangle were considered as asymmetric. This was the case in 39% of all valves. There was no correlation between the aortic wall thickness and P_n values.

Results of microscopic studies did not reveal any significant difference in the elastic fiber content in cases of "strong" and "weak" valves. On the other hand, there was a marked difference in the pigs fed naturally and artificially. In the previous ones the elastic fibers of the aortic wall are tightly packed and have a regular pattern, while in the latter their number is smaller, the pattern is irregular, and there is a marked increase in the amount of collagen.

It seems logical to assume that the value of pressure at which an unstented valve remains competent may be used as a criterion for the classification of valve suitability as a heterograft. Although the stent may change the P_n value by limiting the distention of the valve, a natural valve competent at higher pressures seems to be preferable to a valve made competent by an artificial construction, which the stent is – no matter how – sophisticated.

The choice of pressure values was somewhat arbitrary, but it seems logical to implant a valve competent in an unstented state at pressure double the normal load. In view of inevitable valve deterioration following the implantation, providing such a reserve seems to be a sound approach.

The first elimination of some donors, based on such simple criteria as sex and weight, can be introduced at the moment of harvesting. Another conclusion is that as there is a twofold higher probability of finding a valve proper for heterograft manufacturing in pigs fed naturally, harvesting of the valves limited to this group must have an economic impact and probably these valves will be more durable after implantation.

Contrary to expectations there was no correlation between the elastic fiber content and the P_n values. On the other hand, the influence of the method of feeding on the aortic wall structure is evident and the problem needs further study.

Finally, a correlation between the behavior of aortic dimensions in pressures up to 120 mm Hg and the P_n values seems to have theoretical and probably practical implications. This finding requires investigation on a larger material and will be used as a working hypothesis in the prospective studies. This hypothesis, if confirmed, would allow prediction of the P_n value after testing the valve with physiologic pressures, which cannot be deleterious for the valve structure and mechanism.

In view of the absence in the literature of reports on related problems, we believe that our findings may be of value for those considering the manufacturing of valve heterografts.

References

1. Trenkner M (1974) Aortic homo- and heterografts: a complex study. Medical dissertation, Medical Academy of Gdańsk
2. Trenkner M, Raczyński S, Gutkowski R (1976) Optimal diameter of the stent for aortic valvular grafts. J Thorac Cardiovasc Surg 72:613

Surgical Treatment of Rheumatic Tricuspid Stenosis

S.Tarbiat, M.Ataii, R.Ghazvinian, and A.Sheikh-Zadeh*

It has been pointed out that tricuspid stenosis (TS) occurs much more frequently than was recognized. However, its high incidence in pathological reports, 30% in seven series collected by Kitchen and Turner (11) and 16% in surgical reports by Baily and Bolten (1), is not surprising, in contrast with a modest incidence in most clinical reports. This discrepancy can be explained by the lack of an inital clinical index of suspicion, the difficulty of diagnosis in the presence of atrial fibrillation (13), and the inadequate appreciation of the whole spectrum of organic tricuspid valve disease (6).

Also unrecognized TS may worsen the results of mitral and/or aortic valve surgery, giving rise to unforeseen complications during and after operation (15). The purpose of this communication is to report the surgical results and pre- and postoperative clinical and hemodynamic findings in 73 patients with chronic rheumatic TS, and some surgical points of view.

Material and Methods

Out of 936 patients with rheumatic valvular disease in a period of 70 months, 73 patients with TS underwent open heart surgery with a mean follow-up period of 38 months. All patients had a complete physical examination with particular attention to jugular venous, hepatic pulsation, and auscultation. A 12-lead electrocardiogram and chest roentgenogram were performed on all patients. A phonocardiogram was recorded on a 12-channel E and 6-channel Phillips (Honeywell) UV recorder at a paper speed of 50 and 100 mm per second. The recordings were usually obtained in the expiratory phase. A complete right and left heart catheterization was performed on all patients in fasting state and without premedication. The simultaneous pressures were recorded from the right ventricle and right atrium using two end hole venous catheters, one positioned in the right ventricular cavity and the other in the main right atrial cavity. The pressures were recorded using equisensitive transducers (Model p23 Statham). The recordings were taken from the same baseline. The cardiac output was measured by this principle, and mitral and tricuspid valve areas were calculated hemodynamically from the measurements using the Gorlin formula (7). The criteria of Killip and Lukas (10) were used for hemodynamic diagnosis.

*The Departments of Adult Cardiology, Cardiovascular Surgery and Anesthesiology Cardiovascular Medical and Research Centre, Teheran, Iran

Follow-up studies were performed on all patients. Fifty-two patients had complete hemodynamic studies postoperatively; 21 patients refused the hemodynamic studies. The catheterized patients were divided into two groups: group I (46 cases) had tricuspid commissurotomy, group II (6 cases), tricuspid valve replacement.

Results

Of the 73 patients with TS, 30 were male, and 43 female. These patients constituted the 6% of the total patients with rheumatic heart disease who underwent surgical procedures. Their ages ranged between 14 and 48 years with a mean of 29 ± 11.2 years. All patients had other associated valvular lesions, among which the combination of TS and mitral stenosis was the most common, followed by association of TS and mitral stenosis and tricuspid regurgitation. In two patients all four valves were involved. The majority of patients were clinically in functional class III and IV of the New York Heart Association classifications (Fig. 2).

Large A waves were present in all patients, with sinus rhythm and presystolic liver impulse recordable in 32 patients. Jugular vein pulses showed a tall A wave in patients with normal rhythm and a small V wave and slow Y descent and occasionally an h(d) wave, especially in patients with sinus bradycardia as reported by Holldack and Wolf (9). The auscultatory findings are summarized in Table 1 as well as characteristic changes in both systolic and diastolic tricuspid murmurs that were observed during phases of respiration in all cases (Fig. 1). Increased intensity of the systolic murmur during inspiration in patients with TS dominant over tricuspid regurgitation was present in 12 cases, as also reported by Kitchen and Turner (11). The electrocardiographic findings showed that 42 patients had normal sinus rhythm, whereas 31 patients were in atrial fibrillation. In all patients with sinus rhythm P wave amplitude was more than 3 mv. The peaked P waves in lead 2 had a mean amplitude of 4.98 ± 1.64 mv with a range of 3.5-11.5 mv. The chest X-ray showed a prominent lower right cardiac border; there was, however, no correlation between right atrial bulging and severity of TS; other findings were consistent with associated diseases. All patients underwent open heart surgery. The type of procedures performed are summarized in Table 2.

At surgery we found two types of valve changes. In type I the tricuspid valve are severely thickened with disappearance of the chordae and attachment of the papillary muscles to the cusps. The commissures are not appreciable and the valves are immobile. In type II the valve is mobile, the cusps are thickened, and the commissures are fused with relatively good appreciable chordae and papillary muscles. The type I

Table 1. Auscultatory and phonocardiographic features in 73 patients with rheumatic tricuspid stenosis

	Number of patients	percent
Tricuspid mid-diastolic murmur	68/73	86
Tricuspid regurgitant murmur	72/73	98.6
Tricuspid presystolic murmur	35/73	48
Tricuspid opening snap	48/73	65.1
Large jugular A waves	42/73	57.5

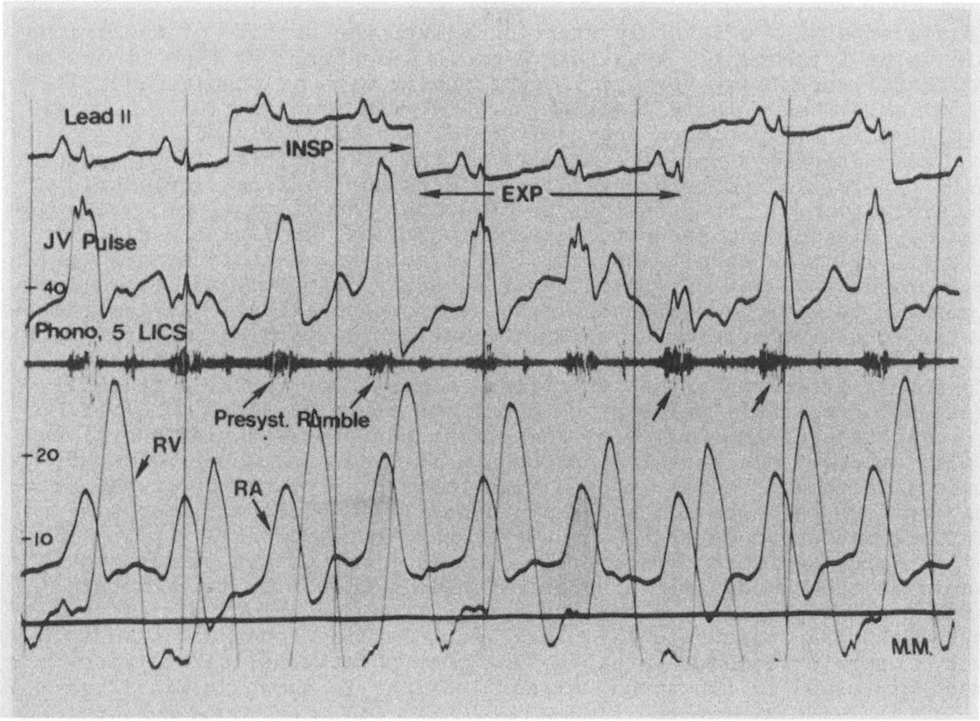

Fig. 1. Typical electrocardiogram, jugular venous pulse, phonocardiogram, and simultanous pressure curve in right atrium and ventricle. Note the effect of inspiration

Table 2. Types of operative procedures performed on 73 patients with rheumatic tricuspid stenosis

Type of procedures	Number of cases
Tricuspid valve replacement and mitral valve replacement	10
Tricuspid valve replacement, mitral valve replacement, and aortic valve replacement	3
Tricuspid commissurotomy and mitral commissurotomy	27
Tricuspid commissurotomy and mitral valve replacement	12
Tricuspid valve repair and commissurotomy and mitral valve replacement	9
Tricuspid valve repair and commissurotomy and mitral commissurotomy	12

is almost always a severely stenotic valve; the orifice of the tricuspid valve is generally less than 8 mm in diameter. The type II can be moderately or mildly stenotic, occasionally with tricuspid regurgitation; this was so in 16 cases at surgery. The right atrium was hypertrophied in all patients (severely in 45 and mildly in 28).

The preferred surgical technique at the present time is to open anteroseptal and posteroseptal commissures and to repair tricuspid regurgitation, if it preexists or develops. The valve is bicuspid. One may dissect and separate attached chordaes, or divide papillary muscles if it is at all necessary. Tricuspid valve replacements were performed in 13 patients because of severely deformed, stiffened, and immobile valves. Two patients were lost postoperatively (2.7% mortality), one with triple valve replacement in low cardiac output, and the other with cardiac tamponade and arrhythmias. One patient died 37 months after surgery in functional class IV of the NYHA classification, of multiple pulmonary and peripheral embolism.

Six cases of embolism were seen; four patients with peripheral emboli, necessitating surgical procedure in one, and two of pulmonary emboli which was lethal in one. Mild tricuspid regurgitation was present in four patients and moderate in one. Mild tricuspid stenosis in three cases and moderate in one were seen after surgery.

The pre- and postoperative hemodynamic findings are summarized in Table 3. The hemodynamic studies revealed a reduction in pulmonary artery wedge pressure, pulmonary artery pressure, right atrial pressure, and mean tricuspid valve gradient. Cardiac index and tricuspid valve area increased remarkably. The postoperative clinical improvement expressed in functional classifications is shown in Fig. 2.

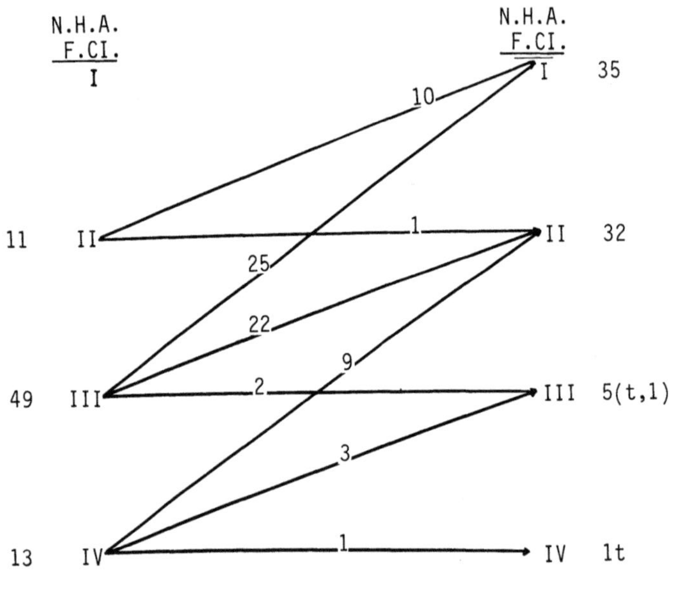

Fig. 2. Pre- and postoperative class (NYHA) of 73 patients with tricuspid stenosis. The numbers on the lines represent the clinical improvement

Table 3. Hemodynamic findings in 73 patients with chronic rheumatic tricuspid stenosis (all values expressed are mean ± 1 SD)

	Preoperative	Postoperative group I (46 pts)	Postoperative group II (6 pts)
RA pressure mm Hg	14 ± 7	5.2 ± 2	8.2 ± 2.4
RVEDP mm Hg	5 ± 3	4.9 ± 1.08	4.8 ± 2
PA pressure mm Hg	S. 68 ± 26 D. 37 ± 15 M. 48 ± 21	32 ± 11 21 ± 7 19 ± 13	37 ± 13 25 ± 9 21 ± 12
PAW pressure mm Hg	28 ± 9	6 ± 2.1	5.8 ± 2.7
Mean DTG	10.9 ± 1.7	2.21 ± 92	3.8 ± 0.21
CI $l/min/m^2$	2.152 ± 0.9	3.5 ± 0.7	3.68 ± 1.2
TVA cm^2	0.887 ± 0.43	3.8 ± 0.9	3.2 ± 0.7

CI, cardiac index; *D*, diastolic pressure; *DTG*, diastolic tricuspid gradient; *m*, mean pressure, pulmonary artery; *PAW*, pulmonary artery wedge; *RA*, right atrium; *RVEDP*, right ventricular end-diastolic pressure, systolic pressure; *TVA*, tricuspid valve area.
Group I = 46 patients with tricuspid commissurotomy or reconstruction
Group II = 6 patients with tricuspid valve replacement

Discussion

The severe TS almost always has a rheumatic origin, but can also have other etiologies (11). The association of TS with mitral stenosis and other cardiac lesions due to rheumatic fever has been known for some time (5, 16). The clinical findings and diagnostic values of auscultatory features are extensively discussed by Sheikhzadeh et al. (14).

Whenever the diagnosis of TS is suspected, by even a single clinical sign, it must be confirmed by simultaneous measurement of the right ventricular diastolic and right atrial pressures by cardiac catheterization using Killips hemodynamic criteria (10). The postoperative findings expressed in Table 2 show that our experience with the surgical treatment of the rheumatic valvular lesions including tricuspid has been extremely favorable.

Our experience also shows that if tricuspid commissurotomy is feasible it is preferable to tricuspid valve replacement. In patients with tricuspid commissurotomy there is a lower tricuspid valve gradient postoperatively than in patients with tricuspid valve replacement, but tricuspid valve regurgitation may occur, necessitating tricuspid annuloplasty in some. From a surgical point of view, we think opening the above-mentioned commissures is quite satisfactory; however, opening of the anteroposterior commissure increases the change of tricuspid regurgitation. If the tricuspid valve is stiffened, fixed, and severely deformed, one may have to replace it with a prosthetic valve. This was the case in 13 patients, although in the last 2 years, with our increasing experience with commissurotomy and repair, no patient required a prosthetic valve. Only two patients had pulmonary emboli, which may have originated from the prosthetic valve. Postoperative clinical follow-up of all patients showed marked clinical improvement in 96% of the cases. These results are in contrast to those reported by other workers (2, 3, 4, 12, 8).

The reason for this discrepancy and for the very low mortality and morbidity of our patients with tricuspid valve replacement or commissurotomy with repair is not quite clear. However, we believe that the young age of our patients and the dominant TS over tricuspid regurgitation with consequent better right ventricular performance might explain the encouraging results. In other series the patients were older and had mostly tricuspid regurgitation and impaired myocardium.

Conclusion

We conclude that 1) Rheumatic tricuspid stenosis is a frequently seen lesion, at least in our part of the world. 2) Clinical diagnosis needs careful attention. If a single clinical sign exists, it must be confirmed by simultaneous measurement of right ventricular diastolic and right atrial pressure. 3) The surgical results are quite encouraging even in prosthetic valve replacement. 4) Whenever possible, tricuspid commissurotomy is the preferred method. 5) The younger age of the patients as well as better right ventricular myocardium by dominant TS might explain the encouraging results.

Summary

The surgical results and pre- and postoperative hemodynamic and clinical findings of 73 patients with rheumatic tricuspid stenosis (TS) are presented. It is concluded that TS is relatively frequent and that clinical diagnosis needs careful attention and must be confirmed by simultaneous measurements of the right ventricular and right atrial pressures. The surgical results are encouraging even in prosthetic valve replacement. Tricuspid commissurotomy is the favored method and has less gradient, but in some cases reconstruction or repair must be carried out. Surgical mortality was 2.7% and postoperative clinical improvement was present in 96% of the cases.

References

1. Baily CP, Bolten HE (1956) Criteria for and results of surgery for mitraloslonosis. NY State J Med 56:649, 825
2. Carpentier A, Deloche A, Hanania G, Forman I (1973) Surgical management of acquired tricuspid valve disease. J Thorac Cardiovasc Surg 67:53-65
3. De Vega NG (1971) La anulosplastia selectiva reguable y permanente. Rev Esp Cardiol 25:6-17
4. Dubost C (1968) Surgery of acquired tricuspid cardiopathies in patients with multivalvular lesions. Ann Chir Thorac Cardiovasc 7:557-564
5. Durosiez P (1968) Du retrecissement de la tricuspid. Gaz Hosp Paris 41:310-315
6. El-Sharif N (1971) Rheumatic tricuspid slonosis. A hemodynamic correlation. Br Heart J 33:13-16
7. Gorlin R, Gorlin S (1951) Hydraulic formula for calculation of the area of the slenotic mitral valve, other valves and central circulatory shunts. Am Heart J 41:1-29

8. Grodin P, Meer C, Limit R, Lopez-Besco L, Delcan JL, Revera R, Carpentier A, De Vega NG (1975) Anuloplasty, the end of tricuspid challenge. J Thorac Cardiovasc Surg 70:825-85
9. Holldack K, Wolf D (1966) Atlas und kurzgefaßtes Lehrbuch der Phonokardiographie und verwandte Untersuchungsmethode. Thieme, Stuttgart, p 165
10. Killip T III, Lukas DS (1957) Tricuspid stenosis physiologic criteria for diagnosis and hemodynamic abnormalities. Circulation 16:3-13
11. Kitchen A, Turner R (1964) Diagnosis and treatment of tricuspid stenosis. Br Heart J 26:354-379
12. Ruiz E (1973) Results of tricuspid surgery. Arch Mal Coeur 66:1369-1380
13. Sanders CA, Harthrone JW, De Sanedis RW, Austen WG (1966) Tricuspid: a difficult diagnosis in the presence of atrial fibrillation. Circulation 33:26-33
14. Sheikhzadeh A, Tarbiat S, Paydar D, Shakibi J (1978) Rheumatic tricuspid stenosis. A clinical overview. Acta Cardiol (Brux) 33:431-442
15. Watson H, Lowe K (1962) Severe tricuspid stenosis revealed after aortic votomy. Br Heart J 24:241-244
16. Wood P (1954) An appreciation of mitral stenosis. Br Med J 1:1113

In Vitro Comparison of Heart Valves With Plane and Curved Pendulum Discs

J. Köhler*

Introduction

The most common pendulum valves as heart valve substitutes are the *Björk-Shiley (BS)* and the *Lillehei-Kaster (LK)* valves. Their discs are flat (Fig. 1). As has been shown by the author in earlier investigations, a disc curvature can favor the opening behavior of a pendulum valve in comparison to that of a valve with plane disc. The disadvantages of the flat disc are an incomplete opening and a strong asymmetric distribution of the flow with flow separation and a high risk of thrombus formation behind the valve ring.

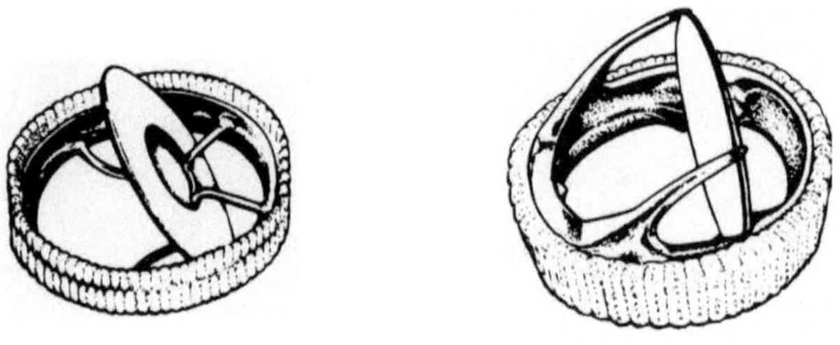

Björk-Shiley (BS) **Lillehei-Kaster (LK)**

Fig. 1. Two types of heart valve prostheses as pendulum valves

The effective opening angle depends on the turning moment of the main flow into the opening direction and two other mechanisms effecting an opposite torque in the closing direction (negative). They are 1) the jet against the small lever of the disc and 2) the vortex behind the disc (see Fig. 2).

Therefore the *Björk-Shiley* valve in mitral position has a small equilibrium opening angle of about 50 degrees accompanied by an unnecessary high pressure loss.

The following report summarizes three steps of investigation:

1) Flow observations with eight different curved discs in an open water channel to determine best disc shapes,
2) measurements of the turning moment and of the pressure loss with eight three-dimensional models in steady flow, and
3) measurements of the pressure loss of two new commercially available pendulum valve types *(Björk-Shiley-cc* and *Omni Science)* in the pulsating flow of a model circulation.

---

*Aerodynamisches Institut der RWTH Aachen, Wüllnerstr. 5-7, D-5100 Aachen

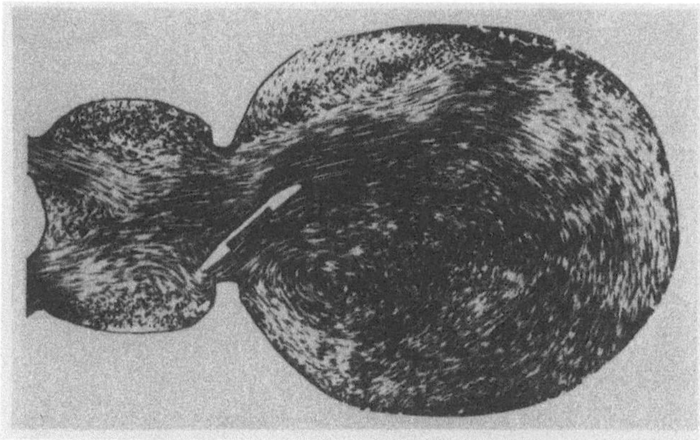

Fig. 2. Simulated flow through the model of a *Brörk-Shiley* mitral valve in a water table with aluminum powder on the water surface. Equilibrium opening angle: $\alpha_g \approx 50^o$

Flow Observations

In order to increase the equilibrium opening angle α_g, where the flow-induced turning moment on the disc vanishes, two valve prototypes have been developed with a plane-convex and a concave-convex disc ([1], see Fig. 3).

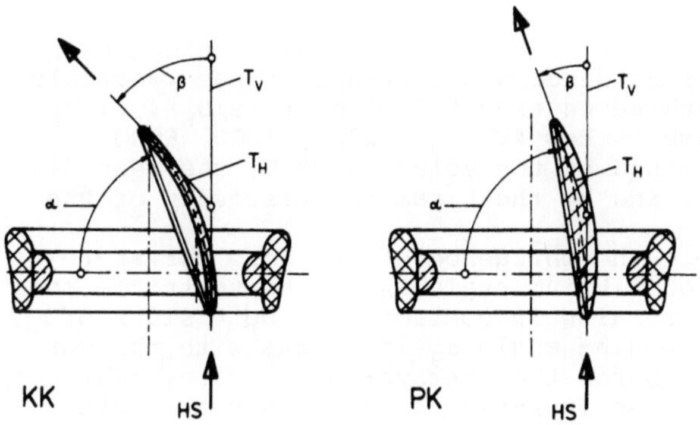

Fig. 3. Two model valves with concave-convex (KK) and plane-convex (PK) disc

The major portion of the stroke volume passes the valve during the main flow phase. In order to compare different valves, the flow therefore can be studied under steady conditions [2].

The curved disc is mounted into the valve ring, so that the bloodstream is guided opposite to the turning direction α of the opening motion. The angle β between the tangents T_V and T_H is greater than zero.

The circular arch was chosen as the basic form of eight different discs for flow visualization. With $r/D_K = 0.02$ and the curvatures $\varphi = f/D_K = 0.031$, 0.05, 0.075, and 0.1, four plane-convex (PK) and four concave-convex (KK) discs were manufactured in a scale 3:1 (Fig. 4). In the model of the atrioventricular region, sieves were used to simulate the dilatation of the ventricular wall during diastole in an open water table. Aluminum powder on the water surface made the flow visible, so that the paths of the particles were reproduced as short lines on photographs.

In the flow model the outer diameter of the valve ring (90 mm) was equivalent to a mounting diameter of about 30 mm. One-half of each disc was fixed at a lever with highly movable pivot bearing. Thereby

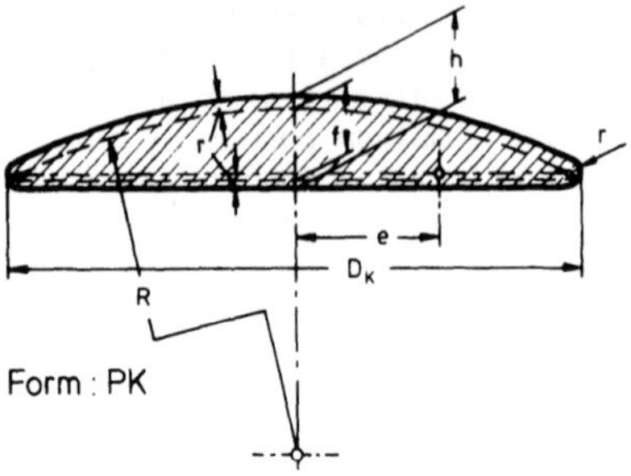

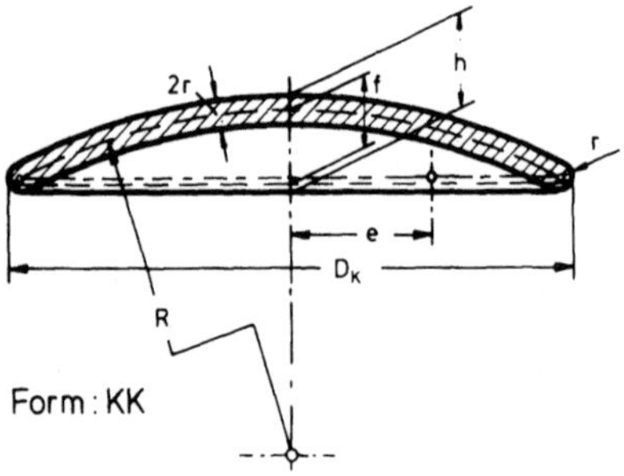

Fig. 4. Geometry of the model valve disc

the different discs were balanced to their equilibrium opening angle α_g by the flow. Each of the eight discs was tested in three ventricles of different sizes (K,M,G) with seven excentricities $\varepsilon = e/D_K$ (0.1 up to 0.4) and three Reynolds numbers $Re = 4\dot{V}/\pi D_o \nu$ (2000, 4000, 6000). The Reynolds number was determined by the volume flow $\dot{V}$, the mean diameter of the mitral ostium D_o, and by the kinematic viscosity of the fluid.

Figure 5 shows as an example the influence of the disc curvature on the flow pattern and on the equilibrium angle α_g in the ventricle model of average size (M). The flow remains in contact with both sides of each of the eight discs. The opening angle α_g increases with the curvature and reaches higher values for the concave-convex discs (KK) than for the plane-convex disc (PK). An increase of α_g appears also with increasing excentricity ε and with increasing Reynolds number as shown earlier [1].

Torque and Pressure Loss in Steady Flow

A three-dimensional model of the left atrium and the left ventricle which is used for torque and pressure loss measurements is shown schematically in Figure 6. The excentricity of the turning axis of the valve disc was $\varepsilon = e/D_K = 0.25$. The Reynolds number $Re = 4800$ corresponded to a volume flow $\dot{V} = 340\ cm^3/s$ in vivo during the main filling phase under normal conditions. The dilatation of the ventricle during diastole was simulated by a textile bag as the ventricle wall. The torque on the valve disc caused by the steady air flow was determined by the torsion angle of a spring wire torque balance and the pressure loss $\Delta p_v = p_1 - p_3$ by the pressure difference between the atrium and the ventricle near the wall (see Fig. 6). A similar model of the outflow tract of the left ventricle and of the ascending aorta was used for valve models in aortic position.

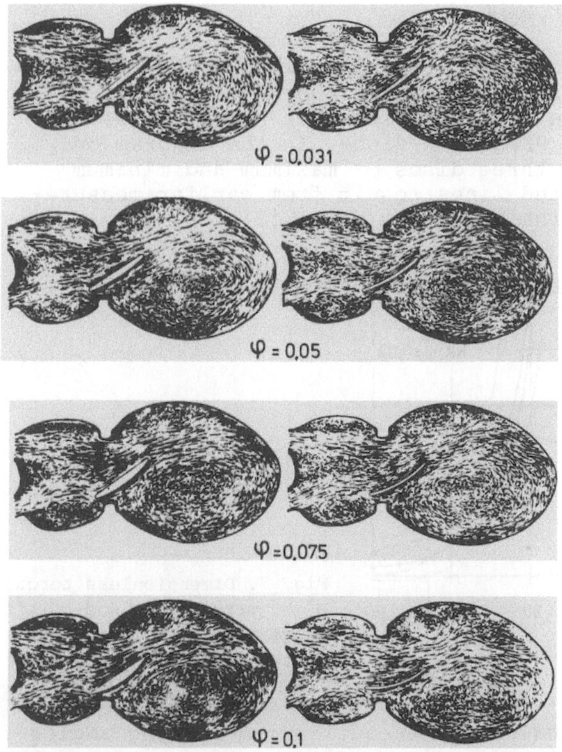

Fig. 5. Highly movable plane-convex and concave-convex discs of different curvature φ in the steady water table flow. Mitral position. Excentricity $\varepsilon = 0.25$; $Re = 6000$

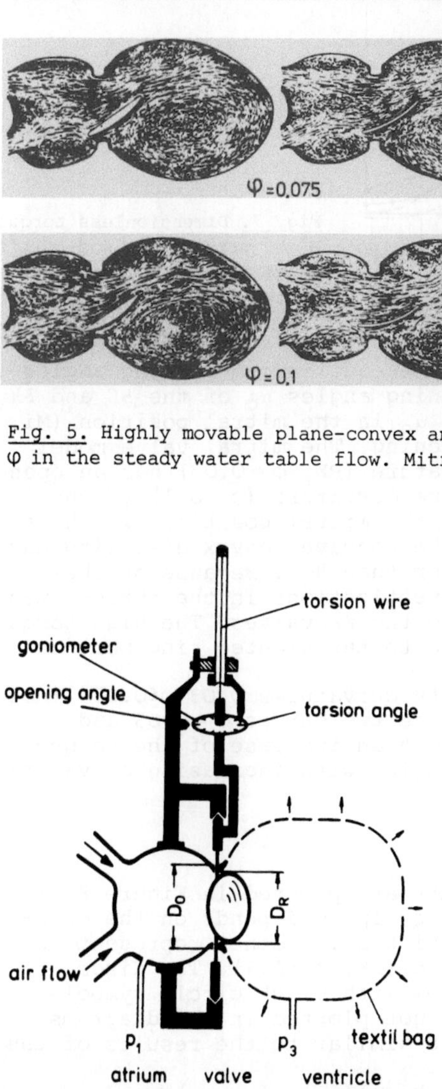

Fig. 6. Three-dimensional atrioventricular model with spring wire torque balance for steady air flow

Turning Moment

In Figure 7 the dimensionless torque $M^+ = M/q_e\,A_o$ (with $q = \rho\dot{V}^2/2A_o^2$ = dynamic pressure of the volume flow $\dot{V}$ in a section $A_o = \pi D_o^2/4$) is plotted versus the opening angle α. The solid lines show the results of the torque measurements with PK and KK discs. In the diagram only the results obtained for two or three discs of maximum and minimum curvature are depicted. The dotted lines result from earlier measurements with *BS* and *LK* valves in the same flow model [3].

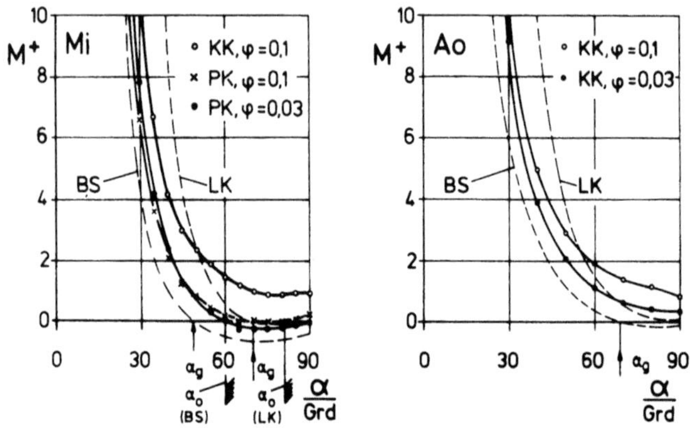

Fig. 7. Dimensionless torque M^+ of mitral (Mi) and aortic valve models (Ao) depending on the opening angle α (exp)

The arrows in the diagrams indicate the equilibrium opening angles α_g and the dashed areas the maximum opening angles α_o of the *BS* and *LK* valves. For both valves α_g is less than α_o in the mitral position (Mi, left) corresponding to an incomplete opening. The mitral valve model with plane-convex disc of smallest curvature (PK, $\varphi = 0.03$) has an opening angle $\alpha_g \approx 60°$. The PK disc of maximum curvature ($\varphi = 0.1$) reaches an equilibrium opening angle $\alpha_g \approx 70°$ in the mitral position, which is higher than that of the *LK* valve. For the concave-convex disc with maximum curvature (KK, $\varphi = 0.1$) α_g is greater than 90°. Because of these better results for the KK discs, the investigations in the three-dimensional aortic flow model were limited to the KK valves. The high torque values of the *LK* valve for $\alpha < 40°$ are due to the slanted ring bore and its smaller inner diameter.

The torque values of the KK discs with curvatures $0.03 < \varphi \leq 0.075$ (not plotted in the diagrams) range between the two curves $\varphi = 0.03$ and $\varphi = 0.1$. In general the measurements showed an increase of the torque values and of the equilibrium opening angles with increasing curvature.

Pressure Loss

Some results of the pressure measurements are plotted in Figure 8. The dimensionless pressure loss coefficient $\zeta = \Delta p_v/q$ depends on the opening angle α and on the disc type. The thick solid lines represent the concave-convex discs of maximum curvature (KK, $\varphi = 0.1$). The discs of minimum curvature correspond to the lines with black circle symbols. The results of the other curved discs – not plotted in the diagrams – range between the full lines in Figure 8 similar to the results of the torque measurements.

Comparing the full lines with the broken lines of the *BS* and *LK* valves of the same textile ring diameter D_o, a considerable decrease of the pressure loss becomes evident for the opening angles $\alpha_o = 60°$ *(BS)* and 80° *(LK)*.

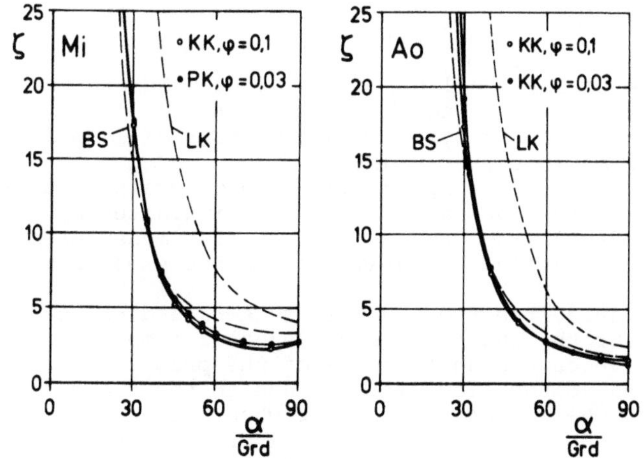

Fig. 8. Pressure loss coefficient ζ of mitral (Mi) and aortic valve models (Ao) depending on the opening angle α (exp)

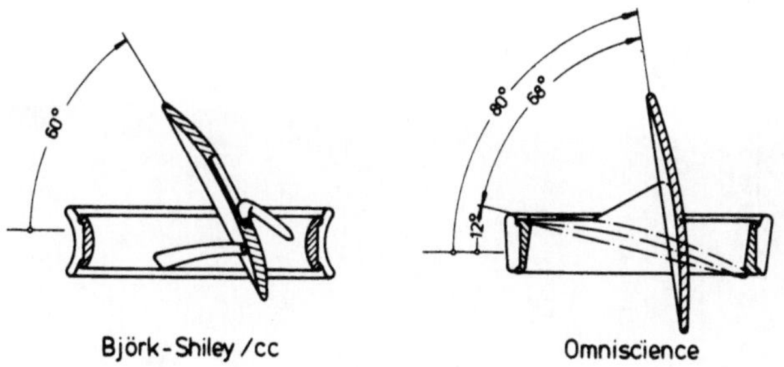

Fig. 9. Two new commercially available prosthetic heart valves with curved discs

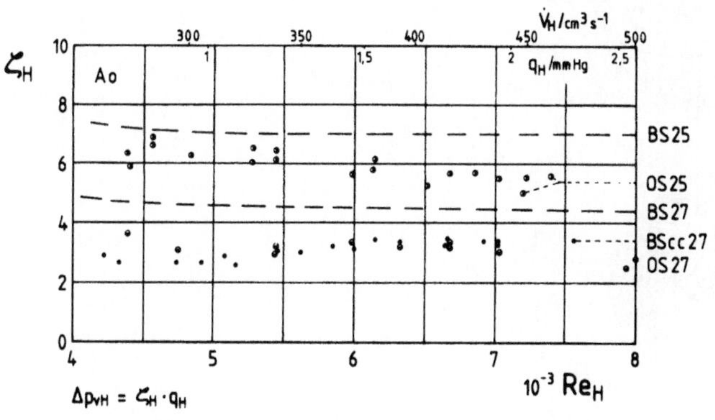

Fig. 10. Pressure loss coefficient ζ_H of *Björk-Shiley* valves (---) and of the two new valves with curved disc *(BS*-cc and *Omni Science)* in pulsating aortic flow of a mock circulation depending on the Reynolds number Re_H

Pressure Loss in Pulsating Flow

The two investigated commercially available types of pendulum valves with curved disc are the *BS-cc valve* and the *Omni Science valve* (*OS*, Fig. 9). They were mounted in aortic position of an artificial, pulsating ventricle with an elastic aortic model [2].

The pressure loss coefficient ζ_H – again the ratio of pressure loss to kinetic energy – is valid for the main flow phase, indicated by the index "H" (Fig. 10). The dotted lines result from earlier measurements with *BS* valves of different textile ring diameters in the same mock circulation.

Compared with former models, the two new valves *BS-cc* and *OS* lead to a smaller heart load over the whole range of Reynolds number or volume flow. The *BS-cc* valve causes an increase of the pressure loss coefficient with increasing volume flow. This is due to the two different positions which the *BS-cc* disc can take up when opened. The *OS* valve shows an increase of the opening angle with increasing volume flow, so that its pressure loss coefficient decreases with increasing Reynolds number.

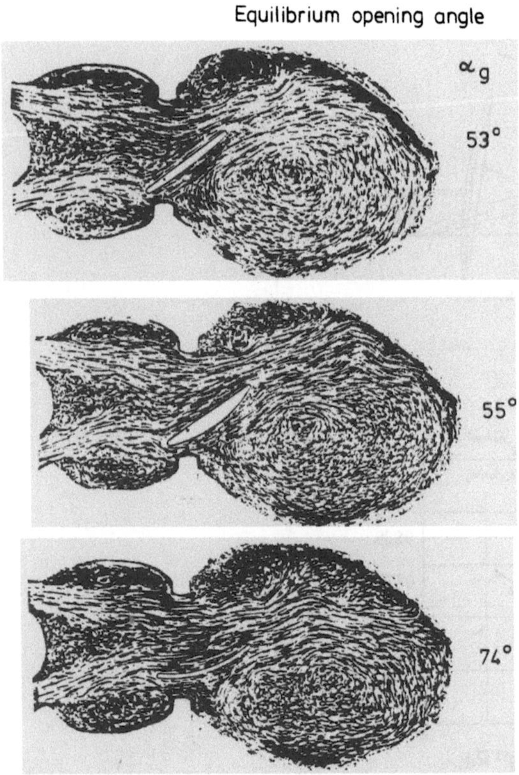

Fig. 11. Comparison of the flow pattern for different highly movable discs in the water table

Conclusion

The results of the flow observations with movable discs in an open water table as well as the torque diagrams of the model valves underline the hypothesis that the equilibrium opening angle α_g of pendulum valves can be increased by a disc curvature as shown in Figure 3. This results in a decrease of the pressure loss, directly caused by the disc shape (for a fixed opening angle, see Fig. 8), and indirectly caused by an increase of the effective opening angle (Fig. 7). In this way the valve disc becomes an insignificant obstacle for the flow. This becomes obvious in the comparison of the three flow patterns with three different disc shapes in Figure 11.

The pressure loss results of steady and pulsating valve flow confirm the advantage of a curved disc shape too (Figs. 8 and 10). The kinetic energy q_H in vivo varies from 1 up to 6 mm Hg. The decrease of the pressure loss to be expected when changing from a *Björk-Shiley* valve to a *BS-cc* valve or to an *Omni Science* valve of the same mounting diameter amounts to more than 10 mm Hg. In the case of high cardiac output the Omni Science valve would be somewhat more favorable.

References

1. Köhler J (1978) Künstliche Herzklappe mit gewölbtem Schließkörper. Thoraxchirurgie 26:209-213
2. Köhler J (1978) Dynamik künstlicher Herzklappen. Dissertation, University of Aachen
3. Köhler J. (1975) Opening angle and torque of the Björk-Shiley and Lillehei-Kaster heart-valve prosthesis. Proc Eur Soc Artif Organs 2:33-35

Valvular Surgery II

Chairman: C. M. G. Duran, Santander; Co-Chairman: M. I. Ionescu, Leeds

Invited Lecture
Biological Valves in Cardiac Surgery

D. N. Ross*

The use of biological valves as a substitute for the diseased heart valve is not a new concept and indeed goes back to 1962 when we inserted the first aortic valve homograft. Since that time, although mechanical valves of one type or another have been in continuous use, homografts have been confined to two or three centres and it is only over the past 5-7 years that there has been a resurgence of interest in the biological valve principle. This has chiefly been brought about by Hancocks's foresight in commercializing the product, fixing the valve to a frame for ease of insertion, and making it readily available.

Nevertheless interest in biological valves fluctuates as cardiac surgeons are attracted to the obvious advantages of their superior flow characteristics and lack of thromboembolisms and at the same time they are deterred by the disadvantages of questionable durability and the difficulty of achieving a surgically acceptable level of sterility. Also there is the neglected problem of immunological rejection when dealing with a biological membrane.

First we need to define our terms in what is becoming an increasingly complex field. To start with we should recognise that any of these valves may be naturally occurring *(made by God)* or *man-made* (wholly manufactured). Also biological valves can either be autologous, that is from the patient's own tissue (pulmonary valve, pericardium, or fascia lata), homologous (allograft) taken from a dead individual of the same species (e.g., homograft), or heterologous (xenograft, for example, a pig valve, or one from say calf pericardium).

Autologous valves (autograft) from patient's living tissue	pulmonary autograft (God made) fascia lata valves (hand made)
Homologous valve (allograft) derived from a human cadaver	aortic homograft (God made) dura mater (hand made)
Heterologous (xenograft) from another species	porcine xenografts (God made) pericardial xenografts (hand made)

This covers the *main range* of biological valves available today and we have had some clinical experience of all of the valves listed here.

Next we should state clearly that while we believe we should conserve the patient's own heart valve wherever possible we at the National Heart Hospital in London also believe that the best substitute for

*National Heart Hospital, Westmoreland Street, London W1, Great Britain

the excised aortic valve is another aortic valve sewn in place free-hand in the orthotopic subcoronary position. There can be no denying the superior design features of this flexible centrally opening valve together with the overwhelmingly important fact that it is entirely free of embolic complications (Fig. 1).

While no one can dispute the ease and speed of insertion of a mechanical valve prosthesis, I believe we as doctors too readily dismiss the ever-present threat of embolism hanging like a Sword of Damocles over the patient with a mechanical prosthesis. There are also the dangers inherent in the use of anticoagulants, estimated to carry a mortality as high as 1% per year. In addition the patient is condemned to an umbilical cordlike lifelong attachment to a department of haematology for thrombotests.

Quite early in my cardiac surgical career I noted the contrast between the *quality* of life enjoyed by prosthetic valve patients compared with those with a biological valve living a life liberated from the routine of regular visits to the doctor's office and usually without medication of any sort. The trouble is that *quality* of life is difficult to quantitate and does not come to light in statistical surveys.

The many virtues of the aortic homograft valve were obscured in our early experience by the problems of avoiding aortic regurgitation. This has largely been solved by one technical innovation or another including the more recently introduced method of inserting the whole aortic root as a composite structure with re-anastomosis of the coronaries (Fig. 2). Now valve durability emerges as the most worrying problem with aortic homografts and this problem applies to all biological valves.

At the same time we have come to recognise that failure or degeneration in an aortic homograft is a slowly progressive problem very similar to the evolving natural history of valve disease. This means there is plenty of time for a safe planned second operation and as a consequence valve-related deaths are comparatively rare amongst homograft patients (Fig. 3).

With mechanical valves on the other hand valve-related complications, when they occur, are generally acute in onset and devastating in their effects, and not infrequently present as sudden unexplained deaths. This contrast between the slow deterioration of biological

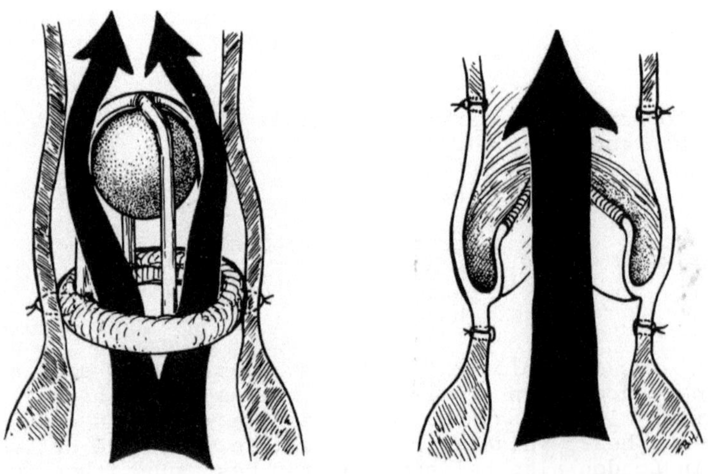

Fig. 1. Comparison of the flow pattern through a mechanical valve on the left, and a tissue valve on the right

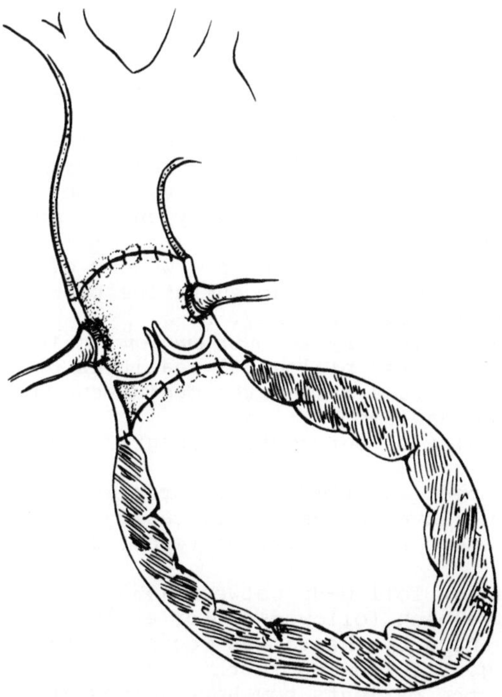

Fig. 2. Diagram of the left ventricle and aorta showing aortic root replacement with reanastomosis of the coronary arteries

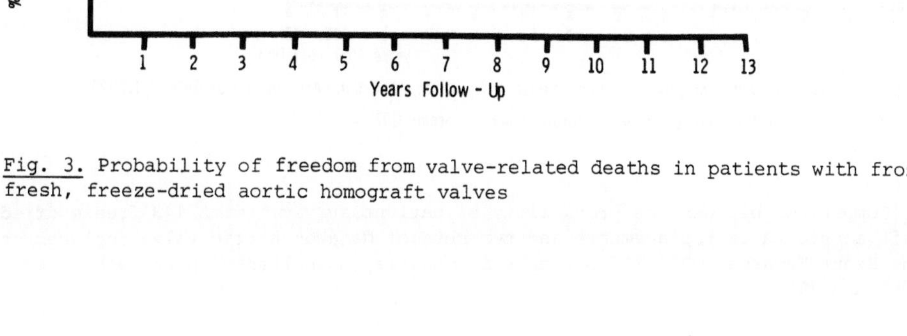

Fig. 3. Probability of freedom from valve-related deaths in patients with frozen, fresh, freeze-dried aortic homograft valves

valves and the sudden events relating to mechanical valves has not been evident from previous reports in the literature.

It is, for example, interesting to compare some of our long-term homograft survivors with those of a comparable series of mechanical aortic valve replacements over a similar period of time (Fig. 4).

From a study of these results it becomes apparent that although the mechanical valve may have the potential to last a hundred years or so, the patient may well not be there to accompany the valve on its triumphal progress! having been carried off prematurely by one or another form of sudden valve-related death.

Furthermore although the mechanical valve represents a wonder of modern technology it is certainly not immune from degenerative processes and complication as many examples will testify.

This is not surprising when one compares the *workshop environment* in which these valves are tested with the harsh biological realities of their true biological environment which is a salt-water medium swarming with macrophages and defensive mechanisms.

We have studied the long-term results of our aortic homograft valves over a period of about 15 years.

About 1500 homograft valves have been inserted but in order to reduce variables as much as possible we have analysed only cases of *isolated* homograft aortic valve replacement and all valves reported here were inserted by the same surgeon.

There are 522 patients available for follow-up between 1965 and 1977, which means that all cases have been followed-up for at least 3 years and are therefore not influenced by the valves recently inserted and not work-tested. The longest follow-up in this series is therefore 13 years although some of the patients now have valves in for up to 16 years. Operative mortality has fallen with the well-recognised learning curve from 16% in the first 5 years to an average of 3.5% over the last 5 years, making this operation comparable with all other forms of aortic valve replacement (Fig. 5).

Subsequent actuarial analysis has been focused on *patient survival* and *late valve complications* after homograft insertion.

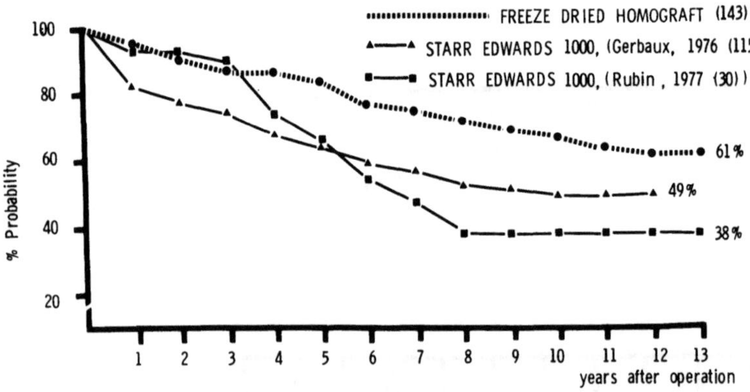

Gerbaux, Hanania, Letteron, Valty, Magnier, Penther, Bensaid, Assouline, & Belfont: Arch Mal Coeur (1976) 69,117-129

Rubin, Moore, Hillson, Ellison: Amer J Cardiol (1977) 40, 345-354

Fig. 4. Comparison between the probability of patient survival with 143 freeze dried homograft aortic valve replacements and two sets of data on aortic valve replacement with the Starr Edwards 1000 (115 patients in one set, 30 patients in the other) between 1963 and 1967

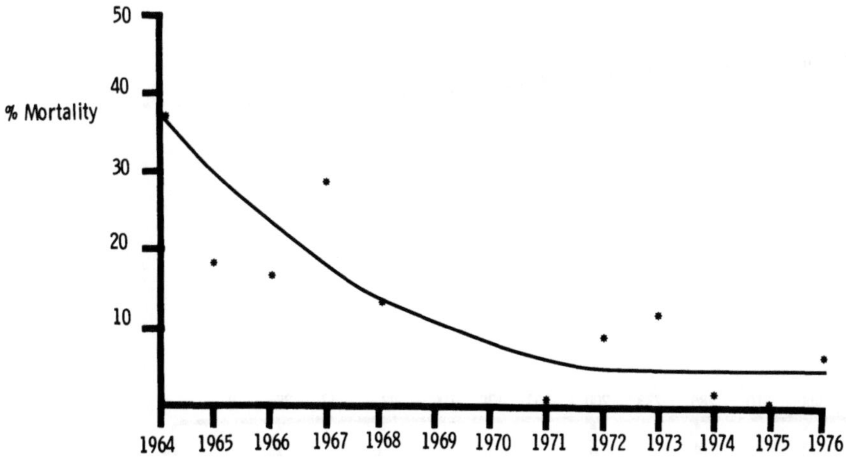

Fig. 5. A 12 year study of annual hospital mortality for patients with allograft valves. The average operative mortality over the last 5 years is 3.5%

On this basis the actuarial probability of a *patient* surviving an aortic homograft replacement at 5 years is 93 ± 3% and 87 ± 3% after 10 years, and remains steady at 85 ± 4% at the end of 13 years (Fig. 6). This is an overall view for *all* aortic homografts, and not unexpectedly even better figures result from improved methods of valve preservation and storage. *This relative freedom from late valve-related deaths, as has already been mentioned, is a strong argument in favour of the biological (homograft) valve and is also a source of considerable comfort to the patient.*

An additional interesting feature of the aortic homograft which has only recently come to light from a study of their application to valved conduits is the relative freedom from early cusp calcification and dysfunction in children. We consequently reviewed all our isolated aortic homografts inserted in children under 16 years of age. Out of 96 children, there have only been 5 cases of proven valve calcification (although calcification in the wall of the aorta has been common). This contrasts with the increasingly common reports of early valve calcification encountered in *porcine* xenografts in children (Fig. 7).

Complications or late malfunctions of the valve have been analysed under the following headings: infective endocarditis, thromboembolism, and degeneration. These are problems common to all forms of valve replacement whether mechanical or biological but immediately we can say that thromboembolism has not been encountered in over 1500 of these aortic valve replacements. Also endocarditis is rare. This leaves degeneration as the one outstanding problem still unsolved.

On an actuarial basis our findings are that there is a 6% probability of degeneration of the inserted valve after 5 years, and about 60% of patients are free of degenerative changes after 13 years (Fig. 8). This figure varies with the different types of valve preparation, but as far as we can assess degeneration affects *all homograft valves* irrespective of the method of sterilisation and storage, and is likely to be a continuing trend. On this basis it is anticipated that few of our present homografts will continue to function for 20 years.

This aortic homograft experience has been invaluable and has set us standards by which to judge other biological valves.

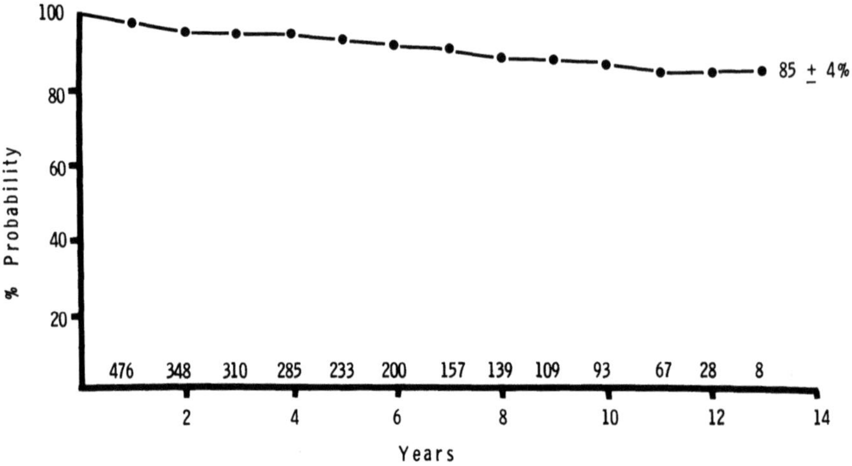

Fig. 6. Actuarial probability of patient survival with an aortic homograft replacement up to 13 years postoperative

	No.	Calcified Cusps
Aortic Valve Replacement	26	3
Aortic Root Replacement	13	0
Homograft Reconstruction (autograft)	10	0
RVOT Conduit Replacement	57	2
	96	5

Fig. 7. The relative freedom from calcification in the homograft valve in children under 16 years old

Ideally what we are looking for as surgeons is a *permanent* biological valve which is unfailingly durable, or like our own living tissue, replaces and repairs itself to counteract the effects of wear and tear.

This ideal has in fact been achieved on a limited scale by the autotransplantation of the patient's own living pulmonary valve to the aortic position as a living transplant. About 200 of these valves have been transplanted and persist as living structures. While these pulmonary autografts continue to function without evidence of failure or degeneration over a 14-year period, the operation unfortunately has a

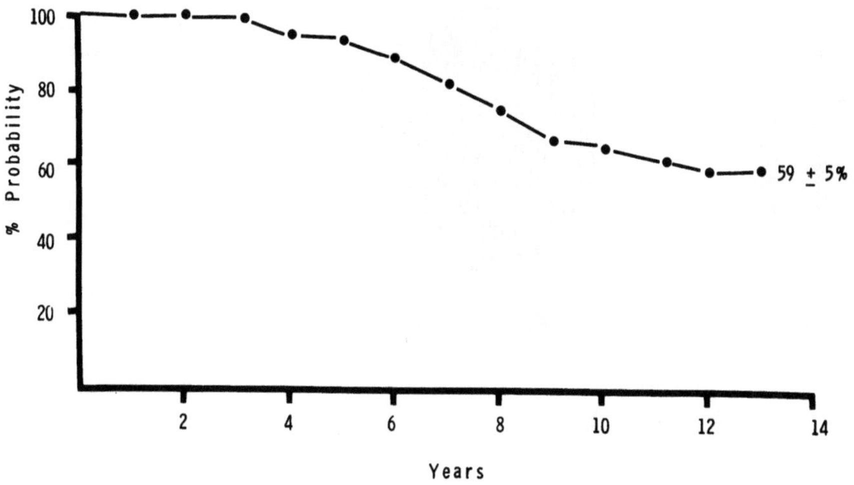

Fig. 8. Actuarial curve of probability of freedom from degeneration of homograft aortic valve replacements over a period of 13 years

limited application to young people with isolated aortic valve disease. Nevertheless it represents an important goal we should all aim at in our valve surgery.

However, living autologous valves made at the time of surgery from the patients' own fascia lata do not persist and function like the pulmonary autograft so that in planning an ideal biological valve other considerations like design criteria are involved and not only the presence of living tissue.

Nowadays the porcine xenograft or mounted pig valve incorporates most of the features pioneered by the early aortic homografts and, coupled with their ready availability and ease of insertion, make them attractive practical alternatives for a valve replacement without the tiresome problem of valve collection and processing which applies to homografts.

However, once a sewing ring or semi-rigid stent is incorporated we lose some of the advantages of the original fully flexible non-obstructive homograft and incur some of the disadvantages of the mechanical prosthesis. For this reason the term bioprosthesis introduced by Carpentier (1) is particularly apt to describe this hybrid.

Other *dis*advantages of a frame-mounted biological valve relate to the degree of rigidity of the frame and its physical structure since it has been shown that some plastics will deform permanently under certain conditions of stress to make the device obstructive, while on the other hand rigid frames throw a strain on the area of cusp attachment with a tendency for the cusp to become avulsed. This has been a particular feature of Zerbini's (2) vast experience with dura mater valves in the aortic area and we can confirm this.

Turning to the mitral we are immediately on much more controversial ground. In the first place we need to remind ourselves that the anatomical features and haemodynamic stresses acting on the mitral valve are very different from those acting on the aortic valve. In fact they differ in almost every respect (Fig. 9).

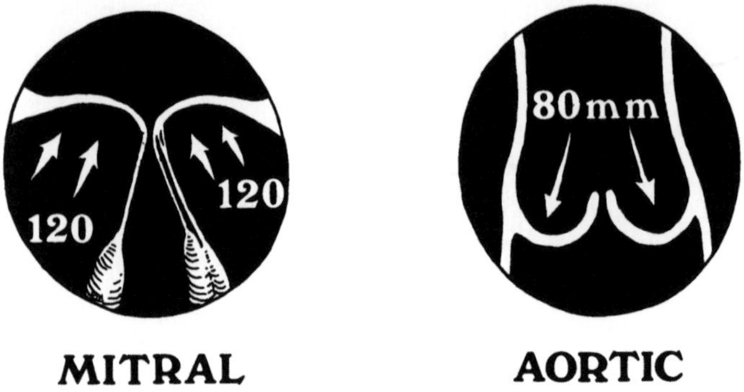

Fig. 9. Diagram of a mitral valve and an aortic valve to show the different anatomical features and haemodynamic stresses acting upon them

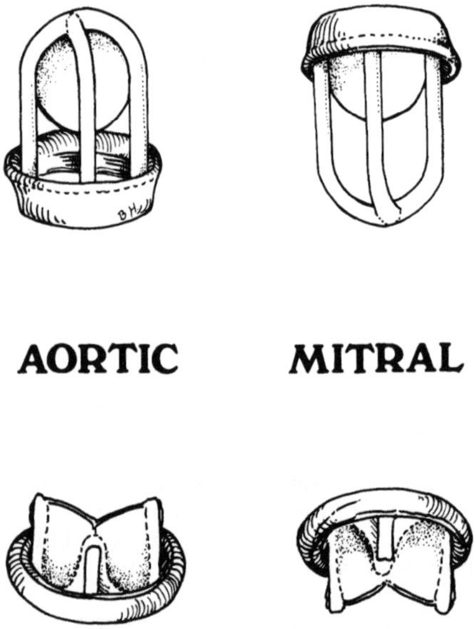

Fig. 10. The mechanical valve (above) and tissue valve (below) used in the aortic and mitral positions are essentially the same valves

In spite of this knowledge we continue to turn the perfectly satisfactory aortic substitute valve upside-down, change the label, and call it a mitral valve (Fig. 10). Certainly the aortic homograft when turned upside-down and fitted in the mitral area on a rigid frame failed more rapidly than an aortic homograft in the aortic area of the same patient. This was also our experience with fascial and dura valves in the mitral area.

Basically we need to rethink and redesign our mitral valve replacements and in this respect the tilting disc type of mechanical or non-biological prosthesis approaches more closely to the natural mechanism than does our present generation of biological valves.

The tilting disc valves, however, suffer from the thromboembolic propensity common to all mechanical valves. Consequently until a more perfect biological valve is developed there is general agreement among most surgeons that we should *conserve* the patient's own *mitral* valve wherever possible and for as long as possible, rather than use a less than perfect valve replacement *of whatever type*.

Where a mitral valve replacement *is* obligatory we at present favour a biological valve in women and young adults but in children we are cautious since most biological valves except possibly the homograft calcify rapidly during periods of rapid bone growth.

In choosing a biological valve for mitral valve replacement this should offer the maximum valve orifice available to ensure a low diastolic opening pressure and, judging from our earlier experiences with rigid-framed homografts, they should probably also have a flexible mounting to minimise the possibility of cusp avulsion and failure (Fig. 11).

Ionescu-Shiley's hand-made pericardial valve undoubtedly offers superior flow characteristics over the mounted pig valve and we currently favour such a valve design for the mitral area. However, the ring is rigid and immobile and at present we make similar pericardial xenografts ourselves but with a *flexible* mounting.

In the tricuspid and pulmonary valve areas there is much less room for controversy. Although most surgeons try to avoid tricuspid valve replacement wherever possible, when it is obligatory there is general agreement that a biological valve with its low opening pressures is more acceptable than a mechanical valve, which is likely to thrombose and is in any event certainly always obstructive.

The right ventricular outflow, however, represents the area where the biological valve principle is unchallenged. The first biological or homograft valve conduit was inserted in the right ventricular outflow in 1966 in a case of pulmonary outflow atresia, that is about 14 years ago. In spite of a number of variations on the theme there has been no convincing evidence that anything has been developed which would influence surgeons to replace the biological valved conduit with a mechanical one.

Also there is mounting evidence that the porcine conduit is not only more obstructive (Fig. 12) than the homograft but is probably liable to earlier calcification and degeneration. The general impression emerging from the recent World Congress of Pediatric Cardiology in London was that the homograft conduit had more to offer and that homograft valves in general were worthy of clinical re-evaluation.

In summary, the biological valve offers a realistic replacement at all four valve sites and our clinical experience and follow-up now extends halfway through the second decade. Their centrally-flowing non-

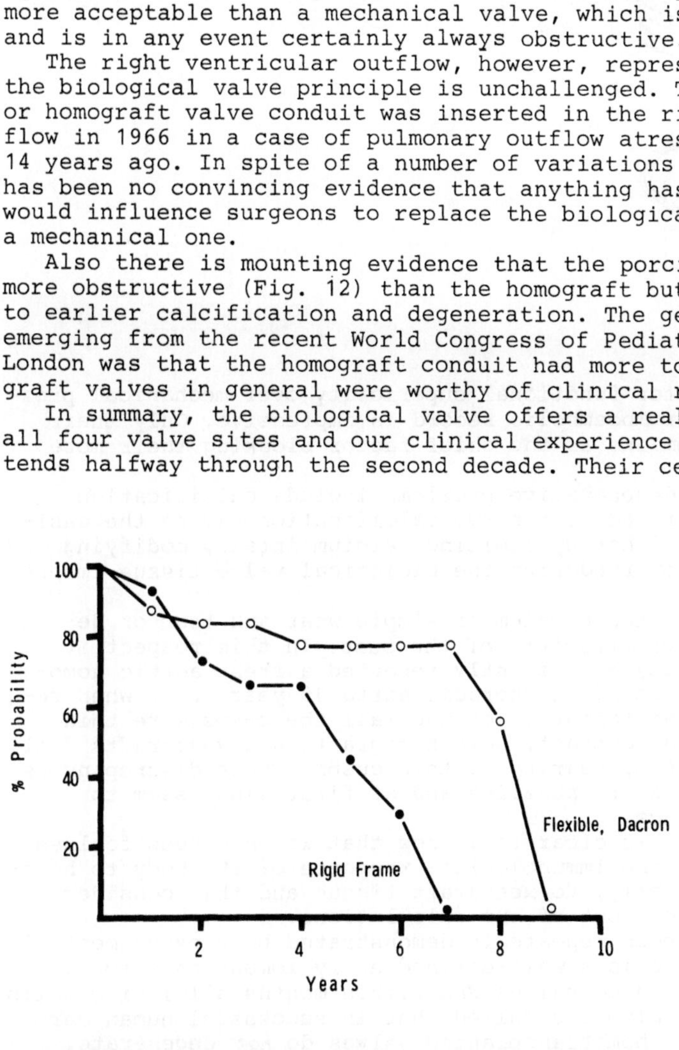

Fig. 11. Comparison between rigid frame-mounted and flexible Dacron supported homograft valves. The flexible valve has a significantly better complication-free performance

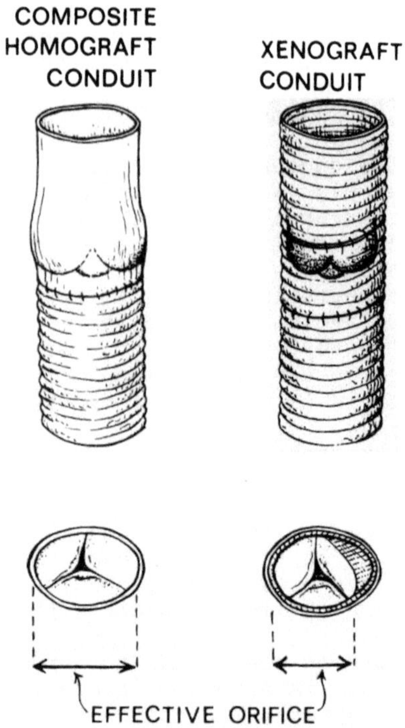

Fig. 12. Comparison of the effective orifices in the composite homograft conduit and xenograft conduit of similar external diameters

obstructive features offer functional superiority over mechanical prostheses and their low thromboembolic record is impressive. Only their uncertain durability remains as the chief factor blocking their more widespread application.

Their durability or degenerative problems include calcification and simple wear and tear and of the two calcification may be the easiest problem to control either by limiting calcium intake, modifying calcium deposition, or by rendering the biological valve tissue impervious to calcium salts.

This does not obviate the problem of simple wear and tear or destruction of the collagen structure of the cusp. In this respect it is of interest that Cooley has recently reported a fresh aortic homograft inserted in the descending thoracic aorta 19 years ago. When removed because of aneurysm formation of the wall the cusps were thin and fully functional. In contrast, some homografts and xenografts fail early with calcification or tearing of thin cusps. These discrepancies and unpredictable results are puzzling and at first sight seem to follow no logical sequence.

On the other hand, it is clear to me now that we have been foolish in failing to allow for the immunological response of the body to homologous or, more particularly, to xenograft tissue and this consideration can no longer be left out of our calculations.

For example, it has been repeatedly demonstrated both experimentally and clinically that there is a well-defined early immune reaction in the cusps of all transplanted valves and within months all living cells have disappeared. It is also recognised that in successful human cardiac transplantation the homotransplanted valves do *not* degenerate. On this evidence there is a clear message that we have to take measures to block the immune response probably with low-dose immunosuppression if we are to expect our biological valves to persist in an immunologically hostile environment. This argument should apply even more emphatically to xenografts. With this in mind we are currently evaluating both experimentally and clinically the possibility of low-dose immunosuppression as a means of prolonging the working life of our homografts and possibly of xenografts also.

In the past, ladies and gentlemen, we have had a simple choice between the robust mechanical supervalve and the gentle but less durable homograft. For the future we can look forward to the perfect marriage combining the best features of mechanical man and Miss Piggy – perhaps under a golden umbrella of immunosuppression. I hope for all of us that it will be a happy and long-lasting marriage.

On a more serious note, I believe the balance of evidence is still in favour of the biological valve principle and encourages us to continue with our efforts to improve the durability of the biological valve membrane.

References

1. Carpentier A (1969) Evolution of concepts and techniques of valvular heterografts. Ann Surg [Suppl] 172:1
2. Zerbini EJ, Puig LB (1979) Experience with dura mater allograft. Long term results. In: Sebening F, Klovekorn WP, Meisner H, Struck E (eds) Bioprosthetic cardiac valves. Deutsches Herzzentrum Munich, p 179

Mitral Valve Surgery in Syria

S. S. Kabbani and T. Bashour*

Rheumatic heart disease is the commonest reason for cardiac operations in the Middle East, and of the varieties of rheumatic involvement that require surgical correction, *mitral valve disease* is the most prevalent.

Between January 15, 1976 (when our open-heart program started at Damascus University), and January 15, 1980, i.e. a period of 4 years, a total of 269 patients with symptomatic mitral valve disease were operated on at the Damascus University Cardiovascular Center.

The purpose of this report is to analyse the data obtained from these cases with a view to discerning the major characteristics of this common disease entity in Syria.

As shown in Table 1, there is a female preponderance in our group of patients with the male/female ratio at 0.63. Another tendency for rheumatic disease in our country is for it to affect patients at an early stage in their lives. The mean age of our patients was 25.6 with about 1/3 of the patients under 20 years.

Table 2 reveals our cardiologist's estimate of the NYHA functional classification of our patients just before operation. Most patients fell in Classes III-IV.

Table 1. Operations on the mitral valve

Total	269 Patients
Male	104
Female	165
M/F Ratio	0.63
Age Range	6-60 years
Mean	25.6 years
Males below 20:	36%
Females below 20:	33%

Table 2. Preoperative functional classification

Class II	37 (14%)
Class II-III	43 (16%)
Class III	68 (25%)
Class III-IV	62 (23%)
Class IV	59 (22%)
	269

One hundred ninety-six (73%) of patients had complete right and left heart catheterization. Those that were not catheterized were mainly the younger patients who underwent closed mitral commissurotomy in the earlier period of our experience.

*Damascus Medical School, P.O.Box 2837, Damascus, Syria

One-half of the catheterized patients had proven mitral stenosis, 11% had mitral insufficiency, and 39% had combined stenosis and insufficiency. Associated lesions were aortic and tricuspid in the proportions shown in Table 3. As expected only a fraction of the tricuspid lesions and less than the entire number of aortic lesions had to be corrected.

Most of our patients had advanced disease with severe pulmonary hypertension. The mean pulmonary pressure averaged 45 and the mean wedge pressure 23 mm Hg (Table 4).

The operations we performed are listed in Table 5. Closed commissurotomy (CC) was done in the earlier stages of our experience when facilities for extracorporeal circulation were not sufficient to meet the patient load. Now we do it more sparingly and resort mainly to the "open" method preferring the more accurate repair it offers.

Table 3. Operations on the mitral valve

Preoperative diagnosis Total patients catheterized: 196		Associated lesions	
Pure mitral stenosis	98 (50%)	Tricuspid insufficiency (functional)	30 (15%)
Pure mitral insufficiency	22 (11%)	Tricuspid stenosis	2 (1%)
Combined mitral stenosis and insufficiency	76 (39%)	Aortic insufficiency	46 (23%)
	196	Aortic stenosis	14 (7%)

Table 4. Preoperative catheterization data

Mean pa pressure		Mean wedge pressure		LV Function	
Average	45 mm Hg	Average	23 mm Hg	Good	40%
Highest	110 mm Hg	Highest	50 mm Hg	Adequate	45%
		(higher than 25 in 52% of the patients)		Poor	15%

Table 5. Operations

Closed commissurotomy (CC)	83
Open commissurotomy (OC)	73
(OC) + Aortic valve replacement (AVR)	2
Mitral annuloplasty (MA)	1
(MA) + (AVR)	1
Mitral valve replacement (MVR)	73
MVR + Tricuspid commissurotomy	2
MVR + Tricuspid annuloplasty	3
(MVR) + (AVR)	30
(MVR) + (AVR) + Tricuspid valve replacement	1
	269

Open commissurotomy (OC) was performed in 75 cases, 2 of whom had concomitant aortic valve replacement (AVR). Two cases had mitral annuloplasty, one with AVR. Mitral valve replacement (MVR) was carried out in 109 cases, 5 of whom had tricuspid commissurotomy or annuloplasty, and 30 had concomitant AVR. One case had triple valve replacement.

For our extracorporeal circulation we use disposable bubble oxygenators primed with lactate/Ringer's solution for complete hemodilution. Our blood requirement during and after operation has averaged 1100 cc/patient. We use moderate hypothermic perfusion with low flow rates averaging 45 cc/kg/min for adult patients.

The aorta is continuously cross-clamped and we have used surface cooling together with cold potassium solution cardioplegia for myocardial preservation over the past 2 years. The Björk-Shiley prosthesis was used in all valve replacements except four in whom the Carpentier-Edwards porcine valve was implanted.

Results were considered very good with improvement by two or three functional classes in 66% of survivors (Table 6). Twenty-eight (28%) improved by one functional class and 6% did not improve. Most of those who did not benefit had mitral regurgitation following commissurotomy as a postoperative complication, but in none of them have we yet had to replace the valve.

Hospital mortality for the varying procedures on the mitral valve was a little over 5% (Table 7).

Most of the causes of fatalities had to do with low-output states [either due to LV failure or fixed pulmonary artery resistance (Table 8)].

Table 6. Results

Very good	168	66%
Good	72	28%
Poor	15	6%
Total	255	Survivors

Very Good:	Functional improvement by two or more classes
Good:	Functional improvement by one class
Poor:	No improvement or deterioration

Table 7. Mortality

		Operative mortality	Late mortality
Closed commissurotomy	83	2	-
Open commissurotomy (± AVR)	75	2	-
Mitral annuloplasty (1 with AVR)	2	-	-
MVR (± tricuspid procedure)	78	6	4
MVR + AVR	30	4	1
MVR, AVR, and TVR	1	-	-
	269	14 (5%)	5

Table 8. Causes of hospital mortality

Low-output (left ventricular failure)	6
Low-output (high pulmonary artery resistance)	5
Bleeding-perforation of calcified annulus	1
Myocardial infarction	1
Acute renal failure	1

Follow-up on our patients was adequate in about 80% of patients, and we know of five cases who died suddenly 2 months to 3.5 years after mitral valve replacement, presumably of thrombus-occluded valves. Four of those were definitely not properly anticoagulated and from remote areas of Syria.

Table 9 shows a list of the major early and late complications following the aforementioned procedures on the mitral valve. In spite of the young age of our operative group there were only two rheumatic exacerbations and three occasions of restenosis in our postcommissurotomy patients. It is fair to say, however, that our operative mortality and complications figures have significantly improved as our team was acquiring increasing experience in handling these patients during and after operation.

A decreasing operative time (Table 10), better attention paid to myocardial preservation, and better postoperative care have all been factors that helped decrease operative mortality and morbidity.

Table 9. Postoperative complications

Post-commissurotomy insufficiency	5
Post-commissurotomy restenosis	3
Rheumatic exacerbation	2
Bacterial endocarditis	1
Bleeding requiring reexploration	2
Late bleeding due to anticoagulants	2
Trachial stenosis	1
Major coronary air embolism	1
Cerebral air embolism	0
Pneumonia	3
Pericardiotomy syndrome	6
Significant wound infection	1
Major cautery skin burn	1

Table 10. Average aortic cross-clamp time (min)

	1977	1978	1979
Open mitral commissurotomy	27.25	22.17	19.15
Mitral valve replacement	52.00	46.15	38.05
Mitral and aortic valve replacement	79.25	79.34	76.41

Over the past 6 months we operated on 43 patients with rheumatic mitral disease, 3 of whom had had closed commisssurotomy 2-4 years earlier, with only one mortality in the case of a patient with fixed pulmonary vascular resistance, and another in a moribund patient with bacterial endocarditis (Table 11).

Table 11. Recent operations (Jan. 15, 1980 - June 15, 1980)

		Operative mortality
Open commissurotomy (OC)	12	1
(OC) + AVR	4	-
M: Annuloplasty + AVR	1	-
MVR	20	1
MVR + AVR	6	-
Total	43	2

We have learned from our experience that rheumatic mitral valve disease starts early in life in Syria and progresses rapidly to severity, but that this fact should not deter us from aggressive surgical treatment, since the frequency of rheumatic reactivation is not as great as was previously believed. Most of these patients require no greater procedure than mitral commissurotomy since pure stenosis seems to form the most common pathological condition.

Choice of the implanted valve remains a problem. We now feel that porcine valves have a place in women about to have children, and in patients coming from underdeveloped and remote areas where adherence to a strict regimen of anticoagulation is very difficult. We are also awaiting more data on the long-term results of such new prosthetic valves as the St. Jude's medical and the concave-convex variety of the Björk-Shiley.

Finally, we have learned that despite the severity of mitral valve disease in Syria, surgery can provide adequate palliation at a very low operative risk.

Eight Years Experience With the Björk-Shiley Prosthesis Implanted in 733 Patients

G. A. Tolis, A. Michalis, A. Pouliou, G. Papas, and C. Stathatos*

From 1 January, 1972 through 31 December, 1979 the Björk-Shiley prosthesis was used exclusively for cardiac valve replacements in 733 patients. The 30-day postoperative mortality was 9% (66 deaths). For single valve replacement in 566 patients (216 aortics, 342 mitrals, 8 tricuspids) the postop mortality was 6% (34 deaths). For multiple valve replacements in 167 patients (140 aortic-mitrals, 20 mitral-tricuspids, 1 aortic-tricuspid, 6 triple replacements) the postop mortality was 19.1% (32 deaths). The late mortality was 10.6% (78 deaths). Of those who survived the operation, 88.3% were alive at the end of the 8-year study. Fifteen patients developed peripheral emboli, and one died. Seven patients thrombosed their prostheses (five mitral, two aortic), and three died. No early postop death was caused by thromboembolism. Anticoagulation treatment was started on the 2nd postop day with Coumadin. Hemorrhage from anticoagulation was responsible for two late deaths. We think that the Björk-Shiley prosthesis is a dependable cardiac valve substitute.

*Evangelismos Hospital, Athens, Greece

Cardiac Valve Replacement With the St. Jude Medical Prosthesis: Clinical, Echocardiographic and Biological Results

E. Baudet, G. Fel, R. Roudaut, D. Gibson, X. Roques, and J. F. Garbe*

From June 1978 to February 1980, 139 patients underwent valve replacement with the St. Jude Medical Cardiac Valve Prosthesis (SJMP): 107 aortic (AVR), 22 mitral (MVR), and 10 double replacements (DVR). Intraoperative transvalvular pressure gradients were always within 10 mm Hg. There were four (2.8%) non-valve-related operative deaths. Out of the two late deaths (1.4%), one occurrred in a DVR patient not maintained on anticoagulants and was due to a mitral SJMP thrombosis.

Sixty-two patients, in sinus rhythm, did not receive anticoagulants from July 1978 to July 1979; five of them (8%) developed thromboembolic episodes. Three patients, not reoperated on, have been successfully treated with fibrinolytic drugs. There has been no incidence of valve thrombosis or thromboembolism in patients maintained on Coumadin.

Clinical, echocardiographic, and biological data have been obtained from the first 94 patients, with a follow-up from 5 to 19 months (mean, 10 months). Of these patients, 93.6% have returned NYHA class I. Pulsed doppler echocardiography in patients with AVR showed absence of turbulences. The effects of the SJMP in the mitral position upon left ventricular (LV) filling characteristics (peak rate of increase of LV dimension during diastole and duration of the rapid filling period), assessed echocardiographically, indicate that it approximates closely to normal. Reticulocyte count, platelet count, hemoglobin level, and bilirubin level were unchanged from preoperative values, but haptoglobin was under the inferior normal level and serum LDH was slightly elevated (250 IU/liter), suggesting infraclinical hemolysis; red cell filterability has also been found to be impaired (increase of filtration time).

Thrombogenicity on anticoagulants and durability will be assessed only with time, but hemodynamically the SJMP seems, especially in the small sizes, to represent a step forward in prosthetic cardiac valve replacement.

*Hôpital Cardiologique, Université de Bordeaux II, 33604 Bordeaux-Pessac, France

In Vitro Comparison of Björk-Shiley and St. Jude Medical Valvular Prosthesis in Aortic Position in a new Pulse Duplicator

M. G. Gottwik, R. Tessari, K. Neumeier, S. Langsdorf, P. Robens, J. Fricke, K. Kramer, F. Hehrlein, and M. Schlepper*

In vivo testing of artificial valves is complicated by the lack of standardisation of technique in different laboratories. Furthermore a continuing variation of the most important parameters, i.e. flow and heart rate, makes it a difficult task to evaluate the hemodynamic qualities of different valves from single measurements in different patients. However, the clinician in his decision process leading to an engagement with a clinical trial is dependent on such data with respect to any new valvular prosthesis, since preclinical testing of any new device is performed usually by the designing laboratory or more frequently by a promoting industrial firm, with the result that data of valves that could serve as comparison in the literature as a rule have been established under nonidentical experimental conditions.

In 1978, when a clinical trial of the St. Jude Medical prosthesis was stated in cooperation with the Department of Cardiovascular Surgery of the University of Giessen, exactly this problem presented itself. Based on technical data the St. Jude valve could be expected to show better hemodynamic results because of its effective valve area.

Therefore it was decided to perform a small pilot study in which 20 patients received Björk-Shiley and St. Jude valves in aortic position alternatively. The analysis of the data was reported in the literature (1, 2) and did not reveal significant differences between the two models under the testing conditions that were available in the clinical catheterisation laboratory.

In order to further examine possible reasons why the clinical results did not appear to correspond with the technical data of the preclinical testing period a pulse duplicator was constructed in a cooperative effort including the Max Planck Institute for Experimental Cardiology and the Fachhochschule for Biomedical Engineering Giessen that provided a facility to test and compare prosthetic devices under well-defined pulsatile pressure and flow conditions.

Methods

The pulse duplicator was constructed in three parts and consisted of an atrium, a ventricle and a proximal aorta all of which were machined from a block of plexiglass to facilitate optical, echocardiographic, and laser optical observation of mechanical function of the valves and of the flow profiles. The ventricular pump function was performed by fluid displacement from the rigid ventricle by rhythmic inflation and deflation of rubber balloons in the interior, without the necessity

*Max Planck Institute, Dept. Exp. Cardiology, Kerckhoff-Clinic, D-6350 Bad Nauheim, and Fachhochschule, Dept. Biomedical Engineering, Dept. Cardiovasc. Surg., D-6300 Giessen

to expand them. This proved to be a very important feature at high stroke volumes and frequencies. The pump used was a specially adapted animal respirator that permitted variation of stroke volume between 40 and 90 ml and frequencies between 40 and 120 cycles per minute and showed linear relations of flow and frequency in this range ($r \geqq 0.9$) (3).

In mitral position an M25 Björk-Shiley valve was used. In aortic position a Björk-Shiley standard valve and a St. Jude Medical valve with equal inner diameters of the ring (21 mm) were used for comparison, at different stroke volumes and frequencies.

Pressures were measured with Statham DB23 transducers, amplified and recorded on photographic paper with an electronics for medicine direct writer. An electric flow meter was built in the proximal aorta in order to record anterograde and retrograde flow in normal and defective valves. For the experiments presented a 36% glycerol-water mixture was used to simulate blood viscosity consistent with a hematocrit of 42% or 3.4 cp. The pressure difference between aorta and left ventricle was subtracted electronically and recorded on a separate channel against time.

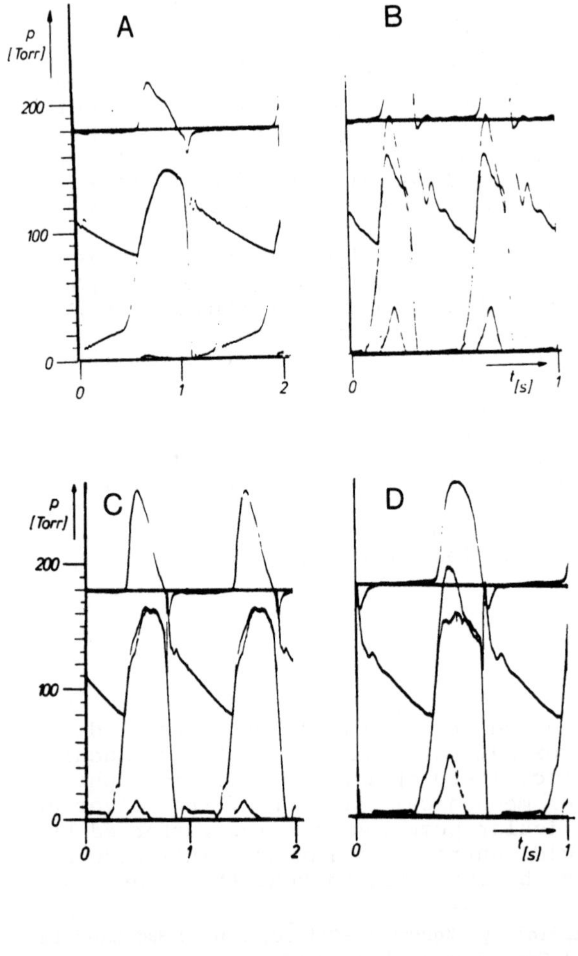

Fig. 1

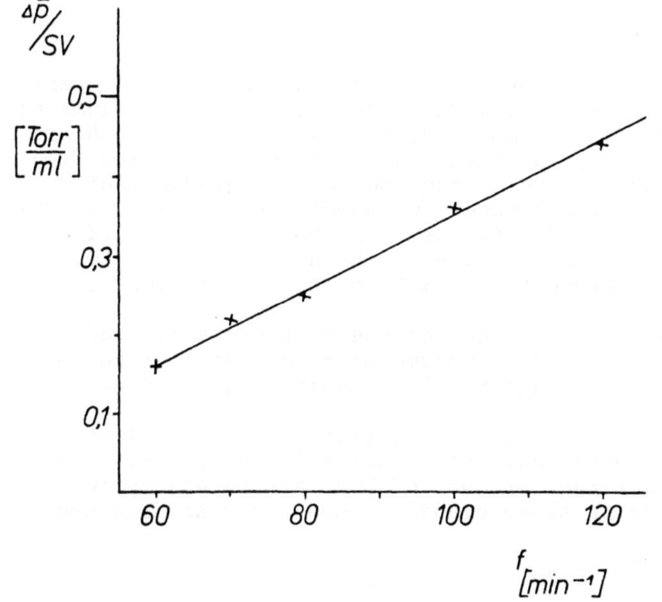

Δp̄/SV
[Torr/ml]
0,5
0,3
0,1
60
80
100
120
f [min⁻¹]

Fig. 2a

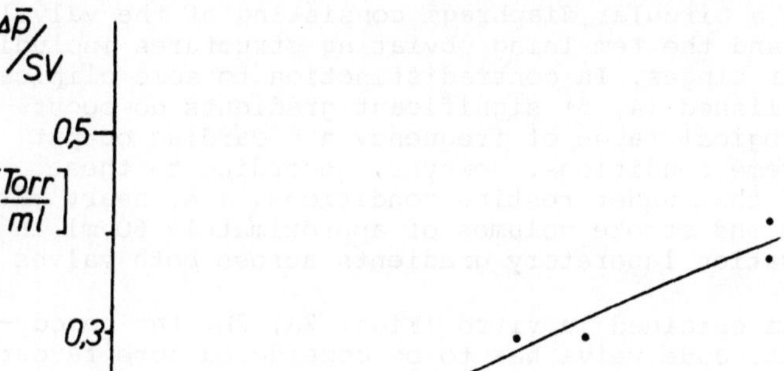

Δp̄/SV
[Torr/ml]
0,5
0,3
0,1
60
80
100
120
f [min⁻¹]

Fig. 2b

Results

Figure 1 is a composite of four original tracings. In the upper panel on the left (A) represents the St. Jude valve with a stroke volume of 45 ml and a frequency of 48 cpm. No gradient was observed. On the right upper panel (B) the same valve with the same stroke volume at a frequency of 136 cpm is shown. At this frequency a peak gradient of 40 mm Hg was measured. The lower panel (C) shows the Björk-Shiley valve at a stroke volume of 50 ml and a frequency of 50 cpm on the left. No gradient could be observed. An increase of the heart rate to 100, however, produced a gradient close to 45 mm Hg on the right lower panel (D).

Figures 2a and 2b show correlations of the mean pressure gradient across valve, divided by the stroke volume plotted against frequency for the Björk-Shiley (Fig. 2a) and St. Jude Medical valve (Fig. 2b) in aortic position.

The regression lines show linear correlations for both valves ($r \geqq 0.9$) with parallel slopes indicating that a larger stroke volume, a higher frequency, or a larger product of both are necessary for the St. Jude valve to produce pressure gradient equal to that obtained for the Björk-Shiley valve.

Discussion

The data show that both valves produce pressure loss across the outflow track that is caused by a circular diaphragm consisting of the valvular ring, the suture ring, and the remaining obviating structures including the obturators and their hinges. In contradistinction to some clinical data that have been published (4, 5) significant gradients do occur well within the physiological range of frequency and cardiac output and not only under extreme conditions. However, according to these data it can be expected that under resting conditions, i.e. heart rates of approximately 60 bpm and stroke volumes of approximately 60 ml in the clinical catheterisation laboratory gradients across both valves may not be observed.

According to the data obtained in vitro (Figs. 2a, 2b) the hemodynamic function of the St. Jude valve has to be considered more favourable. However, the differences that have been observed between the two valves are of a magnitude that in the clinical laboratory, in situ, even under optimal standardisation of the procedure can hardly be demonstrated.

References

1. Hehrlein FW, Gottwik MG, Fraedrich G, Mulch J (1980) First clinical experience with a new all pyrolyte carbon bileaflet heart valve prosthesis. J Thorac Cardiovasc Surg 79:632-636
2. Thormann J, Gottwik MG, Schlepper M, Hidajat H (1980) Ein Vergleich belastungsinduzierter hämodynamischer Änderungen nach Aortenklappenersatz mit Björk-Shiley und SJM Prothesen. Z Kardiol 69:100-109
3. Neumaier K, Tessari R (1979) Simulatoruntersuchungen zur Erfassung der Druck- und Strömungsverhältnisse bei Björk-Shiley- und SJM-Aortenklappenprothesen. Diplomarbeit, Fachhochschule Giessen

4. Chaux A, Gray R, Sustaita H, Matloff JM (1979) Single valve replacement using porcine xenografts. Hemodynamic performance, incidence of thromboembolic complications and analysis of survival as compared to other nonbiologic prostheses. In: Sebening F (ed) Bioprosthetic cardiac valves. Deutsches Herzzentrum, Munich, pp 243-254
5. Gray R, Chaux A, Matloff J, Raymond M (1979) Early postoperative hemodynamic comparison of St. Jude valve prostheses and porcine xenografts at rest and with stress. Circulation 60/4:II/867

Long-Term Results of Emergency Surgery for Active Infective Endocarditis of the Aortic Valve

P. Blondeau, S. Chauvaud, R. Nottin, P. Menasche, A. Piwnica, A. Carpentier, and C. Dobust*

Valvular surgery for active endocarditis is rare but could be life-saving. In spite of the high risks of emergency valvular replacement during the acute period of the endocarditis, the results are favorably influenced by rapid indication for surgery. But little is known of the long-term results, especially of the functional status. The aim of this study is the appreciation of the long-term follow-up regarding the incidence of reoperation, late mortality, and functional improvement.

Material and Methods

From 1966 to 1978, 481 patients had been operated on for an aortic valve lesion secondary to endocarditis. Seventy-nine were operated in emergency and were at the active phase of infection. The criteria for active infective endocarditis were patients at least one of the following: 1) positive valve culture, 2) positive blood cultures within 1 month preoperatively, or 3) fever or infectious manifestations within 48 h preoperatively. All patients were receiving antibiotics.

Sixty-four patients were male and 15 were female. The age is 15 to 77 years, mean 47. Sixty patients (76%) were operated on for progressive heart failure only, 4 patients (5%) for resistant organisms, and 15 patients (19%) for hemodynamic reasons associated with nonsterilized endocarditis. Blood culture and/or valve culture was positive in 65% of the cases (52 patients). Twenty-seven patients had viridans streptococcus, 11 enterococcus, 8 staphylococcus (aureus 5, epidermidis 3), and 6 gram-negative. Infectious emboli were associated in 10 cases: brain abscess 3 cases, pulmonary abscess 1 case, limbs emboli 6 cases.

A previous cardiac lesion was found in 37 cases (47%), aortic for 31 patients and mitral for 6 patients. Eighteen had acquired valvular disease and 19 congenital lesions; 42 patients were free of valvular disease before the endocarditis. Endocarditis on prosthetic cardiac valve has not been included in this study.

Aortic valve replacement was performed in all patients. A mitral replacement was associated in 27 cases (35%). A triple valve replacement was performed for one patient. Aortic ring abscess was present in 19 cases and associated with abscess of the interventricular septum in 15 patients. A ventricular septal defect was closed in three cases. A sinus of Valsalva aneurysm was found in two cases. The duration of antibiotic treatment after the operation was at least 4 weeks.

*Clinique Chirurgicale Cardiovasculaire, Hôpital Broussais, 96, rue Didot, 75674 Paris Cedex 14, France

Results

The hospital mortality is 35% (28 patients), 23% for isolated aortic valve replacement and 44% for multiple replacement. Fifty-one patients had been followed for 1 to 13 years (mean 5.6 years). Twelve patients (15% of the 79 patients and 23% of the surviving patients) died after dismissal from the hospital. Four patients died during the first year postoperatively. The causes of the late mortality are related to the first operation for four patients (Table 1): septicemia (one patient, different organism than the endocarditis), chronic renal failure (one patient), reoperation (two patients). Six patients died at home and because no autopsy was performed, no precise cause was found.

The actuarial curve of survival (Fig. 1) indicates that 47% of the patients are alive at 5 years and this rate is stable from 5 to 10 years. The functional status was estimated for 30 patients; 22 are in functional class I (New York Heart Association), 7 are in class II, 1 in class III, and none in class IV.

Fifteen patients had signs of paravalvular leak: 13 aortic valve dehiscence and 2 mitral valve dehiscence. One patient had severe aortic insufficiency immediately after the operation and died from heart failure without reoperation. Five patients had mild and well-tolerated paravalvular leak. Nine patients underwent a reoperation. One patient died after the second operation; one patient died at home from unexplained causes; two patients had a good result without sign of heart failure; five patients had recurrence of paravalvular leak. One is well tolerated and four experienced a third operation. One patient died after the third operation; one has a good functional result; two had recurrence of aortic insufficiency. One is well tolerated and one had to be reoperated. The results of this fourth operation are now satisfactory. No patient with paravalvular leak had recurrence of endocarditis. The technical problems of reoperation could be difficult and are related to the weakness of the remnant annulus structure. One

Table 1. Late deaths after emergency surgery for infective endocarditis of the aortic valve

Interval since surgery	Cause of death
5 months	Unknown
6 months	Unknown
6 months	Unknown
1 year[a]	Staphylococcal septicemia
1.5 year	Cerebral tumor
1.5 year	Unknown
2 years[a]	Reoperation
3 years[a]	Ionic disturbances (hemodialysis)
3.5 years	Carcinoma
4 years	Unknown
4 years	Unknown
5 years[a]	Reoperation

[a]Related to the endocarditis (4)

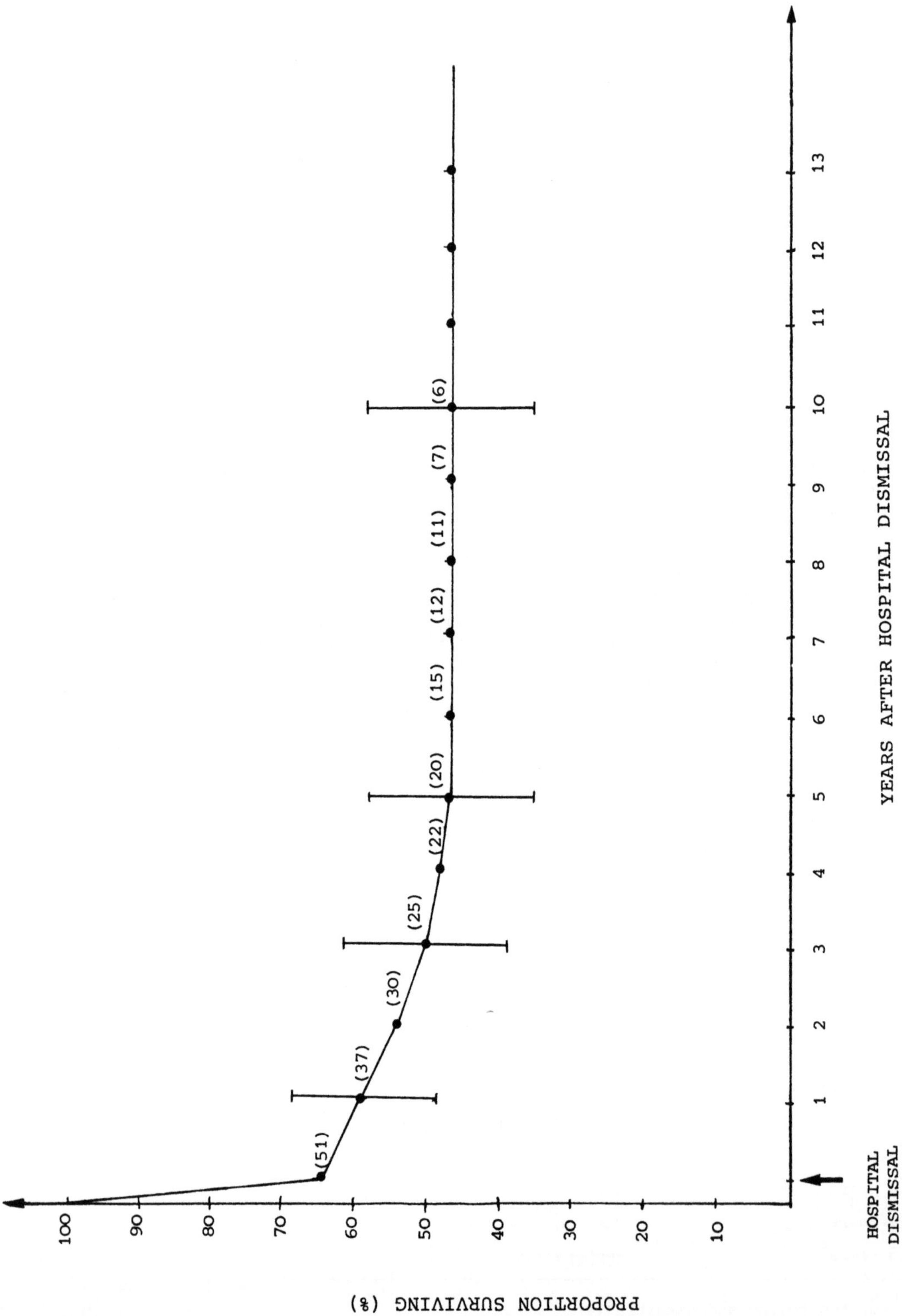

Fig. 1. Survival curve

patient had an aortic valvular replacement using a Dacron conduit with a Björk valve inserted in the aortic root below the coronary arteries.

Discussion

Active endocarditis still has a high operative risk, but the surgical therapy seems to be better than medical treatment (2). The factors of hospital mortality are miscellaneous and it is difficult to make an analysis since the methods of myocardial protection had varied from the beginning of this study. The presence of severe heart failure at the time of the operation is a determining factor. The hospital mortality for patients with pulmonary edema is 50% compared with 25% in the absence of pulmonary edema. This suggests that early surgery could lower the operative risks when the operation is performed before cardiogenic shock. There is no correlation of the hemodynamic deteriorations and the late results.

In our series the presence of a valvular disease before the onset of endocarditis does not influence the operative risk. The late mortality for patients with previous aortic disease is 20%, compared with 9% for patients without valvular disease before the endocarditis. This could explain some of the sudden deaths occurring a long time after the operation in the absence of paravalvular leak and due to the evolution of myocardial damage. Reoperation for periprosthetic dehiscence is directly correlated with the presence of aortic annulus abscess. Of 15 patients having periprosthetic leak, 9 had destruction of the aortic ring or abscess in the interventricular septum. Fifty per cent of the aortic annulus destruction is secondary to staphylococcus infection as pointed out by other authors (1).

Conclusions

This study suggests that emergency surgery for acute aortic endocarditis provides good functional results on a long-term basis. No cases of recurrent endocarditis have been encountered. The survival rate is highly influenced by valvular disease prior to the endocarditis.

References

1. Rapaport E (1978) The changing role of surgery in the management of infective endocarditis. (Editorial) Circulation 58:598
2. Richardson JV, Karp RB, Kirklin JW, Dismukes WE (1978) Treatment of infective endocarditis: a 10 years comparative analysis. Circulation 58:589

Decision-Making Aspects in Valve Surgery for Active Bacterial Endocarditis

R. Hetzer, N. Papagiannakis, D. Dragojevic, H. Oelert, K. Gahl, and H. G. Borst*

At present, bacterial endocarditis (BE) can be cured by antibiotics in the majority of cases (7, 8). There is, however, a certain number of patients who develop systemic or local life-threatening complications of valvular infection during medical treatment (12, 14). In this subset of patients valve replacement has become a very successful kind of treatment, even in the presence of active BE in spite of the basic surgical principle not to implant artificial material into infected tissue.

In the vast majority of operated patients BE can be definitely cured once normal valve function is restored. However, the serious problem of prosthetic infection is more prevalent in these patients than in those undergoing valve replacement in non-infective valve disease (11). Thus, decision-making for surgery appears to be dominated by the weighing of the presumable outcome under conservative regime and the risk of prosthetic infection.

The purpose of this study was to analyze our patient collective with valve replacement in active BE in order to answer the following questions:

1. When is surgery indicated in the presence of hemodynamic deterioration?
2. What is the incidence of postoperative prosthetic infection and which patients are at risk of such?
3. Are there appropriate means to cope with the predisposition of prosthetic infection?
4. What is the adequate mode of treatment in "jet" lesions of the mitral valve secondary to aortic regurgitation?

Patients and Clinical Courses

Between 1969 and June 1980, 69 patients underwent valve replacement in the presence of active BE. There were 53 men and 16 women, patient age ranging from 15 to 65 years ($\bar{x} = 42.8$). More than half of these operations were performed during the last 3 years whereas valve replacement in active BE was a more rare case before this period.

In 48 patients indication for surgery was progressive heart failure irresponsive to medical treatment. These patients all presented in clinical stage IV NYHA; however, they were not in shock. Operative mortality in this group was 8% (4 patients). Emergency operations were performed in 21 patients who had developed cardiogenic shock with

*Klinik für Thorax-, Herz- und Gefäßchirurgie, Medizinische Hochschule Hannover, Karl-Wiechert-Allee 9, D-3000 Hannover 61

pulmonary edema and oliguria/anuria. Six patients in this group died at or early after surgery (28%).

Five of the shock patients were operated in a state of highly septic toxicity. Mortality was particularly high; three patients died (60%).

Nine patients out of the whole collective had suffered systemic embolization in addition to hemodynamic deterioration prior to surgery. Causes of hospital death were shock sequelae (three), septic myocarditis (two), myocardial infarct (two) and septic prosthetic thrombosis in one instance. Two patients suffered early prosthetic disruption and died at or early after reoperation.

The predominant BE lesion was aortic regurgitation (60 patients) which was accompanied by mitral lesion in 12 patients. There were only nine patients with isolated mitral regurgitation. Isolated aortic valve replacement was performed in 47 patients; operative mortality was 15%. One patient died after isolated mitral valve replacement (11%). In nine patients both aortic and mitral valves were replaced; all these patients survived. In four patients aortic valve replacement was combined with mitral reconstruction; two of these patients died.

As a rule, operative survivors displayed dramatic hemodynamic improvement. In the 59 survivors long-term follow-up was complete ranging from 1 month to 9 years ($\bar{x} = 3.0$ years). There were eight late deaths (13.5%) 3 months up to 5 years after surgery ($\bar{x} = 2.8$ years). These were due to valve thrombosis (two), "sudden death" (two), and myocardial infarct (one). One patient died at reoperation for prosthetic leak and there were two deaths not related to cardiac causes.

Persistent Infection

Seven patients were reoperated for persistent prosthetic infection, five with paraprosthetic leak and two without. In six cases the aortic prosthesis was infected and the mitral valve in one. All five paraprosthetic leaks occurred in aortic prostheses and all these patients had displayed anular or subanular abscess at the time of operation (five out of 12 patients with aortic anular abscess). There was no prosthetic disruption in the 48 aortic valve patients who had not shown anular abscess formation. Difference of disruption incidence was statistically significant in these two groups ($p < 0.01$).

Prostheses subject to leak were: Starr-Edwards (one out of seven), Björk-Shiley (two out of 21), Hancock (two out of 22). There was no paraprosthetic leak in seven Lillehei-Kaster and in two St. Jude Medical prostheses.

Anterior Mitral Leaflet "Jet" Lesions

In 15 patients with aortic regurgitation "jet" lesions of the anterior mitral leaflet were observed. In severe aortic incompetence, particularly in the right coronary and the noncoronary leaflet area, regurgitant blood in diastole hits the opened anterior mitral leaflet (1, 4), the chordae and sometimes the papillary muscles (Fig. 1) resulting in chordae rupture or leaflet perforation or only vegetations on these structures (3). In nine of the patients with significant leaflet perforations and chordae involvement, including one case with papillary muscle rupture due to abscess, aortic and mitral valve replacement was performed. All patients survived; one had to undergo mitral redo for valve thrombosis and survived. In four patients mitral leaflet repair was performed in the presence of perforation. Two patients died after

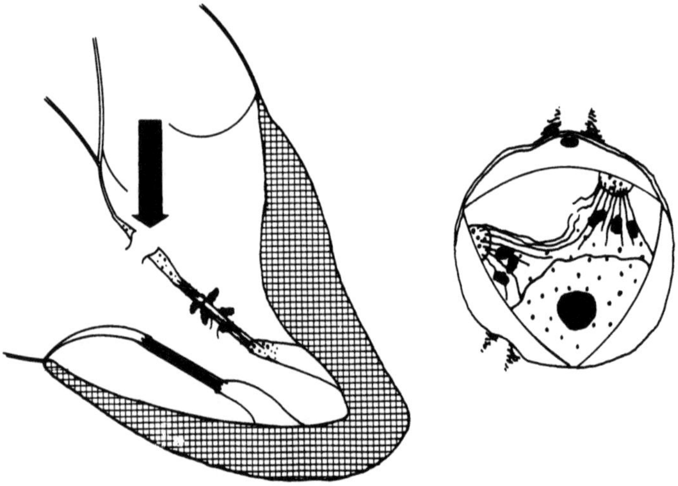

Fig. 1. "Jet" lesion of mitral valve secondary to aortic incompetence in bacterial endocarditis. In diastole the regurgitant blood hits the opened anterior mitral leaflet (left). Transaortic view (right)

surgery; one patient had to be reoperated because of mitral incompetence and survived. In two of the cases mitral repair broke down early after surgery.

In two patients who demonstrated only minor vegetations on the mitral leaflet surface without leaflet defect, no mitral surgery was performed. Three-and-a-half and one year after operation these two patients do not show any signs of infection or mitral incompetence.

Discussion

Although valve replacement in the presence of active BE was first reported by Yeh et al. (15) as early as 1964 it took a decade until this form of treatment became generally accepted, predominantly due to the reluctance of both physicians and surgeons to consider prosthetic implantation in infected media. Since surgery was often not performed until the patient was in an extremely deteriorated hemodynamic condition early results of surgery were less favorable (5, 6, 9, 13).

Progressive hemodynamic deterioration even under adequate medical treatment almost always has a fatal outcome (8, 10, 14). When surgery is performed once first signs of progressive heart failure are observed despite vigorous medical therapy, results in our series were similar to those in valve replacement for noninfected valvular disease. When surgery was delayed until the patient was in cardiogenic shock hospital mortality was substantially higher; almost one-third of such patients died. The direct relationship between hemodynamic state and operative outcome is also illustrated by the large proportion of shock sequelae such as respiratory and renal failure among hospital death causes and has been similarily reported by other teams (12). The improving results during the most recent 3 years in our series are mainly attributed to a smaller proportion of patients operated in cardiogenic shock. This fact and the increasing number of cases referred would illustrate the growing readiness of physicians to consider surgery in the course of active BE. The most unfavorable results were obtained in patients who had to be operated in a highly toxic, septic state characterized by continuous multiple septic microembolism, delirium, renal failure, high fever, and shock. Three out of five such patients died immediately after surgery, a proportion similar to that reported by Utley et al. (13).

Those patients who survive surgery demonstrate a dramatic recovery and often resume full physical activities since the hearts in general do not suffer from the irreversible changes secondary to long-lasting valve disease. Late death was due to cardiac causes in six of eight cases, in three instances presumably as a result of persistent infection (valve thrombosis, reoperation for prosthetic leak). At present 51 patients are alive up to 9 years after surgery. Without surgery, most likely they all would have died.

The most serious problem of valve replacement in active BE is persistent infection of the implanted prosthesis. When living and aggressive bacteria are found at the site of prosthetic implantation the prosthesis must be considered infected. Surprisingly, in the vast majority of cases, endocarditis may heal under a prolonged postoperative course of antibiotics provided that no prosthetic disruption occurs. At present, we would keep the patients after surgery on well-tested antibiotics for at least 6 weeks or until blood sedimentation rate is normalized.

Seven patients were reoperated for persistent prosthetic infection, five with paraprosthetic leak. This incidence of prosthetic infection of 10.1% is in sharp contrast to the rate of reoperation for prosthetic infection following primarily sterile valve replacement at our institution which is 14 out of 2150 equaling 0.7%.

According to our experience the finding of anular or subanular abscess at surgery is an ominous predisposition for later-on prosthetic infection and disruption. All five patients who developed paraprosthetic leaks had shown abscess whereas no leak occurred when the anulus was intact.

The choice of prosthesis in active BE is controversial particularly in regard to biological valve substitutes. In our series there was no predominance of leak related to any of the used prostheses. While a slightly higher incidence of early prosthetic infection was reported for the porcine heterograft leaflets (11) we did not observe any such case. Furthermore, up to now we have not observed accelerated porcine valve degeneration as was shown for infected valves (16). The broad sewing ring of the commercially available heterograft allowing for tight wedge-like fixation appears to be an even favorable feature for the use in questionable anulus.

Whereas prosthetic disruption may be prevented in mild forms of anular destruction by using special suture techniques such as circumferential transaortic wall fixation as suggested by Stinson (12), severe forms would ask for more extensive surgical techniques. Supra-anular valve implantation as first reported by Danielson et al. (2), has been used for cases of recurrent prosthetic infection in three instances at our institution with one long-term survivor (Fig. 2). Although up to now, this type of operation has been reserved for desperate situations it appears to be a feasible method primarily in active BE when dealing with severely destructed anulus precluding safe orthotopic valve replacement.

In 15 patients we observed so-called jet lesions of the anterior mitral leaflet and/or the tension apparatus secondary to aortic regurgitation. The relatively large proportion of concomitant mitral involvement would indicate the need of careful examination of the mitral valve once the aortic valve is excised. When significant destruction of the mitral valve was present, best results were obtained by mitral replacement at the time of aortic valve replacement.

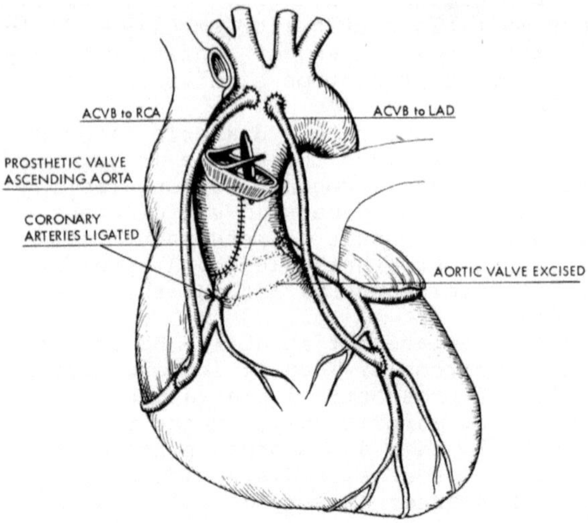

Fig. 2. Supraanular implantation of prosthetic valve in case of severe abscess destruction of aortic anulus according to Danielson et al. (2)

In four cases repair of mitral leaflet perforations was attempted resulting in early repair breakdown in two. When a structural defect of the mitral valve is observed, we now would replace the valve in the first instance. Minor vegetations on the anterior leaflet surface without defect may heal when aortic incompetence is corrected as shown in two patients.

In this report only a few problems of the challenging field of surgery in active BE could be elucidated. At present, the place of this type of surgery has been well delineated by the experience of several groups which is in agreement with ours. It appears that valve replacement should be considered early when hemodynamic deterioration occurs since a substantial number of patients can be saved who otherwise would be subject to an almost certain fatal outcome.

In a relatively small subset of patients prosthesis infection is a serious hazard that needs further technical achievement and advanced bacteriological and immunological knowledge of the disease.

Summary

In 69 patients valve replacement was performed in the presence of active bacterial left heart endocarditis and heart failure (aortic valve replacement in 47 patients, mitral valve replacement in nine patients, and double valve replacement in 13 patients). Hospital mortality was 28% in 21 patients who were in cardiogenic shock and 8% in 48 patients with progressive heart failure.

After operation seven patients developed prosthetic valve infection, five with paraprosthetic leak. All cases with leak had shown subanular abscess at the first operation whereas there was no leak in 48 patients with intact anulus. In 15 patients with anterior mitral leaflet "jet" lesions secondary to aortic incompetence best results were obtained by aortic and mitral replacement.

It is concluded that valve replacement should be considered early in the course of active BE when hemodynamic deterioration is observed. The presence of aortic anular abscess asks for more extensive surgical techniques in order to avoid paraprosthetic leakage. Structural changes of the mitral valve secondary to aortic incompetence appear to be an indication for mitral replacement.

References

1. Daniel W, Walpurger G, Lichtlen P (1976) Diagnostische Wertigkeit der mitralen und septalen echocardiografischen Veränderungen bei der Aorteninsuffizienz. Kardiologie 65:590
2. Danielson GK, Titus JL, Du Shane JW (1974) Successful treatment of aortic root abscesses by insertion of prosthetic valve in ascending aorta and placement of bypass grafts to coronary arteries. J Thorac Cardiovasc Surg 67:443
3. Edwards JE, Burchell HB (1958) Endocardial and intimal lesions (jet impact) as possible sites of origin of murmurs. Circulation 18:946
4. Gouley BA (1941) Aorta valvular lesions associated with Austin-Flint murmur. Am Heart J 22:208
5. Hancock EW, Shumway NE, Remington JS (1971) Valve replacement in active bacterial endocarditis (Editorial). J Infect Dis 123:106
6. Hetzer R, Dalichau H, Borst HG (1975) Herzklappenchirurgie bei bakterieller Endocarditis. Thoraxchirurgie 23:427
7. Kaye E (1973) Changes in the spectrum, diagnosis and management of bacterial and fungal endocarditis. Med Clin North Am 57:941
8. Lerner PI, Weinstein L (1966) Infective endocarditis in the antibiotic era. N Engl J Med 274:199
9. Manhas DR, Mohri H, Hessel EA, Merendino KA (1972) Experience with surgicall management of primary infective endocarditis: A collected review of 139 patients. Am Heart J 84:738
10. Robinson MJ, Ruedy J (1962) Sequelae of bacterial endocarditis. Am J Med 32:922
11. Rossiter SJ, Stinson EB, Oyer PE, Miller DC, Shapira JN, Martin RP, Shumway NE (1978) Prosthetic valve endocarditis: A comparison of heterograft tissue valves and mechanical valves. J Thorac Cardiovasc Surg 76:795
12. Stinson EB (1979) Surgical treatment of infective endocarditis. Prog Cardiovasc Dis 22:145
13. Utley JR, Mills I, Hutchinson IC, Edmunds LH, Sanderson RG, Roe BB (1972) Valve replacement for bacterial and fungal endocarditis. Circulation [Suppl 3] 47,48:42
14. Weinstein L, Schlesinger JJ (1974) Pathoanatomic, pathophysiologic, and clinical correlations in endocarditis. N Engl J Med 291:832
15. Yeh PJ, Hall BP, Ellison RG (1964) Surgical treatment of aortic valve perforation due to bacterial endocarditis: A report of six cases. Am Surg 30:766
16. Zuhdi N (1976) The porcine aortic valve prosthesis. Ann Thorac Surg 21:573

Session II Vascular Surgery

Extra-anatomic Bypass

Chairman: K. Kremer, Düsseldorf; Co-Chairman: N. L. Browse, London

Review of Indications for Extra-anatomic Bypass

S. Ekeström*

In most centres for vascular surgery, the indications for extra-anatomic bypasses are sufficiently limited. In some places, however, the number of extra-anatomic bypasses is surprisingly large. The reason for this seems to be unacceptably broad indications for the extra-anatomic procedure. It may thus be of interest to discuss the indication for one type of extra-anatomic bypass, the axillofemoral, which is performed in high risk patients due to its simplicity and safety. The most common type of high risk patients in vascular surgery reported in the literature are the following: high risk not suitable for aorto-iliac reconstruction, cardiopulmonary disease, cancer, massive abdominal adhesion, poor risk for laparotomy, advanced age, infected synthetic grafts, and poor general condition. In practically all reports there is a lack of detailed information of the type and degree of high risk. It seems as if the justifications for selecting a patient as a high risk and therefore as a candidate for extra-anatomic bypass procedure are rather loose. It gives the impression that the choice is made in order to allow the use of an extraordinary operative procedure.

The number of extra-anatomic bypasses performed at different clinics varies immensely. One could, in fact, observe surprising differences between neighbouring clinics where such variations of the panorama of diseases should not exist. At one cardiovascular clinic at the Scandinavian peninsula during a long period, only one axillofemoral bypass was performed, while the General Surgical Clinic nearby had a 20% incidence of extra-anatomic bypasses. The reason for the discrepancy seems to be a different opinion of the indication for extra-anatomic bypass. The indications for the procedure were at this clinic advanced age in 7 cases, infected graft in 11, and other grave diseases in 43 patients. The three most commonly reported indications for axillofemoral bypasses are advanced age, infected synthetic graft, and other grave diseases.

Advanced Age

Analysing the indication of advanced age one may notice first that the age over 20 years is no longer a hindrance to aortocoronary bypass or cardiac valve replacement. Furthermore, in elective surgery, in 66 patients with aortic abdominal aneurysm at an age over 80 years, O'Donnel and collaborators reported a primary operative mortality of 4.5%. This mortality is equal to that reported in much younger age groups. Biologic rather than chronologic age should determine operability in aortic abdominal aneurysm. Thus it may perhaps be concluded that advanced age per se is not a poor risk for reconstructive surgery due to an

*Thoraxkirurgiska kliniken, Karolinska sjukhuset, Stockholm, Sweden

improved selection of patients and improved preoperative treatment. Secondly, techniques for anesthesia and surgery and thirdly postoperative intensive care have been improved.

Infected Synthetic Grafts

Another poor risk in vascular surgery is the infected synthetic graft after previous reconstructive arterial surgery. In case of infection in a synthetic graft in the aortic bifurcation or the iliac arteries, the patient is threatened by rupture of the anastomoses with a risk of a perfuse bleeding and/or septicaemia. It is a general agreement that an infected graft is the most serious complication in vascular surgery. To save the patient's life it is essential to remove the graft; thereafter the arterial incision should be closed with a monofilament suture to avoid bacterial growth along the suture. The infected area should be well drained and strong antibiotics should be administered. The incidence of the infected synthetic graft is according to the literature 1% - 22% in various reports. A rather high mortality rate (25% - 75%) has been reported in case of infected synthetic graft. As a secondary procedure, extra-anatomic bypass may be used to save the leg if it is threatened – which is not always the case.

Other Grave Diseases

The third indication which is not used for extra-anatomic bypass procedures is other grave disease. Many severe cardiopulmonary diseases may influence the selection of a surgical procedure for arterial reconstruction. However, to be classified as a poor risk, the cardiac patient must belong to groups III or IV according to NYHA classification. It indicates symptoms on slight effort or at rest. The benefit of vascular surgery for such a patient may be dubious. In case of severe aortic stenosis or grave angina pectoris a poor risk exists as long as the cardiac disease is not cured or improved by cardiac surgery. In case of severe aortic valvular stenosis with a pressure difference between the left ventricle and the aortae of 100 mm Hg or more and symptoms of angina pectoris or syncope a very high risk exists. An aortic valvular replacement is strongly indicated and will eliminate the high risk for vascular surgery. A left main coronary artery stenosis with more than 50% decrease of the lumen area implies a high risk – the elimination of the stenosis is essential and should be given priority, whereafter the patient is no longer poor risk. Thus, the treatment of grave cardiac diseases demands priority, if sufficient methods for treatment exist. Severe pulmonary diseases that contraindicate vascular reconstructions are dubious candidates for extra-anatomic bypass procedures.

Conclusion

1. In conclusion it has to be stressed that *advanced age* per se is not a poor risk.
2. An infected synthetic graft is a very high risk to the patient and the basic treatment is its removal.
3. The patients belonging to NYHA, groups III and IV include uncertain candidates for vascular surgery. Some other grave cardiopulmonary diseases demand priority.

Revascularization of Lower Limbs Using the Axillary Artery. Early and Late Results of 98 Bypass Grafts

C. Devolfe, P. Adeleine, F. Violet, and J. Descotes*

The axillofemoral bypass was introduced in 1962 by Blaisdell and Hall (2), and also by Louw (9) as a substitute for conventional arterial reconstruction in high risk patients with severe aortoiliac occlusive disease. With the passage of time and increased experience with this procedure, the indications were expanded to include management of infected abdominal aortic grafts (1) and a limited trial of extra-abdominal bypass of abdominal aortic aneurysms (3).

However, considerable doubt exists as to the ability of this procedure to maintain long-term patency, and for many vascular surgeons, its place in relation to the more traditional anatomic approaches remains uncertain. In order to provide further information on this question we have analysed the immediate and late results of the axillofemoral grafts especially with regard to graft patency, limb salvage, and patient survival for which a life-table analysis according to standard statistical methods was performed (6, 12).

Material and Methods

Between January 1971 and June 1979, 98 procedures of revascularization of 128 lower limbs were carried out using the axillary artery in 93 patients. There were 88 men and 5 women ranging in age from 39 to 89 years with a mean age of 67.8 ± 8.7 years.

Indications for operation were severe occlusive disease in 81 patients – 62 with rest pain or gangrene, 4 with acute aortic occlusion, and 15 with disabling claudication – bypass of an abdominal aortic aneurysm in 10 patients and infectious complication of previous aortoiliac reconstruction in 2 patients.

Seventy-three patients were considered to be poor candidates for conventional surgery because of advanced age or severe associated disease. In 30 patients the procedure was used because of unfavourable local conditions – previous aortoiliac reconstruction in 19, calcifications or dysplasia in 8, and previous abdominal surgery in 3.

The operative techniques employed were essentially those originally reported by Blaisdell and Hall (2) for the unilateral procedure, and by Sauvage and Wood (14) for the bilateral procedure. Thirty axillobilateral femoral, 62 axillounilateral femoral, and 6 axillounilateral popliteal grafts were performed. The prosthetic materials used were woven Davron in 78 grafts, knitted Dacron in 15 grafts, and knitted Dacron velour in 5 grafts. All grafts were 8 or 10 mm in diameter.

*Department of Vascular Surgery - Dr. Descotes - Hopital Edouard, Herriot 69374, Lyon Cedex 2, France

Results

There were eight deaths within 30 days of the operation for a postoperative death rate of 8.2%. Five deaths occurred in patients with acute aortic occlusion (2/4) or with aortic aneurysm (3/10) and two in patients with subsequent amputation. There were 35 late deaths, or from 1 to 38 months after operation. The cumulative patient survival rate was 63.5% at 1 year, 48.1% at 2 years, 34.8% at 3 years, and 31.3% at 4 years (Fig. 1).

Twenty-five of 98 grafts at risk occluded. Seventeen of these grafts occluded early or within the first 6 months after operation and eight grafts occluded late or from 6 to 38 months after operation. Ten occlusions were managed with a new graft procedure, 13 required an amputation, and 2 required no further therapeutic intervention. The overall cumulative graft patency rate was 73.4% at 1 year, 63.4% at 2 and 3 years, and 52.8% at 4 years (Fig. 2). When the graft patency curve and the patient survival curve are compared it becomes apparent that the cumulative mortality rate exceeded the cumulative thrombosis rate. There was no statistically significant difference in patency rates between axillounilateral femoral and axillobilateral femoral grafts. Patency rates with the grafts when used with anticoagulation were better than those obtainable with no anticoagulation within the first 6 months ($X^2 = 4.14 - p < 0.05$).

Twenty-nine of 128 limbs at risk were lost to major amputation. Twenty-eight amputations were above the knee and one was below the knee. In 19 cases the limb loss was subsequent to graft thrombosis – to original graft thrombosis in 11, and to new graft thrombosis in 8. In eight cases the graft was patent at the time of the amputation and in two cases the amputation was subsequent to graft infection. The cumulative limb salvage rate was 72.4% at 1 year, 63.7% at 2 years, 58.4% at 3 years, and 51.1% at 4 years (Fig. 3). Comparison of the graft patency curve with the limb salvage curve shows that they are almost identical.

The only major complication was graft infection which developed in three patients from 1 to 4 months after implantation. The overall incidence was 3.2%, but two infections resulted in limb loss and subsequent death. In one patient an acute graft infection with involvement of the entire subcutaneous tunnel required complete graft removal following severe bleeding at the site of the distal anastomosis. In the other two patients with a localized infection in the groin a segmental graft removal was performed with a subsequent iterative bypass; in one patient a recurrent graft infection led to complete removal.

In two patients a pseudoaneurysm occurred in the groin at 20 months and 6 years after implantation. They were managed successfully without further morbidity.

Comments

Does the axillary-femoral procedure achieve a low operative mortality rate in high risk patients? Several reported series have confirmed an operative mortality rate between 7% and 10% (4, 7, 8, 10, 11). Although this rate appears high, most of the patients died for reasons indirectly related to the axillary-femoral procedure. In our series of 62 patients operated on for claudication, rest pain, or gangrene, there were only three postoperative deaths for a rate of 4.8%. On the other hand, of

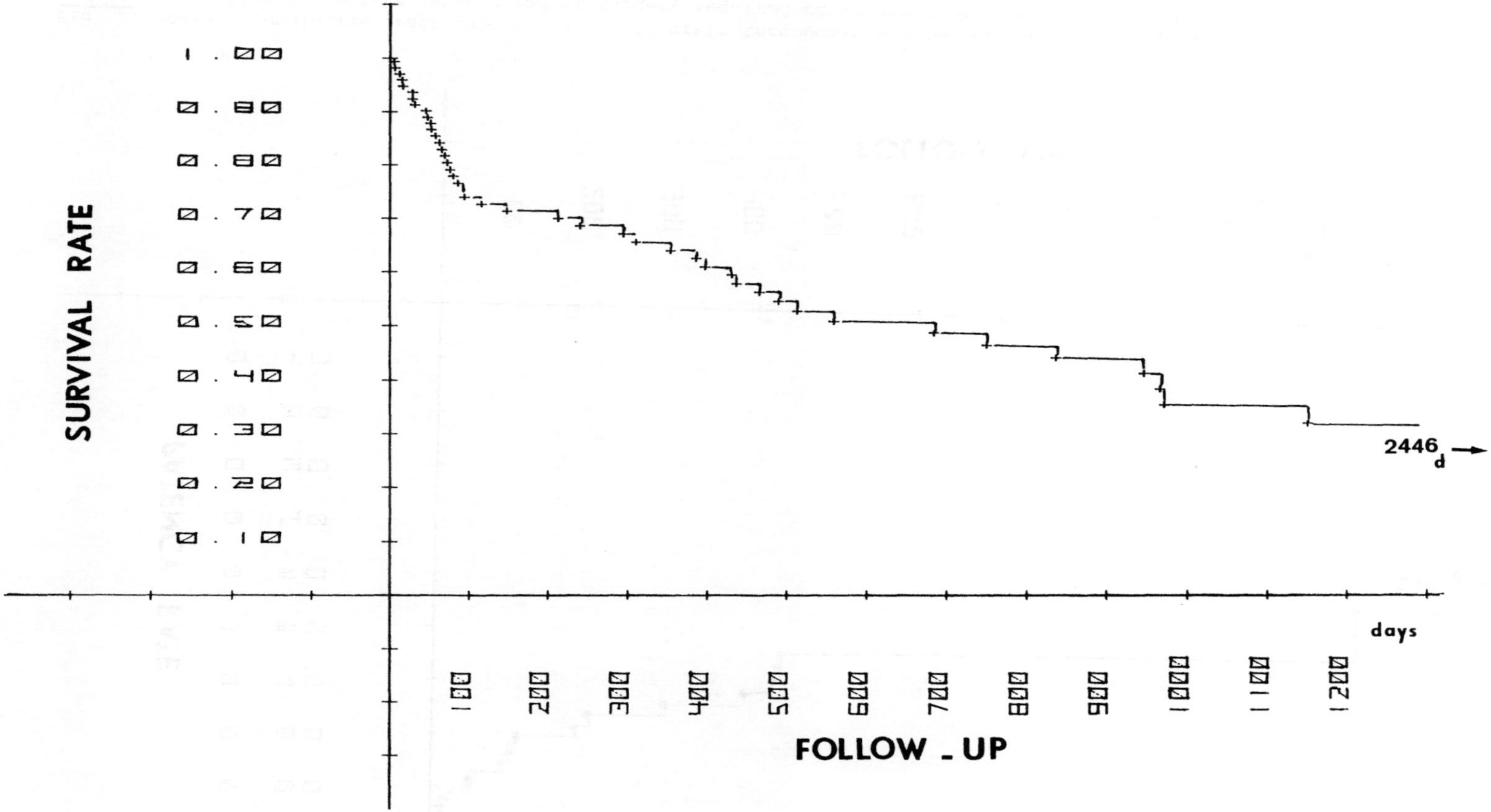

Fig. 1. Cumulative patient survival curve

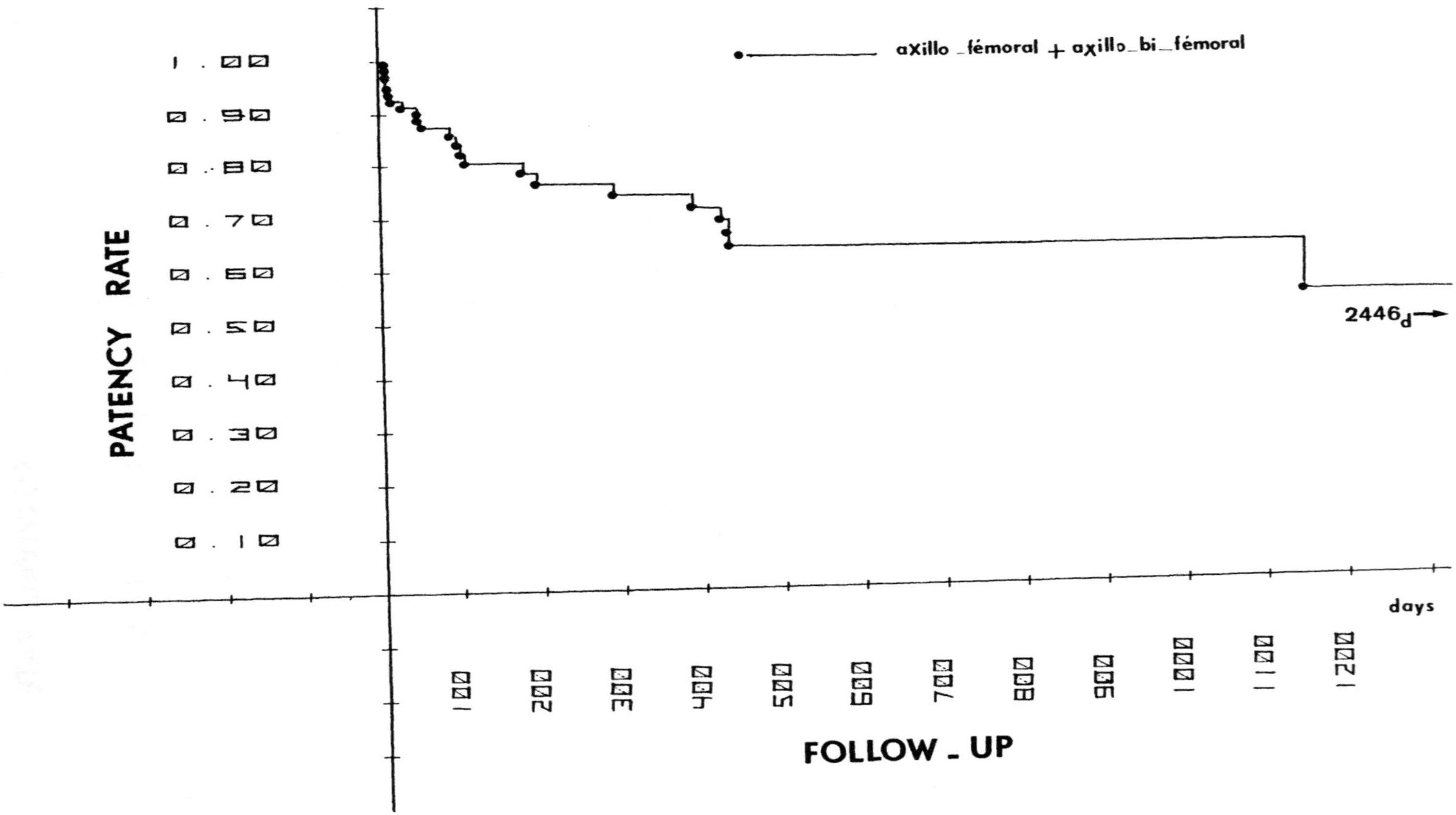

Fig. 2. Overall cumulative graft patency curve. If graft thrombosis was managed successfully by thrombectomy the graft was scored continually patent. When remedial surgery required replacement of the initial conduit the original graft was scored non-patent and the new graft was not placed at risk

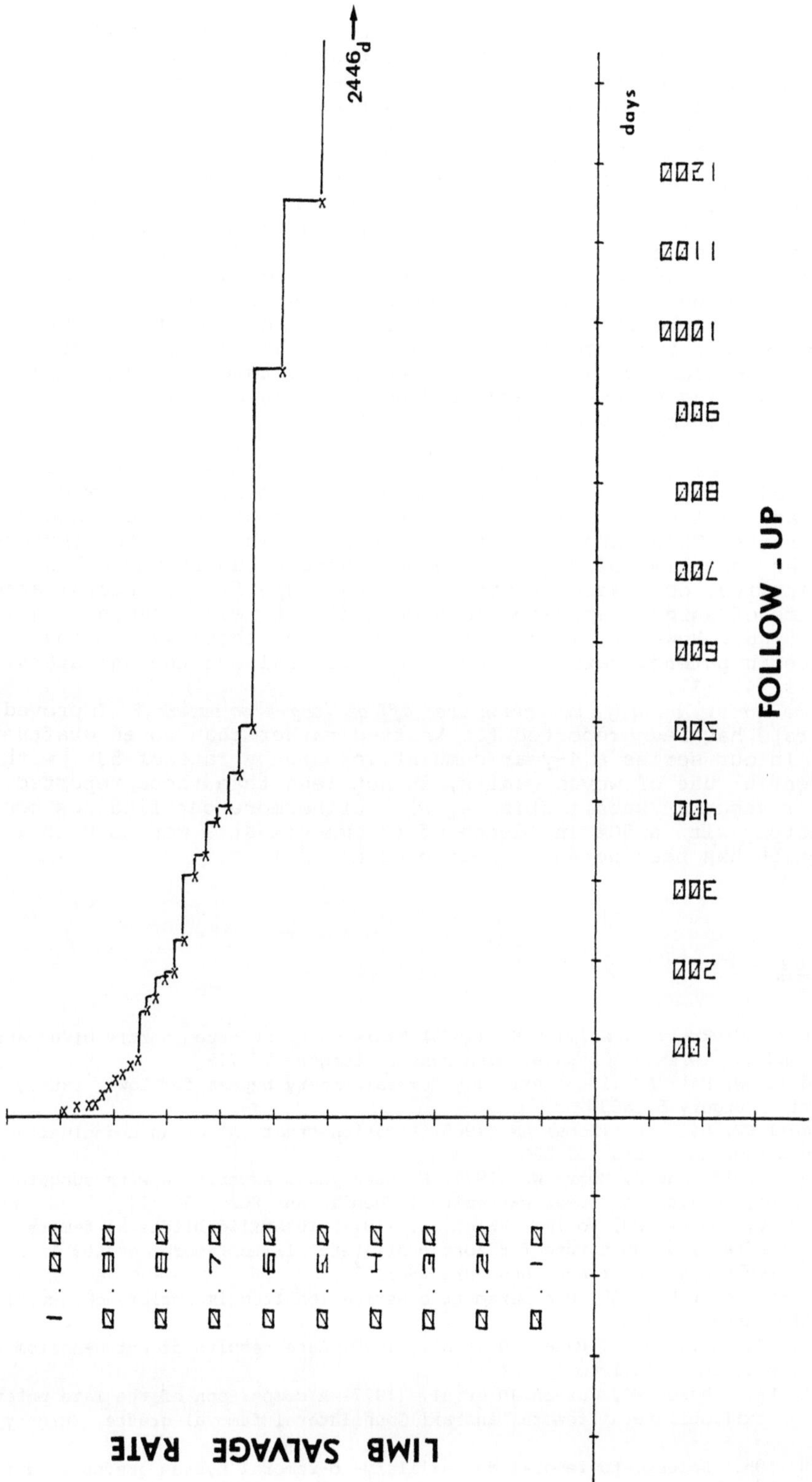

Fig. 3. Cumulative limb salvage curve

27 patients with a subsequent limb loss, 8 died within 1 month of the amputation for a rate of 29.6%. The fact that the cumulative patency rate exceeds the cumulative survival rate reflects the high risk patients who made up the majority of the series (4, 7, 11).

Is there an explanation for the common occurrence of early graft thrombosis? In our series a 6-months cumulative thrombosis rate of 22.2% was noted, but in almost one-half of cases a reoperation was successful in restoring grafts to long-term patency. Of concern to some authors is the vulnerability of the long limb of the graft to compression (5, 8, 10). Also evidence has been presented to suggest that after the first postoperative months the tendency for the graft to occlude in response to compression may be considerably lessened because of endothelialization of the lining of prostheses (13, 15). Furthermore a relatively stiff fibrous capsule forms around the graft during the same period of time and endows the graft with a greater capacity to tolerate temporary periods of bending stress. These findings may explain the early role of anticoagulant therapy which we have noted.

Does the concept of attaching the graft to both femoral arteries represent a real advance in term of further improvement of long-term patency? Logerfo et al. (8) reported a 3-year patency rate improving from 37% to 74% when axillobilateral femoral grafts were done instead of axillounilateral femoral grafts. This superior late rate was attributed to the increased flow in the long limb of the graft when a second runoff vessel is added. Likewise, occlusion or patency of the superficial femoral artery at the time of surgery appeared to have a direct relationship on graft patency (5, 8). However, in some reported series there was no obvious difference in patency rates between the bilateral and the unilateral procedures (4, 11).

Does the variety of graft materials used affect long-term patency? Improved patency rate has been reported for knitted rather than woven grafts (4, 11). In our series a 4-year cumulative patency rate of 53%, with a preferential use of woven grafts, is not less than those reported with other vascular substitutes (4, 8). Furthermore our findings contrast sharply with a 50% incidence of thrombosis at 9 months with woven Dacron which has been noted by Eugene et al. (4).

References

1. Becker RM, Cockroft D, Poirier NL (1975) Excision of infected aortic bifurcation graft and axillofemoral bypass: Case report. Surgery 77:718
2. Blaisdell FW, Hall AD (1963) Axillary-femoral artery bypass for lower extremity ischemia. Surgery 54:563
3. Blaisdell FW, Hall AD, Thomas AN (1965) Ligation treatment of an abdominal aortic aneurysm. Am J Surg 109:560
4. Eugene J, Goldstone J, Moore WS (1977) Fifteen years experience with subcutaneous bypass grafts for lower extremity ischemia. Ann Surg 186:177
5. Johnson WC, Logerfo FW, Vollman RW et al. (1977) Is axillo-bilateral femoral graft an effective substitute for aortic-bilateral iliac/femoral graft? An analysis of ten years experience. Ann Surg 186:123
6. Kaplan EL, Meier P (1958) Non parametric estimation from imcomplete observations. J Am Stat Assoc 53:456
7. Livesay JJ, Atkinson JB, Baker JD et al. (1979) Late results of extra-anatomic bypass. Arch Surg 114:1260
8. Logerfo FW, Johnson WC, Corson JD et al. (1977) A comparison of the late patency rates of axillobilateral femoral and axillounilateral femoral grafts. Surgery 81:33
9. Low JH (1963) Splenic-to-femoral and axillary-to-femoral bypass grafts in diffuse athero-sclerotic occlusive disease. Lancet 1:1401

10. Mannick JA, Williams LE, Nabseth DC (1970) The late results of axillofemoral grafts. Surgery 68:1038
11. Moore WS, Hall AD, Blaisdell FW (1971) Late results af axillary-femoral bypass grafting. Am J Surg 122:148
12. Peto R, Peto J (1972) Asymptotically efficient rank test procedures. J R Stat Soc 135:185
13. Reichle FA, Stewart GJ, Essa N (1973) A transmission and scanning electron microscopic study of luminal surfaces in Dacron and autogenous vein bypasses in man and dog. Surgery 74:945
14. Sauvage LR, Wood SJ (1966) Unilateral axillary bilateral femoral graft: A procedure for the poor risk patient with aortoiliac disease. Surgery 60:573
15. Sauvage LR, Berger K, Beilin LB et al. (1975) Presence of endothelium in an axillary-femoral graft of knitted Dacron with an external velour surface. Ann Surg 182:749

Analysis and Follow-up of 186 Alternative Bypasses

D. Raithel*

Primarily poor risk patients, or patients with infection of the prosthesis, presented the indication for an extra-anatomic bypass, both in the aortoiliac region and in lesions of the subclavian artery (1, 2, 5, 6, 10). Long-term observations have proven that compared with the direct reconstruction the femorofemoral and the carotidosubclavial bypass achieve the same good results in the long run with a significant decrease of operative risk (1, 3, 7-9).

Like many other teams, we have also expanded our indication for an extra-anatomic bypass (3, 8, 9).

Materials and Methods

At the Surgical Clinic of the University of Erlangen, we implanted 186 extra-anatomic bypasses, mainly in the carotidosubclavian axillofemoral, and femorofemoral position, up until the end of 1974.

Carotidosubclavian Bypass

Of 49 carotidosubclavian reconstructions 35 were done with a PTFE prosthesis and 14 with a Dacron prosthesis, each of them 8 mm in diameter. These patients were of an average age of 58 years. In the beginning the indication for reconstruction was given in the case of a higher operative risk. Today, we almost always use the carotidosubclavian reconstruction principle in lesions of the subclavian artery.

Axillofemoral Bypass

In four patients we implanted an axillofemoral, in five other patients an axillobifemoral bypass. The indication for reconstruction was in three cases an infection; six patients were "high risk patients". For the reconstruction we used only Dacron prostheses, 8 mm in diameter. These patients were of an average age of 69.2 years.

Femorofemoral bypass

One hundred and twenty reconstructions in the femorofemoral position were done with 8-mm prostheses; 30 of these were Dacron prostheses. In recent years we have used only PTFE prostheses (90 patients). The

*Chirurgische Universitätsklinik, Maximiliansplatz, D-8520 Erlangen

patients were of an average age of 62.5 years, the youngest patient being 28 and the oldest 80 years of age.

The indication for the femorofemoral bypass in 47% was a higher operative risk; 11% were emergency operations, in which, because of acute ischaemia, the aortoiliac region could not be reconstructed transfemorally (Table 1). In 17% a direct reconstruction was not possible, because of earlier operations or infections.

For various reasons, such as adipositas etc., in 4% we reconstructed the aortoiliac region with a femorofemoral bypass. In 27% we expanded the indication for the operation for younger patients, referring to the studies of Davis et al. (3).

Table 1. Graft patency in femorofemoral procedures

Study		No. of Proced.	Mortality within 1 month	Patency (%) Follow-up (years)
Brief et al.	1976	57	-	80.8 (8 years)
Eugene et al.	1977	33	15	53 (4 years)
Preston-Flanigan	1978	80	3.8	83 (5 years; prim. proc.) 65 (5 years; sec. proc.)
Sauvage et al.	1978	51	-	75.6 (5 years)
Blaisdell	1978	-	-	75 (5 years)
Own study	1980	120	1,7	75.4 (5 years)

Indication	n	%
Direct correction not possible	20	17
poor risk patient	47	39
good risk patient	32	27
Emergency	16	13
Other reasons	5	4
Total	120	100

Results

The mortality of the operation for the carotidosubclavian and axillofemoral bypass was 0%. The mortality of femorofemoral reconstruction was 1.7%. One patient died postoperativity of acute "tourniquet shock", the other of the consequences of an infection of the prosthesis.

Carotidosubclavian Bypass

After an average follow-up time of 48 months and maximum of 144 months (Fig. 1), 47 of 49 carotidosubclavian bypasses are still functioning. Using the life-table method the patency was 92.6% after 6 years.

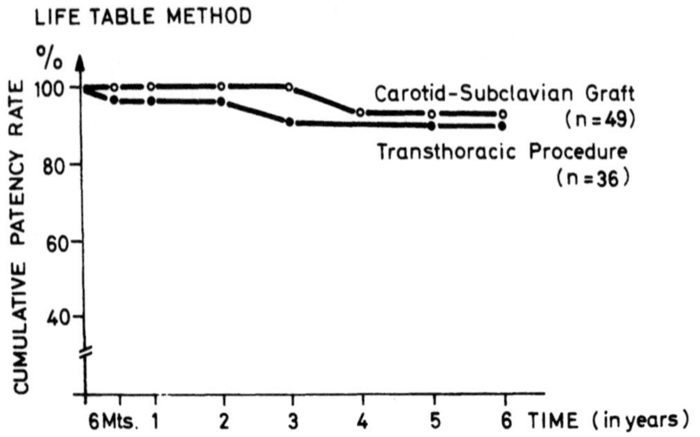

Fig. 1

Axillofemoral Bypass

During a follow-up of 6 years (average 42 months), two unilateral and one bilateral prostheses reoccluded. In the meantime one patient had died of an infection of the prosthesis leading to sepsis, 4 1/2 years after the operation though the transplant was still patent. This means a patency rate of 67%.

Femorofemoral Bypass

Within this series there were four acute, three early, and six late occlusions. Seven of these 13 reocclusions were successfully treated by thrombectomy. These rethromboses in the early postoperative period were caused by technical errors or hypotensive crises, the late reocclusions by run-off problems.

Using the life-table method this series results in a patency of 89.5% at the end of the first year, and 75.4% after 5 years (Fig. 2). In spite of occlusion of the graft, some of these extremities could be saved. Thus the cumulative limb salvage rate was 86%. Three patients with a femorofemoral bypass suffered claudication in the donor leg, this being caused in two cases by a stenosis of the femoral donor anastomosis.

Discussion

Our good long-term results with extra-anatomic bypasses give us reason to use them in the carotidosubclavian and femorofemoral positions (1, 3, 8, 9). The results in *axillofemoral* position in our small series are also good, and comparable to the results of other authors. Today, however, we prefer to use the axillofemoral bypass only in the case of an infection of the abdomen that excludes a direct reconstruction of the aortic occlusion. Furthermore, there are methods of anaesthesia today which enable us to make bilateral reconstructions of the aorto-iliac arteries even in high risk patients.

Comparing our operative results following *femorofemoral* bypass with those of other authors we are convinced that this method achieves the same good long-term results as the direct reconstruction of the aorto-iliac region (Fig. 3) (1, 3, 8). The operation itself carries an ac-

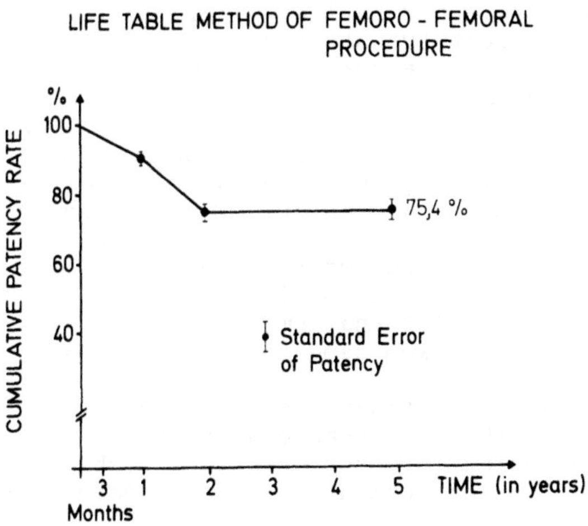

Fig. 2

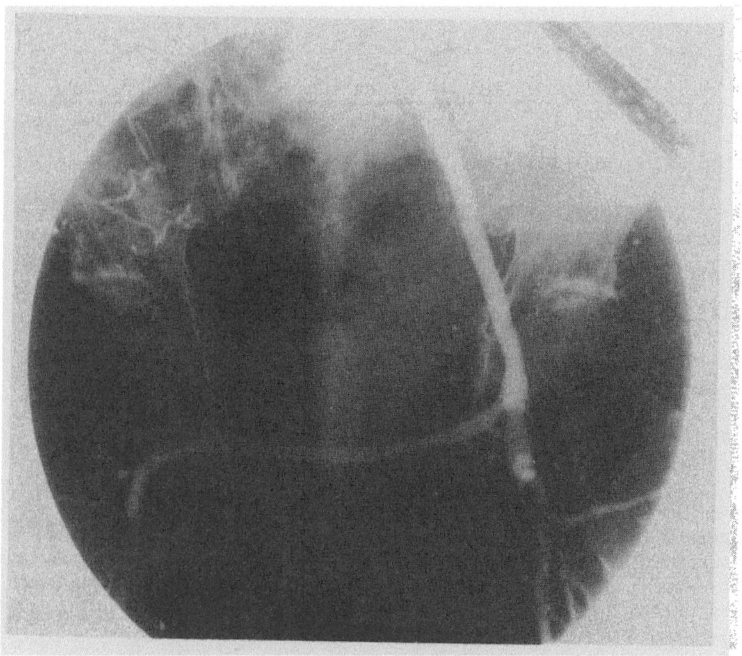

Fig. 3

ceptably low risk. Our cumulative patency after 5 years was 75.4%, i.e. comparable to those rates reported by other authors.

Even stenosis of the aortoiliac run-in region did not diminish the good long-term results. Some authors, however, advise not to implant a femorofemoral bypass in case of a stenosis of more than 50% (4).

A very commendable indication for the femorofemoral bypass is the unilateral occlusion of the prosthesis of the bifurcation. In this case the femorofemoral bypass, combined with correction of the run-off of the profunda femoral artery, is the method of choice. We used this procedure in 20 patients. An analysis of the late results showed only a small loss in the long-term success for this group, compared with the simple femorofemoral bypass of patients who had not been operated earlier. The carotidosubclavian bypass in our patients achieves results that are comparable to those of the direct transthoracic correction of a lesion of the subclavian artery. For the latter method the mortality was 5.5%, the patency after 6 years 91.4%.

Because of these good late results with a very low mortality (0% in our series), we now almost always use the extrathoracic approach for correction of subclavian lesions. The primary and secondary morbidity was also lower than that of the transthoracic correction. Regarding the material for the prosthesis, we have successfully used the 8 mm PTFE prosthesis during the past few years. We would not recommend this prosthesis, however, to be used in the axillofemoral position. There is a risk of tearing out prostheses at the axillar anastomosis, as seen in the course of two reoperations of patients who came to us from other hospitals.

In conclusion, it can be said that the extra-anatomic bypasses achieve very good long-term results with a remarkable decrease in mortality, given narrow indication and using an exact operative technique. We therefore recommend a broadening of the indication for the carotido-subclavian and femorofemoral graft.

References

1. Blaisdell FW, Carson SN (1979) Alternatives to direct surgery of aortoiliac disease. In: Bergan JJ, Yao JST (eds) Surgery of the aorta and its body branches. Grune & Stratton, New York
2. Blaisdell FW, De Mattei GA, Gauder PJ (1961) Extraperitoneal thoracic aorta to femoral bypass graft as replacement for an infected aortic bifurcation prosthesis. Am J Surg 102:583
3. Davis RC, O'Hara ET, Mannik JA, et al. (1972) Broadened indications for femorofemoral grafts. Surgery 72:990
4. Flanigan DP, Pratt DG, Goodreau JJ, et al. (1978) Hemodynamic and angiographic guidelines in the selection of patients for femorofemoral bypass. Arch Surg 113:1257
5. Freeman NE, Leeds FH (1952) Operations on large arteries. Calif Med 77:229
6. Hafner CD (1976) Subclavian steal syndrome; a 12-year experience. Arch Surg 111:1074
7. Logerfo FW, Mannick JA, et al. (1977) A comparison of the late patency rates of axillobilateral femoral and axillounilateral femoral grafts. Surgery 81:33
8. Raithel D (1980) Analysis of 81 femorofemoral grafts. Vasc Surg 14:73
9. Raithel D, Meister R (1979) Spätergebnisse nach Korrektur von uni- und bilateralen Beckenarterienverschlüssen mittels extraanatomischer Umleitung. In: Hild R, Spaan G (eds) Therapiekontrolle in der Angiologie. Witzstrock, Cologne
10. Vetto RM (1962) The treatment of unilateral artery obstruction utilizing femorofemoral graft. Surgery 52:342

Extra-anatomic Bypasses. Clinical and Hemodynamic Results

J. Matesanz, F. Acin, and S. Tamames*

Introduction

Aortoiliac occlusive disease is often the cause of disabling claudication and/or rest pain. At other times it can be an important contributing factor to the presence of ischemic ulcers and gangrene in the lower extremities.

Throughout the years revascularization procedures at the aortoiliac level by means of endarterectomy or bypass grafts have gained popularity and general acceptance in view of their good long-term results. They are therefore in our opinion the surgical techniques of choice. However, direct aortic surgery carries a considerable operative morbidity and mortality if the patient is old and/or has severe concomitant diseases such as chronic pulmonary insufficiency, coronary arteriosclerosis, renal insufficiency, arterial hyptertension, etc. On other occasions the presence of retroperitoneal sepsis make the conventional direct aortic approach unfeasible.

Under those circumstances – poor surgical risk or intra-abdominal sepsis – extra-anatomic routes to bring blood to the ischemic lower extremities have been used with acceptable results and lower mortality and morbidity. The most commonly used of these techniques are the cross-femoral grafts, introduced in 1962 by Vetto (1), to treat unilateral iliofemoral occlusive disease, and the axillofemoral or bifemoral grafts introduced in Europe by Lewis (2) in 1961, and popularized in the United States by Blaisdell and Hall (3) in 1963. Since those early times several reports have spoken in favor of these extra-anatomic surgical alternatives in the treatment of selected cases of aortoiliac occlusive diseases (4-8).

In this paper we are going to present the results obtained in 50 consecutive extra-anatomic procedures performed in our service in a 3-year period starting in January 1977.

Material

The hospital records of 48 patients in whom 50 extra-anatomic procedures were performed in the period of time from January 1977 to December 1979 have been carefully analyzed.

The total number of cases were classified in two groups: (A) femorofemoral (35 cases) and (B) axillofemoral or bifemoral (4 and 11 cases;

*Catedra de Patologia y Clinica Quirurgicas (Prof. S. Tamames), Hospital Clinico de San Carlos, Facultad de Medicina, Universidad Complutense, Madrid, Spain total 15). The mean age of the femorofemoral group was 63 years and of the axillofemoral group 64 years. All the patients were male.

The clinical status, using the classification of Fontaine, of these patients is outlined in Table 1, separated into the two above-mentioned groups A and B. In group A, more than half of the patients (58.8%) were in Stage II, that is claudication. The rest of the patients had either rest pain and/or trophic changes and gangrene.

Table 1. Clinical classification (Fontaine)

Group A: Femorofemoral grafts		Group B: Axillofemoral grafts	
Stage II	20 (58.8%)	Stage II	0 (0%)
Stage III	7 (20.5%)	Stage III	6 (42.8%)
Stage IV	7 (20.5%)	Stage IV	8 (57.1%)

Conversely in group B (axillofemoral), all the patients were in Stages III and IV. That obviously means that in our service we have been doing axillofemoral grafts only in cases with advanced degrees of arterial insufficiency, to relieve rest pain or to save an extremity from impending gangrene. About the indications for cross-femoral grafts we have been a lot more liberal, doing as shown more than half of the cases in patients with claudication only.

There is a discrepancy between the number of patients and the number of cases that deserves specific explanation. One was a patient with an axillofemoral bypass who presented with thrombosis of the graft 5 months after insertion. He came to the hospital 1 week after thrombosis; an immediate thrombectomy was attempted but the graft rethrombosed 24 hours later. A contralateral graft with a cross-femoral extension was placed with an additional extended profundoplasty. This graft was considered in our study as a new graft at a different risk period.

The other case was a patient who had a functioning axillofemoral graft 6 months after insertion when he developed obstruction of the contralateral iliofemoral segment. A cross-femoral graft was placed from the patent axillofemoral graft to the contralateral common femoral artery. This graft was considered in this study as a separate femorofemoral graft with a different risk period.

There is also another patient who deserves special mention. He was a 62-year-old diabetic male who had undergone a successful aortoiliac reconstruction by means of an aortobifemoral bypass graft 5 years earlier and came to a follow-up visit with thrombosis of the left limb of the graft. A thrombectomy of the occluded limb was attempted without success; therefore a cross-femoral graft was inserted from the contralateral patent limb of the graft to the profunda femoral artery in the occluded side. This case was considered as a femorofemoral bypass graft in our study.

It is also important to point out that in group A, 44.1% of the patients had severe arteriosclerotic heart disease and 5.8% had severe respiratory insufficiency. In group B, 85.5% had severe arteriosclerotic heart disease, 35.7% had important respiratory insufficiency, and 7.1% had septic contamination of the classic intra-abdominal route.

Results

We have analyzed the immediate clinical results, the long-term patency rate, and the hemodynamic results. The immediate clinical results are outlined in Table 2. We did not have any deaths in the operative period (30 days after surgery). We realize that this very low figure must be partially due to fortune and we expect to have a figure more realistic than 0% as we continue doing more of these cases.

Table 2. Early clinical results

Thrombosis	4 cases	(8%)
Infection of the graft	1 case	(2%)
Amputation	3 cases	(6.3%)
Healing of limited amputation	6 cases	(12.5%)
Limb salvage	12 cases	(25%)
No improvement with functioning graft	6 cases	(12.5%)
Pulmonary embolism (not lethal)	1 case	(2%)
Deaths	0 cases	(0%)

The early thrombosis rate of 8% is comparable to that presented by other authors. We had a 6.2% amputation rate in three cases in which the procedure failed to save the extremity. In six cases (12.5%), the procedure helped to reduce the amputation level to the foot with good healing. It is important to mention that in six cases (12.5%) there was no clinical improvement in spite of a successful grafting procedure. In all patients who had concomitant femoropopliteal occlusive disease a subsequent vascular procedure at this level was required.

All the cases were performed with 8 mm Dacron velour prostheses and additional profundoplasty was performed whenever significant stenotic lesions of the profunda femoral artery were found either arteriographically or at the time of the intervention.

The long-term patency rates were calculated separately in both groups and are outlined in Tables 3 and 4. In the femoral-femoral group the patency rate after 36 months of follow-up was of 79.8%. In the axillofemoral group at 24 months the patency rate was 62.1%. We think that this figure is artificially low and that it does not really reflect the outcome of these grafts, since the patency rate of each period is a lot higher. However, since the total number of cases is very low, a solitary failure lowers considerably the final figure that we expect to improve substantially as the number of cases increases and the follow-up period is somewhat prolonged.

Figures 1 and 2 represent the improvement of ankle systolic pressure after the insertion of the graft.

An attempt was also made to determine whether any steal phenomena could be demonstrated in the donor extremities. Ten donor extremities that were considered normal preoperatively were studied between 4 and 8 weeks after surgery in each of the groups, that is a total of 20 extremities.

In the axillofemoral group the brachial systolic pressure (Doppler) at rest was recorded and compared with the value obtained after exercise in the treadmill to obtain maximum flow through the graft. Also,

Table 3. Accumulated patency rate — femorofemoral group

Interval (months)	No. of grafts	Termination	Deaths	Occlusions	Patency (%)	Accumulated patency (%)
3	35	7	1	2	94.3	94.3
6	26	4	0	0	100	94.3
12	22	10	0	1	95.4	89.9
18	11	2	0	0	100	89.9
24	9	6	0	1	88.8	79.8
36	2	2	0	0	100	79.8

Table 4. Accumulated patency rate — axillofemoral group

Interval (months)	No. of grafts	Termination	Deaths	Occlusions	Patency (%)	Accumulated patency (%)
3	15	4	1	1	93.3	93.3
6	9	4	0	1	88.8	82.8
12	4	2	0	1	75	62.1
24	1	1	0	0	100	62.1

in the femorofemoral group the ankle systolic pressure (Doppler) in the donor side was recorded before and after treadmill exercise.

The results obtained can be seen in Figures 3 and 4. It can be seen that no changes after exercise were demonstrated in the axillofemoral group. In the femorofemoral group there were three cases with significant drop in systolic pressure after exercise. It could be seen in all these three cases on retrospective review that there were stenotic lesions in the donor iliac artery proximally to the anastomosis that had been overlooked preoperatively.

Conclusions

We think that extra-anatomic revascularization procedures of the lower extremities by means of cross-femoral and axillofemoral grafts are valid alternatives to treat symptomatic aortoiliac occlusive diseases when the conventional direct aortic surgery cannot be performed due to poor general condition of the patient or presence of sepsis in the peritoneal cavity.

The immediate clinical results, long-term patency rate, and hemodynamic postoperative improvement prove the validity of these techniques. It is also our feeling that femorofemoral grafts can be used safely in cases with unilateral iliofemoral occlusive disease and claudication only.

It is important, however, to point out that a careful evaluation of the donor iliac artery should be carried out before surgery in order to avoid embarrassing signs of steal phenomenon postoperatively.

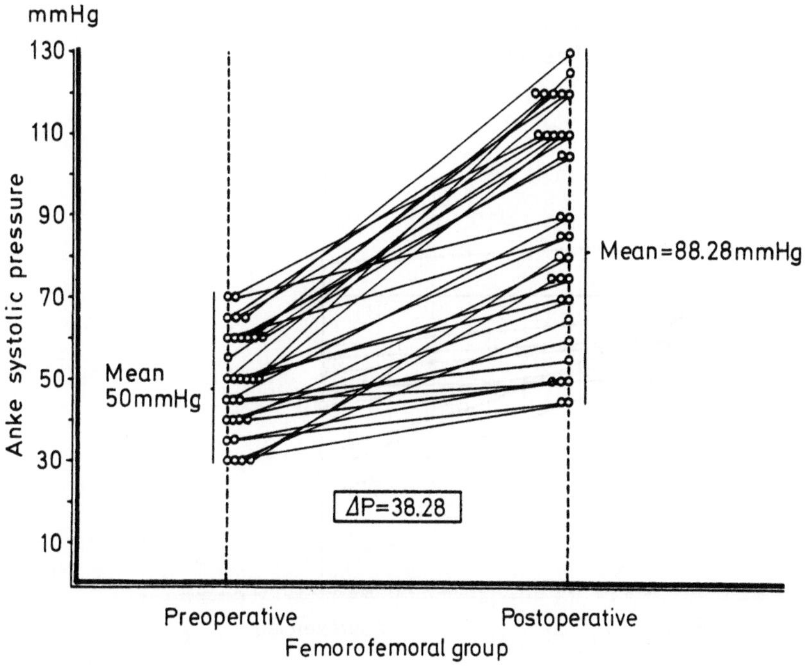

Fig. 1. Hemodynamic results. Femorofemoral group

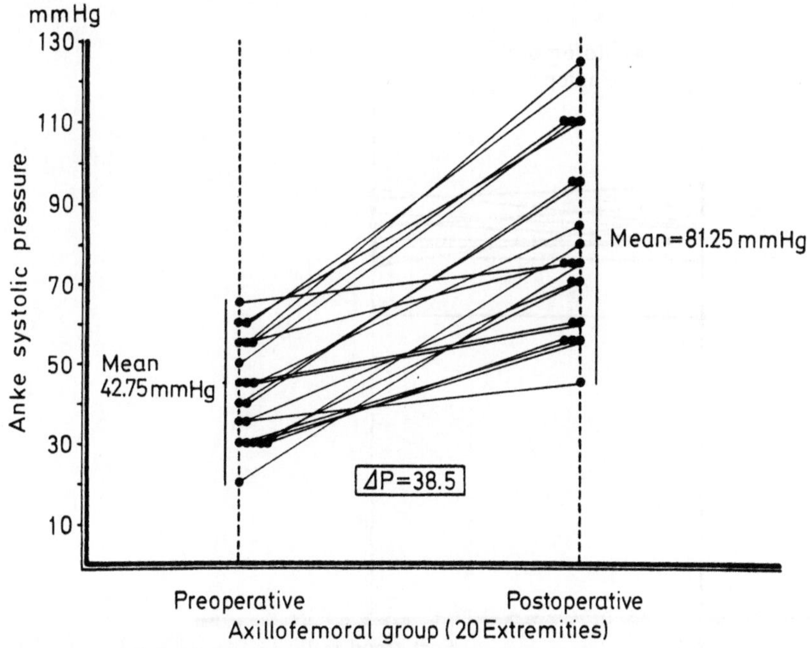

Fig. 2. Hemodynamic results. Axillofemoral group

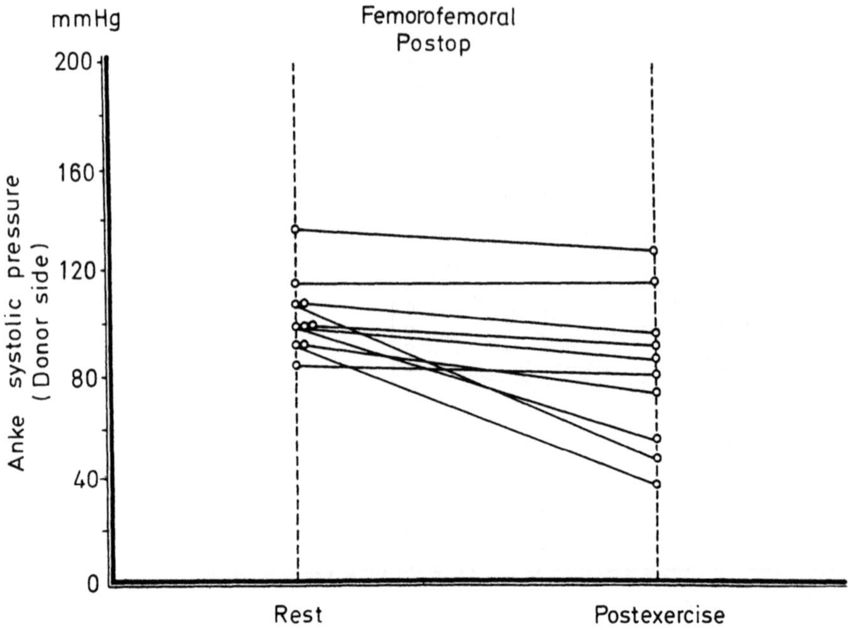

Fig. 3. Femorofemoral group. Postoperative evaluation of the donor extremity

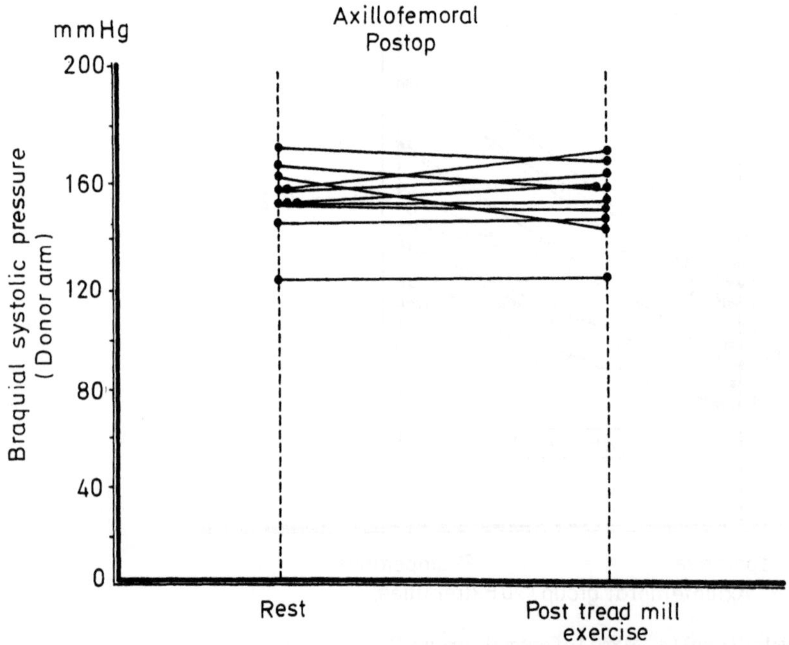

Fig. 4. Axillofemoral group. Postoperative evaluation of the donor extremity

Summary

Our experience with 50 cases of extra-anatomic bypass procedures in the treatment of aortoiliac occlusive disease has been presented. The early clinical results are good. The patency rate after 36 months of follow-up in the femorofemoral group was 79.8% and after 24 months in the axillofemoral group was 62.1%.

It is our feeling that these techniques can be used safely in selected cases of symptomatic aortoiliac occlusive disease with low morbidity and mortality, and satisfactory clinical and hemodynamic results.

References

1. Vetto RM (1962) The treatment of unilateral iliac artery obstruction with a transabdominal, subcutaneous, femorofemoral graft. Surgery 52:342
2. Lewis CD (1961) Subclavian artery as means of blood supply to lower half of the body. Br J Surg 48:574
3. Blaisdell FW, Hall AD (1963) Axillary-femoral artery bypass for lower extremity ischemia. Surgery 54:563
4. Blaisdell FW, Hall AD, Lim RC, Moore WC (1970) Aortoiliac arterial substitution utilizing subcutaneous grafts. Ann Surg 172:775
5. Brief D, Alpert J, Parsonnet V (1972) Crossover femorofemoral grafts: compromise or preference. Arch Surg 105:889
6. Johnson WC, Logerfo FW, Vollman RW, Corson JD, Mannick JA (1977) Is axillo bilateral femoral graft an effective substitute for aortic bilateral iliac femoral graft? Ann Surg 186:123
7. Mannick JA (1971) Are there practical alternatives to aortoiliac reconstruction? Am J Surg 122:344
8. Moore WS, Hall AD, Blaisdell FW (1971) Late results of axillo femoral bypass grafting. Am J Surg 122:148

Axillofemoral Bypass: An 8 Year Follow-up

S. Weimann and G. Flora*

In high risk patients with arterial circulatory impairment of the lower extremity in stages III or IV, Blaisdell and Hall (1) described in 1963 the subcutaneous axillofemoral bypass as therapy of choice which was often described and substantiated in the following years (2-4, 6-8, 10, 11, 14, 17-19, 20).

From 1972 to 1980 axillofemoral vascular reconstructions were carried out by the Vascular Surgery Department of the First University Clinic of Surgery in Innsbruck on 44 patients, 39 males and 5 females. Thirty-five suffered from arterial circulatory impairment of the lower extremity in stage IV and nine in stage III. The average age at operation was 70 years. Angiographically an infrarenal occlusion of the aorta was noticed in 10 cases and in 34 we found infrarenal stenosis and bilateral pelvic vessel stenosis which all were combined with stenosis or occlusion in the femoropopliteal area.

The risks of cardiac decompensation (18), obesity (10), bronchial asthma (2), diabetes mellitus (6), hypertension (3), malignant tumor (7), reduced general condition (6), coronary heart disease (10), tuberculosis (1), and condition after multiple previous abdominal operations (1) were a hinderance to the direct reconstructive surgery in the aortoiliac region. Seventeen times we performed a right axillofemoral, 15 times a left axillofemoral bypass, 7 times a right axillobifemoral bypass, and 5 times on the left side the same (Fig. 1).

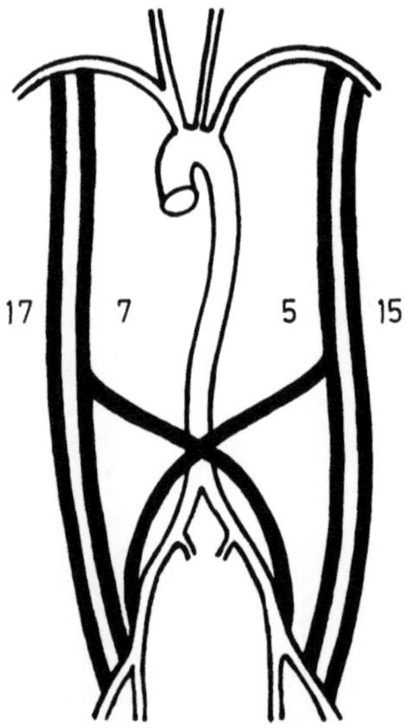

Fig. 1. Operative methods

*Vascular Surgery Department, First University Clinic of Surgery, Anichstr. 35, A-6020 Innsbruck

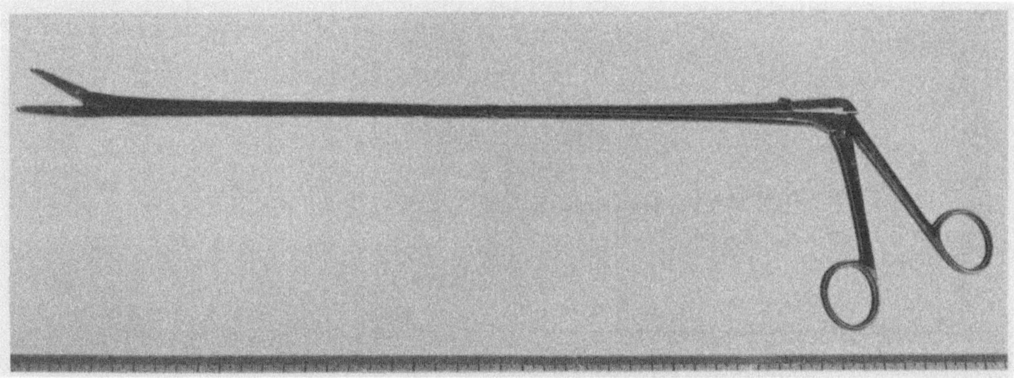

Fig. 2. Specially built instrument for through passage of the graft

If possible we prefer to operate with two teams using general anaesthesia. Preoperatively we check for sufficient flow in the a. axillaris using an angiogram if necessary. The anastomosis at the a. axillaris is laid as centrally as possible proximal to the origin of the a. subscapularis (6). An 8-mm knitted Dacron graft is most satisfactory. For through passage of the graft we use a specially built instrument which saves us an extra incision (Fig. 2). The distal anastomosis is usually done in form of a distal or extreme distal profundoplastic (Fig. 3).

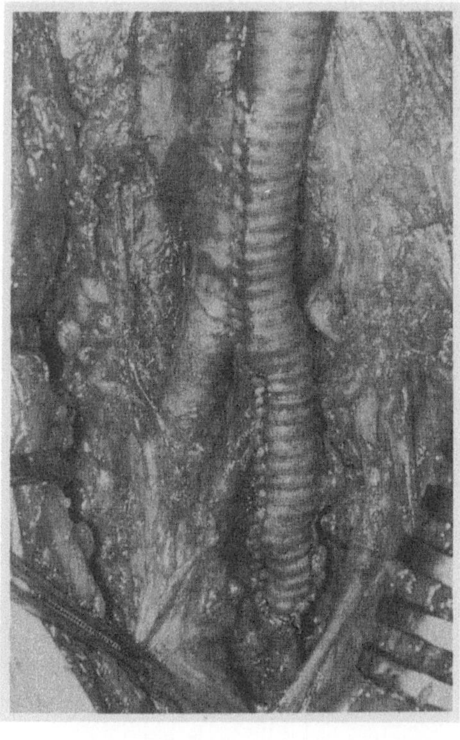

Fig. 3. Distal anastomosis in the form of a profundoplastic

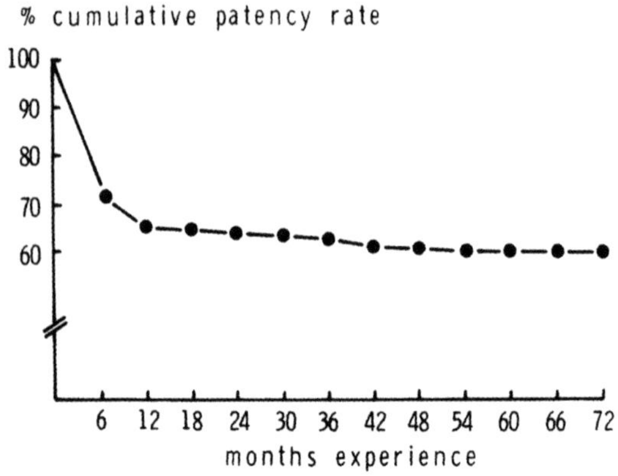

Fig. 4. Patency rate

The results of the 44 patients show that 9 died within a month of whom 5 were of myocardiac attack, 2 of malignant tumor, 1 of cardiac decompensation, and 1 of gangrene. One patient died 18 months later during open reconstruction. Of the remaining 34, 6 could not be contacted, leaving 28 which were reexamined. Of these, 17 had open and 11 had closed reconstruction. In the 17 open reconstructions, 6 had to be reopened in 11 successful relapse operations in the form of a thrombectomy; 9 of them had to be carried out in the first 12 months. Eleven remained open without relapse operation. Thirteen patients showed substantial improvement in arterial circulation, and in 4 cases no improvement was observed despite open reconstruction. In the closed reconstruction group, seven relapse operations were carried out without success. We had to perform four amputations of the lower limb; in two patients the bypass became infected, in one case with the development of a pseudoaneurysm in the proximal anastomosis area which ultimately made an extirpation of the bypass necessary although this did not affect the extremity concerned as in the five remaining cases.

Further complications were wound healing impairment with no influence on the function of the bypass; these healed conservatively. The ischaemia syndrome in the donor vessel region mentioned in the literature was not observed in our study (5, 9, 10, 12, 16, 20).

The cumulative patency rate in a maximal observation period of 72 months shows a percentage of 60%, where, analogous to the numbers indicated in the literature, the first year is of great importance for the prognosis of the patency rate (4, 15). Other factors contributing to a long-term patency are increased graft flow and good peripheral runoff.

De Laurentis (4) therefore found an excellent patency rate in all those cases where he combined axillofemoral bypass with femoropopliteal bypass. In our patients this was not possible because of complete femoropopliteal occlusion. We could not observe a difference between axillobifemoral and unilateral bypass as reported by Moore et al. (15) and Logerfo (13). Since we exclusively use an 8-mm knitted Dacron graft, we can by means of our case histories also say nothing about the assumption that the 10-mm knitted Dacron graft increases the patency rate significantly (15).

Naturally, long-term anticoagulant therapy in patients with axillofemoral bypass is very problematic because of the high risk factors and advanced age. Only eight of our patients received anticoagulants, all others antiplatelet agents. No difference of the patency rate was noticed between these two groups. Janisch et al. (8) found that the number of occlusions during anticoagulant therapy was even higher than in the groups compared (Fig. 4).

In comparison to the very much higher success rate after direct reconstruction in the aortoiliac region within the same observation period, the 60% patency rate is a rather modest result. Considering that every single open reconstruction in most cases means the rescue of the extremity from amputation which again is burdened by a mortality rate of 20%-40%, this represents a certain success.

References

1. Blaisdell FW, Hall AD (1963) Axillo-femoral-arteria bypass for lower extremity ischaemia. Surgery 54:563-569
2. Bürger K, et al. (1971) Der axillo-femorale Bypass als Notoperation. Zentralbl Chir 96:1761-1768
3. Campbell CD, Brooks DH, Siewers RD, Peel RL, Bahnson HT (1979) Extra-anatomic bypass with expanded polytetrafluorethylene. Surg Gynecol Obstet 148:525-530
4. De Laurentis DA, Sala LE, Russell E, McCombs PR (1978) A twelve year experience with axillofemoral and femorofemoral bypass operations. Surg Gynecol Obstet 147:881-887
5. Ehrenfeld WK, Harris JD, Wylie EJ (1968) Vascular "steal" phenomenon. An experimental study. Am J Surg 116:192
6. Gorman JF, Douglass FM (1965) Axillary-femoral artery bypass. Arch Surg 91:509-512
7. Gruß JD, Stojanovic R, Kuhn H (1967) Extraanatomische Umleitungsoperationen in der rekonstruktiven Gefäßchirurgie. MMW 118:1527-1532
8. Janisch K, Bürger K, Hübner R (1974) Spätergebnisse nach axillo-femoralem Bypass. Zentralbl Chir 99:78-81
9. Kerstein MD, Stansel HC (1974) Ischemia and subsequent amputation of the upper extremity following axillofemoral bypass. Angiology 25:305
10. Krüger HJ, Stockmann U, Witte C (1971) Der axillofemorale Bypass; ein therapeutisches Verfahren bei Risikopatienten mit chronischer Verschlußkrankheit der Arterien im Beckenabschnitt. Thoraxchirurgie 19:493-496
11. Kuhlgatz G (1974) Gliedmaßenerhaltende gefäßchirurgische Noteingriffe bei arterieller Verschlußkrankheit im Becken-Beinbereich. Zentralbl Chir 99:929-934
12. Lewis CD (1961) A subclavian artery as the mean of blood supply to the lower half of the body. Br J Surg 48:574-579
13. Logerfo FW, Johnson WC, Corson JD, et al. (1977) A comparison of the late patency rates of axillobilateral femoral and axillo unilateral femoral grafts. Surgery 81:33-37
14. Louw JH (1964) The treatment of combined aortoiliac and femoro-popliteal occlusive disease by spleno-femoral and axillo-femoral bypass grafts. Surgery 55:387
15. Moore WS, Hall AD, Blaisdell FW (1971) Late results of axillary femoral bypass grafting. Am J Surg 122:148-153
16. Müller JHA, Heyn G (1969) Der axillo-femorale Bypass. Thoraxchirurgie 17:297-308
17. Parsonnet V, Alpert J, Brief DK (1970) Femorofemoral and axillofemoral grafts — compromise or preference. Surgery 67:26-33

18. Raithel D, Knecht H (1978) Spätergebnisse nach extraanatomischen Umleitungsverfahren in der Gefäßchirurgie. Chirurg 49:436-439
19. Staudacher M, Weisskirchner R, Bardach G (1979) Extraanatomische Gefäßumleitungen bei Risikopatienten. Wien Klin Wochenschr 91:610-614
20. Thiele H, Altstaedt F, Kersting KH (1978) Extraanatomische Umgehung beim aorto-iliacalen Verschluß. Chirurg 49:752-756

Late Results of Extra Anatomical Bypass Methods

H. Imig, S. Horsch, H. Erasmi, and H. Pichlmaier*

The reconstruction of the aorta and pelvic arteries in arteriovascular disease cannot always be done in the conventional way although the indication for operation is absolute. Age, general condition, and number of risk factors limit the operation possibilities. This shows a comparison of vascular, bone, and abdominal surgery in our clinic in 1 year.

1. In 990 vascular, 408 bone, and 1573 abdominal surgical patients, an age peak of over 60 was seen in the vascular surgery patients.
2. The general condition of the patients was divided into five groups: normal, slightly reduced, very reduced, severely reduced, and moribund. In both abdominal and bone surgery patients, most of the patients were in normal general condition, whereas in our vascular surgical patients we operated mostly patients in slightly reduced condition, then patients in very reduced general condition, and least frequently patients in normal general condition.
3. The comparison of risk factors in the three groups showed the highest percentage of cardial risk in vascular surgery patients.
4. Operations lasting longer than 4 h were found almost exclusively in the vascular surgery group.

Summarized, vascular surgery is performed on older patients in poorer condition, with greater risk factors, and longer operation times.

So, if the vascular operation is already marked by a greater operation risk, this applies to the high risk patient in vascular surgery to a much greater degree and the extra-anatomical bypass is a limb-saving alternative.

From 1974 to 1980, at the University Clinic of Cologne we performed 106 femorofemoral bypasses with a hospital mortality of 4% and 136 axillofemoral bypasses (54 of these were bifemoral) with a hospital mortality of 14%. The long-term (from 6 months to 5 years) results should answer the following questions.

1. How does the extra-anatomical bypass improve the symptomatic staging (as from Fontaine) on the long term?
2. How high is the amputation rate and long-term mortality?
3. How high is the revision rate?
4. How high is the cumulative patency after extra-anatomical bypass?

From 242 patients who received an extra-anatomical bypass we can report on the long-term results in 219.

*Chirurgische Universitätsklinik, Josef-Stelzmann-Str. 9, D-5000 Köln 41

Femorofemoral Bypass (Table 1)

The late results of 102 patients could be evaluated. An improvement of the preoperative condition (stage) was found in nearly all patent bypasses. Twenty patients died (most due to cardiac causes), 18 patients were lost in the study, and 14 in the meantime needed an amputation. The revision rate was 12%.

Axillofemoral Bypass (Table 2)

Also here we found an improvement on the preoperative condition. Thirty-three patients died, 19 patients were lost, and 9 patients needed amputation. The revision rate here, as opposed to that of the femorofemoral bypass, was 30%.

Table 1. Late results of 102 patients with femorofemoral bypass

	preop	pop
II b	4	42
III	25	2
IV	21	6
Amputation	-	14
Deaths	-	20
Unknown	-	18
Revisions		12

Table 2. Late results of 117 patients with axillofemoral bypass

	preop	pop
II b	10	41
III	23	10
IV	23	5
Amputation	-	9
Deaths	-	33
Unknown	-	19
Revisions		33

Looking at the cumulative patency in atypical bypass methods we can state the following (Fig. 1): The femorofemoral bypass is generally better than the axillofemoral bypass, and the axillofemoral bypass shows better results than the unilateral bypass. This agrees with the findings of most other authors.

In summary, we can answer our original questions as follows:

1. The extra-anatomical bypass greatly improves on the preoperative condition.
2. The late thromboses after axillofemoral bypass of 30% and after femorofemoral bypass of 12% is high, as are the amputation and mortality rates.

A comparison of the long-term results of extra-anatomical bypasses and standard operative procedures in arteriovascular diseases of the aorta and pelvic arteries shows the extra-anatomical bypass only as the "ultimo ratio" treatment (last resort). These operations are indicated only in patients with high risk factors.

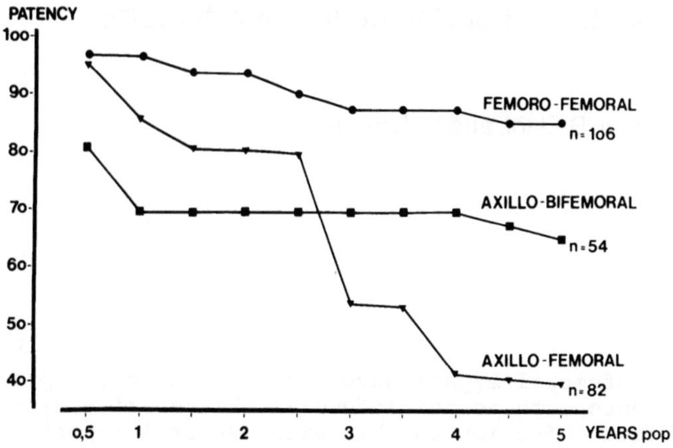

Fig. 1. Cumulative patency of 242 atypical bypasses

References

1. Johnson WC, Logerfo FW, Vollmann RW, Corson JD, O'Hara ET, Mannick JA, Nabseth DC (1977) Is axillo-bilateral femoral graft an effective substitute for aortic-bilateral iliac/femoral graft? Ann Surg 186:123-129
2. Pratschke E, Schäfer K, Becker HM (1980) Der gekreuzte suprapubische femoro-femorale By-pass. ANGIO 1/2:31-36
3. Zehle A, Stücker FJ, Gehl H (1974) Atypische Umleitungsverfahren in der rekonstruktiven Gefäßchirurgie. In: Heberer G (ed) Indikation zur Operation. Springer, Berlin Heidelberg New York, pp 166-174

Axillo-femoral Bypass – A Method of Choice in Aorto-femoral Obliterative Disease

E. Ribbe, A. Broomé, J. T. Christenson, B. Eklöf, and L. Norgren*

Reconstructions with axillofemoral bypass have become an accepted procedure for poor risk patients with aortoiliofemoral obliterative disease and patients with graft infection in this area. Several reports on good long-term results have been published during the last years (1-8).

In this report our experience in Lund and Helsingborg, Sweden, during a 5-year period is reviewed in order to provide further information concerning long-term patency of axillofemoral grafting using both velour-Dacron grafts and expanded PTFE grafts (Gore-Tex).

Material

During 1973-1978, 61 patients have been reconstructed with axillofemoral bypass. Mean age of the patients was 66 years (range 45-82 years). There were 51 men and 10 women. Velour-Dacron grafts (8-10 mm) were used in 30 patients and in another 31 patients expanded PTFE grafts (Gore-Tex 8 mm) were used. No differences concerning age and sex distribution were noticed between the two groups. Fourteen patients in the velour-Dacron group and six patients in the PTFE group had previous vascular reconstructions. The indication for axillofemoral bypass was severe ischemia (rest pain and/or gangrene) in 54 patients (89%) and disabling intermittent claudication in 7 patients (11%).

In 17 patients an axillounilateral femoral bypass was performed, while in 44 cases axillobilateral femoral bypass was used. The velour-Dacron grafts were preclotted, a procedure that was unnecessary for the PTFE grafts. The patients were given 5000 units of heparin intravenously during the operation. Twenty-six patients received preventive antibiotics, dicloxacillin (Diclocila). All patients were given 500 ml dextran 40 (Rheomacrodex) daily during the first 5 postoperative days. All patients have been followed until December 31, 1979, or until death.

Results

During the early postoperative course five patients died, two due to sepsis and three due to cardiac failure (Table 1). Four patients had a graft infection. None of the infected patients had received preventive antibiotics. A transient renal insufficiency occurred in one patient. In 8 patients with early graft thrombosis, 16 thrombectomies

*Department of Surgery, Lasarettet, S-221 85 Lund

Table 1. Early postoperative complications after axillofemoral bypass operations

Complications	Velour-Dacron	PTFE	Total
Postoperative mortality	4	1	5
Graft infection	3	1	4
Graft thrombosis	6	2	8
Amputation	1	2	3

were performed, in 10 of them with successful outcome. Six patients had early graft failure and three of these patients were amputated unilaterally.

Later, during the follow-up, another nine patients died. Six more patients were amputated below the knee joint and graft thombosis was seen in 12 cases (Table 2).

Graft patency rate after 4 years was 75%. No difference between velour-Dacron and PTFE grafts was seen (Fig. 1). Limb salvage rate among the patients with severe ischemia was 90%.

Table 2. Late complications after axillofemoral operations

Complications	Velour-Dacron	PTFE	Total
Mortality	6	3	9
Graft thrombosis	9	3	12
Amputation	4	2	6

Discussion

Axillofemoral bypass is an acceptable method to reestablish the blood flow to legs with severe ischemia in poor risk patients. Our patency rate and limb salvage rate combined with a low frequency of postoperative complications verify this statement. The procedure also seems justified as a method of choice in poor risk patients with disabling claudication. Our findings indicate that there are no differences between the use of velour-Dacron grafts and expanded PTFE grafts concerning patency rate. There is, however, a lower frequency of both early and late graft thrombosis and a higher success rate of late thrombectomies when the PTFE graft is used. We therefore recommend this graft for axillofemoral bypass reconstruction.

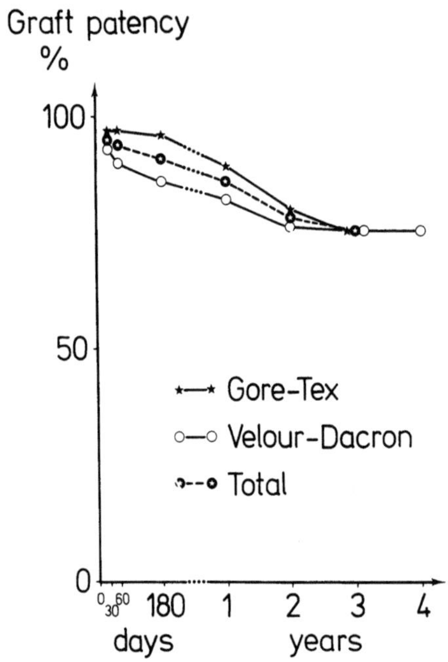

Fig. 1. Graft patency concerning the PTFE group, velour-Dacron group, and the total material for 4 years in axillofemoral bypass

References

1. Absalon KB, Freant L, Newsome D, Kim SC, Obbler A (1975) Extrathoracic axillary-iliac bypass. Substitution of a resected descending thoracic aorta. Surgery 77:275-278
2. Bliss BP, Barrett GS (1972) Axillofemoral and axilloprofunda bypass grafts. Ann R Coll Surg Engl 50:268-271
3. Christenson JT, Einarsson E, Eklöf B, Norgren L (1978) Synthetic arterial grafts III. The outcome in 22 patients with synthetic axillo-femoral bypass grafts. Scand J Thorac Cardiovasc Surg 12:121-124
4. Johnson WC, Logerfo FW, Vollman RW, Corson JD, O'Hara ED, Mannick A, Nabseth DC (1977) Is axillo-bilateral femoral graft an effective substitute for aortic-bilateral iliac/femoral graft? An analysis of ten years experience. Ann Surg 138:387-393
5. Mannick JA, Williams LE, Nabseth DC (1970) The late results of axillofemoral grafts. Surgery 68:1038-1041
6. Moore WS, Hall AD, Blaisdell FW (1971) Late results of axillary femoral bypass grafting. Am J Surg 122:148-152
7. Taheri A (1970) Axillofemoral bypass graft for poor risk patients. Angiology 21:682-685
8. Whitte C, Krüger BJ, Stockman U (1974) Axillary femoral bypass grafting: A report on 52 patients. Langenbecks Arch Chir 337:848-851

Extra-anatomical Bypass Through the Obturator Foramen

L. T. Cotton*

The need for this route of extra-anatomical bypass is limited to those cases of massive aneurysmal dilatation in the thigh where the only alternative would be ligature of the common or external iliac artery followed by a very high above knee amputation. The first cases using this route were described by Shaw and Baue in 1963 (1); later MacPherson added a case history in 1967 (2), and Spiro and I described three cases in 1970 (3). This paper describes another five cases, a total of eight in a 10-year experience.

In Table 1 the indications for the operation are listed; seven were for aneurysm of the common femoral artery and one for an aneurysm of a homograft inserted 10 years ago as a femoropopliteal bypass. Two of the common femoral aneurysms were atherosclerotic. Of the two mycotic aneurysms, one followed the insertion of a femoral artery line for cardiac bypass for an emergency pulmonary embolectomy. The other appeared in a drug addict who was in the habit of injecting his femoral artery with a wide variety of drugs dissolved in unsterile water. Of the three false aneurysms, one followed cardiac bypass for the emergency treatment of a dissecting aneurysm, and another followed cardiac catheterisation through the femoral artery in a patient who was taking antiplatelet drugs; the last case followed aortofemoral bypass. In all, the appearance was of a massive pulsating swelling extending from the groin to the knee with evidence of infection in two cases. In two patients the false aneurysm had ruptured subcutaneously and three showed leakage of blood through an inguinal wound.

Table 1. Indications for obturator canal bypass

I. Aneurysm of common femoral artery		
	Atherosclerotic	2
	Mycotic - after cardiopulmonary bypass	1
	- after drug abuse	1
	False - after cardiopulmonary bypass	1
	- after cardiac catheterisation	1
	- after aortofemoral bypass	1
II. Aneurysm of femoropopliteal homograft		1
	Total	8

*King's College Hospital, Denmark Hill, London S.E.5., Great Britain

In Figure 1 a diagram of the operative technique is shown. The operation is usually an emergency procedure. The bladder is emptied by catheter. A transverse incision is made in the iliac fossa to achieve transperitoneal exposure and control of the common iliac artery and its bifurcation. The abdominal wall is strongly lifted up to expose the bottom of the pelvis, exposure assisted by having the feet of the patient elevated above the level of the head. The peritoneum is incised with a long-handled knife, taking care to be as far away as possible from the obturator nerve and vessels. Sometimes the membrane can be disrupted by a finger, but often is so extremely tough that a knife must be used.

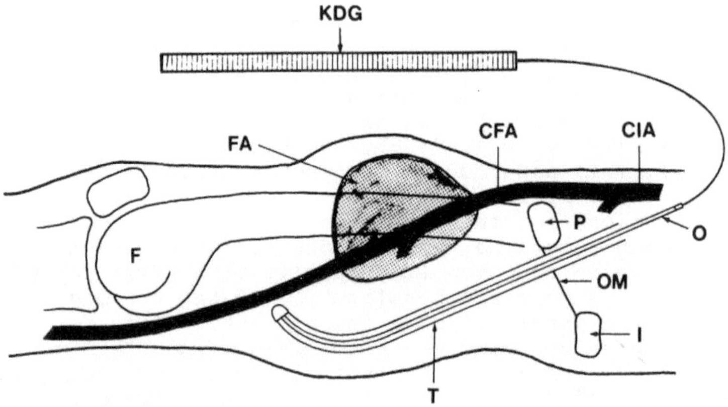

KDG	**Knitted Dacron graft**	**P**	**Pubis**
FA	**Femoral aneurysm**	**I**	**Ischium**
F	**Femur**	**T**	**Tunneller**
CFA	**Common femoral artery**	**O**	**Obturator**
CIA	**Common iliac artery**	**OM**	**Obturator membrane**

Fig. 1. Diagram of operation for obturator canal bypass

An essential tool is a tunnelling device (Fig. 2), a simple home-made steel tube of 10 mm bore with a handle. The end of the tube is slightly curved forward at its distal end. The obturator has a blunt nose attached to a moderately flexible rod. The end of the rod is drilled to provide a hole through which a suture can be passed to which the graft can be attached. Once the tunneller is through the membrane it can be pushed into the muscles of the posterior compartment of the thigh.

An incision is now made over the inner aspect of the lower third of the thigh well away from the aneurysm. The wound is deepened subsartorially to expose the lower end of the femoral and upper end of the popliteal arteries. When the thigh is lifted the nose of the tunneller can be felt through the muscles of the back of the thigh. With pressure on the handle of the tunneller above, its nose can be directed by external pressure on the back of the thigh into the adductor canal. With blunt dissection the finger can be passed along the adductor canal until the nose of the tunneller can be felt and it can be negotiated to lie alongside the lower part of the femoral artery.

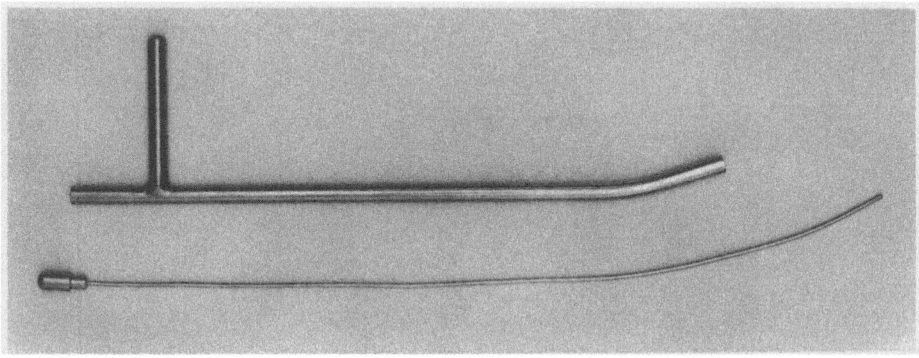

Fig. 2. Tunnelling instrument and flexible obturator (reversed)

A knitted Dacron graft, size 8-10 mm, is preclotted and attached to the proximal end of the obturator by a long thread stitch (Fig. 2). By withdrawing the obturator distally the graft can then be drawn through the tunneller slowly to avoid twisting. The tunneller is then withdrawn.

Anastomoses are performed proximally, either end to end, or end to side, with either the common iliac or preferably the external iliac artery, which is ligated distal to the anastomosis. Distally an end-to-side anastomosis is performed with ligation of the femoral artery proximal to the anastomosis to cut off retrograde arterial flow. The wounds are closed with suction drainage. After the wounds have been sealed off with dressings the aneurysm in the groin is incised and evacuated of clots. Specimens are taken of the clot and the blood present for evidence of infection. Any infected part of a prosthesis is removed. Bleeding can still occur from the deep femoral artery so the cavity is packed with 10 cm wide gauze roll which is removed after 2-3 days. In all cases it has been possible to route the graft without entering the aneurysmal cavity. Healing of the cavity may take up to 6-8 weeks, but has given rise to no problems.

In Table 2 the results of the procedure are described. In the cases of atherosclerotic aneurysm one graft occluded at 18 months, leaving the patient with intermittent claudication. The other has remained patent for 6 years. One graft for mycotic aneurysm occluded after 18 months, leaving the patient with claudication. The other patient, the drug addict, died due to septicaemia and general disintegration of both his mind and body. The three grafts for false aneurysm have remained patent. The graft performed for disruption of the femoropopliteal homograft occluded after 1 year; in her the run-off was so bad that an above-knee amputation had to be performed.

In summary, of eight patients one died and one lost a leg, but six limbs were saved that otherwise could only have been amputated at a very high level. Lastly, it is essential to stress that the operation is only simple if a tunnelling instrument is available. The same tunneller is also very useful in both axillofemoral and femoropopliteal grafting. An additional help then is to have a straight tube so that the appropriate instrument can be used.

Table 2. Results of obturator canal bypass

Lesion in thigh	Result	Months
Atherosclerotic aneurysm	Occluded[a]	18
	Patent	72
Mycotic aneurysm	Occluded[a]	12
	Died	-
False aneurysm	Patent	60
	Patent	6
	Patent	12
Aneurysm homograft	Occluded[b]	12

[a] Claudication after occlusion

[b] Above-knee amputation after occlusion

References

1. Shaw RS, Baue AE (1963) Management of sepsis complicating arterial reconstructive surgery. Surgery 53:75-86
2. MacPherson AIS (1967) Ileofemoral arterial bypass through the obturator foramen. Br J Surg 54:946-947
3. Spiro M, Cotton LT (1970) The obturator canal as a route for iliofemoral bypass. Br J Surg 57:168-172

Poor Risk Patients Selection in the Management of Aorto-iliac Occlusions: Extra-anatomic Bypass Versus Extra-peritoneal Procedures

G. Agrifoglio, G. Vercellio, and G. Lorenzi*

Since 1962, when Blaisdell (2) performed the first axillofemoral bypass graft, a large number of extra-anatomic subcutaneous grafts have been reported by several authors. Indication to these operations was originally limb salvage in poor risk patients or the presence of an infected aortic prosthesis. Recently some surgeons have encouraged the use of such procedures as an alternative to the aortoiliac-femoral bypass or endarterectomy. A review of our experience in the surgical management of aortoiliac atherosclerotic occlusions in high risk patients suggests a less extended indication.

Clinical Material

Between 1971 and 1980, 855 aortoiliac-femoral vascular reconstructions were carried out. One hundred and seventeen of them were performed in high risk patients; in 101 cases an extraperitoneal approach was used to perform a thromboendarterectomy or a bypass graft, whereas in the other 16 cases an axillofemoral or a femorofemoral graft was carried out (Table 1). In seven patients an axillofemoral bypass graft was performed for management of infected aortic prosthesis but they were not included in this study because they are not comparable, in regard to risk factors, to the patients of the other group.

In the extraperitoneal group severe claudication was present before surgery in 80% of cases (Table 2). By contrast, in patients submitted to extra-anatomical operations the primary indication for surgery was limb salvage in the majority of the cases (88%) and in only two patients (12%) was severe claudication present before operation.

Table 1. Operations for aortoiliac occlusive disease

Total aortoiliac-femoral reconstructions (1971-1980)	855
Extraperitoneal procedures in high risk patients	101
Extra-anatomical procedures in high risk patients	16
Extra-anatomical procedures for infected aortic prosthesis	7

*Institute of Vascular Surgery, University of Milan, Milan, Italy

Table 2. High risk patient selection

	Extraperitoneal	Extra-anatomical
Mean age	60 years	70 years
Claudication (severe)	80%	12%
Rest pain and gangrene	20%	88%

In this group the average age was 70 years compared to 60 years in the extraperitoneal series. Patients selected for axillofemoral and femorofemoral bypass graft (Table 3) presented the association of two, three, or more severe diseases. Particularly, the association of four severe diseases was present in nine patients. As severe diseases were considered myocardial ischemia, renal failure, advanced respiratory insufficiency, hepatic failure, malignant hypertension, cerebrovascular insufficiency, and cancer; advanced age (70 years or more) was considered only an important risk factor. Preoperative angiography was carried out in only six cases; in the other patients it was decided not to add an adjunctive risk to vascular reconstruction.

Unilateral axillofemoral graft was performed in seven patients (Table 4), bilateral axillofemoral graft in three, femorofemoral bypass graft in two. An 8-mm Dacron prosthesis was used for grafting in all cases. When an extraperitoneal approach was preferred, the semiclosed thromboendarterectomy was the technique of choice in most of the cases. In 16 cases we performed an aortobifemoral bypass.

Table 3. Association of severe diseases (extra-anatomical group)

Association of five severe diseases	1 patient
Association of four severe diseases	9 patients
Association of three severe diseases	3 patients
Association of two severe diseases	3 patients

Results

Postoperative patency rate (Table 5) was high in both extra-anatomical and extraperitoneal groups (87.5% and 91.1%, respectively). Mortality rate was very low in the series of extraperitoneal operations: 2% compared to 12.5% in the extra-anatomical series. Cause of death was myocardial infarction in one case of iliac-femoral bypass graft, in one case of iliac-femoral thromboendarterectomy, and in one case of axillofemoral graft; one patient with an axillofemoral graft died of cirrhosis. The long-term patency rate, analyzed by the life-table method (Fig. 1), shows a decrease in the first 2 years from 87.5% to 65.6% after extra-anatomical reconstructions; this value does not change from the second to the third year. The percentage is higher in the extraperitoneal group both at the second and third year, with 88.3% and 78.7%, respectively.

Table 4. Surgical procedures

Extraperitoneal	
Bilateral aortofemoral bypass	16
Unilateral aortofemoral and iliac femoral bypass	18
Iliac-femoral thromboendarterectomy	67
Extra-anatomical	
Unilateral axillofemoral bypass	7
Bilateral axillofemoral bypass	3
Femorofemoral bypass	6

Table 5. Immediate results

	Good	Poor	Death
Extraperitoneal Group: 101	92 (91.1%)	[a]7 (6.9%)	[b]2 (2.0%)
Extra-anatomical Group: 16	14 (87.5%)	-	[c]2 (12.5%)

[a]Six amputations
[b]Myocardial infarction
[c]Myocardial infarction and cirrhosis

Table 6. Complications

	Extraperitoneal group	Extra-anatomical group
Infection	1 (0.9%)	2 (12.5%)
Early thrombosis	7 (6.9%)	2 (12.5%)
Late thrombosis	7 (6.9%)	2 (12.5%)
Hemorrhage	-	-
Upper extremity ischemia		-

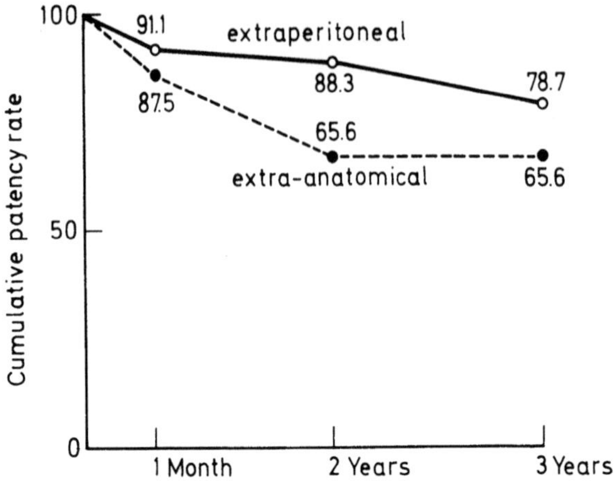

Fig. 1. Life-table method for extraperitoneal and extra-anatomical procedures

Infection (Table 6) occurred in two patients with subcutaneous grafts (12.5%); four patients who presented early and late thrombosis of axillofemoral grafts were successfully operated with simple thrombectomy. We have never observed upper extremity ischemia.

Discussion

In reviewing the results of the two series, we can attribute the difference in the mortality rate to a larger incidence of risk factors and above all to the association of more than two of them in the extra-anatomical group. The clinical stage at the time of surgery appears to be in direct relationship to late patency rate; in fact, in the extra-anatomical group the majority of patients presented rest pain and gangrene and were operated for impending limb loss, whereas in the extraperitoneal group claudication, although severe, was the indication for surgery in 80% of cases. In conclusion, extraperitoneal thromboendarterectomy and bypass can achieve, in our experience, a low mortality rate even when performed in high risk patients and appear to be the procedure of choice whenever possible. Extra-anatomical bypass grafts can obtain good results with regard to patient survival and limb salvage, but in our opinion they are only to be performed for impending limb loss in patients in whom the association of risk factors absolutely contraindicates an extraperitoneal approach.

References

1. Ayvazian VH, Auer AI, Hershey FB (1972) Limb salvage by extended femorofemoral bypass. Surg Gynecol Obstet 135:737-741
2. Blaisdell FW, Hall AD (1963) Axillo-femoral artery bypass for lower extremity ischemia. Surgery 54:563
3. De Laurentis DA, Sala LE, Russell E, McCombs PR (1978) A twelve years experience with axillofemoral and femorofemoral bypass operations. Surg Gynecol Obstet 147:881-887

4. Foley WF, Dow RW, Fry WJ (1969) Crossover femoro-femoral bypass grafts. Arch Surg 99:83-87
5. Johnson WC, Logerfo FW, Vollman RW, Corson ID, et al. (1977) Is axillo-bilateral femoral graft an effective substitute for aortic-bilateral iliac/femoral graft? Ann Surg 186:123-128
6. Moore WS, Hall AD, Blaisdell FW (1971) Late results of axillary-femoral bypass grafting. Am J Surg 122:148-154
7. Raithel D (1979) Late results after extra-anatomic bypass routes. J Cardiovasc Surg 20:487-492

Indications and Results of Femoro-femoral Bypass

R.C. de Sobregrau, E. Viver Manresa, J.M. Callejas, J.A. Gutierrez, and A. Martorell*

The femorofemoral bypass was proposed by Vetto in 1962 as an alternative treatment for isolated obliterations of unilateral iliac artery. The good results and the simplicity of the technique are the reasons why this operation is carried out in some patients with special conditions.

Since 1970, 115 femorofemoral bypasses have been performed for obliterations of the unilateral iliac artery: in 112 patients for arteriosclerosis and in three for traumatic lesions of the iliac artery. In 39 cases the saphenous vein was used and in 76 a Dacron graft.

The associated pathology and topography of the lesions and the risk factors are analysed. The system of exploration and the indications for femorofemoral bypass are discussed.

Good postoperative results have been achieved in 90.4% of the cases. The late results are shown and compared with the aorto- or iliofemoral unilateral bypass.

In conclusion the authors consider femorofemoral bypass an elective procedure in management of unilateral iliac artery obliteration in aged or high-risk patients and in some patients with previous abdominal operations.

*Ciudad Sanitaria de la Seguridad Social "Francisco Franco", Barcelona, Spain

The Femoro-femoral Cross-over-Bypass: An Alternative Treatment of Unilateral Artery Obstruction

H.F. Welter, E. Pratschke, F. Utz, K. Schäfer, H. Stiegler, and H.M. Becker*

The extra-anatomic, suprapubic femorofemoral crossover bypass was first described by McCaughan and Kahn in 1960 (6). Later on Vetto described 10 patients with unilateral iliac artery obstruction who were treated successfully by this method (12).

Material and Procedure

Between 1969 and June 1980, 160 femorofemoral bypass procedures were performed in 152 patients with a unilateral iliac artery obstruction and a poor general condition (Table 1). In 87.5% rest pain or gangrene necessitated this minor operation. The patients' ages ranged from the fourth to the ninth decade of life (Fig. 1).

A high mortality rate following other bypass procedures revealed the high risk of arteriosclerotic patients undergoing this crossover bypass procedure to prevent amputation of a limb. The poor risk of these patients is also proved by an analysis of life expectancy following the femorofemoral bypass procedure (Fig. 2).

Table 1. Risks of patients undergoing femorofemoral bypass procedures (n = 152)

Heart failure	69.8%
Diabetes and disorders of lipometabolism	34.2%
Arterial hypertension	28.4%
Impaired pulmonary function	20.1%
Obesity	11.9%
Other risks	2.2%

In 54% common and external iliac arteries were occluded, while in 18.7% the common iliac artery alone was occluded and in 9.9% only the external iliac artery. In 13% femorofemoral crossover bypass grafting was performed following unsuccessful endarterectomy of the iliac artery. The rare reasons for performing this procedure were occlusion following radiation and trauma (Table 2). In 65 patients (40.6%) additional obstructions of the femoral artery were observed on the obstructed side, whereas in 82 patients (51.3%) they were contralateral on the donor side.

*Department of Surgery, University of Munich, D-8000 Munich

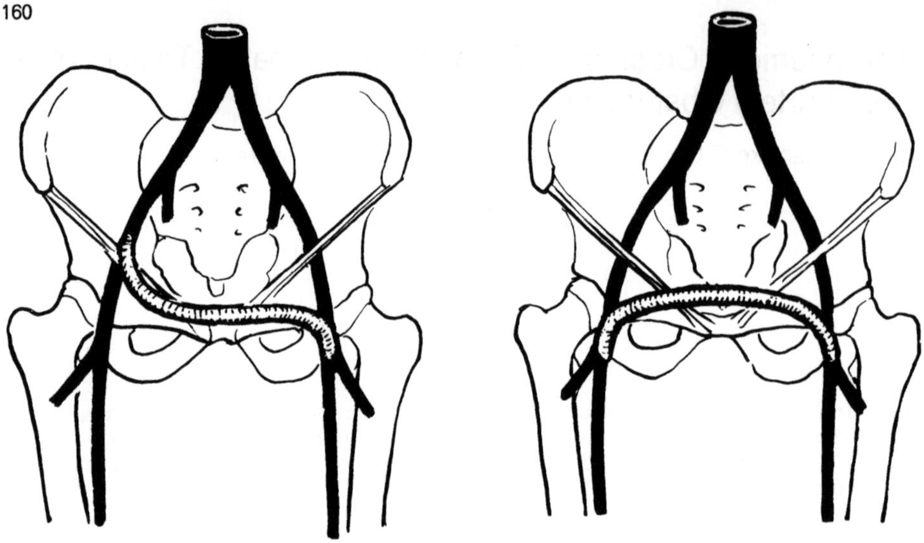

Favourable

Fig. 1. Different curves chosen in femorofemoral bypass procedures. The S-like curve on the left has been favoured since 1974. The femorofemoral crossover bypass on the right is grafted like a roman arch. This form was used prior to 1974

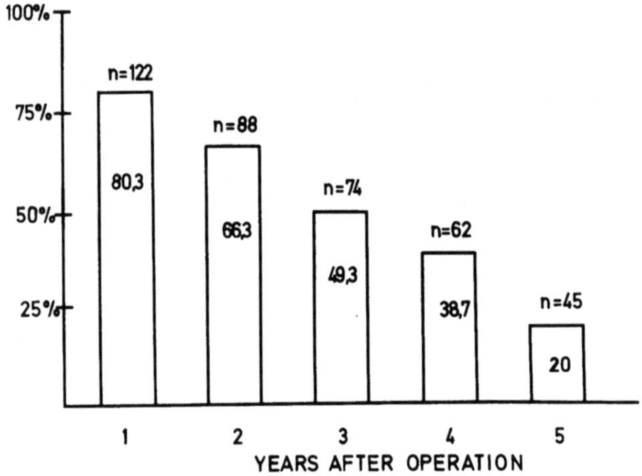

Fig. 2. Cumulative life-table method following femorofemoral bypass procedures. The poor risk of patients undergoing this operation is demonstrated by a high mortality rate

Operation Procedures

Operations were performed 39 times under local anesthesia and 121 times under general anesthesia. Dissection is first begun over the common femoral artery on the obstructed side. The prosthesis is anastomosed to this artery and must be pulled through a subcutaneous tunnel to the donor artery on the good side. While in the first years the preclotted

Table 2. Indications for femorofemoral crossover bypass procedures in poor risk patients (n = 152)

Indications	n	%
Obstruction of common and external iliac artery	87	54.0
Obstruction of common iliac artery	30	18.7
Obstruction of external iliac artery	16	9.9
Obstruction following iliac endarterectomy	21	13.0
Obstruction following radiation	3	1.9
Obstruction due to trauma	4	2.5

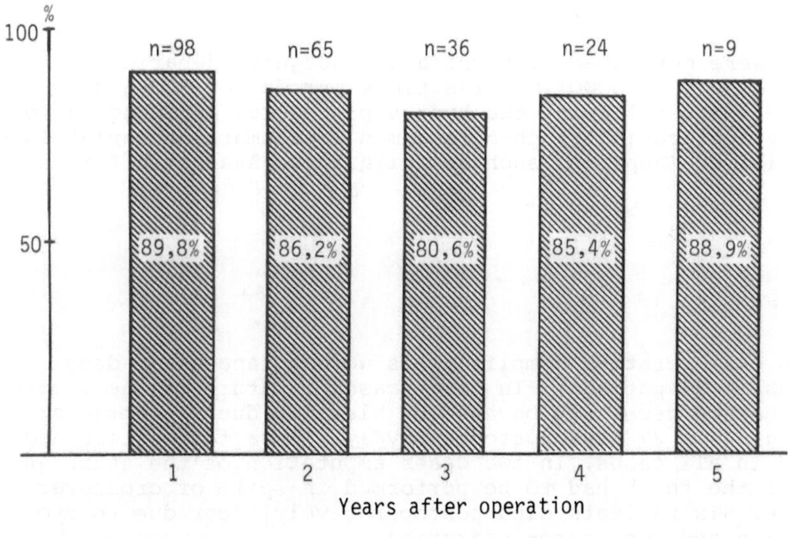

Fig. 3. Patency rates at time of annual follow-up examinations. In contrast to other studies, results are not summarized cumulatively; therefore patency rates showed an increasing tendency after the third year following grafting

prostheses were grafted from the donor to the obstructed side like a roman arch, since 1974 grafting has been performed in an S-like form as shown in Figure 3.

Anastomoses were sutured using a typical end-to-side technique. In the first period lightweight prostheses (Weavenit, n = 66, 41.2%) were employed. In the last four years Dacron double-velour prostheses 6 mm in diameter have been preferred (n = 67, 41.8%). To summarize, 133 Dacron prostheses were used during 83% of cases undergoing femorofemoral bypass surgery. Xenogeneic, allogeneic, and autologous materials did not yield any advantage when compared with the Dacron prostheses.

In 66 patients (41.2%) additional procedures were performed to improve inflow or outflow. The most frequent operation performed was the retrograde endarterectomia of the external iliac artery. On the other side 12 patch grafts were implanted at the junction of the obstructed profunda femoris artery and also 12 femoropopliteal grafts were implanted for improvement of arterial outflow (Table 3).

Table 3. Summary of necessary additional operations in femorofemoral bypass surgery (n = 152)

a) Improvement of arterial inflow	n
Retrograde endarterectomy of the external iliac artery	33
Open endarterectomy of the common iliac artery	4
Iliac-popliteal bypass procedures	9
Aortofemoral bypass procedures	5
b) Improvement of arterial outflow	
Endarterectomy of common femoral artery	8
Roof patch over the profunda femoris artery	12
Femoropopliteal bypass procedures	12

All patients were mobilised at night after surgery. Heparin was administered in a dosage of 5000 IU three times per day or 300-500 IU per hour over 3-5 days following the bypass procedure. Anticoagulation was continued by application of phenprocoumon (Marcumar) or a platelet-aggregation inhibitor (aspirin) such as Colfarit or Asasantin for example.

Results

The most common postoperative complications were cutaneous or deep wound infections in 24 patients. In three cases ligature of the femorofemoral bypass became necessary because of bleeding due to septic arrosion occurring 14 to 27 days postoperatively. The affected limb had to be amputated in all cases. In two cases amputation of the shank and in two others of the thigh had to be performed in spite of crossover bypass procedure. Six patients died postoperatively, four due to myocardial infarction and two to re-infarction.

In seven cases early occlusion of the bypass occurred, in two patients technical failures caused occlusion and in four cases thrombendarterectomia was successful. In two cases aortofemoral bypass procedures became necessary and were performed successfully.

Late Results

All patients who left the university hospital after successful bypass surgery were invited for an annual follow-up examination. Patients who did not come were examined by the family doctor, or facts regarding the patient were obtained from other hospitals or members of the family.

Patency rates following bypass procedure amounted to 89.8% after 1 year, to 80.6% after 3 years, and to 88.9% after 5 years (Fig. 4). An increasing rate after 3 years is due to differences in patient groups at the different times of examination. One patient was followed-up over 7 years until he died with a patent femorofemoral crossover bypass in 1979.

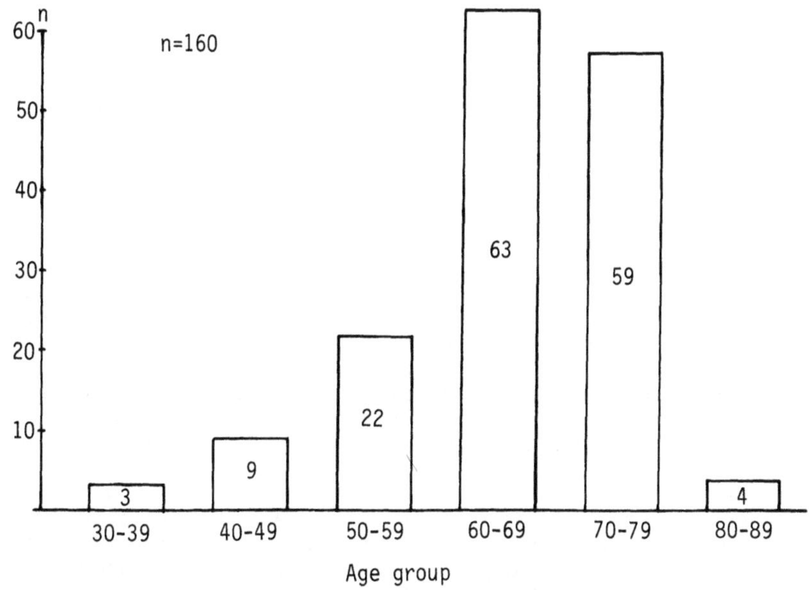

Fig. 4. Frequency of femorofemoral bypass procedures in the different decades of life. Most patients have been operated in the seventh and eighth decades

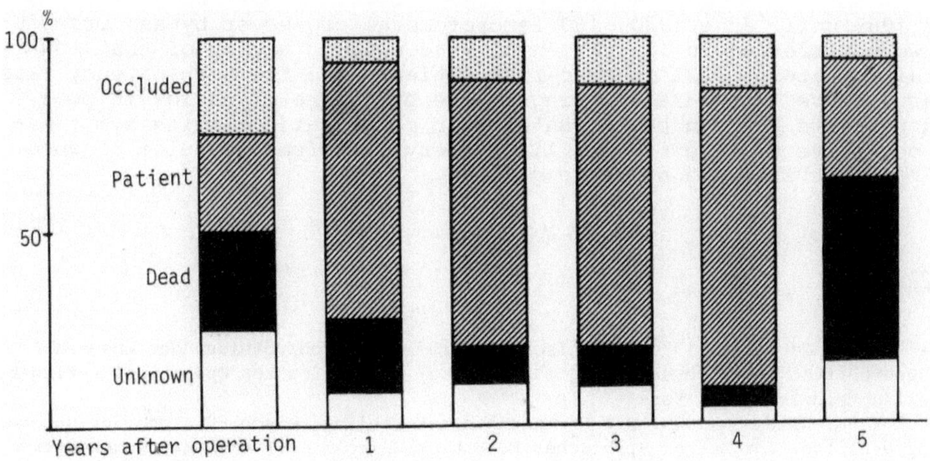

Fig. 5. Results of annual follow-up examinations. Occluded and patent grafts are summarized as well as dead patients and patients who for various reasons could not be examined

In Figure 5 patency and mortality rates after 1 to 5 years are summarized. In 84% patients were relieved from rest pain and gangrene and in 10% even claudication disappeared.

Discussion

Death following the operation amounted to 4.2% of all cases and became comparable with that observed following endartectomia of iliac arteries but remained lower than in other extra-anatomic bypass procedures which was about 7% (1, 2, 4). The 1-year patency rate is similar to that described in the literature (3, 5, 7, 9, 13) and is shown in Figure 3. The reported patency rate after 4-5 years is comparable to that following orthotopic bypass grafting and ranges from 73% to 93% (11).

Therefore femorofemoral bypass procedures can be performed not only in elderly, poor risk patients but also in younger patients with disabling aortoiliac occlusive disease. This procedure can be performed successfully if a) the arterial inflow is sufficient and b) the outflow along at least one femoral artery is also sufficient.

If there are additional obstructions at the junction of the profunda femoral artery re-establishment with a roof-patch graft should be performed. Peripheral occlusions should be treated by femoropopliteal procedures if possible.

Late occlusions of the graft were due to multiple peripheral obstructions on the side of the iliac obstruction. A steal syndrome of the better side could not be observed in any case (10). Until 1974 the proximal part of the bypass was implanted, as shown above, ascending; later the descending S-like arch was performed.

Summary

From 1969 until June 1980, 160 femorofemoral crossover bypass procedures were performed in 152 patients. We consider in view of that low mortality rate of 4.2% in poor risk patients and the high patency rate after 5 years that this grafting is the procedure of choice in poor risk patients but can be chosen also in other patients with symptomatic occlusive disease of one iliac artery if a femoral pulse of good quality exists in the opposite groin.

References

1. Becker HM, Jabour A (1974) Chronische arterielle Verschlußleiden der unteren Körperhälfte. In: Heberer G, Hegemann G (eds) Indikation zur Operation. Springer, Berlin Heidelberg New York
2. Becker HM, Witte J (1978) Die chronischen arteriellen Verschlußleiden der unteren Körperhälfte. In: Zenker R, Deucher F, Schink U (eds) Chirurgie der Gegenwart. Urban & Schwarzenberg, Munich Vienna Baltimore
3. Brief DK, Alpert J, Parsonnet V (1972) Cross-over femoro-femoral grafts. Compromise or preference: A reappraisal. Arch Surg 105:889
4. Levinson SA, Levinson HJ, Halloran LG (1973) Limited indications for unilateral aorto-femoral or ilico-femoral vascular grafts. Arch Surg 107:791
5. Mannick JA (1971) Are there practical alternatives to aorto-iliac reconstruction? Am J Surg 122:344
6. McCaughan JJ Jr, Kahn SF (1960) Cross-over graft for unilateral occlusive disease of the iliofemoral arteries. Ann Surg 151:26
7. Raithel D, Knecht H (1978) Spätergebnisse nach extraanatomischen Umleitungsverfahren in der Gefäßchirurgie. Chirurg 49:436
8. Salerno TA, Ayeni DR, Blundell PE, Chui RC (1978) Femoro-femoral bypass: a valuable procedure. Can J Surg 21:112

9. Sethi GK, Crawford FA, Scott SM, Takaro T (1975) Femoro-femoral bypass graft: Choice or compromise? Am Surg 41:61
10. Thiele H, Altstaedt F, Kersting KH (1978) Extraanatomische Umleitung beim aorto-iliacalen Verschluß. Chirurg 49:752
11. Utz F (1978) Früh- und Spätergebnisse beim alloplastischen Gefäßersatz. Medical-dissertation, University of Munich, p 97
12. Vetto RM (1962) The treatment of unilateral iliac artery obstruction with a transabdominal, subcutaneous, femoro-femoral graft. Surgery 52:342
13. Vetto RM (1966) The femoro-femoral shunt. An appraisal. Am J Surg 112:162

Acute Ischemia of the Upper Limb Following Extra-anatomical Bypass

J. Natali, P. Jue Denis, A. C. Benhamou, E. Kieffer, M. Maraval, and J. F. Tricot*

Since the first description of axillary-femoral artery bypass (AFB) published by Blaisdell and Hall in 1963 (1), numerous authors have described the indications and results of this method, as well as its complications. But acute ischemia of the upper limb following AFB or other extra-anatomic bypasses (EAB) have been rarely recorded (6, 7).

Between 1970 and 1980, nine complications of this type were observed; these complications are the subject of this paper.

Material and Method

Nine patients were operated on: seven men and two women, their ages averaging 61.2 years. Seven axillary-femoral bypasses were carried out because local or general contraindications existed for direct aorto-iliac surgery, in six cases for ischemia of the lower limb, and in one case for aneurysm of the abdominal aorta. One interaxillary bypass was built for ischemia of the upper limb, and one intersubclavian bypass for thrombosis of the innominate artery with certebro-basilar insufficiency.

Surgery Performed

Simple thrombectomy was successful in only one case. Thoracic sympathectomy was resorted to as a secondary measure because of residual claudication of the upper limb after efficacious medical treatment. In all other cases it was necessary to provide revascularisation, starting either from the controlateral axillary artery (two cases), from the homolateral subclavian artery (two cases), or from the endarterectomized trunk of the brachiocephalic artery (two cases), the distal anastomosis being applied on the lower axillary artery or the humeral artery. Dacron was used in five cases, Gore-tex in two cases.

Results

Three postoperative deaths were due to a severely deficient general condition (one myocardial infarct and two acute respiratory distresses). In one case the upper limb had to be amputated from the start because of irreversible ischemia. In all other cases the recuperation

*Service de chirurgie vasculaire. Centre hospitalo-universitaire Pitié-Salpêtrière, 47 boulevard de l'Hôpital 75651 Paris Cedex 13, France

of the upper limb was complete and persisted after 26 months, despite thrombosis of one bypass.

Discussion

Frequency

The frequency of acute ischemia of the upper limb in extra-anatomical bypass seems very low compared with the incidence of thrombosis and infarctus. Kerstein and Stansel (7), in 1974, reported the first case published in the literature after a right axillofemoral bypass, ending with amputation of the upper limb. In 1978, Kempezinski and Penn (6) reported another case which regressed partly under heparin therapy. In 1979, Lagneau et al. (9), for a series of 266 axillary-femoral artery bypasses, reported 11 cases including an amputation. In our own series of 200 axillary-femoral artery bypasses performed between 1970 and 1980 (11), we recorded seven cases of ischemia of the upper limb (3.5%), a frequency identical with that of false aneurysm.

Mechanism

Thrombosis or ligation of the proximal axillary artery is usually well tolerated due to the rich collateral circulation present especially in the periscapular circuit. Conversely, when the thrombosis proceeds downstream at the level of the axillofemoral junction, or when extensive atheromatous lesions are present, ischemia of the upper limb becomes a major risk.

In our series, two causes have been found responsible for this complication: extensive thrombosis of the extra-anatomical bypass in the axillohumeral arc (six cases), and ligation of the axillary artery (three cases). This had to be done twice to permit excision of a bypass, and once because of a technical problem (out of 13 axillary artery ligations following excision of a bypass, we record two cases of ischemia of the upper limb, i.e., 15%).

Treatment

Preventive treatment must consist in a better selection of the indications for bypass through as thorough as possible an appreciation of the condition of the giving artery (murmur, blood pressure of the upper limbs, Doppler) and also by a strict surgical technique (implantation on the lower part of the proximal axillary artery, suture without tension, and preservation of the maximum number of collaterals). When removing an EAB, it is preferable to close the arteriotomy over a patch rather than to ligate the giving artery.

Curative treatment is based essentially on cervical bypass. Conservative treatment is rarely possible, specially when the site of the initial operation is at some distance.

Our preference, therefore, is for homolateral cervical bypass – sometimes starting from the subclavian artery – but its course is sometimes difficult to follow and an internal cleidectomy may become necessary; in addition, the risk of injury to the phrenic artery is not to be disregarded. So we rather start from the homolateral common carotid artery which is easier to reach and allows a good tolerance of the bypass from the hemodynamic viewpoint, provided that both the common carotid and internal carotid arteries are free from atheromatous stenosis. The late patency rate of this bypass is excellent, the rates of morbidity and mortality are low (between 4.5% and 6%), and the neurological hazard is negligible.

Sometimes, when dealing with an urgent case, the surgeon ignorant of the state of carotid arteries is reluctant to do a clamping and prefers to resort to interaxillary bypass, a procedure which can be accomplished easily without endangering the cerebral circulation. As for thoracotomy, this should be exceptional and applied only when dealing with patients to whom direct surgery has been denied from the start.

Summary

Acute ischemia of the upper limb following EAB is not an exceptional complication (3.5% in our series of 200 AFB). With EAB, we risk a healthy limb to save an endangered one, a fact which must be taken in consideration when examining the indications for EAB which should be carried out only when direct surgery is impossible. Let us stress the interest of carotido-axillary and interaxillary bypasses in this type of complication.

References

1. Blaisdell FW, Hall AD (1963) Axillary femoral artery bypass for lower extremity ischemia. Surgery 54:563
2. Craxford S, De Bakey ME, Morris GC, Howell JF (1969) Surgical treatment of occlusion of the inomminate, common carotid and sub-clavian arteries. A ten years experience. Surgery 65:17-31
3. Dietrich E, Gerret ME, Ameriso J, Crawford ES, El Bayer M, De Bakey ME (1967) Occlusive disease of the common carotid and subclavian arteries treated by carotid subclavian bypass. Am J Surg 114:800-808
4. Johnson WC, Logerfo FW, Follman RW, et al. (1977) Is axillo-bilateral femoral graft an effective substitute for aortic-bilateral iliac femoral graft? Analysis of ten years experience. Ann Surg 186:123
5. Jausseran JM, Reggi MP, Courbier R (1976) Interêt du pontage carotido-humeral dans certaines revascularisations du membre supêrieur. Nouv Presse Mêd 38:2550
6. Kempezinski MD, Penn MD (1978) Upper extremity complications of axillo-femoral graft. Am J Surg 136:209-211
7. Kerstein MD, Stansel HC (1974) Ischemia and subsequent amputation of the upper extremity following axillo-femoral bypass. Angiology 25:305
8. Kieffer E, Laurian C, Surugue P, Natali J (1976) Pontage veineux fêmoro-fêmoral par le pêrinêe (6 observations). Chirurgie 102:420
9. Lagneau P, Bailly M, Cormier JM (1979) Les pontages axillo-femoraux dans les ischêmies aigües et subaigües des membres infêrieurs. J Mal Vasc (Paris) 4:15-17
10. Shumaker UB (1973) Carotid axillary bypass graft for occlusions of the proximal portion of the subclaviant artery. Surg Gynecol Obstet 136
11. Tricot JF, Kieffer E, Maraval M, Benhamou AC, Natali J (1978) Pontages axillo-femoraux, technique complications et rêsultats. J Chir (Paris) 115/6/7:329-336

Reconstructive Surgery of the Supraaortic Main Trunks: Extra-anatomic (-thoracic) Versus Transthoracic Procedures

H. Hamann, J. Vollmar, and K. Geissler*

Surgery for occlusive arterial diseases of the supraaortic branches is mainly concerned with the repair of carotid artery lesions at the level of the *carotid bifurcation*. From 1970 to 1979, only 77 of 534 patients, i.e. 14%, needed surgical repair for stenotic lesions of the supra-aortic *main trunks*.

Only patients with the involvement of all three supraaortic main trunks (brachiocephalic trunk, left common carotid artery, left subclavian artery) were considered as candidates for a *transthoracic approach*. In this group the patients showed neurological symptoms of carotid or vertebro-basilar insufficiency; two patients had ischemic symptoms of the upper extremities.

Via median sternotomy a *bypass procedure* from the aortic arch to the postocclusive supraaortic branches was the preferred surgical repair (1-4, 6, 8, 9, 14, 15, 17, 21; Fig. 1). Simultaneous interventions were necessary in four patients: endarterectomy of the internal carotid artery in two cases; retrograde ring desobliteration of the right subclavian artery in one, and open endarterectomy of the brachiocephalic trunk in another patient.

Postoperative *complications* occurred in five patients (Table 1): two grafts failed, one for early thrombosis and one following infection of a Dacron prosthesis. Two patients died 4 and 6 weeks postoperatively from myocardical infarction and from hemorrhage due to graft infection.

Table 1. Reconstructive surgery of the supraaortic main trunks

Transthoracic procedures (No. of patients = 14)	
Op. Morbidity = 36% (5 patients)	
Graft thrombosis	n = 1
Graft infection	n = 1
Pneumonia	n = 2
Sternal dehiscency	n = 1
Op. Mortality = 14% (2 patients)	
Myocardial infarction	n = 1
Graft infection (hemorrhage)	n = 1

All survivors have been followed-up 3 months up to 9 years postoperatively. The evaluation includes palpation and auscultation of the supraaortic branches, blood pressure measurements, and Doppler sono-

*Department of Surgery, University of Ulm (II), D-7900 Ulm

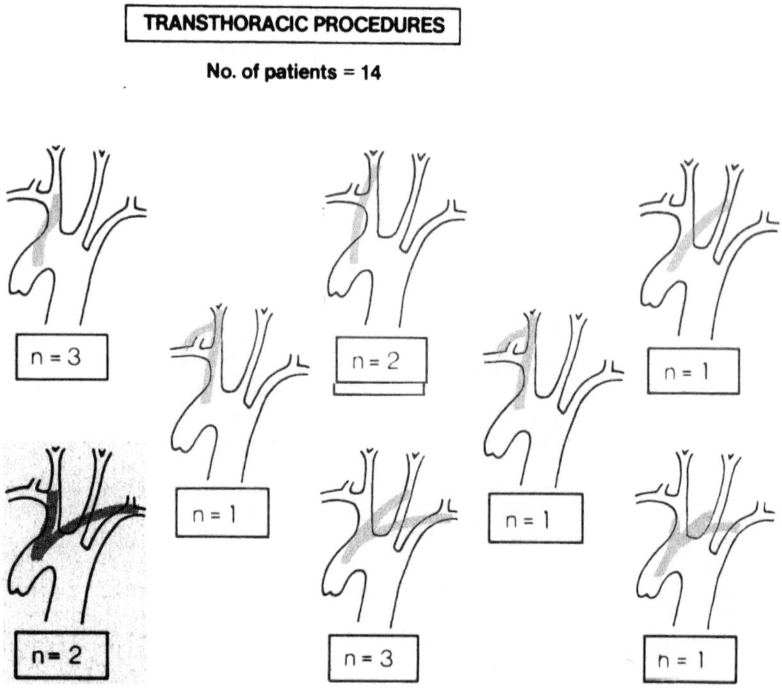

Fig. 1. Transthoracic bypass procedures in patients with occlusive lesions of the supraaortic main trunks

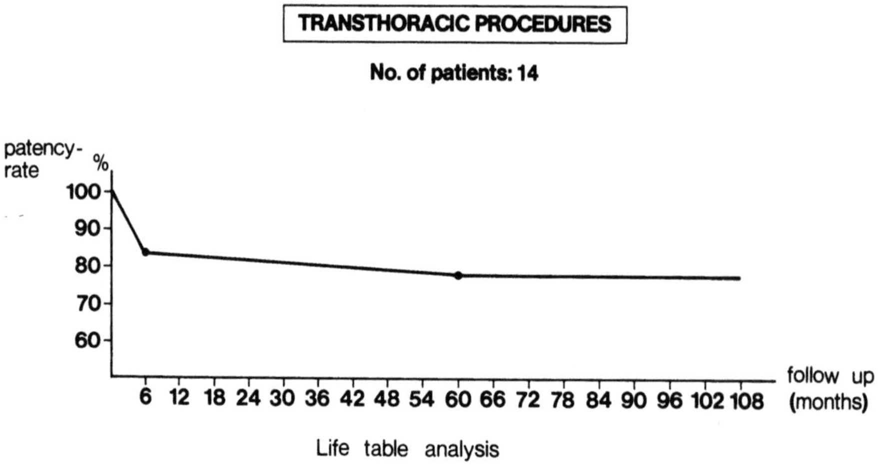

Fig. 2. Long-term results of transthoracic bypass repair: patency rate = 78%

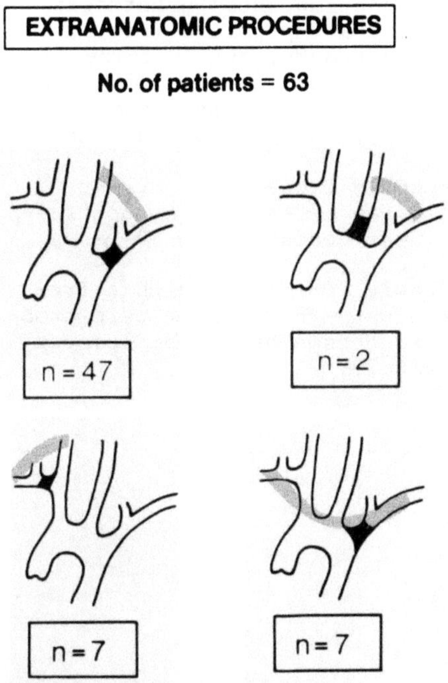

Fig. 3. Extraanatomic (-thoracic) bypass procedures in patients with occlusive lesions of the supraaortic main trunks

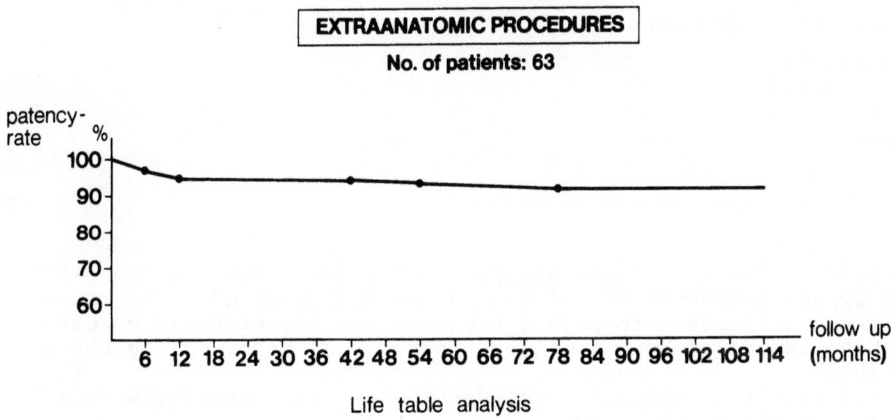

Fig. 4. Long-term results of extrathoracic bypass repair: patency rate = 92%

graphy. In the follow-up of 9 years, 78% of the implanted prostheses were still patent and 83% of the patients were asymptomatic (Fig. 2).

In patients with one (or more) patent main trunks, an *extrathoracic bypass procedure* was the favoured reconstructive approach. *Main indications* for surgery were complaints and signs of *vertebro-basilar insufficiency* due to a *subclavian steal syndrome* (5, 10, 13, 16, 19), in 7% combined with ischemia of the upper extremities.

The various techniques applied are listed in Figure 3. A bypass graft between the common carotid and subclavian arteries was most frequently used. Additional vascular repairs were necessary in 10 cases (Table 2).

There was *no postoperative death*; the operative *morbidity*, with a frequency of 8%, is listed in Table 3. Two early *graft thromboses* were probably due to technical faults. Two Dacron prostheses had to be removed for *late infections* 1 and 4 years postoperatively.

Table 2. Reconstructive surgery of the supraaortic main trunks

Extraanatomic procedures (No. of patients = 63)	
Simultaneous operations	
Thoracic sympathectomy	n = 5
Carotid endarterectomy	n = 3
Brachial embolectomy	n = 1

Table 3. Reconstructive surgery of the supraaortic main trunks

Extraanatomic procedures (No. of patients = 63)	
Op. morbidity = 8% (5 patients)	
Graft thrombosis	n = 2
Vocal cord paralysis	n = 1
Plexus brach. lesion	n = 1
Pneumonia	n = 1
Op. Mortality = 0%	

According to the life table analysis the patency rate of the extrathoracic bypasses amounts to 92% during the follow-up of 9 1/2 years (Fig. 4). All patients with patent bypasses are asymptomatic concerning cerebral insufficiency as well as ischemic symptoms of the upper extremities.

Compared with transthoracic procedures the *extraanatomic bypass repair* showed the following *advantages*:

1. Lower operative morbidity and mortality (7, 12, 18),
2. shorter operation time,
3. shorter hospitalisation.

Steal phenomena following carotid-subclavian bypasses could not be observed in the postoperative follow-up. The same is true for axilloaxillary crossover grafts, which is easily done especially in patients with infection of the supraclavicular area.

The small number of axilloaxillary grafts in our study (n = 7) does not allow a comparison with the carotid-subclavian bypass procedures (n = 56) as to comfortability, long-term patency rate, and operative morbidity. It should be considered, however, that an axilloaxillary bypass makes a median sternotomy difficult and should be avoided therefore in patients with coronary heart disease, who are potential candidates for an aortocoronary bypass (20).

Conclusions

1. The *extrathoracic bypass repair* includes convincing advantages, both in terms of operative mortality (0%) and of patency rate (92%) (11).
2. As a consequence, this type of extraanatomical repair for occlusive lesions of the supraaortic main trunks should no longer be restricted to poor risk patients or to special indications such as deep wound infections.
3. The favourable clinical results compared with those of the transthoracic approach justify its use as the *method of choice* also in good risk patients.

References

1. Berger RL, Sidd JJ, Ramaswamy K (1967) Retrograde vertebral-artery flow produced by correction of subclavian-steal-syndrome. N Engl J Med 227:64
2. Blakemore WS, Hardesty WH, Bevilacqua JA, Tristan TA (1965) Reversal blood flow in the right vertebral artery accompanying occlusion of the innominate artery. Ann Surg 161:353
3. Bryant LR, Spencer FC (1966) Occlusive disease of subclavian artery. JAMA 196:123
4. Cohen A, Manion WC, Spencer FC, Czarnecki SW, De Bakey ME (1962) Occlusive lesions of the great vessels of the aortic arch. Arch Surg 84:628
5. Contorni L (1960) Il circolo collaterale vertebro-vertebrale nella deliterazione dell'arteria succlavia alla sua origine. Minerva Chir 15:268
6. Craddock DR, Logan A (1966) The subclavian steal syndrome and its surgical management. Br J Surg 53:926
7. Crawford ES, De Bakey ME, Morris GC, Howell J (1969) Surgical treatment of the occlusion of the innominate, common carotid and subclavian arteries. A 10-year experience. Surgery 65:17
8. Daicoff GG, Lancaster JR, Ranniger K, Houlder PV (1965) Rational for aorta-subclavian artery bypass. J Thorac Cardiovasc Surg 49:945
9. Dumanian AU, Frahm CJ, Pascale LR, Teplinsky LL, Santschi DR (1965) The surgical treatment of the subclavian steal syndrome. J Thorac Cardiovasc Surg 50:22
10. Editorial (1961) A new vascular syndrome: The subclavian steal. N Engl J Med 265:912
11. Fields WS, Lemak NA (1972) Joint study of extracranial arterial occlusion. VII. Subclavian steal: A review of 168 cases. JAMA 222:1139
12. Hagmüller GW, Denck H (1977) Taktisches Vorgehen beim zentralen Subclaviaverschluß. Vasa 6:43
13. Harrison P (1829) The surgical anatomy of the arteries of the human body. In: Dublin, Hodges, and Smith (eds)
14. Javid HJ, Julian WS, Dye WS, Hunter JA (1965) Management of cerebral arterial insufficiency caused by reversal of flow. Arch Surg 90:634
15. Lee RH, Kieraldo JH, Jamplies RW (1967) Surgical treatment of the subclavian steal syndrome. Am J Surg 114:308
16. Liston RL (1838) Aneurysm of the right subclavian artery (ligature of the subclavian and carotid arteries). Lancet 2:668
17. Müller JHA, Münster W (1967) "Seitenumkehr eines Subclavian-Steal-Effect" nach Gefäßrekonstruktion bei Truncusobliteration. ROEFO 107:284
18. Raithel D (1979) Late results after extra-anatomic bypass routes. J Cardiovasc Surg 20:487

19. Smyth AW (1866) Successful operation in a case of subclavian aneurysm. New Orleans Med Rec 1:4
20. Thompson BW, Read RC, Campbell GS (1980) Operative correction of proximal blocks of the subclavian or innominate arteries. J Cardiovasc Surg 21:125
21. Vollmar J, Elbayar M, Kolmar D, Pfleiderer T, Diezel PB (1965) Zerebrale Durchblutungsinsuffizienz bei Verschlußprozessen der A. subclavia (subclavian steal effect) Dtsch Med Wochenschr 90:8

Our Experiences With Extra-anatomical Bypass Operations in the Supraaortic Area

J.D. Gruß, D. Bartels, E. Tsafandakis, H. Straubel, and T. Ohta*

Introduction

While extraanatomic bypass operations are the exception for the reconstruction of aortoiliac arteries, for instance if there are cumulative serious risks, an infection or a distinct X-ray damage in the inguinal region, or if the patient has an anus praeter, extraanatomic bypass operations on the supraaortal field can be considered as routine operations today. A summary of literature has shown that, within the past 10 years, still more than 50% of all occlusions of the large supraaortic main branches were directly, i.e. transthoracically, corrected. Today, there is an evident tendency for the extrathoracic, i.e. extraanatomic, procedure in all vascular surgery centres (2, 3). The operation lethality in case of the axillofemoral bypass is indicated as 7% in the literature (4, 6); for the extraanatomic bypass operations in the supraaortic area it amounts to 0.7%. The low mortality and morbidity rate as well as the relatively positive treatment results encouraged us to extend the indication for an extraanatomic procedure in case of occlusions of the brachiocephalic trunk of the common carotid arteries and the subclavian arteries more and more, and also to include younger patients in this treatment.

Material and Methods

From July 1, 1971, to January 31, 1980, among 4751 vascular-surgical operations 96 extraanatomic bypasses were made in our department. Fifty-nine of these 96 operations were in the supraaortic area; 37 operations were necessary for the revascularization of ischemic lower extremities. Forty-seven of our 59 patients were male, 12 female. The average age was 65 years (6). Ten of the 59 patients showed only cerebral symptoms of stage II or IIIa, 17 only brachial symptoms of stage II to IV, and 32 a combined cerebrobrachial symptomatic. Angiographically or pathological-anatomically we found 47 occlusions of a subclavian artery, 7 occlusions of the brachiocephalic trunk, and 5 occlusions of a common carotid artery.

In 31 cases carotido-subclavian bypasses or subclavio-carotideal bypasses were accomplished, in 5 cases the reconstruction was made by carotido-carotideal bypass, in 23 cases a subclavio-subclavian bypass was done.

*Kurhessisches Diakonissenhaus, D-3500 Kassel

Indication for Operation and Technique

As we had transient ischemia attacks in two cases after carotido-subclavian bypasses and this because of advanced stenoses of the internal carotid artery, today we prefer the subclavio-subclavian bypass to the carotido-subclavian bypass. Still, most of the occlusions in the supra-aortic area are located at the carotid bifurcation, so it is probable that later there will be alterations in case of a patent carotido-subclavian bypass. In the vast majority of cases, the indication for operation was based on cerebrovascular complications in stage II, in a few cases in stage IIIa. The brachial symptomatic varied from claudication to rest pain to digital necroses. There are no asymptomatic patients and prophylactic operations in this group. All 47 patients with subclavian occlusions showed the typical signs of a subclavian steal syndrome. Here no patients are listed who had direct reconstructive operations, for instance a thrombendarterectomy or subclavian reimplantations. Of course, we also left out the patients who were directly corrected, that is transthoracically. Usually, the subclavio-carotideal bypasses were done from a supraclavicular approach.

Reconstructive Procedures	Extra-anatomic Bypasses		
4751	96	supra-aortic	59
		aortoiliac	37

(July 1, 1971 - January 31, 1980)

Fig. 1

59 patients	47 male	
	12 female	

The average age: 65 years

(July 1, 1971 - January 31, 1980)

Fig. 2

No. of patients	Symptoms: only cerebral	only brachial	combined
59	10	17	32

(July 1, 1971 - January 31, 1980)

Fig. 3. Symptoms of 59 patients with extra-anatomic supra-aortic reconstructions

1.	Tr. brachiocephalicus	7
2.	A. subclavia	47
3.	A. carotis communis	5

(July 1, 1971 - January 31, 1980)

Fig. 4. Localization of the occlusions in 59 patients with extra-anatomic supra-aortic reconstructions

A. carotis com.	⇄	a. subclavia:	31
A. carotis com.	→	a. carotis com.:	5
A. subclavia	→	a. subclavia:	23
(July 1, 1971 - January 31, 1980)			

Fig. 5. Type of extra-anatomic bypass procedures in 59 patients with supra-aortic lesions

No. of patients	⊞ early	⊞ late
59	1	8
(July 1, 1971 - January 31, 1980)		

Fig. 6. Mortality of 59 patients with supra-aortic extra-anatomic bypass procedures

No. of patients	permeable	occluded		
50	44	6	1	subclavio-subclavian
			1	carotido-carotideal
			4	carotido-subclavian
(July 1, 1971 - January 31, 1980)				

Fig. 7. Results of 50 extra-anatomic supra-aortic bypass procedures

For the subclavio-subclavian bypass we use two symmetric infraclavicular incisions. The subclavian artery is dissected after stump separation of the clavicular part from the sternal part of the major pectoral muscle, at the medial edge of the small pectoral muscle. The anastomosis of the transplant is done obliquely end-to-side on both sides. Either 8-mm double velour Dacron grafts or PTFE prostheses are used as transplant material.

Results

One of our 59 patients died of a myocardial infarction during the first postoperative days. Eight other patients died within the follow-up period; however, the exact causes of death are unknown. We also do not know if the transplants were still intact until death. So we can report about 50 patients who had extraanatomic bypass operations in the supra-aortic area. Forty-four of them are postoperatively still in function 6 months to 8 years after the operation. Six transplants are occluded; this applies to one carotido-carotideal and to one subclavio-subclavian bypass each, and to four carotido-subclavian bypasses. The carotido-carotideal transplant had to be removed because of a bilateral infection of the prosthesis. Both carotid arteries were closed by direct sutures. The neurological symptomatic remained constant. Two anastomotic stenoses after subclavio-subclavian bypasses ought to be mentioned. Both stenoses were noticed due to a reoccurred brachial symptomatic and an increasing blood pressure difference. In the meantime, these two stenoses could be corrected by patch plastic.

Discussion

Extraanatomic bypass operations in the supraaortic area are routine operations with a relatively comprehensive indication. This is also verified by the survival rate in comparison to the axillofemoral bypass. While the 5-year survival rate of 87% (according to a summary of literature) after extraanatomic correction in the supraaortic area is strikingly high, 50% of the patients died within 2 years after an axillofemoral bypass. Compared with this, the survival rate after thrombendarterectomy of the internal carotid artery amounts to 66%. The treatment results after extraanatomic bypass operations can be called "good". Among our own patients, 44 of 50 transplants, that is 88%, are still patent 6 months to 8 years postoperatively. Similar reports are given by Denck (1), who stated 81% of hemodynamically and clinically good results after extraanatomic corrections compared with 62% of good results of direct transthoracical corrections. In comparison to this, the results of the axillofemoral bypass are unfavourable; so Janisch (4) reports about 13% of reocclusions within the first 6 months, and Krüger (5) found a permeability rate of 56.5% after 2 years in a review of literature. The operation lethality during extraanatomic reconstructive operations in the supraaortic area amounts to 4%-6% according to Raithel (8). We ourselves had one case of death in our 59 patients. Compared with this, Denck (1) speaks of an operation lethality of 16% for the transthoracic procedure. The same author does not report any case of death for his extraanatomic corrections. We never noticed a steal symptomatic after a subclavio-subclavian bypass and we never found any information about this in the literature, either (7). As shown by our own summary of literature, the rate of nonlethal general, local, and cerebral complications of 13.4% for the transthoracic procedure is clearly higher than the rate of 1.4% for extraanatomic bypasses (2, 3).

References

1. Denck H (1975) Rekonstruktive Arterienchirurgie an den extrakraniellen Hirnschlagadern bei zerebraler Mangeldurchblutung. Zentralbl Chir 100:1281-1297
2. Gruss JD, Stojanovic R, Kuhn H (1976) Extraanatomische Umleitungsoperationen in der rekonstruktiven Gefäßchirurgie. MMW 118/47:1527-1532
3. Gruss JD, Karadedos C, Kawai S (1978) Long-term results after surgical treatment of the subclavian-steal-syndrome. A report of 931 cases. 27th International Congress of the European Society of Cardio-Vascular Surgery, Lyon, June 28 - July 1, 1978
4. Janisch K, Bürger K, Hübner R (1974) Spätergebnisse nach axillo-femoralem Bypass. Zentralbl Chir 99:78-81
5. Krüger BJ, Stockmann U, Witte C (1971) Der axillo-femorale Bypass; ein therapeutisches Verfahren bei Risikopatienten mit chronischer Verschlußkrankheit der Arterien im Beckenabschnitt. Thoraxchirurgie 19:493
6. Mannick JA, Williams LE, Nabseth DC (1970) The late results of axillofemoral grafts. Surgery 68:1038-1043
7. Mozersky DJ, Sumner DS, Barnes RW, Callaway GP, Strandness DE Jr (1972) The hemodynamics of the axillary-axillary bypass. Surg Gynecol Obstet 135:925-929
8. Raithel D (1975) Extraanatomische Umleitungsverfahren in der rekonstruktiven Arterienchirurgie. Klinikarzt 4/8:319-323

Two-stage Procedures in Cerebrovascular Insufficiency: Combination of Carotid Endarterectomy and Externa-interna Bypass

M. Deutsch, J. Kaliman, G. Kletter, H. Schuster, and E. Valencak*

Combined occlusive disease of the extra- and intracranial portion of the brain vessels represents a special pattern of atherosclerotic cerebrovascular insufficiency (CVI).

Material and Method

At the Neurosurgical and Second Surgical Clinic at Vienna University Medical School, since 1975 600 reconstructive procedures for treatment of CVI have been performed; 274 desobliterations of the carotid bifurcation, 51 kinks and loops, and 26 lesions of arch vessels were corrected. The overall mortality of this extracranial diseased group is 2.5%, the incidence of permanent neurologic deficits 0.9%. Two hundred and forty-six extraintracranial anastomoses (EIA) have been performed with a hospital mortality of 3.5%.

Twenty-five of our patients presented a correctible extra- and intracranial lesion; the hospital mortality of this group was 8%. Among this group diabetes and arterial hypertension have been observed in 76% and 80%, respectively. Transient ischemic attacks (TIAs) were present in seven patients, PRIND and progressive stroke (PS) were each seen once, and the clinical picture of a completed stroke (CS) was observed in 16 patients; four of them had additional TIAs.

Sixteen patients had an occluded internal carotid artery and a contralateral stenosis, two patients had a stenosis of the carotid artery at its bifurcation and an ipsilateral stenosis or occlusion of the middle cerebral artery. Two patients had a stenosis at the carotid syphon and a stenosed carotid artery. Three patients underwent correction of a kinking and demonstrated a contralateral occluded internal carotid artery. In two cases of internal carotid artery occlusion the additionally stenosed external carotid artery was endarterectomized.

Technical Remarks

The technical details of the externa-interna anastomosis have been described extensively (2). As far as the carotid endarterectomy is concerned, all operations have been performed under conditions of general anesthesia. Cerebral protection is maintained by using an indwelling shunt in any case. The arteriotomy is closed performing a patch angioplasty (1).

---

*Department of Neurosurgery and the 2nd Surgical Service of the University Medical School, Vienna, Austria

Results

Among the 22 patients in whom the extracranial repair was performed first, 16 (72%) were clinically improved, five remained unchanged (22%) and one patient died (4.5%). In the small group of three patients who underwent first the EIA procedure and later on had a desobliteration of the carotid artery, two were improved and one died (Table 1).

Table 1. Results of extracranial repair

	Improved	Unchanged	Died
Desobliteration of carotid bifurcation and externa-interna anastomosis			
TIA (6)	5	1	0
PRIND (1)	1	-	-
Progressive stroke (1)	1	-	-
Completed stroke (14)	9	4	1
Externa-interna anastomosis and desobliteration of carotid bifurcation			
TIA (1)	-	-	1
Completed stroke (2)	2	-	-
Total	18	5	2

Discussion

It is our policy to correct first the stenosed extracranial portion, and the EIA is performed in a second procedure if necessary. This sequence has been observed in 22 of our 25 patients. The reverse situation was characterized by a late – at least 6 months after the EIA – appearance of the carotid stenosis, because the patient developed symptoms related to the contralateral hemisphere.

Nevertheless, in the case of concommittant extra- and intracranial lesions it is still a matter of discussion which step should be done first. A few centers in the USA and Europe are doing the EIA routinely as a first procedure. The strongest argument for this timing is that in case of an extracranial carotid stenosis the preexisting EIA would represent a certain degree of cerebral protection of the more threatened hemisphere during the clamping time of the internal carotid artery. This argument is somewhat acceptable if one realizes the impressive enlargement of the diameter of the external carotid artery branch. Otherwise, this rapid adaptation of the externa flow represents a distinct threat to the contralateral stenosed and extracranial internal carotid artery. Due to the changes in flow pattern an acceleration of the occluding tendency of the diseased internal carotid artery may be observed.

We do believe that an EIA done dirst offers a certain amount of cerebral protection, but mostly it cannot replace functionally a rapidly occluding internal carotid artery. A certainly more striking argument for the priority of the extracranial reconstruction is that this procedure may be efficient enough to cure the patient and no further revascularization of the brain may be necessary.

Summary

Twenty-five patients underwent an extra-and intracranial revascularization procedure. Eighteen (72%) patients were improved, five (20%) remained unchanged, and 2 (8%) died. The priority of the extracranial repair is our treatment of choice.

References

1. Deutsch M, Kaliman J, Valencak E (1979) Zur Chirurgie der extrakraniellen Karotisverschlußprozesse. Wien Klin Wochenschr 91:421
2. Kletter G (1979) The extra-intracranial bypass operation for prevention and treatment of stroke. Springer, Vienna New York

Surgical Management of Takayasu-Onishi-arteritis

A. Thevenet

Aortitis syndromes have recently emerged from the confusing disease known as Takayasu's arteritis - pulseless disease, aortic arch syndrome, atypical coarctation, and numerous other names. The first description was made by Savory in 1856 but the disease is associated with Takayasu who in 1908 presented the ocular manifestations and Onishi who, in a discussion of the presentation, mentioned absent brachial pulses. The disease is a nonspecific, inflammatory panarteritis of unknown etiology involving aortic arch, thoracic, or abdominal aorta with segmental occlusion of the major arterial branches.

Three anatomical types have been described: Type I involving the branches of the aortic arch corresponds to pulseless disease with brachiocephalic ischemia. Type II is characterized by stenosis or coarctation of the thoracoabdominal aorta with frequent involvement of the visceral arteries, namely the renal artery. Its clinical manifestation is hypertension. Type III combines the Type I and II with extensive occlusive changes on both segments and manifestations of brachiocerebral insufficiency concurrently with hypertension. A Type IV has been added which may include any other types in addition to the pulmonary artery. Furthermore, coronary artery involvement as well as cardiac has been noted with aortic incompetence.

Different features of vascular lesions are observed: constriction, dilatation, aneurysm, irregularity, total occlusion, and any combination to the above. The stenotic variant is most commonly seen. The multiple and extensive character of certain lesions constitutes a challenge in the surgical management.

The purpose of this paper is to present a personal series of 26 cases, to emphasize the multiple aspects, and to point out the surgical character of the disease.

Clinical Material

Between 1967 and 1979, 26 patients with Takayasu-Onishi arteritis were observed. Twenty-four were submitted to surgery, two of them underwent a second operation at intervals of 4 to 6 years due to progress of the disease, and two others were operated in two stages of different location.

The types of arterial involvement are as follows: Type I comprises 11 patients (42%), Type II 7 (27%), and Type III 8 (31%). No Type IV has been observed.

Age and sex distribution is presented in Table 1. Women were affected in 58% in this series and males in 42%. The disease is seen in

*Hôpital Aiguelongue - C.H.U., 34059 Montpellier Cedex, France

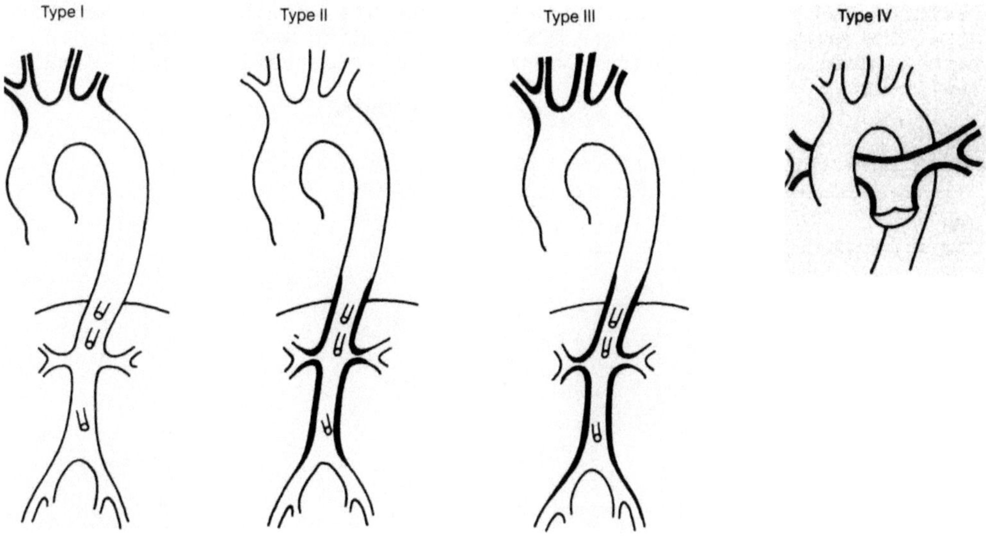

Fig. 1. Anatomical types of Takayasu-Onishi arteritis

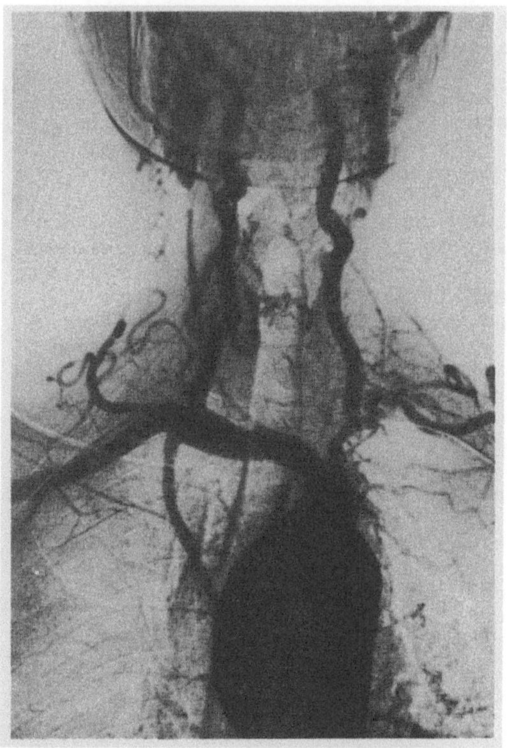

Fig. 2. Aortic arch involvement of a Type III disease: occlusion of right and left common carotid and left subclavian arteries

children and young adults, and 50% of patients were below 30 years of age. The youngest was 5 years old and the oldest was 58 years old, with a mean age of 29 years, lower in males (22 years) than in females (34 years).

Table 1. Age and sex distribution (n = 26)

Age	M	F	
0-10	2	-	2
10-19	2	2	4
20-29	3	4	7
30-39	3	3	6
40-49	1	5	6
50-59	-	1	1
Total	11	15	26
(mean)	(22)	(34)	(29)
	5-44	16-58	5-58

Seventeen patiénts presented with brachiocephalic insufficiency, ten had hypertension, four were admitted with lower limb insufficiency, 20 had weak or absent pulses, in 23, arterial bruits were heard at various sites, cervical or/and abdominal, and seven evidenced a subclavian steal syndrome. Chief complaints related to cerebrovascular impairment were headache, dizziness, vertigo, visual disturbances, syncopal attacks, and hemiplegia. Two patients experienced claudication of masticatory musculature.

Complete aortography is essential to confirm the diagnosis and to outline the type and extent of the lesion as well as the involvement of different branches. The frequency of involvement of the vessels in brachiocephalic arteritis (Types I and II) affecting 19 patients is shown in Table 2. Subclavian arteries were the most commonly affected ones, principally on the left side, followed by vertebrals and carotids. Lesions were isolated in nine patients, bilateral in three, and multiple involving three or more vessels in six. A subclavian steal syndrome was observed in seven patients.

Involvement of the visceral branches of the abdominal aorta, seen in Types II and III (15 patients), is demonstrated in Table 3. The renal arteries were the most frequently affected, 18 times in ten patients, and the superior mesenteric artery in seven patients. Extensive process involved the iliac arteries in six patients.

The pathologic features are those of a panarteritis varying from disruption of elastic fibers to complete loss of normal architecture with inflammatory reaction or replacement by scar. The histologic pattern found in our surgical specimens, according to Nasu's classification, is shown in Table 4. Each lesion mostly consists of a combination of features with a predominance of fibrous thickening of adven--titia, proliferation of vasavasorum into the media and intima, inflammatory cell infiltration, presence of giant cells, disruption of elastic fibers, and replacement by scar tissue into the medioadventitial layers. The stage of the disease may be speculated from the histologic pattern of giant cell granuloma to diffuse proliferative inflammation and fibrous in active lesion. Atheromatous changes and calcifications can be seen in old lesions.

Table 2. Aortic arch branches. Types I-III (n = 19)

Innominate		2
Carotids	right	7
	left	6
Subclavian	right	9
	left	17
Vertebrals		9

Table 3. Abdominal aorta and branches. Types II-III (n = 15)

Renal	18
Sup. mesenteric	7
Celiac	1
Inf. mesenteric	3
Iliac	12

Table 4. Histological pattern (NASU classification)

Type 1 = granulomatous	3
Type 2 = inflammatory infiltration	8
Type 3 = fibrous	13

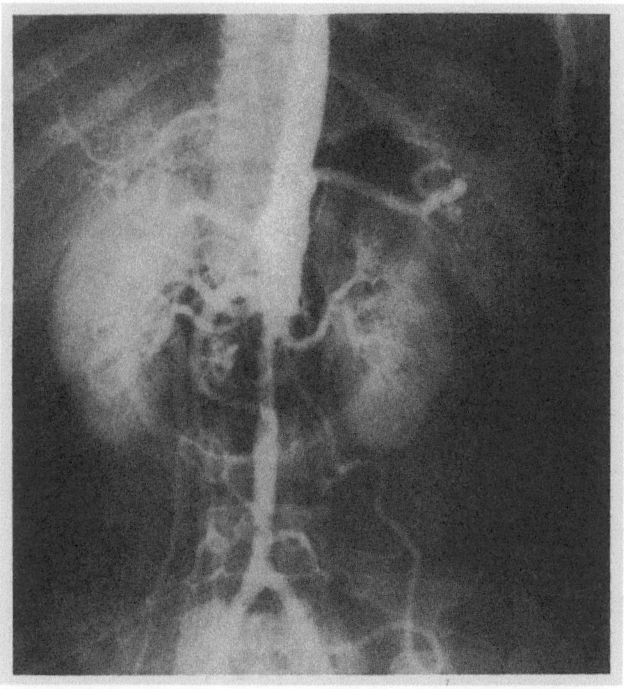

Fig. 3. Abdominal aorta stenosis with hypertension in Type III disease

Surgical revascularization procedures were attempted 28 times in 24 patients. Two patients were operated in two stages of different localizations (Type III). In two cases a second operation was undergone at interval of 4 to 6 years due to progress of the disease (Type I). In multiple involvement of the same type, simultaneous complete corrections of several vessels were performed in one stage. Brachiocephalic reconstructions for Type I and III affected 35 arteries in 19 patients (11 Type I, 8 Type III).

In *isolated lesions* of the subclavian or subclavian-axillary arteries (11 unilateral, 2 bilateral), a cervical approach was used and the different procedures utilized are listed in Table 5. Bypass and grafts were the most commonly used, with saphenous vein in 8, Dacron in 1, and Goretex in 1.

Table 5. Brachiocephalic reconstructions. Isolated lesions (n = 13)

Cervical approach	
Biopsy + Thor. Sympathect.	2
Endarterectomy	3
Carotid-brachial bypass	3
Subclavian-brachial bypass	3
Subclavian graft	2
Carotid-subclavian bypass	2

In *multiple lesions* (Table 6), transsternal revascularization of 20 arteries was performed in six patients. Prosthetic bypass grafting from the ascending aorta to both carotid bifurcation was associated to bypass to subclavian and/or brachial arteries. In addition, a segmental vertebro-subclavian endarterectomy was used in five cases.

Table 6. Brachiocephalic reconstructions. Multiple lesions (n = 6)

Transsternal revascularization	
Aortobicarotid bypass	3
Aortobicarotid-subclavian bypass	3
Associated procedures	
Vertebrosubclavian endart.	5
Carotid-brachial bypass	2
Subclavian brachial bypass	1

Operations on abdominal aorta and its branches (Table 7) were performed in nine patients (seven Type II, two Type III). Aortic reconstruction consisted of endarterectomy (1 case), aortoplasty (2 cases) resection and graft (3 cases), and bypass graft (3 cases). Additional repair of the renal and visceral arteries used identical procedures. Secondary nephrectomy was necessary in one patient due to late thrombosis of a renal artery.

Table 7. Operations on abdominal aorta and branches (n = 9)

Aortic repair	endart	1
	aortoplasty	2
	resection-graft	3
	bypass	3
Renal repair	endart.	3
	reimplant.	4
	graft	4
Nephrectomy		1
Mesenteric repair	endart.	1
	reimplant.	2
	patch graft	2

Results

The *results* are shown in Table 8. One hospital death has been observed in a 22-year-old man due to neurologic coma following an aortobicarotid bypass for an extreme form of occlusion of all the brachiocephalic trunks. This patient had been previously operated upon 6 years before after a hemiplegic attack with a segmental innominate obstruction. Such an extensive involvement is a contraindication to attempt revascularization.

Table 8. Results

Type	I	II	III	Total
Nb patients	11	7	6	24
Hospital mortality	1	0	0	1
Arterial patency	9	6	6	21
Asymptomatic	9	5	5	19
Late death	1	0	0	1
Follow-up (years)	1-15	5-10	1-6	1-15
	(8)	(6)	(3)	(6)

Patients were followed from 1 to 15 years with an average of 6 years. Only one late death not related to the disease (suicide) was noted. Arterial patency, demonstrated by angiographic control, blood pressure, pulses, or Doppler effect, was maintained in 21 patients. Nineteen patients are asymptomatic at an average of 8 years for group I, 6 years for group II, and 3 years for group III.

A second patient has shown in a 4-year period a progressive involvement from a left subclavian-axillary occlusion treated by carotidobrachial bypass to a four-vessel obstruction managed with aortocarotid-subclavian bypass. Patency is maintained at 1 year.

Three patients (two group II, one group III) have persistent hypertension necessitating medical treatment.

Conclusions

1. Takayasu-Onishi arteritis may involve any part of the aorta from the aortic valves down to the iliac arteries as well as any major branches.
2. Total aortography is essential to confirm the diagnosis and to outline the type and extent of the lesion.
3. Two syndromes – brachiocephalic insufficiency and hypertension – are the most frequent indications for surgical treatment.
4. Bypass grafting is the treatment of choice in multiple and extensive lesions. Endarterectomy with or without angioplasty is a useful technique in localized lesions at the sclerotic stage of the disease, or associated with bypass.
5. Clinical and anatomical results are satisfactory with a mean follow-up of 8 years.

References

1. Labauge R, Thevenet A, Tannier C, Rachdi M (1977) Etude évolutive d'un cas de maladie de Takayasu. Oto-Neuro-Opht 49:327-332
2. Nasu T (1963) Pathology of pulseless disease. A systematic study and critical review of twenty-one autopsy cases reported in Japan. Angiology 14:225
3. Onishi (1908) Discussion. Acta Soc Opht Jap 12:554
4. Pokrovsky AV, Tsireshkin DM (1975) Non specific aorto-arteritis. J Cardiovasc Surg 16:181
5. Savory WS (1856) Case of a young woman in whom the main arteries of both upper extremities and of the left side of the neck were throughout completely obliterated. Med Chir Trans 39:205
6. Sen PK (1973) Non specific aorto-arteritis. A monograph based on a study of 101 cases. McGraw Hill, Bombay New Delhi
7. Takayasu M (1908) A case with unusual changes of the central vessels in the retina. Acta Soc Opht Jap 12:554
8. Thevenet A, Mary H, Boennec M, Benhamou A (1978) Coarctations et dysplasies de l'aorte abdominale. A propos de 9 observations. Ann Chir Thorac Cardiovasc 17:187-196

Session III Cardiac Surgery

Tachycardiac Rhythm Disorders Coronary Disease

Chairman: C. Hahn, Geneva; Co-Chairman: H.H. Bentall, London

Surgical Treatment of Wolff-Parkinson-White Syndrome

G. Guiraudon, R. Frank, G. Fontaine, P. Coumel, R. Slama, Y. Grosgogeat, and C. Cabrol*

Since 1972, 32 patients with Wolff-Parkinson-White syndrome (WPW) have been treated surgically. Nine patients presented with valvular lesions associated with WPW. Malignant ventricular arrhythmia secondary to atrial fibrillation (AF) was present in 14, and reciprocating supraventricular tachycardia in 18.

Preoperative electrophysiological studies demonstrated in all cases the responsibility of Kent's bundle in the genesis of arrhythmia.

At surgery, the location of Kent's bundle was determined by anterograde ventricular mapping and retrograde atrial mapping. Kent's bundle was located over the left ventricular free wall in 21 patients and over the right ventricular free wall in 2 patients; it had a posteroseptal location in 9 patients. In 3 patients it conducted only retrogradely. In 1 patient conduction disappeared at surgery, so the location was only based on preoperative studies.

Division of Kent's bundle was achieved by A-V disconnection through an endoatrial approach under cardiopulmonary bypass. The division was achieved in 28 patients, obtunded in 2, and missed in 2. Tachyarrhythmias were cured in 30 patients: 3 of the 15 first patients died with low output failure. The last consecutive 17 cases had a safe recovery period since better myocardial preservation has been achieved.

The authors conclude that surgical treatment of WPW can be contemplated in patients with malignant ventricular arrhythmia and/or reciprocating supraventricular tachycardia resistant to medical treatment.

*Department of Cardiology, Hôpital de la Salpêtrière, Paris, France

Surgical Problems Encountered in Interruption of Multiple Anomalous Pathways of Atrioventricular Conduction (Kent Bundles)

W.C. Sealy, and J.J. Gallagher*

Among the 160 patients operated on by the authors for anomalous pathways of atrioventricular conduction (APC), 15 had more than one APC, with 13 having two APCs and 2 having three. Nearly all possible combinations of APC were found. Four patients had Ebstein's anomaly, all four having a right free wall and a septal pathway. The principal surgical problem, the identification of the APC, requires detailed electrophysiologic studies (EPS) before operation and intraoperatively. The suspicion of the presence of other APCs was raised by a wide QRS during reentrant tachycardia (RT) and chaning patterns of RT. Alterations of preexcitation patterns on the ECG during right and left atrial pacing and atrial flutter may denote other APCs. Atrial activation sequences during RT were particularly helpful in finding APC with only retrograde function, as found in four patients, and also in demonstrating septal pathways. Eight of the patients with 17 APCs had the APCs demonstrated before surgery. At surgery, EPS before and after division of the known APC was successful in identifying the additional APC in four patients. Failure to find the additional APCs during preoperative and intraoperative EPS may result from trauma to the pathway, close proximity of a second APC to the known APC, or suppression of the manifestation of one pathway by the other. For these reasons three APCs were not identified until the postoperative period.

Of the 32 APCs, 29 were divided. Eleven patients had one or more APC with lethal potential. One of the missed pathways was in this group. The remaining two APCs not divided, one with only retrograde function and the other in the posterior septal group, were electively left intact. One patient with severe associated cardiomyopathy died after surgery.

Surgery for interruption may require both a right and left atriotomy as well as extensive dissection in the coronary sulcus when there are two ipsilateral free wall pathways.

The identification of multiple APC is the principal surgical problem in effecting their interruption.

*Duke University Medical Center, Durham, North Carolina, USA

Surgical Treatment of Ventricular Tachycardia: Value of Underlying Mechanism

G. Guiraudon, G. Fontaine, R. Frank, K. Ouattara, Y. Grosgogeat, and C. Cabrol*

Sixty-six patients with ventricular tachycardia (VT) were surgically treated on the basis of the underlying mechanism, ventricular mapping, and study of the anatomical lesions.

Twenty-two patients with "idiopathic VT" underwent a simple ventriculotomy (V) at the breakthrough of the VT determined by ventricular mapping. Four patients died after surgery; all four patients in whom VT was not inducible by programmed stimulation relapsed after surgery.

One patient with chronic inducible VT after myocardial infarction (MI) underwent successful V after mapping. Twenty-two patients with chronic inducible VT after MI underwent an aneurysmectomy. Four patients died after surgery, and nine relapsed.

Out of 21 patients with encircling endocardial ventriculotomy, only two relapsed.

EEV is performed after entering the left ventricle. EEV is an almost transmural ventriculotomy perpendicular to the wall along the limits of the endocardial fibrosis which separates the pathological from the healthy myocardium. EEV excludes the septum if involved.

Inducible VTs are considered to be related to a macroreentry circuit mechanism. Successful surgery of WPW syndrome has demonstrated that a reentry circuit can be definitely interrupted at surgery.

Successful V and EEV on inducible VT suggest that reentrant VT can be cured by suitable ventriculotomy after mapping.

The surgical approach in noninducible VT needs further investigations.

*Department of Cardiology, Hôpital de la Salpêtrière, Paris, France

Invited Lecture

Coronary Artery Surgery – Current State of the Art

D.B. Effler*

Direct revascularization surgery utilizing bypass graft techniques is in its 13th year and has become one of the most common forms of elective surgery performed in the USA. From a technical standpoint the concept of bypass graft surgery is basically simple. Many surgeons believe that cardioplegia, hypothermia, coronary artery perfusion, and intraaortic balloon assist are essential for this type of surgery – the author disagrees.

The rationale and the basic technical approaches to direct revascularization surgery are presented. Certain misconceptions in application are discussed (e.g., the more grafts, the better the result). Acceptable mortality and graft patency rates are analyzed. The author's opinions on alternative procedures, such as catheter angioplasty, are presented.

*St. Joseph's Hospital Health Center, Syracuse, N.Y., USA

Patterns of Coronary Artery Distribution: Radiological and Anatomical Correlations

S.P.Allwork* and M.J.Raphael**

Introduction

Appreciation of the disposition of the coronary arteries from coronary arteriograms is mandatory to their identification in patients. This in turn is, of course, mandatory for successful surgical intervention. This knowledge is facilitated by studying casts of the coronary arteries because they represent the substance of the radiographic shadow (1-7).

Anatomy

Examination of a cast of the whole heart reveals that the two coronary arteries occupy the four sulci of the heart. The two interventricular sulci contain the anterior and posterior descending arteries respectively, while the two atrioventricular sulci are encircled by the right and circumflex arteries respectively (Fig. 1).

Angiographic Anatomy

The anterior descending coronary artery originates in the left or anterolateral aortic sinus and passes leftwards as a common trunk, varying in length between about 6 and 26 mm (in adults) before it divides into anterior descending and circumflex branches. The anterior descending branch gives a variable number of branches called diagonal arteries to the left ventricular muscle: some right ventricular branches may also be given (Fig. 1) but these are extremely difficult to identify radiographically as they tend, in most projections, to resemble septal arteries (Fig. 1).

The anterior descending branch gives a variable number of septal coronary arteries which originate from the underside of the anterior descending artery. Their straight passage into the anterior ventricular septum makes them easy to identify in most projections (Fig. 1).

*Department of Surgery, Royal Postgraduate Medical School, Hammersmith Hospital, Ducane Road, London, W12 OHS, Great Britain

**Department of Diagnostic Radiology, Middlesex Hospital, Mortimer Street, London, W.1., Great Britain

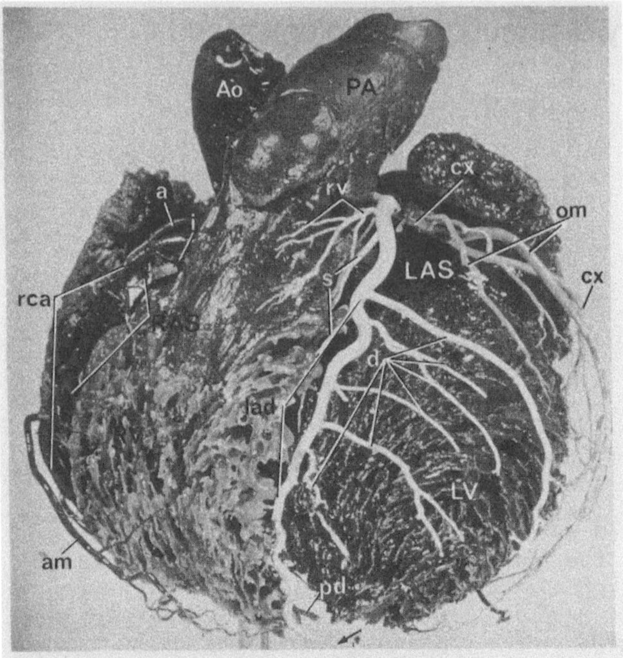

Fig. 1. Cast of the heart. Anterior view. The right coronary artery *(rca)* originates from the right aortic sinus and passes in the right atrioventricular sulcus *(RAS)*. It gives an infundibular *(i)*, an atrial *(a)*, and an acute marginal *(am)* branch. The posterior descending *(pd)* is just visible in the posterior interventricular sulcus. The left main coronary artery is not seen, but the anterior descending *(lad)* branch occupies the anterior interventricular sulcus. It gives septal *(s)*, diagonal *(d)*, and right ventricular *(rv)* branches before passing around the apex to ascend a short distance (arrowed). The circumflex artery *(cx)* occupies the left atrioventricular sulcus *(LAS)*. It gives several obtuse marginal branches, one larger than itself (om) before turning away to the back of the heart. *Ao*, aorta; *PA*, pulmonary artery; *RV*, right ventricle; *LV*, left ventricle

The anterior descending artery may be identified by:
1) Length. It (normally) traverses the apex of the heart to ascend for a variable, though usually short distance on the diaphragmatic surface (Fig. 1). This is significant especially when disease is present, as the anterior descending branch may fill retrograde from the right coronary artery when it (the left) is obstructed proximally (Figs. 2a,b).
2) Position. The anterior descending coronary artery is the most anterior structure in the lateral projection.
3) Septal arteries. The septal arteries take origin from the undersurface of the artery, and in right anterior oblique projection are at right angles to the main vessel (Fig. 2b). In disease, these septal arteries and the characteristic "blush" which their opacification produces may be the best guide to the position of a diseased anterior descending artery. This blush is particularly evident in left anterior oblique projection (Fig. 2a).

The circumflex artery takes origin from the left main coronary artery in the fat between the pulmonary trunk and the left atrial appendage (Fig. 1). It traverses the left atrioventricular sulcus and gives origin to a variable number of obtuse marginal branches. Their origin from the circumflex is usually rather obscure in left or right anterior

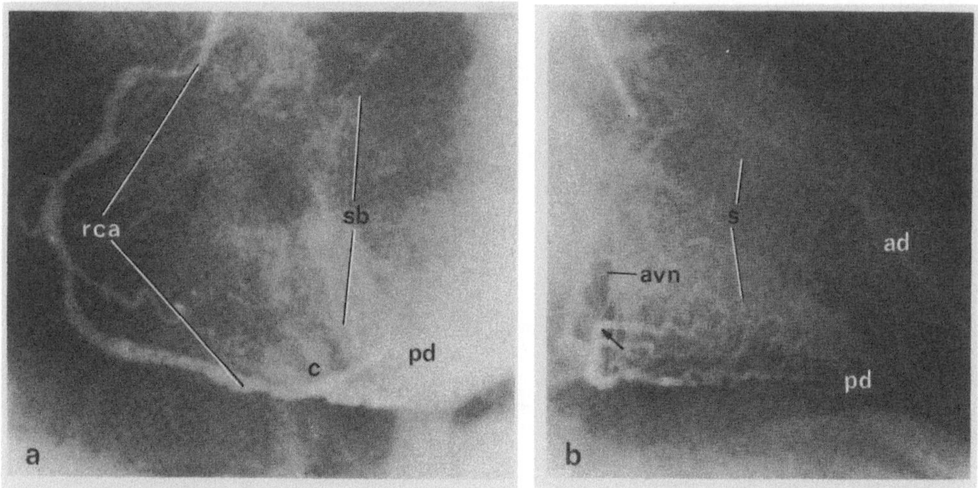

Fig. 2. a Right coronary arteriogram, left anterior oblique projection. The artery *(rca)* which is diseased and irregular in calibre, is well profiled until the crux cordis *(c)* is reached when foreshortening obscures the morphology. The site of the anterior descending artery is marked by the "blush" of septal arteries *(sb)*. Note that the right and anterior descending arteries are parallel in this projection. Abbreviations as before. b Right anterior oblique projection. The diseased rca is faintly outlined for most of its length. The anastomosis of anterior and posterior descending *(ad, pd)* is well seen in this view. The septal arteries also anastomose. *avn*, artery to atrioventricular node from the summit of the loop (arrowed)

oblique views (Figs. 3a,b) but this can be overcome by applying a degree of craniocaudal tilt in the left anterior oblique projection.

The circumflex coronary artery is identified by:

1) Position. It occupies the atrioventricular sulcus and its curve is concave anteriorly (Fig. 3b). It may reach the crux cordis and give the posterior descending artery ("dominant left coronary artery") or it may terminate as an obtuse marginal branch.

2) Morphology. The curve of the circumflex artery is tighter than the obtuse marginal branches, but this is only really apparent in a moving picture.

The obtuse marginal arteries arise from the circumflex artery. They are frequently larger than their parent artery (Fig. 3a), and because they often lie in the muscle, rather than superficially, they may be difficult to find at operation (1). They vascularise the obtuse margin of the left ventricle and (usually) the anterolateral mitral papillary muscle group.

The right coronary artery originates from the right or anteromedial aortic sinus. Its first branch usually passes to the pulmonary infundibulum (Fig. 1) but this little artery quite often originates from a separate ostium in the right aortic sinus. In about 55% of people the second branch passes backwards to the right atrium, where it gives a branch to the sinuatrial node. (In the remaining 45%, this artery is a branch of the circumflex coronary artery).

The artery lies deep in the fat of the right atrioventricular sulcus and gives a variable number of muscular branches to the right ventricle. The most constant of these branches traverses the acute margin of the heart and is called the acute marginal branch (Figs. 1 and 2a). The artery, still in the (now posterior) atrioventricular sulcus, passes to the crux of the heart. (The atrial and ventricular septa

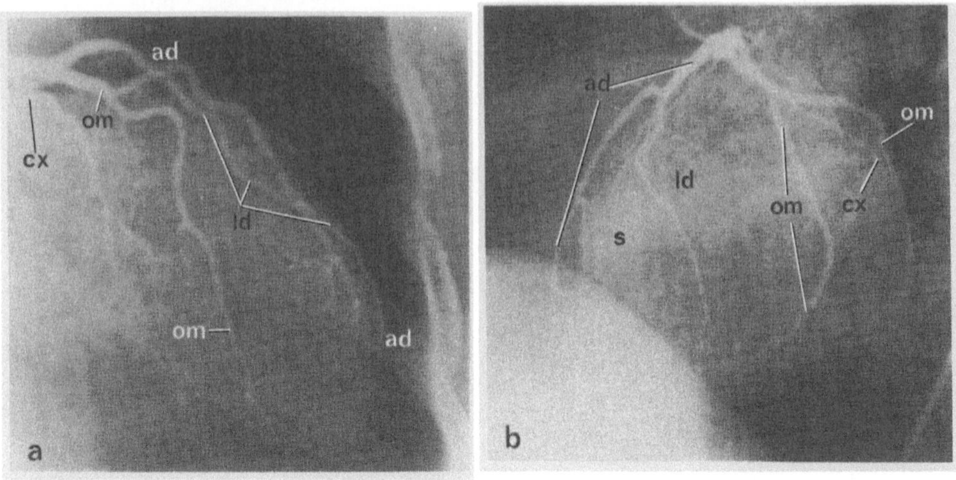

Fig. 3. a Left coronary arteriogram from a normal individual. The origin of the obtuse marginal artery *(om)* from the circumflex *(cx)* is not clear, neither is that of the first diagonal artery *(1d)*. The anterior descending artery is identified by its length and its septal branches. b Same heart. Left anterior oblique projection. As in Fig. 3a, the origin of the circumflex and obtuse marginal branches is unclear, but all the arteries are well profiled distally. The circumflex is recognised by its tighter curve as it traverses the atrioventricular sulcus. These two views of the same heart emphasise the importance of looking at more than one view when examining coronary arteries

meet at the crux or cross of the heart). Here the artery loops into the myocardium and, in most individuals, a small branch passes from the loop to supply the atrioventricular node (Fig. 2b).

In right anterior oblique projection (Fig. 2b) the loop is quite recognisable, but rather foreshortened. The descending limb of the loop divides and gives the posterior descending coronary artery which traverses the posterior (inferior) interventricular sulcus. The posterior descending artery may be identified, like the anterior descending artery, by septal branches passing vertically into the inlet (posterior) ventricular septum (Fig. 2b). The other branch of the descending limb of the loop traverses the crux, leaves the atrioventricular sulcus and terminates as one or more posterolateral left ventricular branches. The posteromedial mitral papillary muscle group is usually vascularised by these. Separation of the posterior descending and posterolateral branches is difficult in both the oblique views because they tend to (a) run parallel in right anterior oblique, and (b) overlap one another (Figs. 2a,b). In left anterior oblique projection the posterior descending branch "approaches" the viewer, and is thus foreshortened (Fig. 2a). In disease, identification may be facilitated by retrograde filling of the anterior descending artery, as in the illustration. Posterolateral branches, though much foreshortened, are easier to identify in left anterior oblique (Fig. 2a).

The wide, gentle curve of the right coronary artery is best seen in the left anterior oblique projection, as it is profiled from the ostium to the crux cordis. Strictures and dilatations are well seen (Fig. 2a), and it is easy to identify the precise location of a stricture or a complete block. Right anterior oblique view shows the origin and proximal 1 or 2 cm of the right coronary artery "en face" and is therefore unsuitable to detect an ostial stenosis.

Summary

Radiographic imaging of the coronary arteries is almost as old as radiology itself, and casts of the heart have been made for about 2 centuries (1).

We have found that comparing casts with radiographs is helpful in understanding radiographic anatomy and well exemplifies the merits and disadvantages of the projections commonly employed at arteriography.

References

1. Allwork SP (1979) A spectrum of normal coronary artery distribution in man. Anat Clin 1:311-319
2. Allwork SP (1980) Angiographic anatomy. In: Anderson RH, Becker AE (eds) Cardiac anatomy. Gower, London, pp 7.1-7.24
3. Allwork SP, Hawtin DR, Raphael MJ (1978) Casts of the heart as an aid to interpretation of arteriograms. J Anat 126:444
4. Allwork SP, Hawtin DR, Raphael MJ (1978) The arteriographic anatomy of the coronary arteries. Br J Radiol 51:156
5. Raphael MJ, Allwork SP (1974) Angiographic anatomy of the left ventricle. Clin Radiol 25:95-105
6. Raphael MJ, Allwork SP (1976) The angiographic anatomy of the right heart. Clin Radiol 27:265-272
7. Raphael MJ, Hawtin DR, Allwork SP (1980) The angiographic anatomy of the coronary arteries. Br J Surg 67:181-187

Coronary Revascularization With Snakegrafts. Experience in 214 Patients

F. Vermeulen, O. Alfieri, S. Ernst, R. de Geest, P. Knaepen, and A. Schaepkens van Riempst*

Between August 1, 1977 and June 30, 1979, 993 coronary revascularization procedures were performed, 214 of which were by "circular" or "snake" grafts.

Except for its terminal end-to-end anastomosis, a snake graft did revascularize all other diseased arteries by side-to-side, mostly diamond-shaped, anastomoses. Only septal arteries were revascularized by separate straight grafts in 14 patients. A total of 1046 anastomoses were constructed (4.9/patient); 31 additional procedures were performed.

Eleven patients (5%) died in hospital, including two with poor left ventricular function, two with combined valvular operations, and one on chronic dialysis. In eight patients (4%) a nonfatal perioperative infarction occurred.

The total graft flow increased with the number of distal anastomoses.

Early postoperative coronary angiography showed a 100% patency in 44 side-to-side and 10 end-to-side anastomoses; 6% of side-to-side anastomoses showed ≥50% stenosis detected at multiple standard, craniocaudal, and special projections to unmask the different anastomotic sites.

At follow-up examination, 95% of the patients were asymptomatic. Two late cardiac deaths occurred, but no postmortem examination was conducted. One noncardiac death occurred.

Late angiographic control in three asymptomatic patients showed a 100% anastomotic patency with 14% anastomotic or vein segment lesion of ≥50%. In six symptomatic patients, a 90% anastomotic patency with 10% additional anastomotic lesions of ≥50% was found.

These data suggest that the continued use of snake grafts for extensive coronary revascularization seems justified in diffuse coronary disease.

*Department of Cardio-Thoracic Surgery and Cardiology, St. Antonius Hospital, Utrecht, The Netherlands

The Immediate Function of Sequential Aorto-coronary Vein Grafts to Closely Adjacent Myocardial Areas

S. Ekeström*

Multiple obliterations of the coronary arteries are in the majority in patients with incapacitating angina pectoris. The surgical treatment of these patients requires aortocoronary bypasses which may be performed as separate vein grafts or/and as a sequential graft (jump graft, etc.). This is referred to as a complete myocardial revascularization which is reported to diminish the operative mortality and improve the long-term results of bypass surgery. The present study deals with the peroperative function of sequential grafts connected to closely adjacent myocardial areas.

Material and Methods

In a series of 48 patients suffering incapacitating angina pectoris and demonstrating multiple coronary artery obliterations, a sequential graft jumping from the aorta to left anterior descending artery (LAD) and a diagonal branch was performed. The saphenous vein and one suitable branch or a perforant branch were anastomosed end-to-side to the LAD and its diagonal branch. After the reconstruction but peroperatively the blood flow was measured in the joint vein graft and in the two branches of the vein perfusing the LAD and the diagonal branch. The blood flow was obtained with the aid of an electromagnetic flowmeter. The influence of a coronary vasodilator (dipyridamole) on joint bypass blood flow and the branch flow was registered.

Results

There was a highly significant difference between the joint graft flow and the branch flow when one of the branches was occluded (Fig. 1). When this branch was continuously kept occluded for 10 min in 11 patients (Fig. 2), the blood flow through the other branch increased insignificantly during this period. However, it never reached the level of the joint blood flow registered when both branches were open.

The effect of a coronary vasodilator (dipyridamole) is demonstrated in Figure 3. The difference between joint graft flow and the branch flow increased under this condition insignificantly.

*Thoraxkirurgiska kliniken, Karolinska sjukhuset, Stockholm, Sweden

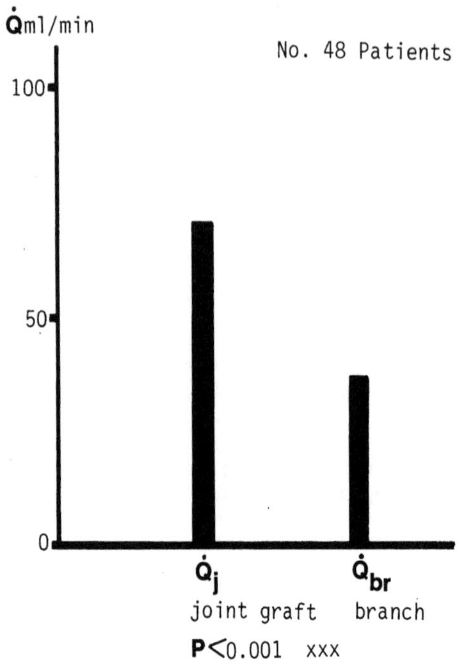

Fig. 1. The blood flow through the joint vein graft was significantly larger than the flow through one branch of the vein graft when the other was occluded

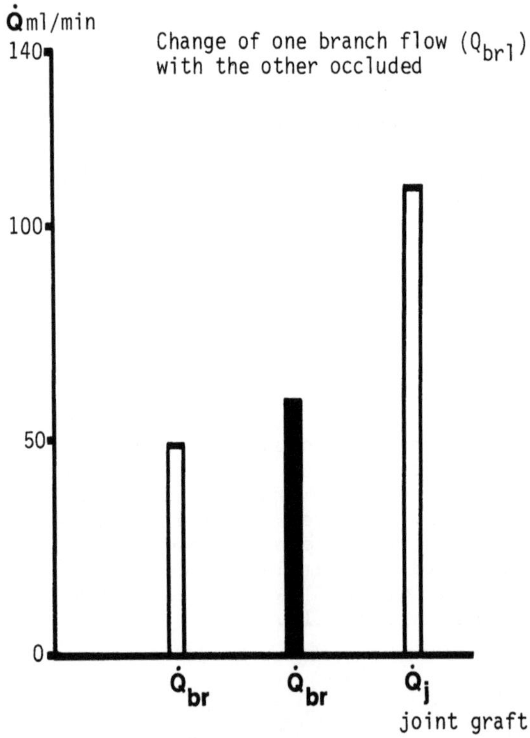

Fig. 2. When one of two branches of a sequential aortocoronary vein bypass was gently occluded over a period of 10 min, the flow through the other branch increased insignificantly and never reached the level of the joint blood flow obtained with both branches open. The filled column represents branch flow after 10 min of occlusion

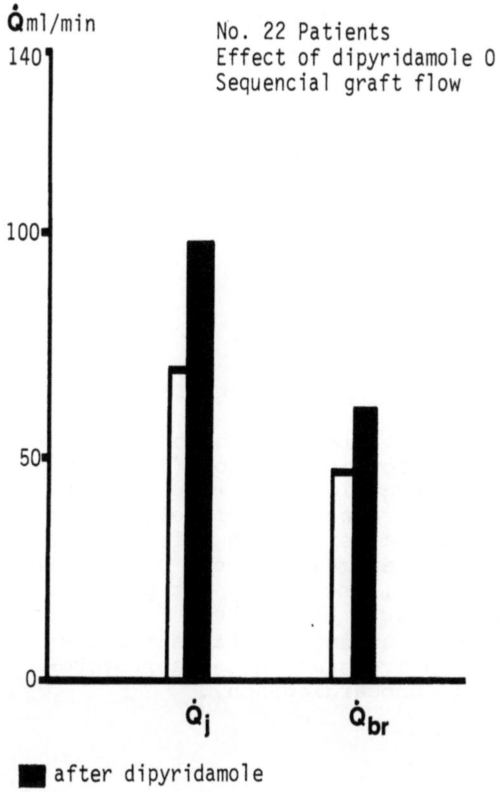

Fig. 3. The effect of a vasodilator (dipyridamole) on joint graft and branch flow. The filled columns show the flow after administration of the vasodilator

Discussion

The need of complete revascularization in case of multiple coronary artery obliterations has been widely accepted for several years. It is based on the assumption that there is an insufficient development of coronary collaterals in these cases.

Two factors seem to be of importance for the development of intercoronary collaterals: (1) pressure difference between two adjacent branches and (2) myocardial hypoxia causing local sustained vasodilation. Since multiple obliterations must cause deeper myocardial hypoxia than an isolated obliteration in one single coronary branch, the local hypoxic vasodilation as a source of collateral development seems less probable.

Severe stenosis or occlusion in two adjacent branches implies little or no pressure difference between them and, thus, no incitement of collateral development. The insufficient collateral system which explains the lower blood flow in one vein branch of a sequential aortocoronary vein bypass than in the joint vein graft is most probably due to the absence of a pressure difference between adjacent coronary branches and not to the lack of myocardial hypoxia in patients with incapacitating angina pectoris and multiple coronary obliterations.

Control of Cardiac Output After Aortocoronary Bypass Surgery in the Early and Late Postoperative Period by Two-dimensional Echocardiography

R. Erbel*, P. Schweizer*, P. Bardos**, B. J. Messmer**, J. Meyer*, and S. Effert*

Introduction

M-mode echocardiography cannot be used in patients with coronary artery disease for evaluation of left ventricular function (3, 5). The methodological limitations of M-mode echocardiography were overcome by two-dimensional echocardiography. Now determinations of left ventricular volume and ejection fraction even in patients with left ventricular asynergy were possible (1, 4, 8). Serial measurements of left ventricular function after open-heart surgery, previously not possible because of septal paradoxical movement, could be started.

The purpose of this study was the evaluation of left ventricular function in the early and late postoperative stage after aortocoronary bypass surgery by two-dimensional echocardiography.

Methods

Heart rate, blood pressure, and two-dimensional echocardiograms were recorded in 31 patients (27 men and 4 women) with a mean age of 51.9 years (range 40 to 63 years) preoperatively. In the mean 2.4 bypass grafts were inserted, 26 to the anterior descending branch of the left coronary artery, 12 to the left circumflex, 6 to the diagonal branch, 11 to the right coronary artery, and 9 to the marginal branch of the right coronary artery.

Early postoperatively (10 to 14 days) in 29/31 patients two-dimensional echocardiograms of acceptable quality could be recorded. Late postoperatively (6 months) 22/31 patients could be studied again. Two-dimensional echocardiograms were done using a phased-array wide-angle (84°) sector-scanner, Varian V-3000. A 2.25 MHz transducer was used. In real-time, two-dimensional echocardiograms were recorded at 30 frames/min on video tape.

Recordings were made by placing the transducer on the apex impulse location and aiming the beam toward the left atrium (Fig. 1). In the four-chamber view left atrium, left ventricle, right atrium, and right ventricle were scanned. The interventricular septum was clearly visualized.

After the images were recorded on video tape, the contour of the left ventricle was traced using a light pen system. Computer-assisted left ventricular volumes were calculated using Simpson's rule. With stop-frame mode and with references to ECG, end-diastolic (peak of R wave) and end-systolic (end of T wave and smallest left ventricular silhouette) frames were defined.

---

*Department of Internal Medicine I, RWTH Aachen, Goethestr. 27/29, D-5100 Aachen
**Department of Cardiovascular Surgery, RWTH Aachen, Goethestr. 27-29, D-5100 Aachen

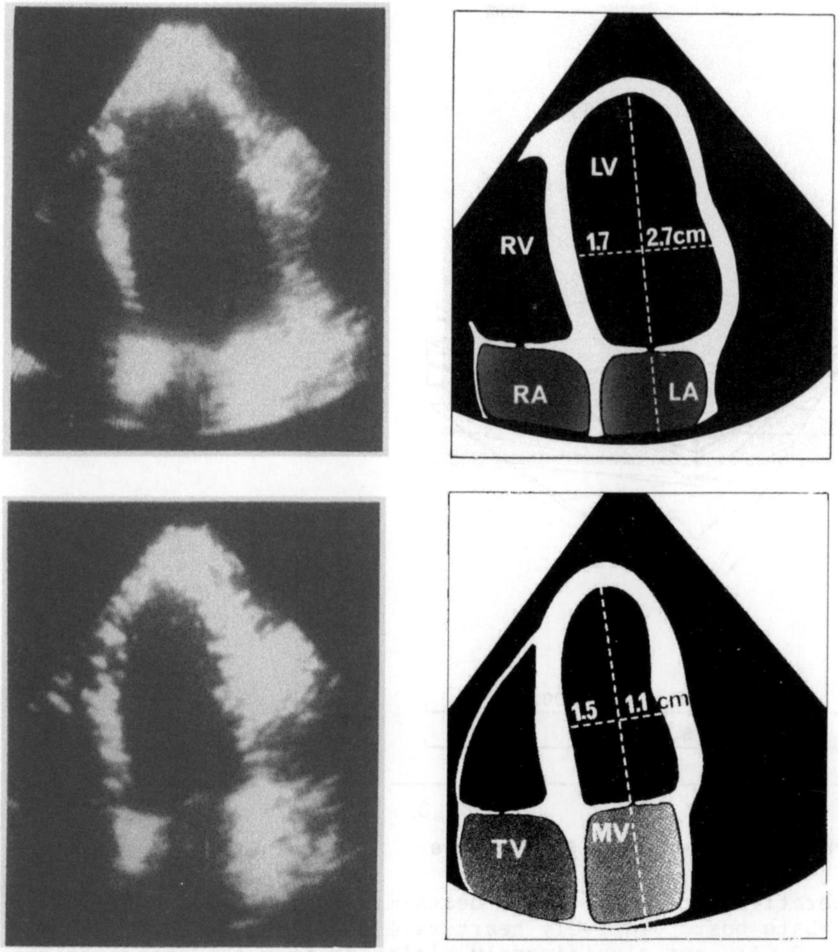

Fig. 1. Four-chamber view of apical two-dimensional echocardiography early postoperatively. Left *(LV)* and right *(RV)* ventricle, as well as left *(LA)* and right *(RA)* atrium are visualized. Interventricular septum and mitral *(MV)*, and tricuspidal *(TV)* valve are illustrated. Left ventricular long axis divided left ventricular diameter (3/8 of the long axis) in a septal and posterior-lateral half-axis. End-diastolic and end-systolic frames can be seen, as well as septal hypokinesis

Calculated left ventricular end-diastolic and end-systolic volumes were corrected using regression analysis, which were obtained from cineangiocardiographic and two-dimensional echocardiographic volume determinations in patients with coronary artery disease (4). These procedures were necessary because a systematic underestimation of left ventricular volume by two-dimensional echocardiography was found compared to cineangiocardiography.

Statistical analyses were made using the student t-test for unpaired data. A p value of <0.05 was found to be significant. All values ±sem. n.s. = not significant.

Results

Early postoperatively 4/31 patients showed a pericardial effusion, which was drained in 2/4 patients. Late postoperatively only 1/4 of the patients had a small pericardial effusion. Heart rate increased

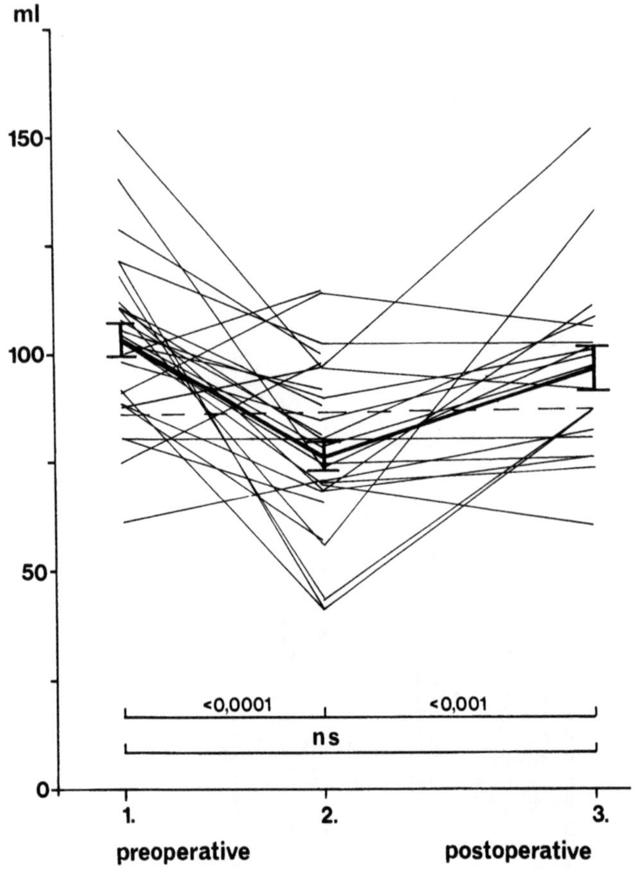

Fig. 2. Left ventricular stroke volume preoperatively *(1.)*, early *(2.)*, i.e., 10-14 days, postoperatively, and late *(3.)*, i.e., 6 months, postoperatively. The mean value and the standard error of the mean are shown as well as all single values. Early postoperatively stroke volume decreased significantly and returned to the starting point late postoperatively.
ns = not significant

early postoperatively from 72.1 ± 2.3 beats/min to 94.8 ± 2.3 beats/min ($p < 0.0001$). Late postoperatively heart rate decreased to 77.6 ± 2.8 beats/min ($p < 0.01$), not significantly different from the preoperative value. Blood pressure was preoperative 131.2 ± 3.7/83.1 ± 2.3 mm Hg, early postoperative 130.2 ± 3.9/85.7 ± 3.2 mm Hg (n.s.), late postoperative 140.5 ± 4.8/89.7 ± 1.7. Only the increase in diastolic blood pressure was significant ($p < 0.05$).

While end-diastolic volume decreased from 172.3±9.1 to 155.8±9.2 ml, end-systolic volume increased from 70.1 ± 8.2 to 77.8 ± 7.8 ml (n.s.). Late postoperatively end-diastolic and end-systolic volumes were not significantly different (155.5 ± 12.5 and 59.9 ± 8.5 ml, respectively) from their starting points.

The changes of stroke volume and ejection fraction are illustrated in Figures 2 and 3. A significant fall of stroke volume (-25 ml) and left ventricular ejection fraction (-9.9%) was found. Six months postoperatively the starting point was nearly reached. Cardiac output remained constant [7.44 ± 0.009 l/min versus 7.39 ± 0.08 and 7.43 ± 0.13 l/min (n.s.), respectively].

Early postoperatively wall motion abnormalities particularly of the septum were observed. For quantitative analysis of wall motion the fractional shortening of the septal and posterior-lateral half-axis were calculated as demonstrated in Figure 1. Early postoperatively septal wall motion decreased significantly from 34.8 ± 3.4% to 14.2 ± 3.2% ($p < 0.01$), whereas posterior-lateral wall motion increased from 24.7 ± 3.2 to 28.9 ± 2.8% (n.s.). Late postoperatively septal wall motion improved significantly (Fig. 4).

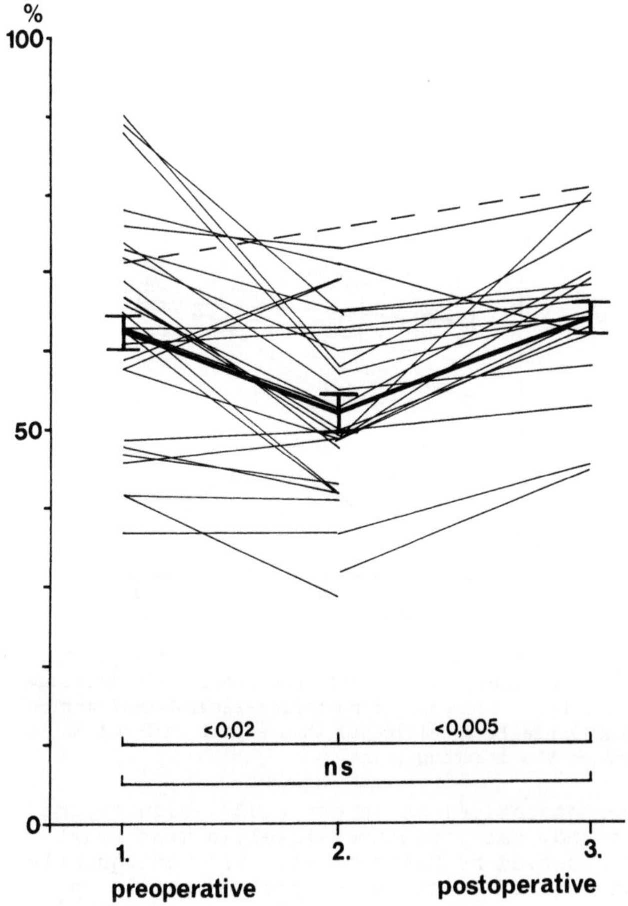

Fig. 3. Left ventricular ejection fraction preoperatively *(1.)*, early *(2.)*, and late *(3.)* postoperatively. Ejection fraction decreased significantly early postoperatively and reached the preoperative value late postoperatively. ns = not significant

Discussion

Apical two-dimensional echocardiography could be performed early postoperatively in 29/31 patients. In four patients a pericardial effusion was detected which was not suspected in 2/4. Apical two-dimensional echocardiography is thus a useful noninvasive method for detecting pericardial effusion even in the postoperative stage. After coronary bypass surgery pericardial effusion has to be expected in 5%-10% postoperatively (10). Based on the two-dimensional echocardiographic images an estimation of the amount of effusion can be obtained. The indication for drainage could easier be decided, taking into account the echocardiographic results.

Even in patients with coronary artery disease left ventricular volume and ejection fraction could be determined by two-dimensional echocardiography (4). Consequently it was used in our study for the evaluation of left ventricular performance after aortocoronary bypass surgery.

End-diastolic volume decreased and end-systolic volume increased slightly postoperative in the early stage. Stroke volume and left ventricular ejection fraction decreased significantly early postoperatively and reached their starting point 6 months later. Similar results were obtained using radiopaque tantalum markers. Mintz et al. (6) reported a significant increase of stroke volume and ejection fraction

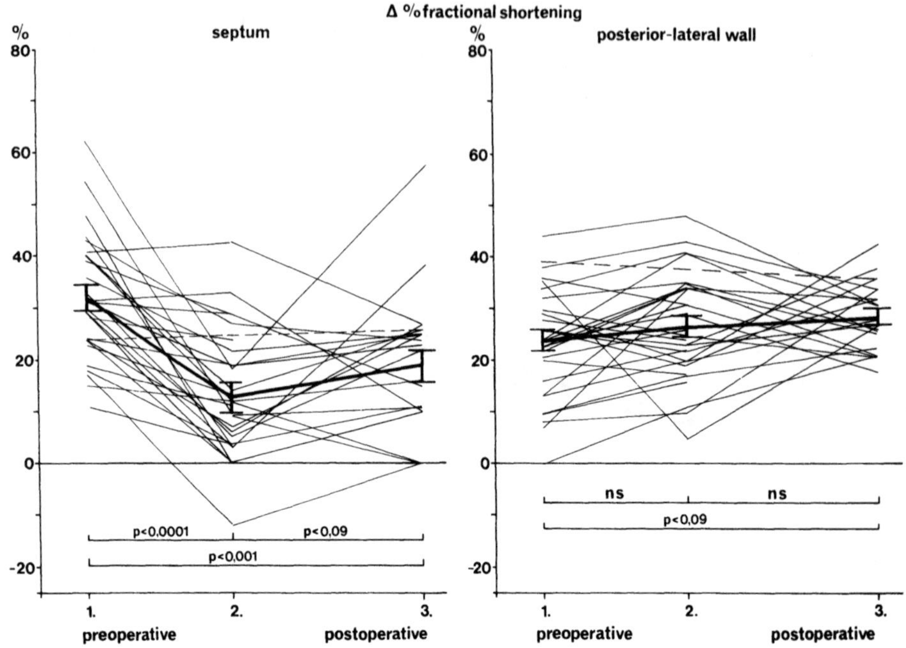

Fig. 4. Fractional shortening of septal and posterior-lateral half-axis preoperatively *(1.)*, early *(2.)*, and late *(3.)* postoperatively. Early postoperatively decrease of septal wall motion is accompanied by an increase of posterior-lateral wall motion. Late postoperatively this increase is nearly significant, when septal wall motion improved significantly without reaching the starting point

between 1 week and 1 year postoperative. As in our study, significant changes in heart rate were found. Early postoperatively a mean heart rate of 91 ± 2 beats/min was observed by Mintz et al. (6). Consequently the main hemodynamic constant – cardiac output – remained nearly unchanged. Our data are in accordance with their results.

Septal wall motion disturbances were the reason for these changes already observed by M-mode echocardiography (2, 7).. But not only the motion but also septal myocardial function was depressed (2, 7). Similar findings were reported from Vignola et al. (10), using M-mode echocardiography and scintigraphy. In our study, these earlier results could be proven by two-dimensional echocardiography. A significant reduction in septal inward movement was found early postoperatively accompanied by a compensatory increase in posterior wall motion, which could not prevent the decrease in stroke volume. In our opinion, the decrease in stroke volume was due to an increase in heart rate and due to reduced septal wall motion. Six months postoperatively septal wall motion had improved. Similar results were obtained with epicardial markers (9). Regional myocardial function improved up to 6 months postoperatively and reached a plateau between 6 and 12 months postoperatively.

Conclusion

Apical two-dimensional echocardiography revealed early postoperatively a depressed septal wall motion causing a decrease in stroke volume. As a compensatory mechanism posterior wall motion increased. Cardiac output remained constant though heart rate increased. Late postoperatively septal wall motion improved, stroke volume increased, and consequently heart rate decreased, cardiac output remained unchanged.

References

1. Carr K, Engler R, Forsythe J, Johnson A, Gosink B (1979) Measurement of left ventricular ejection fraction by mechanical cross sectional echocardiography. Circulation 59:1196-1206
2. Corallo S, Pezzano A, Castognone M, Brusoni B, Ladelli L, Rovelli F (1978) Left ventricular behaviour before and after coronary artery bypass graft. Echocardiographic study. In: Europ. Congr. on Ultrasonic in Medicine. Bologna, Edizioni centro, Minerva Med 287-288
3. Erbel R, Schweizer P (1980) Diagnostischer Stellenwert der Echokardiographie bei der koronaren Herzerkrankung — I. M-mode Echokardiographie. Z Kardiol 69:391-397
4. Erbel R, Schweizer P, Meyer J, Grenner H, Krebs W, Effert S (1980) Bestimmung der Volumina und der Ejektionsfraktion aus dem zweidimensionalen Echokardiogramm bei Patienten mit koronarer Herzerkrankung. Z Kardiol 69:52-61
5. Linhart JW, Mintz GS, Segal BL, Kawai N, Kotler MN (1975) Left ventricular volume measurements by echocardiography: Fact or fiction? Am J Cardiol 36:114-118
6. Mintz LJ, Ingles NB Jr, Daughters GT II, Stinson EB, Alderman EL (1980) Sequential studies of left ventricular function and wall motion after coronary arterial bypass surgery. Am J Cardiol 45:210-216
7. Righetti A, Crawford MH, O'Rourke RA, Schelbert H, Daily PO, Ross J Jr (1977) Interventricular septal motion and left ventricular function after coronary bypass surgery. Am J Cardiol 39:372-377
8. Schiller NB, Acquatella H, Ports TA, Drew D, Goerke J, Ringertz H, Silverman NH, Brundage B, Boswell R, Carlsson E, Parmley WW (1979) Left ventricular volume from paired biplane two-dimensional echocardiography. Circulation 60:547-555
9. Serruys PW, Brower RW, ten Kate HJ, Brand vd M, Hugenholtz PG (1978) Early myocardial depression after coronary artery bypass surgery. In: Roskamm H, Schmuziger M (eds) Coronary heart surgery. Springer, Berlin Heidelberg New York, pp 349-354
10. Vignola PA, Boucher CA, Curfman GD, Walker HJ, Shea WH, Dinsmare RE, Pohost GM (1979) Abnormal interventricular septal motion following cardiac surgery: Clinical, surgical, echocardiographic, and radionuclide correlates. Am Heart J 97:27-34

Assessment of Aortocoronary Bypass Graft Patency by Means of Thallium-201 Myocardial Scintigraphy

B. Lösse, D. Rafflenbeul, H. Krönert, C. van Lierde, L. E. Feinendegen, W. Bircks, and F. Loogen*

Coronary angiography is generally accepted as the most reliable method to assess aortocoronary bypass graft patency. But since it is an invasive method, several attempts have been made to look for a noninvasive method of sufficient accuracy. Recent studies on the use of thallium-201 myocardial scintigraphy for assessment of bypass graft function have yielded conflicting results (2, 4, 5, 8, 10-13). This study, based on a series of 50 unselected patients, will contribute to the problem of how far myocardial scintigraphy can be used to predict bypass graft patency.

Patients and Methods

The study consists of 50 unselected patients, 42 males and 8 females, 27 to 68 years of age. Postoperative studies including myocardial scintigraphy and coronary angiography were performed 3 to 12 months after myocardial revascularization. The time delay between scintigraphy and angiography averaged 5 weeks. All scintigrams were performed after iv injection of 1.7 to 2.0 mCi thallium-201 during maximal bicycle ergometer exercise in supine position. Images were routinely obtained in four projections: anterior, 30° right anterior oblique, 45° left anterior oblique, and left lateral. Images were qualitatively evaluated at the scope of the computer system (Intertechnique Cine 200). The postoperative scintigrams were compared with the preoperative scintigrams and were visually interpreted to show improvement, no change, or deterioration of thallium uptake in the myocardial regions supplied by aortocoronary bypass grafts. After complete evaluation, the scintigraphic results were compared with the angiographic findings. Graft patency was confirmed by selective angiography. Graft occlusion was considered if only the stump was seen or if the graft was not visualized on an aortic root angiogram.

Results

Table 1 shows the distribution of coronary artery involvement and the number of aortocoronary bypass grafts in all 50 patients. It can be seen that in the group of two- and three-vessel disease there was a considerable number of patients with incomplete revascularization, i.e., fewer bypass grafts than angiographically demonstrated stenosed

*Med. Klinik B der Universität, Moorenstr. 5, D-4000 Düsseldorf

Table 1. Distribution of coronary artery involvement and number of aortocoronary bypass grafts in 50 patients with coronary artery disease

	Number of patients	Number of aortocoronary bypass grafts 1	2	3	4
One-vessel disease	10	7	3	-	-
Two-vessel disease	18	4	10	4	-
Three-vessel disease	22	-	7	11	4
Total	50	11	20	15	4

main coronary arteries. This is explained by two reasons: 1) In some cases the periphery of a centrally stenosed coronary artery was unsatisfactory for bypass grafting. 2) In other cases the area of a stenosed or occluded coronary artery was scarred and, therefore, thought to draw no benefit from a bypass graft.

There was a total number of 112 aortocoronary bypass grafts (Table 2), 89 (79%) of which could be visualized on angiography. Patency rate was not dependent on the number of bypass grafts per patient.

Table 2. Patency rate of aortocoronary bypass grafts in 50 patients in relation to the number of bypass grafts per patient

Number of patients	Number of aortocoronary bypass grafts Per patient	Total	Patent
11	1	11	9 = 82%
20	2	40	32 = 80%
15	3	45	34 = 76%
4	4	16	14 = 88%
50		112	89 = 79%

Clinical symptoms improved in 90% of the 30 patients whose bypass grafts were all patent (Table 3). But the majority of 18 further patients, whose bypass grafts were in part occluded, showed clinical improvement, too. About one-third (13 of 40) of the clinically improved patients had at least one occluded bypass graft. There were only two patients with no bypass graft patent. Both worsened clinically.

The myocardial scintigram improved in 71% of the 89 myocardial regions supplied by patent bypass grafts (Table 4), whereas 13% showed no change, and 16% a deteriorated thallium uptake. It should be noted that only 12% of the well-revascularized myocardial regions completely normalized after operation. Of the 23 myocardial regions supplied by occluded bypass grafts, 57% showed a deteriorated thallium uptake, 17% no change, and, surprisingly, 26% an improved thallium uptake. All these improvements were found in six patients who had, besides the occluded graft, one to three further well-perfused bypass grafts to adjacent myodardial regions.

Table 3. Postoperative changes in clinical status in relation to patency rate of aortocoronary bypass grafts

Clinical symptoms	Aortocoronary bypass grafts All patent (n = 30)	Partially occluded (n = 18)	All occluded (n = 2)
Improved	27 = 90%	13 = 72%	0 = 0%
Unchanged	3 = 10%	4 = 22%	0 = 0%
Deteriorated	0 = 0%	1 = 6%	2 = 100%

Table 4. Postoperative scintigraphic changes in 112 myocardial regions supplied by aortocoronary bypass grafts, 89 of which were patent and 23 of which were occluded in control angiography

Myocardial scintigram	Aortocoronary bypass Patent (n = 89)	Occluded (n = 23)
Improved (normalized)	63 = 71% (11 = 12%)	6 = 26%
Unchanged	12 = 13%	4 = 17%
Deteriorated	14 = 16%	13 = 57%

Starting from the scintigraphic evaluation, Table 4 demonstrates that 90% (63 of 69) of the scintigraphically improved regions were supplied by a patent bypass. On the other side, 75% (12 of 16) of scintigraphically unchanged regions and even 50% (14 of 27) of further deteriorated regions were supplied by a patent bypass graft, too.

Discussion

It has been shown that 80% to 90% of aortocoronary bypass grafts are patent 3 to 12 months after operation (3, 6), in most cases accompanied by clinical improvement. Bypass graft patency can, however, not be exactly predicted from clinical status, since a number of patients clinically improve in spite of occluded bypass grafts (6). Coronary angiography is the most reliable proof of bypass graft patency.

Myocardial visualization with thallium-201 is mainly dependent on myocardial perfusion and mass of viable myocardium. Since thallium-201 myocardial imaging at maximal exercise offers satisfactory reproducibility (7), this method should enable the assessment of bypass graft patency by comparing pre- and postoperative scintigrams. Published reports have, however, yielded conflicting results. The majority of authors stated that thallium scintigraphy is highly reliable in the prediction of individual bypass graft patency and occlusion (2, 4, 8, 10, 11). Another report concluded that, in the case of multivessel disease, myocardial scintigraphy is not able to differentiate between patency and occlusion of particular bypass grafts (12).

Our results demonstrate that an improved thallium uptake in a particular myocardial region is highly indicative of a patent bypass to that proper region. Sixty-three of 69 (90%) scintigraphically improved myocardial regions were supplied by patent bypass grafts (Table 4). The remaining six improved regions, supplied by occluded grafts, were found in six patients who had besides the occluded graft one to three further well-perfused bypass grafts. Thus, the scintigraphic improvement may be explained 1) by an overlap with a successfully revascularized adjacent region, or 2) by improved perfusion of the unsuccessfully revascularized region through collaterals from adjacent regions supplied by patent bypass grafts. Until now, we have not seen a scintigraphic improvement in patients who received only one bypass being occluded at control angiography.

A completely normalized thallium uptake indicating a normalized perfusion was, however, found only in a relatively low percentage (11 of 89, i.e., 12%) of well-revascularized regions. This is in agreement with other reports (2, 13) and indicates that in most cases of coronary artery disease disseminated scar tissue is present which persists, of course, after operation irrespective of bypass graft patency.

As can also be seen from our findings, patency of an aortocoronary bypass graft is, however, not necessarily reflected by an improved thallium uptake in the corresponding region. A considerable number of successfully revascularized myocardial regions showed either no change (12%) or a deterioration in thallium uptake after operation. The same observation has been reported by other investigators, too (2, 10, 11). There are several causes for explanation: 1) A progression of coronary artery disease may have occurred in the meantime and led to a worsened perfusion. 2) Perioperative myocardial injury may have occurred and led to myocardial scars (1, 9, 10) which take up no thallium. 3) In case of multiple bypass grafts the perfusion may be improved to a different degree. This may, for example, lead to a marked improvement in the preoperatively worst perfused regions and a slight improvement in the formerly less ill-perfused regions. Since thallium scintigrams yield relative perfusion patterns, the latter slight improvement may erroneously impress as deterioration in relation to the other markedly improved regions.

Consequently, a regionally deteriorated scintigram is in our experience no reliable indicator of bypass graft occlusion. Of 27 scintigraphically worsened regions, only one-half (13 regions) was supplied by an occluded graft, whereas the other half (14 regions) was supplied by patent grafts.

In conclusion, our results suggest that a scintigraphic improvement predicts with high probability a patent graft to the corresponding or, in rare cases, at least to an adjacent myocardial region, whereas an unchanged or further deteriorated scintigram is not reliably indicative of bypass graft occlusion.

Summary

Fifty unselected patients supplied with 112 aortocoronary bypass grafts postoperatively underwent thallium-201 myocardial scintigraphy and angiography. Postoperative myocardial scintigrams were compared with the preoperative scintigrams to predict bypass graft patency. The results were compared with the angiographic findings. The results suggest that a regional scintigraphic improvement is highly indicative of a patent bypass to that region, whereas an unchanged or further deteriorated scintigram is no reliable indicator of bypass graft occlusion.

References

1. Bulkley BH, Hutchins GM (1977) Myocardial consequences of coronary artery bypass graft surgery. The paradox of necrosis in areas of revascularization. Circulation 56:906-913
2. Eichstädt H, Gauss A, Andrasch R, Feine U, Kochsiek K (1979) Noninvasive perfusion control by thallium-201 myocardial scintigraphy after coronary artery bypass surgery. Cardiovasc Radiol 2:243-248
3. Fitzgibbon GM, Burton JR, Leach AJ (1978) Coronary bypass graft fate. Angiographic grading of 1400 consecutive grafts early after operation and of 1132 after one year. Circulation 57:1070-1074
4. Hirzel HO, Nuesch K, Luetolf UM, Gruentzig A, Horst W, Krayenbuehl HP (1980) La scintigraphie du myocarde au thallium 201 dans l'évaluation du succès d'une intervention revascularisatrice soit par pontage aorto-coronarien soit par dilatation coronarienne. Arch Mal Coeur 73:651-660
5. Kolibash AJ, Call TD, Bush CA, Tetalman MR, Lewis RP (1980) Myocardial perfusion as an indicator of graft patency after coronary artery bypass surgery. Circulation 61:882-887
6. Lichtlen P, Liese W, Leitz K, Borst HG (1978) Postoperative Klinik nach aortokoronarem Venen-Bypass in Relation zum Ausmaß der Revaskularisation. Z Kardiol 67:83-91
7. McLaughlin PR, Martin RP, Doherty P, Daspit S, Goris M, Haskell W, Lewis S, Kriss JP, Harrison DC (1979) Reproducibility of thallium-201 myocardial imaging. Circulation 55:497-503
8. Murphy A, Bonet J, McLaughlin P, Feiglin D, Morch J (1979) Noninvasive assessment of early postoperative bypass graft patency. Circulation [Suppl 2] 60:237
9. Righetti A, Crawford MH, O'Rourke RA, Hardarson T, Schelbert H, Daily PO, DeLuca M, Ashburn W, Ross J Jr (1977) Detection of perioperative myocardial damage after coronary artery bypass graft surgery. Circulation 55:173-178
10. Ritchie JL, Narahara KA, Trobaugh GB, Williams DL, Hamilton GW (1977) Thallium-201 myocardial imaging before and after coronary revascularization. Assessment of regional myocardial blood flow and graft patency. Circulation 56:830-836
11. Robinson PS, Crowther A, Jenkins BS, Webb-Peploe MM, Coltart DJ (1978) Exercise testing and thallium-201 myocardial perfusion imaging in evaluation of aortocoronary bypass surgery. Br Heart J 40:1065
12. Schicha H, Blanke H, Rentrop P, Karsch KR, Kreuzer H, Emrich D (1980) Myokardszintigraphie mit Thallium-201 zur Feststellung der Funktionsfähigkeit aortokoronarer Bypasse bei Mehr-Gefäß-KHK und Mehrfach-Bypassen. Z Kardiol 69:531-535
13. Verani MS, Marcus ML, Spoto G, Rossi NP, Ehrhardt JC, Razzak MA (1978) Thallium-201 myocardial perfusion scintigrams in the evaluation of aorto-coronary saphenous bypass surgery. J Nucl Med 19:765-772

Early Revision of Aorto-coronary Bypass Grafts

K. H. Leitz, K. P. Rentrop, H. Oster, and H. Blanke*

The information concerning revision of aortocoronary bypass grafts is rare in the literature. Therefore six patients with nine occluded grafts are presented in whom early revision of the bypass grafts has been performed.

From April 1, 1979, to May 1, 1980, 218 patients were operated upon for coronary artery disease at the clinic for Thoracic and Cardiovascular Surgery of the University of Göttingen. Twenty-nine percent of these patients had reangiography after 14 days postoperative. The overall patency rate in this patient group was 84%. Six patients were restudied early postoperatively because of new chest pain, which could not be related to the sternotomy and which responded positively on nitromedication. These six patients in whom we performed early revision of the bypass grafts represent the body of this presentation.

These six patients were all men with a mean age of 55 years. Two had inferior and three anteroseptal infarction in their history. They had a normal mean ejection fraction, the mean coronary score – according to Kaltenbach (4) – was 29. Eleven grafts were constructed to the different stenotic coronary arteries and one aneurysmectomy of the anterior wall of the heart was performed.

Four to eight days postoperative, these patients complained of angina of the same intensity and mode as preoperative (Table 1). The CPK determination revealed a positive value only in one patient. None of the patients demonstrated signs of infarction in the newly written ECG. During control angiography – done within 24 h after the onset of new angina – nine of the eleven constructed vein grafts were occluded (Table 1). The striking finding in five patients was the unchanged natural coronary system, only in one patient was the distal LAD occluded, too (Table 1).

One patient (LF) was reoperated. We put him on the heart-lung machine again, opened up the veins, and took out the thrombus. Because we were afraid of loosing thrombotic material into the arterial system, the aorta was not clamped. By the aortic pressure all thrombotic material was washed out. On the coronary site a similar method was used until backflow was visible. The other five patients were not reoperated. After the diagnostic angiography, we infused 2000 units of streptokinase for 70-300 min via an infusion pump. In three patients in whom the lysis of the occluded veins went on slowly, the thrombotic material was passed by a wire to increase the surface in order to support the reaction of streptokinase with the thrombotic material.

The method we used is demonstrated in the following patient (RU). The diagnostic angiography revealed on open graft to the posterolateral branch of the circumflex artery, the graft·to the LAD was occluded but the entire course of the LAD was visible (Fig. 1.). After infusion of streptokinase over 35 and 90 min, the proximal part of the vein was

*Klinik für Thorax-, Herz- und Gefäßchirurgie und Abteilung für Kardiologie der Universität Göttingen, Robert-Koch-Str. 40, D-3400 Göttingen

Table 1. Clinical course of patients with new postoperative angina

Name	Angina pectoris days after OP	CPK	ECG	Reangiography Graft		Cor. system
R.U.	4	32	no change	LAD R. marg. PLA	occl. occl. open	no change
R.W.	5	113	no change	PLA	occl.	no change
L.A.	8	70	no change	RCA	occl.	no change
N.L.	8	54	no change	LAD RCA	occl. occl.	no change
L.R.	5	70	no change	LAD RD	occl. open	no change
L.F.	4	42	no change	LAD CX	occl. occl.	distal LAD occl.

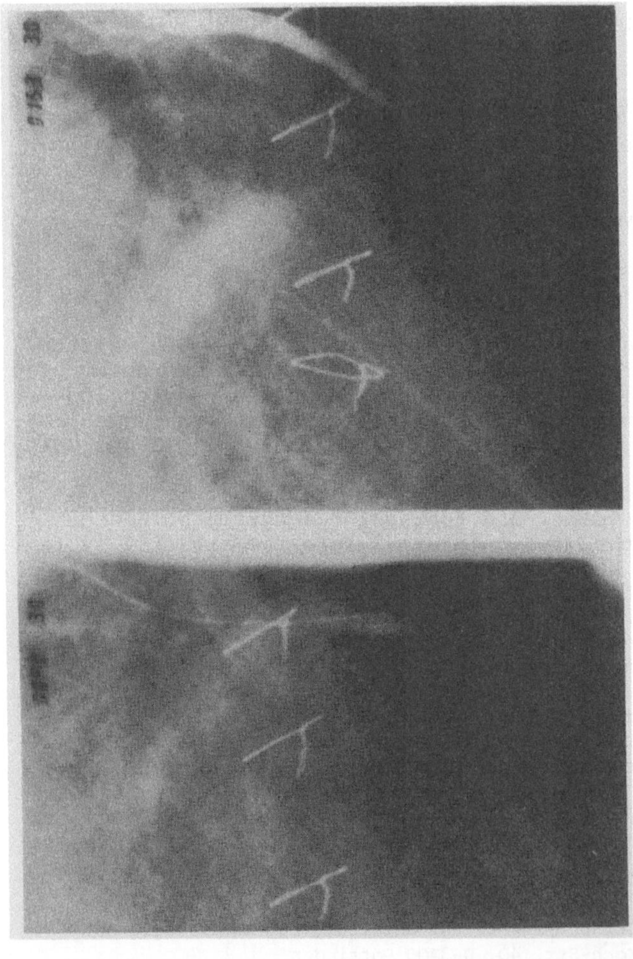

Fig. 1. Patient RU: the graft to the posterolateral branch is open, the graft to the LAD is occluded but the entire course of the LAD is visible

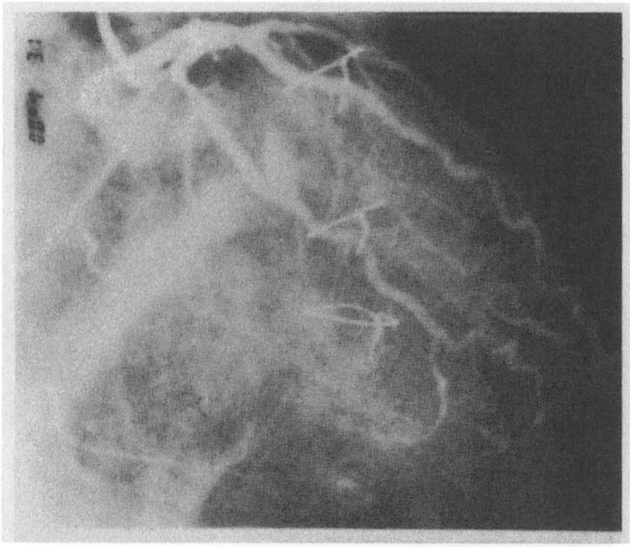

Fig. 2. Patient RU: after infusion of streptokinase over 90 min the proximal part of the vein was visible, after 150 min a wire was advanced

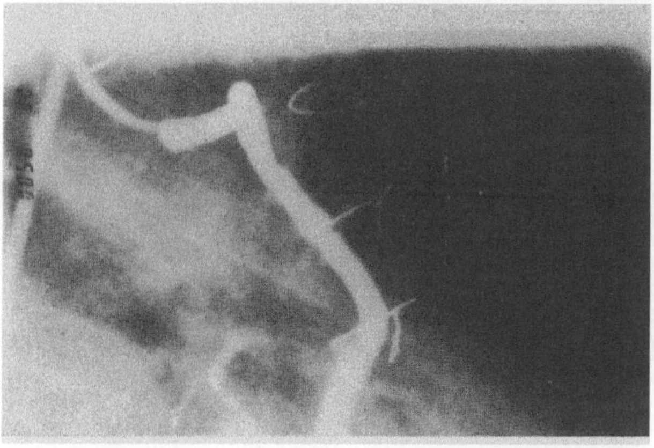

open (Fig. 2). Since after 150 min the lytic process continued slowly, a wire was advanced (Fig. 2). After 220 min a greater part of the vein was outlined and 260 min later the natural coronary artery was filled via the vein (Fig. 3). But watching exactly the inner contour of the vein wall, one realizes that there is still thrombotic material in the vein which disappeared 1 day later on control angiography (Fig. 4).

From the nine occluded grafts, five were opened up by lysis and two by early operative revision (Table 2). All patients became angina-free by our management. Two grafts to small branches of the coronary system remained closed. This fact demonstrates the limitation of the lytic therapy. You have to select the predominant vessel. If you would try to open up all the other occluded vessels, the streptokinase concentration would be too high.

In two patients we observed a pericardial hemorrhage which was indicated by tachycardia during the lytic therapy. In both, the pericardial effusion was documented by echocardiography. Both patients had operative drainage and thereafter an uneventful recovery. Other complications were not seen, especially no bleeding complications. No patient demonstrated on the ECG signs of a new myocardial infarction. All patients were put on anticoagulation therapy. Three months after

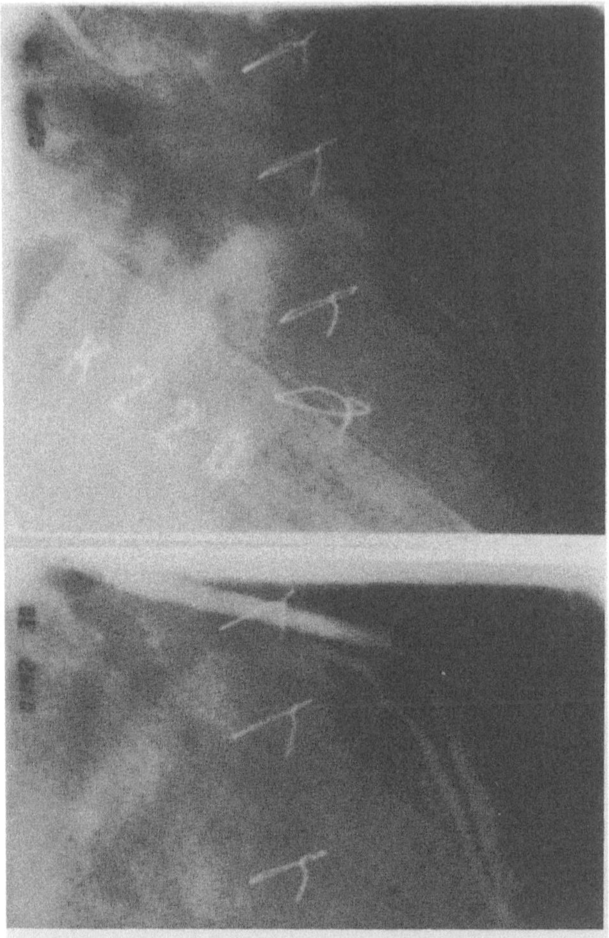

Fig. 3. Patient RU: after 220 and 260 min of streptokinase infusion the natural coronary system is filled via the vein but there is still quite a lot of thrombotic material along the vein wall

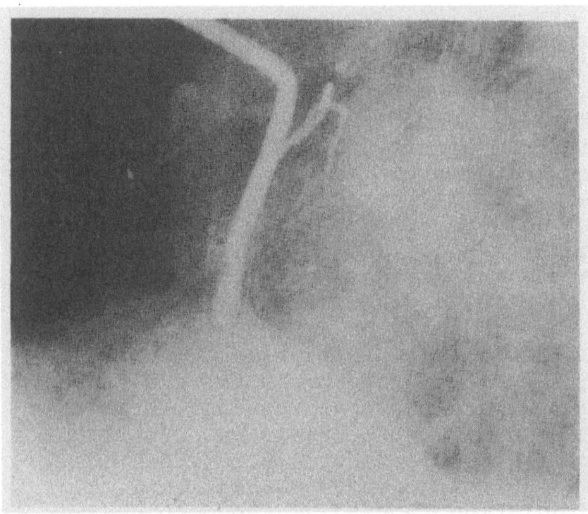

Fig. 4. Patient RU: control angiography 1 day after reopening of the occluded bypass; by streptokinase the thrombotic material has disappeared

Table 2. Results and complications of treatment of postoperative occluded vein grafts

Name	State before lyse		State after lyse		Complications
R.U.	LAD	occl.	LAD	open	
	R. marg.	occl.	R. marg.	occl.	Pericardial tamponade
	PLA	open	PLA	open	
R.W.	PLA	occl.	PLA	open	
L.A.	RCA	occl.	RCA	open	Pericardial tamponade
N.L.	LAD	occl.	LAD	open	
	RCA	occl.	RCA	occl.	
L.R.	LAD	occl.	LAD	open	
	RD	open	RD	open	
L.F.	LAD	occl.	LAD	open	
	CX	occl.	CX	open	
	2 grafts open		2 grafts open		
	9 grafts occl.		7 grafts reopened		
			2 grafts occl.		

the revision every patient had reangiography. All of the seven reopened vein grafts were still open. All the remaining thrombotic material was entirely dissolved. The course of all vein grafts looked perfect.

All great patient groups restudied after 1 to 2 weeks after coronary revascularization demonstrate a graft occlusion rate of 8%-13% (1, 2). By most authors the reason for early graft occlusion is seen in technical mistakes. Therefore no report exists in the literature in which anyone tried to open up occluded vein grafts. An occluded graft has been accepted by the physician and reoperation was only considered if medical medication failed to provide pain relief (3).

With the new method presented here of applying a lytic drug into the occluded graft the possibility exists of opening up occluded vein grafts. Before using this method, the diagnosis of occlusion has to be established. A new pain attack after operation might be the best indicator, but only a small part of patients will suffer angina during bed rest. Therefore more sensitive diagnostic methods have to be elaborated in the future. Maybe the scintigraphic methods applied during rest and stress after operation may help us to find out in which patient the bypass vein is open and in which one it is occluded.

The method used here works only under the condition that the aortic and coronary anastomoses are performed without any technical mistake. The reason for early postoperative graft closure might be clotting disorders, but the real cause is unknown. If technical problems would be the cause, the grafts would reocclude again.

In conclusion, early revision of occluded vein grafts is possible. We prefer doing this with streptokinase. By applying this drug directly to the occluded vein grafts the possibility exists, if the time course is not too long, to dissolve the occluding thrombus. According to our experience the vein grafts so treated stay open.

References

1. Bourassa MG, Lespêrance J, Campeau L, Simard P (1972) Factors influencing patency of aortocoronary vein grafts. Circulation [Suppl 1] 45:79
2. Fowler BN, Jacobs ML, Zir L, Dinsmore RE, Vezeridis MP, Daggett WM (1980) Late graft patency and symptom relief after aortocoronary bypass. J Thorac Cardiovasc Surg 79:288
3. Jrarrazaval MJ, Cosgrove DM, Loop FD, Ennix CL, Groves LK, Taylor PC (1977) Reoperations for myocardial revascularization. J Thorac Cardiovasc Surg 73:181
4. Kaltenbach M (1975) Quantitative Bewertung koronaro-graphischer Befunde mit Hilfe eines Punktsystems (Score). Z Kardiol 64:597

Surgical Treatment of Acute Myocardial Infarction (AMI) Complicated by Septal Rupture (VSR)

G. Semb, N. B. Fjeld, O. Geiran, V. Hansteen, R. Hol, H. Karlsen, E. Sivertssen, E. Søyland, and Østerrud*

The case material consists of 16 patients, 11 men and 5 women, with a mean age of 60 years, suffering manifest shock or preshock from AMI, complicated 1-28 days (average, 9 days) later by VSR. Preoperative IABP was necessary in 11 patients. All were studied by right heart catheterization, left ventricular angiography, and selective coronary angiography. Eleven patients had extensive anteroseptal and five inferior septal AMI with extensive infarction of the right ventricle. All were operated on in the acute stage and had resection of AMI and patch closure of VSR with a special technique. In addition eight patients had 16 aortocoronary bypasses. Fifteen patients needed postoperative IABP for 2-10 days. Ten of the anteroseptal AMI patients survived the operation and eight of these are long-term survivors. All the inferior septal AMI patients died in the postoperative period due to multiple organ failure from irreversible cardiogenic shock. The hemodynamic studies show normalization of all parameters and all survivors enjoy a normal life.

Critically ill patients in cardiogenic shock or preshock from AMI complicated by VSR can be treated surgically with good long-term survival if the lesions are anteroseptal. IABP is of great importance if the patient is to survive.

*Division of Cardiovascular Surgery, Ullevaal Hospital, University of Oslo, Oslo, Norway

Session IV Vascular Surgery

Combined Disease of the Aorto-iliac and Femoro-popliteal Arteries

Chairman: M. Vink, Leiden; Co-Chairman: J. Vollmar, Ulm

Femoral Artery Doppler Waveform Analysis in the Assessment of Combined Iliac and Femoral Artery Disease

P.C. Clifford, R. Skidmore, J.P. Woodcock, D.R. Bird, R.J. Lusby, and R.N. Baird*

Introduction

The functional assessment of incomplete stenosis of the iliac arteries using Doppler ultrasound has developed because routine arteriography may not identify the severity and extent of the occlusive atherosclerosis. The results of both proximal (1, 2) and distal (3) reconstruction can be poor and this has led to the search for better methods of preoperative assessment.

Invasive preoperative tests which predict the presence of X-ray underestimated lesions have failed to gain acceptance. Non invasive Doppler ultrasound studies of the common femoral artery have been used to detect proximal stenosis using pulsatility index (PI) (4, 5) and other techniques of wave-form analysis (6, 7). But in the presence of multisegment disease the accuracy of iliac artery assessment has remained poor. In this study we report the early clinical results using a new technique of Doppler wave-form analysis, termed LT (Laplace transform) damping, to detect iliac stenosis.

Clinical Methods

Two hundred and sixty-three lower limbs of 135 subjects (94 male and 41 female) were studied. Angiographic comparison with Doppler wave-form analysis was possible in 125 limbs of patients with peripheral vascular disease. Femoral artery Doppler wave-form analysis was also performed on 138 limbs of volunteers with no clinical evidence of arterial disease and Doppler ankle/brachial systolic indices of more than 0.98.

Studies were performed in an electrically screened, temperature controlled (21 ± 1°C) laboratory after a 10-min equilibration period. Femoral artery signals were obtained from supine subjects using a 10 MHz continuous wave directional Doppler flowmeter (Fig. 1). To avoid artefacts associated with zero-crossing signal processing the blood maximum velocity/time wave-forms were obtained using a maximum frequency follower constructed in the laboratory. On-line computer calculation of Laplace transform solutions and pulsatility index was performed using a MINC-II digital computer. Due to normal physiological variation between heart beats a 10-consecutive beat average value of LT and PI was calculated.

*Departments of Surgery and Medical Physics, Bristol Royal Infirmary, Bristol BS2 8HW, Great Britain

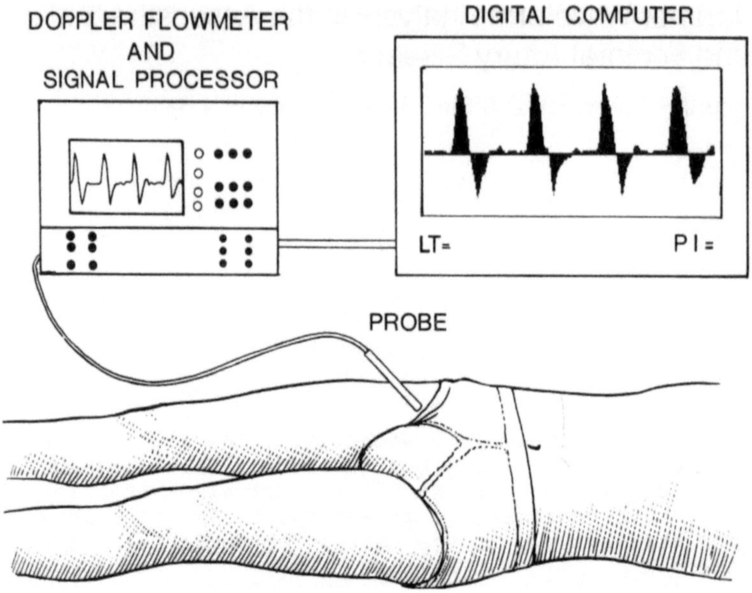

Fig. 1. A 10 MHz Doppler flowmeter and maximum frequency follower were connected to a MINC-II digital computer for on-line calculation of LT damping and PI

The Doppler flowmeter, signal processor and on-line computer produced highly reproducible results in both normal volunteers and patients with arterial disease.

Angiography

Either translumbar or transfemoral aortograms were performed in patients undergoing investigation of arterial disease. Most studies were in a single plane but later biplanar views were obtained. Each was scored independently by two surgeons and one radiologist who made an estimation of stenosis by taking the diameter of the narrowest segment and expressing it as a percentage of the diameter of the nearest normal segment.

Laplace Transform Damping (LT Damping) Derivation

Characterisation of the Doppler wave-form shape by a minimum of parameters reflecting the underlying physiological influence (distal impedance, proximal lumen diameter and arterial wall stiffness) was obtained recently (8). By regarding the arterial pulse as an independent transient phenomenon it is possible to obtain its Fourier transform and by computer aided curve fitting techniques the equivalent Laplace transform.

The three solutions of the cubic equation below

$$\text{Laplace transform } H(s) = \frac{1}{(s^2 + 2\delta w_o s + w_o^2)\ (s + \gamma)}$$

can be expressed graphically (Fig. 2).

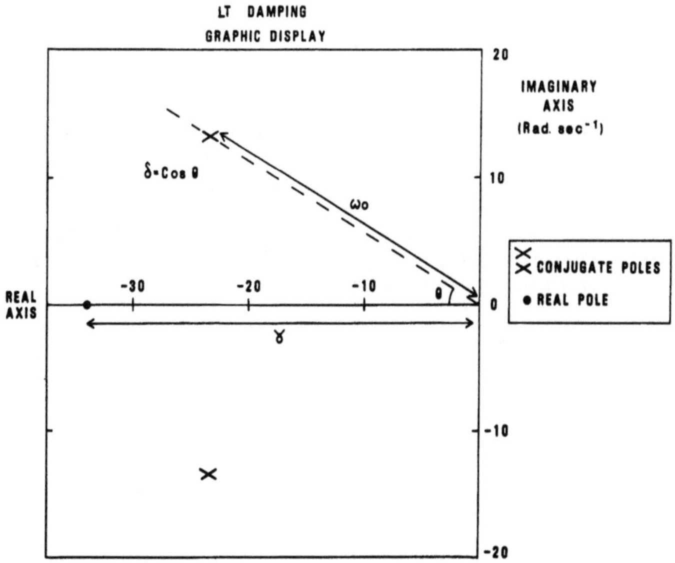

Fig. 2. The solutions of the transfer function equation are displayed on an argand diagram. LT damping δ is calculated from cos θ. w_o relates to arterial wall stiffness and γ to peripheral resistance

The position of the composite conjugate poles, in relation to the two axes, provides a measure related to proximal lumen diameter and arterial stiffness, while the third, the real pole, reflects the degree of peripheral resistance (9-13).

This analytical method has been termed transfer function analysis, and calculation of the damping effect (LT damping δ) of proximal stenoses is made from the position of the conjugate poles. LT damping, increases to unity with increasing lumen stenosis, and values in the region of 0.90-1.0 are associated with total occlusion.

Pulsatility index (PI) was calculated simultaneously using the formula:

$$PI = \frac{\text{Peak to peak velocity}}{\text{Mean velocity}} \quad (4, 5).$$

Comparison of LT Damping and PI

In comparing the results of LT and PI damping, sensitivity and specificity were calculated using receiver operator characteristic (ROC) curves. These were obtained from data of patients undergoing angiography, which was used as the standard. Angiographically significant stenosis was defined as a reduction in vessel diameter by at least 50% equivalent to a cross-sectional area reduction of 75%-80%. An estimation of the true positive and false positive rate in detecting lesions >50% using stepwise "threshold cirteria" of PI and LT damping was plotted on an ROC display. This enabled a comparison of sensitivity and specificity of the two tests without reference to one arbitrary standard.

Results

Normals (138 limbs)

The complex pole, LT damping, had a small range for the 138 age-grouped normal limbs and showed minimal change with age from 0.31 ± 0.04 to 0.37 ± 0.08 (mean ± SD) (Table 1). The normal range was therefore defined as 0.20 ± 0.45 (2 SD about the mean). PI, however, varied widely in these individuals and the mean increased with age from 8.9 ± 3.4 for young normals to 11.8 ± 5.3 subjects aged 50 years and over. The lower limit of normal PI was 3.0 (mean - 2 SD) (Table 1).

Table 1.

Normals (age)	LT damping (M ± SD)	PI (M ± SD)
Under 30	0.31 ±0.04	8.9 ± 3.4
30-39	0.32 ±0.58	9.1 ± 2.5
40-49	0.35 ±0.66	9.5 ± 3.8
50-59	0.33 ±0.06	11.9 ± 4.4
60 and over	0.37 ±0.08	11.8 ± 5.3
Overall	0.33 ±0.06	11.8 ± 4.4

Iliac Artery Stenosis (125 limbs)

Of 65 patients examined following TLA, results from 125 limbs were obtained. These limbs were divided into two groups by arteriographic estimation of iliac stenosis. Sixty-three limbs had 50% or more stenosis and 62 had less than 50%. Twenty-five limbs showed 90% stenosis or were totally occluded. Occlusion of the superficial femoral artery was noted in 65 limbs.

There was a steady increase in LT damping values with increase in percent iliac artery lumen stenosis. The normal controls and each patient group were significantly separated from adjacent groups and there was a highly significant difference between age matched normals and patients with early disease (⩽50% stenosis) $\underline{P} = <0.001$ t test) (Fig. 3). LT damping results lying outside the normal range detected the presence of iliac stenosis in 90% of angiographically positive lesions while with pulsatility index only 23% of lesions fell outside the normal range. Patients with >50% stenosis had LT damping of 0.78 ± 0.16 (mean ± SD) and those with ⩽50% 0.50 ± 0.15, whereas PI values for both patient groups fell within the normal range, ⩽50% PI = 7.4 ± 4.2 and >50% PI = 3.6 ± 1.6 (Fig. 4). LT damping results were not affected in 65 limbs by occlusion of the superficial femoral artery and the good correlation (r = -0.73) with iliac stenosis was unchanged. PI, however, was not correlated with iliac stenosis in the presence of distal occlusion (r = 0.51).

ROC Analysis

The relationship of sensitivity and specificity for the two types of wave-form analysis in detecting 50% stenosis or greater was calculated using ROC curves (Fig. 5). At a threshold value of 0.6 LT damping was

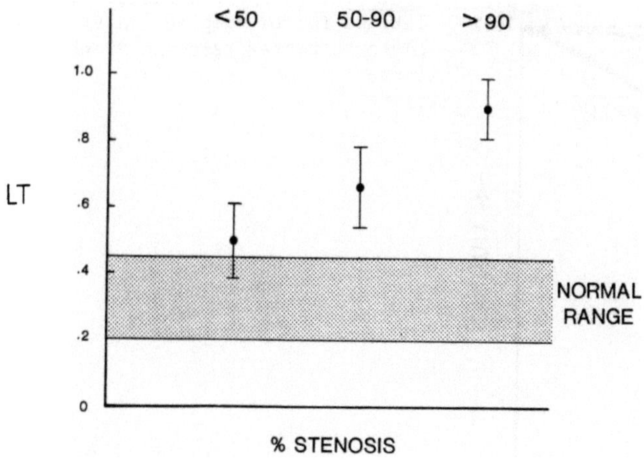

Fig. 3. Femoral artery LT damping (mean ± SD) increases with progressive iliac artery percent stenosis

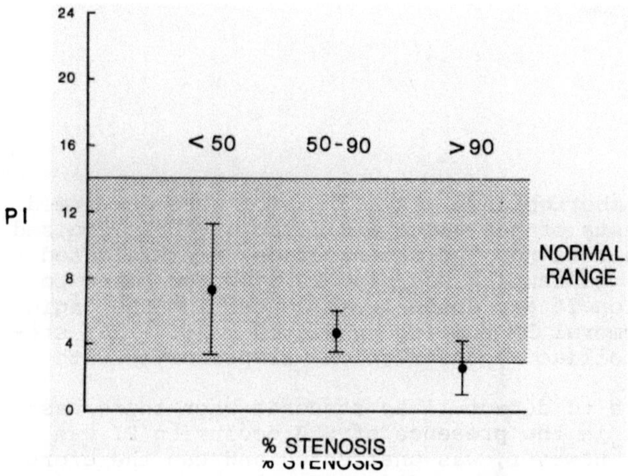

Fig. 4. Femoral PI (mean ± SD) was widely variable and most values fell within the normal range. Only 23% of results in diseased patients were less than the lower limit of normal

the better test and was 85% sensitive and 84% specific while PI (threshold 3) was insensitive (41%) but had a specificity of 94%, the worse test. At other threshold values LT damping always had a higher sensitivity for any given specificity than PI.

Illustrative Case (Fig. 6)

This case illustrates a 65-year-old man with left lower limb rest pain. Calf pulse volume recordings confirmed the presence of severe limb ischaemia. Translumbar aortography revealed an occluded SFA with borderline evidence of proximal disease. Wave-form analysis suggested significant iliac disease (LT damping 0.80). On the basis of this result a proximal reconstruction was performed. Intraoperatively there was a tight iliac stenosis of 2 mm confirming the value of wave-form analysis. An aortobifemoral bypass was performed resulting in postoperative relief of rest pain and claudication.

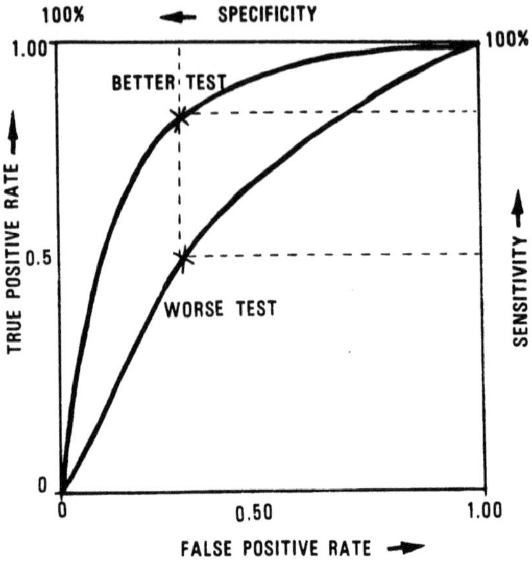

Fig. 5. Stylised ROC curce. Calculations for LT damping and PI showed LT to be better test and PI the worse

Discussion

Arteriography has various shortcomings (14, 15) which were confirmed in this study by taking casts of the aorta and iliac arteries excised during surgery. More often than not the arteriograms underestimated the extent of the disease. LT damping was used in selected cases to aid in the clinical decision if any doubt arose concerning the angiographic appearances. If femoral LT damping predicted major iliac stenosis then a proximal aortoiliac reconstruction was performed with good results.

Both LT and PI were able to detect iliac stenosis when there was a patent distal system but in the presence of SFA occlusion PI was rendered useless (16). LT, however, was unaffected and can therefore be used to assess the input to a proposed femoropopliteal graft as well as to establish that an imcomplete iliac stenosis on X-ray is severe enough to indicate that proximal reconstruction will improve foot perfusion. Although it is only sometimes necessary to implant arterial grafts from the aorta or common iliac artery to popliteal level (17, 18), it should be possible to identify these cases preoperatively with this method.

Preoperative invasive testing by femoral artery pressure measurement during arteriography (15, 19) has failed to gain wide acceptance but non invasive studies are advocated by some authors (2, 6, 20). However, their sensitivity to iliac stenoses has not been fully established.

The ability of LT damping and PI to distinguish the degree of iliac stenosis was tested using ROC curves. These give an independent estimate of the quality of each test. LT damping is much the better test and using a value of 0.6 it was a highly sensitive and specific method of distinguishing stenoses of 50% or more from minor stenoses ($\leq$50%). Using a lower limit of normal 3, PI was insensitive although an individual patient with a PI value <3 has a high chance of having disease (specificity 93%).

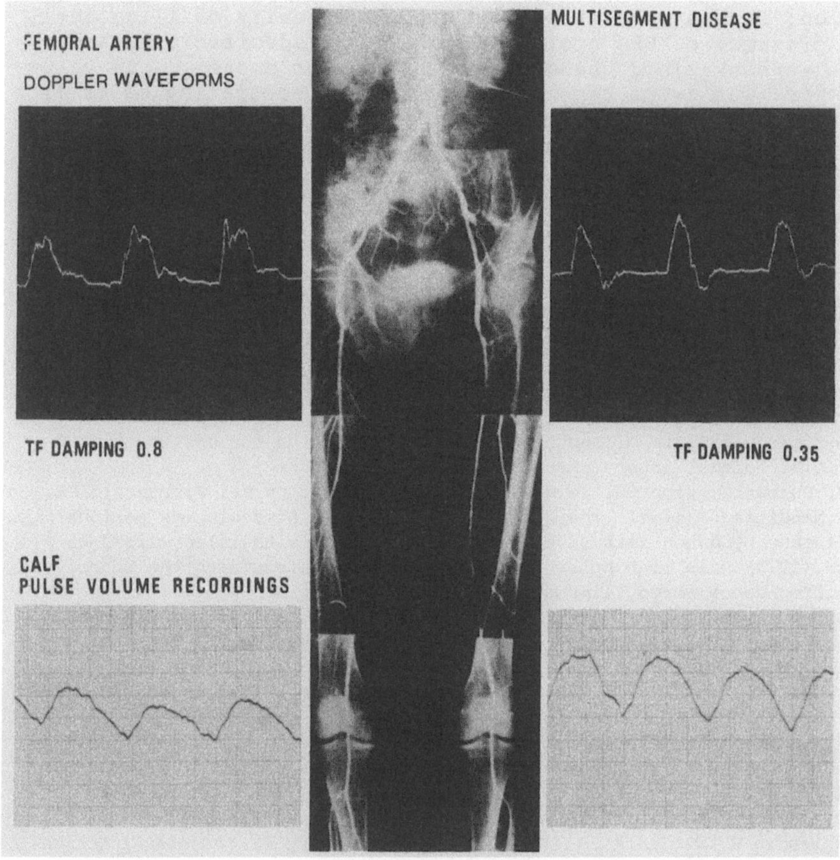

Fig. 6. Translumbar aortogram, pulse volume recordings, and femoral wave-form analysis from a 65-year-old man with left leg rest pain. The arteriogram underestimated an iliac stenosis of 2 mm found at surgery but LT damping (0.8) predicted a severe stenosis

In conclusion these early clinical results suggest that LT damping is a more accurate test than PI for the detection of iliac stenosis. LT damping and other haemodynamic tests may prove to be important complementary techniques to arteriography in the assessment of aorto-iliac disease.

Summary

The functional significance of iliac artery stenosis was assessed non invasively using femoral artery Doppler signals and a new method of blood velocity wave-form quantification. This method, transfer function (LT) analysis, was compared with pulsatility index (PI) on 263 limbs, in patients with iliac occlusive atherosclerosis demonstrated by arteriogram and in normal volunteers. Normal LT damping results ranged from 0.2 to 0.45 with detection of minor iliac stenosis (⩽50%) at 0.50 ± 0.15 and major stenosis (>50%) at 0.78 ± 0.16. LT damping was not affected by raised distal impedance associated with superficial femoral artery

(SFA) occlusion. PI was poor at predicting the severity of iliac lesions in the presence of SFA occlusion. LT and PI specificities and sensitivities were examined using receiver operator curves. At a value of 0.6 LT damping was twice as sensitive as PI in separating major from minor iliac stenoses. This preliminary experience with LT damping analysis suggests that it will reduce the difficulties in the assessment of iliac stenosis in some cases.

References

1. Baird RJ, Feldman P, Miles JT, Madras PM, Gurry JF (1977) Subsequent downstream repair after aorto-iliac and aorto-femoral bypass operations. Surgery 82:785-793
2. Sumner DS, Strandness DE (1978) Aortoiliac reconstruction in patients with combined iliac and superficial femoral arterial occlusion. Surgery 84:348-355
3. Charlesworth D, Harris PL, Cave FD (1975) Undetected aortoiliac insufficiency: a reason for early failure of saphenous vein bypass grafts for obstruction of the superficial femoral artery. Br J Surg 62:567-570
4. Gosling RG, Dunbar G, King DH, Newman DL, Side CD, Woodcock JP, Fitzgerald DE, Keates JS, MacMillan D (1971) The quantitative analysis of occlusive peripheral arterial disease by a non intrusive ultrasonic technique. Angiology 22:52-55
5. Johnston KW (1978) Role of Doppler ultrasonography in determining the haemodynamic significance of aorto iliac disease. Can J Surg 21:319-325
6. Fronek A, Coel M, Berstein EF (1978) The importance of combined multisegmental pressure and Doppler flow velocity in the diagnosis of peripheral arterial occlusive disease. Surgery 84:840-947
7. Blackshear WM, Phillips DJ, Chikos PM, Harley JD, Thiele BL, Strandness DE (1980) Carotid artery velocity patterns in normal and stenotic vessels. Stroke 11:67-71
8. Skidmore R, Woodcock JP (1978) Physiological significance of arterial models derived using transcutaneous ultrasonic flowmeters. J Physiol (Lond) 277:29P-30P
9. Skidmore R, Bird DR, Woodcock JP, Davies PW, Baird RN (1979) Transfer function analysis of common femoral artery Doppler waveforms. Br J Surg 66:883
10. Bird DR, Skidmore R, Woodcock JP (1980) The value of Doppler transfer function analysis in the diagnosis of aorto-iliac occlusive arterial disease. In: Baird RN, Woodcock JP (eds) Diagnosis and monitoring in arterial surgery. Wright, Bristol, pp 121-126
11. Skidmore R, Woodcock JP (1980) Physiological interpretation of Doppler-shift waveforms. 1. Theoretical considerations. Ultrasound Med Biol 6:7-10
12. Skidmore R, Woodcock JP (to be published) Physiological interpretation of Doppler-shift waveforms. 2. Validation of the Laplace transform method for characterisation of the common femoral blood velocity/time waveform. Ultrasound Med Biol
13. Skidmore R, Woodcock JP, Wells PNT, Bird DR, Baird RN (to be published) Physiological interpretation of Doppler-shift waveforms. 3. Clinical Results. Ultrasound Med Biol
14. Moore WS, Hall AD (1971) Unrecognised aorto-iliac stenosis: a physiologic approach to the diagnosis. Arch Surg 103:633-638
15. Udoff EJ, Barth KH, Harrington DP, Kaufman SL, White RI (1979) Hemodynamic significance of iliac artery stenosis: pressure measurements during angiography. Radiology 132:289-293
16. Barrie WE, Evans DH, Bell PRF (1979) The relationship between pulsatility index and proximal arterial stenosis (Abstract). Br J Surg 66:366
17. Dardik H, Ibrahim IM, Harrah M, Sussman B, Dardik L (1979) Synchronous aorto femoral or iliofemoral bypass with revascularisation of the lower extremity. Surg Gynecol Obstet 149:676-680
18. Horton RE, Giddings AEB, Parkes AC (1979) Iliopopliteal dacron grafts as an alternative to amputation. Ann R Coll Surg Engl 61:217-218
19. Leveson SH, Guillou PJ, Terry HJ, Glanville JN, Kester RC (1978) Pulse pressure wave analysis in the diagnosis of aorto-iliac disease. Ann Surg 187:161-165
20. Kempczinski RF, Rutherford RB (1978) Current status of the vascular diagnostic laboratory. In: Rob C (ed) Advanves in surgery, vol 12. Year Book Medical, Chicago, pp 1-52

Numerate Doppler Analysis in the Determination of the Aortoiliac Component of Multilevel Arterial Disease

P. Kitslaar and J. Talmon*

Introduction and Purpose

Distal to an arterial obstruction a diminished *systolic blood pressure* and a less *pulsatile character* of the blood flow can be found (7). Also the *transit time* of the pulse wave over an obstructed segment may be changed, although not so much by degree of stenosis as by changes in vessel wall stiffness or degree of collateral bypass of a total occlusion (4). All these indicators of obstruction can be determined noninvasively with the aid of ultrasonic Doppler equipment. They can be expressed in an objective numerical way and might be called "Doppler parameters".

Information about the condition of the aortoiliac or proximal inflow segment of the leg can be gathered by measurement of the systolic blood pressure below the groin, using a thigh cuff and Doppler meter and by wave form analysis of the Doppler signal of the femoral artery (2, 3). By the simultaneous use of two Doppler probes, one over the aorta and one over the femoral artery, a pulse transit time can be found over the aortoiliac segment. The aim of this study was to determine the relative value of a variety of Doppler parameters in the quantification of aortoiliac obstructions as defined by angiography.

Method

Patients and young healthy volunteers underwent a physical vascular examination, their systolic thigh/brachial pressure indices and aortofemoral pulse transit times were measured, and Doppler signals from their femoral arteries were recorded under resting and hyperemic conditions for subsequent numerate analysis. Some criteria for significant aortoiliac obstruction were derived from all thus-collected parameters and their value in correctly predicting angiographic obstructions was analyzed.

Studied Population

The 100 legs of 10 healthy students (mean age 27 years) and of 40 patients with uni- or bilateral ischemic leg symptoms, all undergoing aortography (mean age 61 years), were studied.

---

*Dept. of Surgery, St. Antoniushospital, J.V.Scorelstraat 2, Utrecht, The Netherlands

Angiographic Score

The single plane aortographies were coded in a so-called *angioscore*. Both the aortoiliac or inflow segment and the outflow vessels in the leg got a score from 0 to 100. For the inflow segment this corresponded with the highest percentage diameter stenosis of the subsegments of aorta, common iliac, or external iliac artery. For the outflow vessels it depended on the condition of the profound and the superficial femoral artery and of the popliteal and crural vessels. Legs in which the common femoral artery had over 50% stenosis were excluded from the study. As well for the inflow as for the outflow segment, an angioscore of over 50 was considered as significant obstruction. The legs of the healthy students – who, of course, had no angiography – got an angioscore of 0 for both the inflow and outflow segments.

Clinical Parameters

The strength of the femoral pulse was determined and graded from 3 (normal) to 0 (nonpalpable). The presence of bruits over iliac or femoral vessels was noted.

Pressure Measurement

The thigh pressure was measured using a pneumatic cuff with an inflatable bladder of 52 x 18 cm placed as near to the groin as possible while the Doppler probe was positioned over a pedal artery. The pressure was given as an index of thigh over brachial pressure.

Hyperemia Test

Femoral Doppler signals were recorded under resting as well as post-occlusion hyperemic condition (5). This last one was created by supra-systolic cuff occlusion at thigh level during 5 min. At 1 and 3 min after release of the cuff the registrations were made.

Doppler Signal Analysis

The audio signals, fully separated into forward and reverse flow components, from a CW Doppler meter (Sonicaid BV 380) were converted to a wave form by spectrum analysis and displayed as a sonagram (Fig. 1). For the femoral artery 7.6 MHz equipment was used and for the aorta 3.7 MHz. The sonagram was analyzed in two different ways. First it got a *sonoscore* by simple visual classification after Thulesius and Gjöres (8). This results in a score from 3 (bi- or trifasic pattern, including reverse) to 0 (nonrecordable).

Also *numerate signal parameters* were derived from each sonagram. To this purpose its maximum frequency envelopes were digitized and fed into a computer which calculated the following ten signal derivatives: maximum forward (F) and reverse (R) frequency, the quotient R/F, the mean height of the forward frequency envelope (M), the acceleration and deceleration times of the systolic peak, the quotient F/M, the pulsatility index (PI) after Gosling and King (4), and the percentages of each cycle without forward flow and of simultaneous forward and reverse flow. Thus for each leg a total of 30 numerate signal parameters were available from signals at rest and during hyperemia.

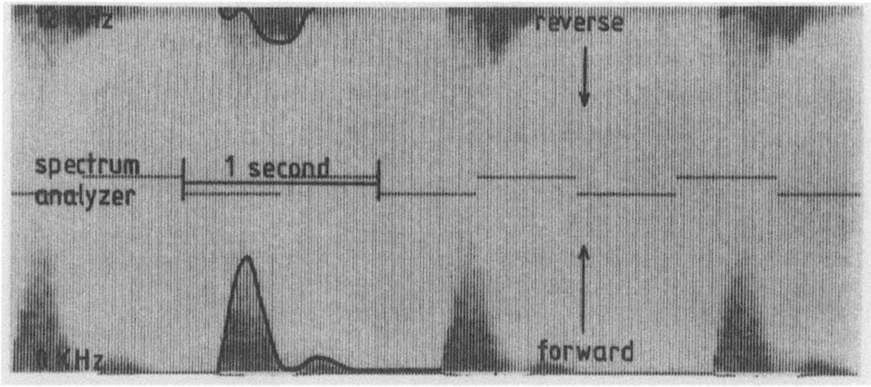

Fig. 1. Sonagram display of a directional Doppler signal of a normal femoral artery, showing four successive heart-beat cycles. The maximum frequency envelopes of the forward (bottom) and reverse (top) component of the second beat have been drawn in this sonagram

Pulse Transit Time

The forward components of an aortic and femoral signal, simultaneously taken with two Doppler probes, were displayed in one sonagram. The foot-foot distances of five consecutive systolic peaks were averaged, giving the transit time of the pulse wave in ms (1, 4).

Criteria Selection

The large number of numerate signal parameters had to be reduced to simplify further analysis. Only that one derivative was selected which gave the best separation between proximal aortoiliac obstruction and patency and was least influenced by the condition of the outflow vessels.

For the selection of the criteria for significant aortoiliac obstruction, all legs were divided into one group with a proximal angioscore of 0-50 ("patent") and another group with a proximal angioscore of 51-100 ("obstructed"). The proportional occurrence of pulsation scores and bruits and of sonoscores as well as means and standard deviations of both thigh pressure index and the selected signal derivative were calculated for each group. The criteria for significant obstruction were derived from the values of the obstructed legs. For the thigh pressure index and the selected signal derivative a dividing line was taken at the mean value plus one standard deviation; for the two scores this line was drawn in such a way that at least two-thirds of the legs with a proximal angioscore above 50 would meet this criterion.

Results

Numerate Doppler Signal Parameter

For none of the 30 computer-calculated signal derivatives was a significant difference found between values for legs with or without outflow obstruction. The best separation between proximal aortoiliac obstruction and patency was possible with the pulsatility index during hyperemia, 3 min after release of the thigh occlusion ($PI_{3'}$). This parameter was the one selected for further evaluation.

Pulse Transit Time

Often a reliable Doppler signal of the aorta was unobtainable due to obesity, bowel movements, or abdominal scars. In 16% of the cases a transit time could not be calculated at all due to these problems. The correlation of the transit time – normalized for age and mean blood pressure (4) – with the proximal angioscores was very poor (Fig. 2). Therefore the transit time was not considered for further evaluation.

Criteria for Significant Aortoiliac Obstruction

The means and standard deviations of thigh pressure indices and $PI_{3'}$, and the proportional occurrences of subnormal pulsation scores and sonoscores for the two proximal angioscore groups are given in Table 1.

The criteria for significant aortoiliac obstruction follow directly from it and are given in Table 2. Only one addition was made: pulsation score 2 is only considered as indicative of significant obstruction if it is found together with a pelvic or femoral bruit.

Application of the Criteria

The criteria were tested for their usefulness by classifying all legs by means of the criteria as legs with and without supposed significant aortoiliac obstruction. The results were compared with the angiography which was considered as the "gold standard". For each criterion the

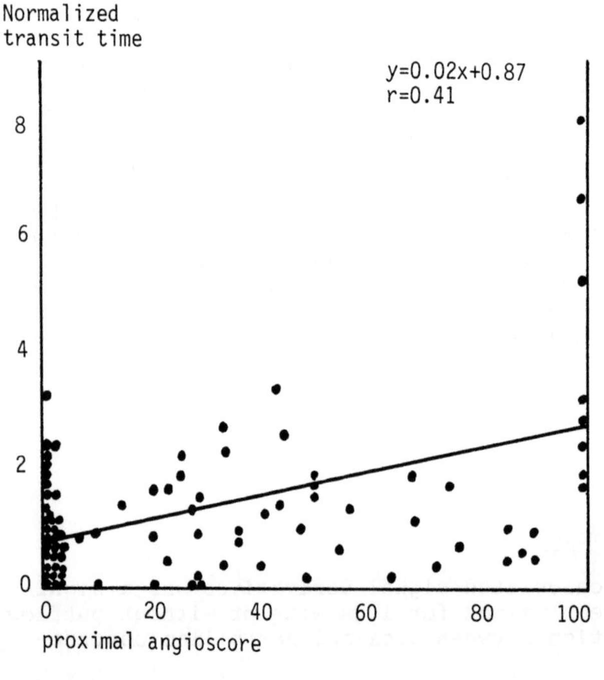

Fig. 2. Correlation between aortofemoral transit times – normalized for age and mean blood pressure after Gosling and King (4) – and proximal angiographic scores

number of correct classifications, of the false positives and of the false negatives was calculated and expressed in terms of accuracy, specificity, and sensitivity (6). The results are given in Table 3. The diagnostic value of the $PI_{3'}$ criterion in predicting aortoiliac obstruction was also calculated separately for legs with and without angiographic outflow vessel obstruction. These results are given in Table 4.

Table 1. Proportional occurrence of subnormal pulsation and Doppler sonoscores and means ± standard deviations of thigh pressure indices and pulsatility indices ($PI_{3'}$) for legs with proximal angioscores ⩽50 and for legs with proximal angioscores >50

Parameters	Proximal angiographic score ⩽50	>50
Pulsation score ⩽2	9%	75%
Doppler sonoscore ⩽2	6%	71%
Thigh pressure index	1.00 ± 0.14	0.62 ± 0.20
Pulsatility index ($PI_{3'}$)	14.7 ± 9.9	3.9 ± 3.0

Table 2. Clinical and Doppler criteria and their values indicating significant aortoiliac obstruction

Criterion	Values
Femoral pulsation score	0-1-2 (with bruit)
Thigh pressure index	⩽0.82
Femoral sonoscore	⩽2
Femoral pulsatility index	⩽6.9

Table 3. Diagnostic value – expressed as accuracy, specificity, and sensitivity percentages – of the criteria for aortoiliac obstruction in comparison to the angiography

Criterion	Accuracy	Specificity	Sensitivity
Pulsation score	89	93	77
Thigh pressure index	88	90	81
Sonoscore	86	90	79
Pulsatility index	85	84	88

Table 4. Diagnostic value – expressed as accuracy, specificity, and sensitivity percentages – of the femoral pulsatility index criterion for aortoiliac obstruction ($PI_{3'}$) in comparison to the angiography and the influence of outflow vessel obstruction on it

Outflow obstruction	Accuracy	Specificity	Sensitivity
No	92	94	86
Yes	71	57	85

Discussion

The results of this study show that the noninvasive detection of significant aortoiliac obstructions is quite well possible with the help of Doppler parameters. The femoral pulsatility index reaches the highest sensitivity, which means that it does not easily miss the pathology of clinical importance in the aortoiliac pathway. On the other hand it does have a reduced specificity, so it seems to attribute pathology to legs which have no significant stenosis on angiography. This might be explained by the well-known fact that single plane aortographies underestimate the severity of aortoiliac lesions, which consequently might be better discovered by numerate analysis of the femoral Doppler signal. However, Table 4 shows that the diagnostic specificity of this signal derivative is considerably reduced (indicating a high number of false positive test results) when the outflow vessels of the femoral artery have obstructions. This suggests that the femoral Doppler pulsatility index is influenced by pathology in both the inflow and the outflow vessels of the femoral artery. So it seems to suffer from the same limitation for the noninvasive diagnosis of aortoiliac obstruction which was already known for the thigh pressure measurement (2). The transit time measurement could not be found of value in quantifying the degree of aortoiliac obstruction.

References

1. Craxford AD, Chamberlain J (1977) Pulse wave form transit ratios in the assessment of peripheral vascular disease. Br J Surg 64:449-452
2. Faris IB, Jamieson CW (1975) The diagnosis of aorto-iliac stenosis: A comparison of thigh pressure measurement and femoral artery flow velocity profile. J Cardiovasc Surg 16:597-602
3. Fronek A, Coel M, Bernstein EF (1978) The importance of combined multisegmental pressure and Doppler flow velocity studies in the diagnosis of peripheral arterial occlusive disease. Surgery 84:840-847
4. Gosling R, King DH (1974) Continuous wave ultrasound as an alternative and complement to X-rays in vascular examinations. In: Reneman RS (ed) Cardiovascular applications of ultrasound. North-Holland, Amsterdam London, pp 266-282
5. Hummel BW, Hummel BA, Mowbry A, Maixner W, Barnes RW (1978) Reactive hyperemia vs treadmill exercise testing in arterial disease. Arch Surg 113:95-98
6. McNeil BJ, Keeler E, Adelstein SJ (1975) Primer on certain elements of medical decision making. N Engl J Med 293:211-215
7. Strandness DE, Sumner DS (1975) Hemodynamics for surgeons. Grune & Stratton, New York San Francisco London, pp 73-119
8. Thulesius O, Gjöres JE (1971) Use of Doppler shift detection for determining peripheral arterial blood pressures. Angiology 22:594-603

Principles of Surgery in Combined Aorto-iliac and Femoropopliteal Occlusive Lesions

B. Heyden, J. Vollmer, and E. U. Voss*

In chronic arterial occlusive disease approximately 75% of all symptomatic patients have multiple arterial lesions in more than one level, classified as ABC. Under all combined lesions the proximale *"two level occlusions"* have undoubtedly the greatest surgical importance. The surgical approach to these combined aortoiliac and femoropopliteal lesions is still controversial and under discussion.

Some vascular surgeons still prefer *total repair* not only of both arterial segments in one or two stages but also of concomitant lesions below the knee. The other approach includes *partial repair*, i.e., revascularization only of the aortoiliac segment in combination with profundoplasty and lumbar sympathectomy. This is a lesser extensive intervention which may be called *triad procedure*. Comparing both surgical approaches a retrospective evaluation of 620 operative interventions was undertaken.

Group I: *Total correction of both segments*. This was the preferred procedure up to 1973. This group includes 72 limbs of 69 patients with a follow-up rate of 91%.

Group II: The *triad procedure* includes 548 limbs of 347 patients with a follow-up rate of 94%.

The *cumulative patency rate* based on the life-table analysis after 9 years was 34% for group I *(total repair)* and 75% for group II *(partial repair)*. This significant difference was also true for limb salvage procedure (stage III and IV). In operations for claudication (stage II) reocclusion occurred in 37% of group I but only 7% of group II.

Recurrent occlusion after total repair (group I) concerned predominantly the femoropopliteal segment. The difference in *reocclusion rate* was even more pronounced in patients who were operated on in stages III and IV. In addition, the *rate of major amputations* following interventions for limb salvage was 30% for group I and 9% for group II.

Following *limb salvage operations*, 38% of the extremities in group II returned to stage I (asymptomatic) and 53% to stage II (mild rest claudications). In 11% of operated patients, revascularization via profundoplasty proved insufficient, necessitating an additional long bypass graft below the knee.

In 52 patients of group II intraoperative electromagnetic *flow measurements* were performed. There was a remarkable increase of flow rate in the deep femoral artery following profundoplasty (126%) and an additional augmentation of 62% immediately after lumbar sympathectomy. Up to now it is unknown if this phenomenon is a persisting one or represents only a transitory hemodynamic effect. Pre- and postoperative volume plethysmography show a continuous increase of *peak flow* up to 24 weeks after operation.

The results of profundoplasty with lumbar sympathectomy but *without reconstruction* of the iliac segment are less favourable: there is a relatively quick decrease of cumulative patency rate up to the ninth post-

*Chirurgische Universitätsklinik (II) Ulm, D-7900 Ulm

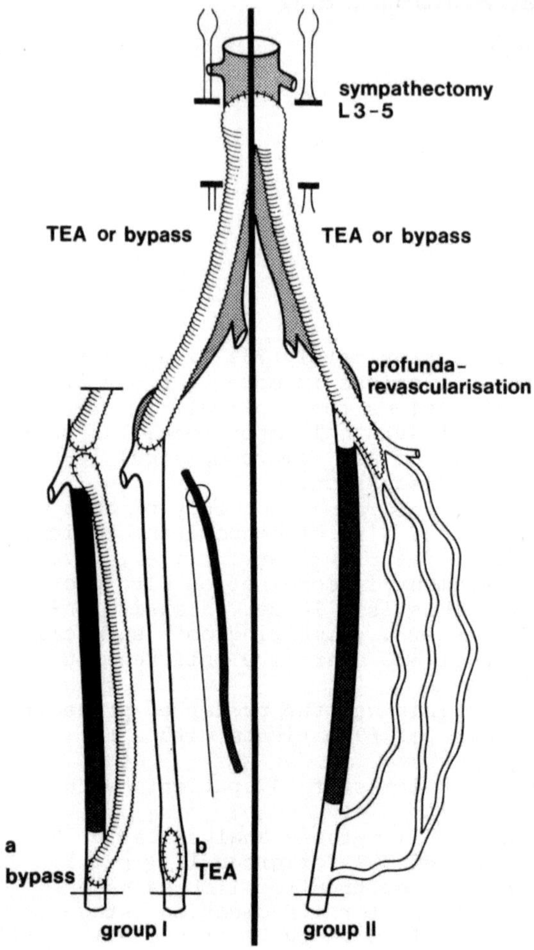

Fig. 1. Principles of surgery in combined aortoiliac and femoropopliteal occlusive lesions, two-level occlusions

operative month, represented by the lined curve in this life-table analysis. Beyond this time the patency rate reaches the same level as in patients with a triad procedure. This early decrease in patency rate is probably caused by incorrect preoperative assessment of the run-in and run-off conditions. In many conventional arteriograms, an unknown percentage of concomitant stenoses in the iliac arteries and the distal run-off vessels escapes the diagnosis. Intraoperative flow measurements favour this explanation. Without reconstruction of the iliac run-in, the increase of flow after profundoplasty was 72% vs 126% in the group with simultaneous aortoiliac reconstruction.

In patients with *distal necrosis* (stage IV) the effect of revascularization following partial repair (triad operation) was sufficient in about 90% for a definitive healing of the ischaemic lesions, preventing major amputation and a return to stage I or II. Following the *IRA principle* one or more weeks after profunda revascularization a border zone amputation was performed with full success.

The technical principle of an *optimal profundoplasty* may be defined as an *optimal conic adaption* of a big run-in vessel (common femoral artery *or graft*) to a small run-off vessel (deep femoral artery). From

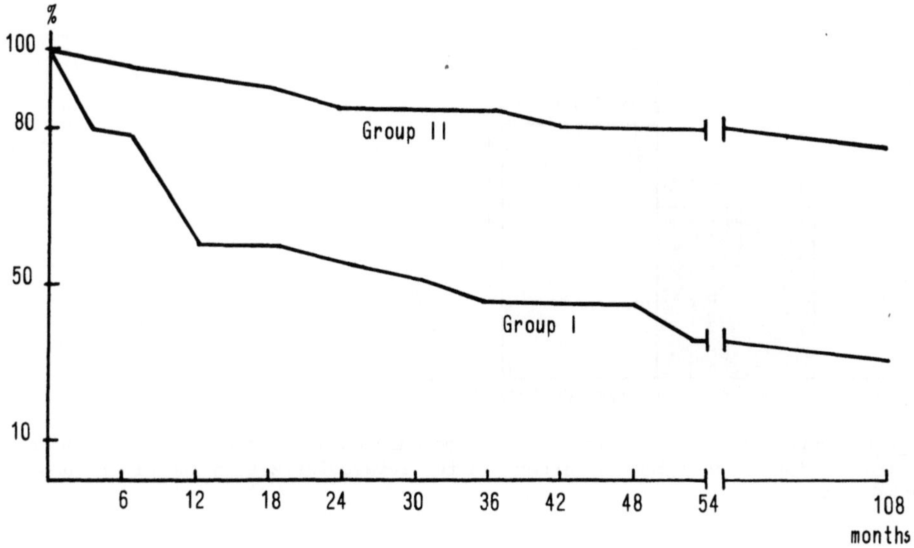

Fig. 2. Cumulative patency rate for both groups of patients operated on in Stages II-IV (August 1970 to December 1979)

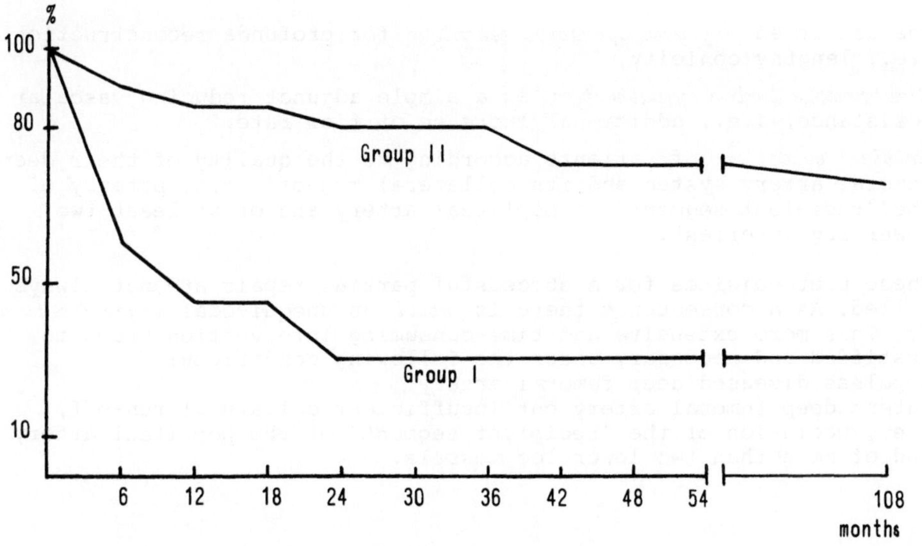

Fig. 3. Cumulative patency rate for both groups of patients operated upon in Stage III and IV (August 1970 to December 1979)

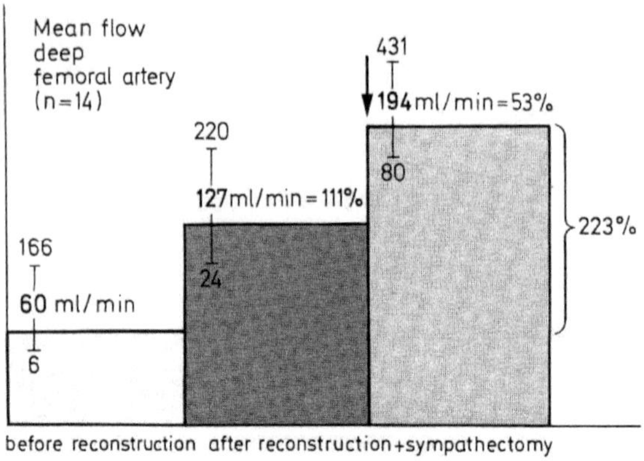

Fig. 4. Intraoperative electromagnetic flow measurements in triad procedure before revascularization of deep femoral artery, after revascularization and after lumbar sympathectomy

a haemodynamic point of view conicity means increase of flow velocity, i.e., an additional protective factor against suture line thrombosis.

The explanation for the impressive better results obtained by the minor intervention of *partial repair* vs combined distal arterial reconstruction may be seen in the following points:

a) The use of an *improved operative technique* for profunda reconstruction, i.e., lengthy conicity,

b) *Simultaneous lumbar sympathectomy* as a simple adjunct reducing vascular resistance, i.e., additional increase of flow rate.

c) *Critical selection* of patients according to the quality of their deep femoral artery system and its collateral run-off (e.g. patency of the "recipient segment" of popliteal artery and of at least two lower leg arteries).

These prerequisites for a successful partial repair are not always fulfilled. As a consequence there is *still* an unequivocal *place for total repair*. This more extensive and time-consuming intervention seems to be justified and necessary under the following conditions:

1. Hopeless diseased deep femoral artery.
2. Patent deep femoral artery but insufficient collateral run-off, i.e., occlusion of the "recipient segment" of the popliteal artery and of more than two lower leg vessels.

Summary

1. The partial revascularization of the aortoiliac segment by *disobliteration* or *bypass* in combination with *profundoplasty* and *lumbar sympathectomy* represents a simple and effective alternative to the previously preferred total repair of both arterial segments. The main advan-

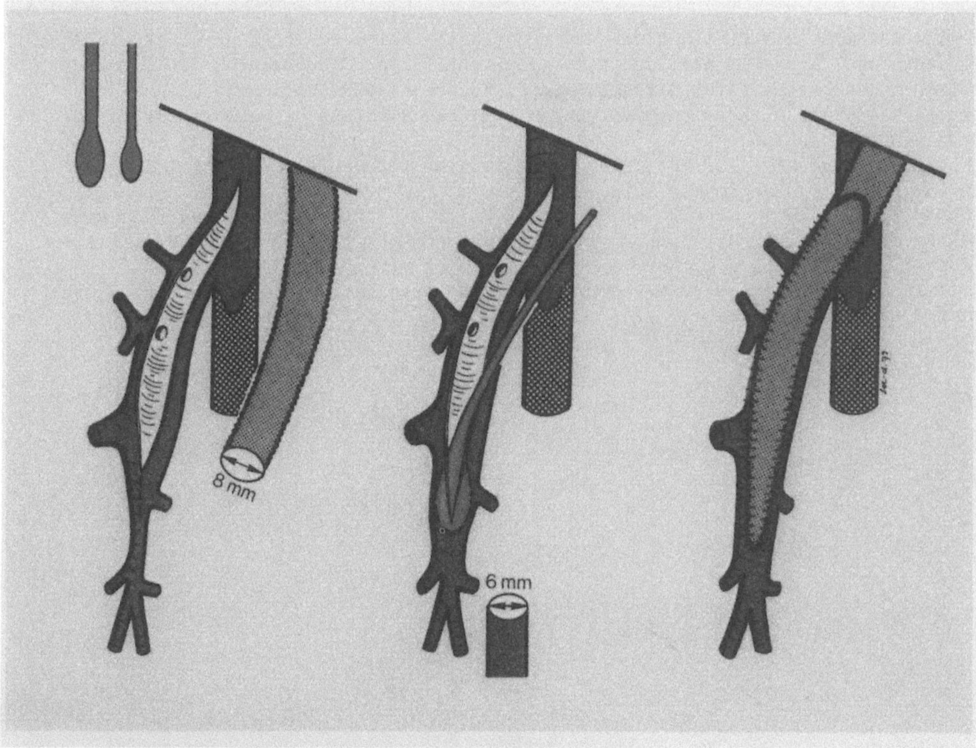

Fig. 5. Technical principles of profundoplasty

tages of this triad procedure may be seen in an improved long-term patency and in a reduced rate of reocclusions, consecutive reoperations and amputations.

2. In addition, the presented results prove that the interventions for femoropopliteal occlusive lesions done for claudication are unnecessary.

3. In the presence of a remarkable high failure rate *distal arterial reconstructions* below the knee should be restricted to a few patients in which a triad procedure is either technical not applicable or has failed. There is sufficient evidence that for many of these patients a *primary below-knee amputation is a preferrable alternative* versus a long graft procedure with questionable outcome. Its early failure results mostly in above-knee amputations and favours disillusionment both of patient and of surgeon.

References

1. Berguer R, Higgins RF, Cotton LT (1975) Geometry, blood flow, and reconstruction of the deep femoral artery. Am J Surg 130:68
2. Fontaine R, Kim M, Kieny R (1954) Die chirurgische Behandlung der peripheren Durchblutungsstörungen. Helv Chir Acta 21:499

3. Heyden B (1976) Die Stellung der Profundaplastik bei der Korrektur von Zweietagenverschlüssen (aorto-iliakal und femoropopliteal). In: Jahrestagung der Österreichischen Gesellschaft für Gefäßchirurgie, Kongreßband 9. Egermann, Vienna
4. Linton RR (1963) Diskussionsbemerkungen. In: Fundamentals of vascular grafting. McGraw-Hill, New York
5. Rocher A, Basyn ML, Joos FE (1975) Blood flow measurements in arterial surgery of lower limb. J Cardiovasc Surg 16:384
6. Schoop W, Aboudan F, Schmidtke I, Zeitler E (1972) Angiographische Befunde nach Reobliteration einer Arterie im Vergleich zum präoperativen Zustand. Herz/Kreislauf 4:144
7. Vollmar J (1980) Reconstructive surgery of the arteries, 3rd edn. Thieme, Stuttgart; Stratton, New York

Surgical Management of the Aorto-iliac and Femoro-popliteal Arteritis Disease

B. Baehrel, B. Brandt, C. Clement, J. M. Marcon, and H. Nicaise*

Surgical indications in atheromatous disease involving the aortoiliac and femoropopliteal segments are difficult to assess: either limit the revascularization to the profunda femoris or extend it to both levels.

This study proposes a comparison between the different revascularization procedures in terms of clinical findings pre-, per-, and postoperative hemodynamic and angiographic assessments.

Material and Methods

One hundred and seventeen patients presenting combined arteritis disease were operated in the Department of Vascular Surgery in Reims from January 1978 to December 1979. Patients' mean age was 61 years, ranging from 38 to 84 years. Sex ratio was 6 women to 111 men. All patients underwent aortography and low extremity arteriography before operation. Noninvasive investigations were always performed: pulse volume recording amplitude, Doppler systolic occlusion pressures, exercise testing on travelling band and segmental plethysmography ("irrigraphy") during the last 6-month period of this study.

Fifty-five of 117 patients presented with claudication (second Fontaine clinical stage), 36 of them had a walking capacity of less than 50 meters. The 62 limb salvage group included 28 patients with rest pain, pregangrene of the foot, marked dependent rubor and petechiae, third stage; 34 patients in fourth stage with focal traumatic tissue loss (IV A = 24) or with infected ulceration and gangrene (stage IV B = 10). Two among them were single limbs.

Procedures and Materials used

The diversity of the techniques used showed the difficulties encountered by the extensive atheromatous disease. At the aortoiliac level, the diffusion of the lesions often contraindicated the endarterectomy that we electively reserved for short and noncalcified stenosis (19 cases = 16.2%). The most frequently employed prosthetic material was Dacron (69.2%). For long bypasses to the popliteal or tibial arteries we used expanded polytetrafluoroethylene (PTFE).

At the femoropopliteal level endarterectomy was limited to very short lesions (three cases). As often as saphenous veins were available, we used venous autografts (seven cases). Four times we extended one branch of an aortobifemoral prosthesis with Dacron bypass to the popliteal. We preferred the better-tolerated PTFE prosthesis especially below the knee (19 cases).

*Department of Vascular Surgery, Hôpital Robert Debré, 51090 Reims Cedex, France

Procedure of Revascularization

In 17 cases (14.5%), the severity of lesions involving the profunda femoris (PF) made its revascularization impossible and imposed the popliteal artery as site of distal revascularization - above the knee 14 times, and below the knee 3 times. In the majority of cases only inflow restoration of the PF was performed (84 of 117 = 71.8%). In 16 cases we associated simultaneous revascularization of the PF and popliteal artery. Seventy lumbar sympathectomies were indicated in addition to profunda revascularization when distal arteries were occluded. Lastly, due to severe cardiopulmonary insufficiency, seven extra-anatomic bypasses (five axillofemoral and two axillopopliteal) were performed.

Peroperative aortoarteriographic control is systematically performed with high definition equipment based on the principle of amply-photography. In the same way we carried out peroperative electromagnetic flow measurements, flow-increase test after vasodilatator injection, estimates of the peripheric resistances, and measurements of segmental pressures above and below the restoration; recently in a few cases we attempted to appreciate the values of resupply and peripheric transfer by means of rheography and distal plethysmography.

On the tenth postoperative day hemodynamic estimation was carried out, similar to the preoperative investigations.

Results

Early Results

The hospital death was 5 percent (six patients with severe cardiopulmonary insufficiency). Nevertheless, repair could be linked to mesenteric infarction after left aortofemoral bypass. Peroperative arteriography helps us in the decrease of early thrombosis. In the four cases recorded, all were repaired with patency and very good results. In one case of gangrene, prosthesis infection made amputation compulsory.

Late Results

The same noninvasive investigations were performed 6 months, 1 year, and 2 years postoperative. In a few cases arteriography was carried out either systematically after endarterectomy or because of worsening of the result. Ninety percent had a follow-up from 6 to 24 months, a 6-month follow-up for 50, 12 months for 37, and 12 to 24 months for 19.

Net Results (Table 1). Net results were satisfactory. One hundred patients were improved or asymptomatic (85%). Correlative to the clinical preoperative stage, a good result could be considered to be the rule in the second stage (93%). Results were more significant in the limb salvage group, with amelioration of 85.7% in the third stage and 73.5% in the fourth stage with only two amputations.

Second Repair. We had to proceed to secondary repair in 11 patients (10.4%) after 5 to 18 months.
a) Underevaluated aortoiliac lesions (three cases): Two iliac and one aortic stenosis were underevaluated; this gave poor results after repair of the femoropopliteal level. Better results were obtained after restoration of the lesions. These three cases confirmed that hemodyna-

mic evaluations of aortoiliac stage must be carried out in all combined lesions.
b) Femoropopliteal lesions (eight cases): In two cases, where popliteal stenosis was aggravated, we had to carry out secondary repair by a lower restoration. In six other cases a complementary distal revascularization was performed, in one case for thrombosis of PF and in five cases for a low output with persistent ischemic lesions. In all cases we obtained secondary a good result.

Results Correlative to the Type of Revascularization (Table 2). Restoration of PF alone in the majority of cases (84) gives good results independent of the ischemic stage (second stage, 93%; fourth stage, 80%). This confirms the hemodynamic value of the PF in the surgical management of the combined aortoiliac and femoropopliteal disease. But in five cases restoration of PF was insufficient (6%) requiring a second repair.

Profunda femoris and popliteal repair: In a few cases of severe distal ischemic tissue loss, we preferred a combined revascularization of both levels to obtain complete restoration with good results in all cases.

Popliteal repair alone: When the PF could not be used, we carried out a direct repair of the popliteal artery alone. This was always done in severe ischemic lesions. In the limb salvage restoration, we obtained good results in the fourth stage in six cases out of ten, in two of them after a secondary repair.

Table 1. Results correlative with clinical stages

Clinical stage	Death or no follow-up	Follow-up 6 to 24 months: Asymptomatic or improved	Status quo or aggravated
55 II	2	51 93%	2
28 III	3	24 86%	1
34 IV	6	25 73.5%	3 (2 amputations)
Total 117	11	100	6

Table 2. Results correlative with surgical procedure

Revascularization site	Clinical stage	Death or no follow-up	Follow-up: Asymptomatic or improved	Status quo or aggravated
84 profunda femoris (PF) alone (72%)	II 44	1	41 93%	2
	III 20	2	17 85%	1
	IV 20	2	16 80%	2
16 PF + popliteal (13.5%)	II 7	-	7	-
	III 5	1	4	-
	IV 4	1	3	-
17 popliteal alone (14.5%)	II 4	-	3	-
	III 3	1	3	-
	IV 10	3	6	1

Discussion

Combined aortoiliac and femoropopliteal lesions set up the choice of the repair level.

Estimation of the Profunda Femoris

Analysis of this study confirms hemodynamic estimation of PF as shown by other authors (1, 9, 18). The PF repair alone gives very good results in the majority of the cases. But this may be insufficient (five cases in our study group) as correlated to Morzeski et al. 20% (11), Edwards and Wright 57% (6). In 8% to 17% of cases (2, 10, 12), a difficult secondary repair is carried out.

Taking into account the failures, some authors (5, 10) carried out combined restoration in the limb salvage group. We discuss this method. In fact, distal revascularization is not always necessary in addition to the fact that it increases the infectious risks. Finally, long-term effects after complete revascularization are far from being satisfactory (3, 4, 9). Sometimes the results declined during the first year when distal revascularization was performed on the popliteal artery below the knee or on the tibial arteries (9, 17). Thus, pre- and peroperative investigations allowed us to evaluate the PF before choosing the type of repair.

Predictive Value of PF

Preoperative tests. The multiplicity of preoperative tests of the PF evaluation reflects their insufficiency and the difficulties in an estimation: segmental systolic pressures measurements with index (7, 8, 15); femorotibial pressure gradient: invasive measurement of femoral and brachial pressure and noninvasive ankle indirect pressure (14).

In the department, we used the following methods: Doppler systolic occlusion pressure, "irrigraphy", invasive femoral artery systolic pressure, and preoperative arteriography. This last method with profile films on the common femoral helps us to appreciate the PF, the quality of revascularization, and the state of popliteal and tibial run-off. Even repair of PF may be dangerous or insufficient due to: extending stenosis or occlusion below first perforating, multiple separate origin of the different branches of PF, stenosis of the collateral which must assure run-off. In our experience these rare cases indicated by long bypasses excluding the PF. On the contrary severe ischemia indicated combined revascularization in case of "blind" popliteal artery because the PF restoration alone is insufficient.

Peroperative Estimations. Revascularization of PF may not be possible in cases of extended calcification or bad retrograde flow after arteriotomy. Peroperative measurements of muscle pH after repair may give an idea about the predictable results (16). Peroperative arteriography allowed us to detect technical failures which could be immediately repaired, controlled once again, and permitted us to appreciate the timing and the quality of popliteal reinjection from the PF (13). Peroperative flow measurements added numerical evidence. We carried out flow measurements in different types of repair. Above a "critical" flow of 130 ml/min, clinical results are good (13). The flow increase test after vasodilatator injection gave better measurements. A 50% flow increase confirmed good peripheric supplying of PF (Table 3).

Table 3. Predictive value of arterial reconstruction and peroperative flow measurements (95 cases)

Surgical procedure	Flow (ml/min)	Results Good	Poor
66 PF	210	66	-
8 PF	130	8	-
16 PF + P*	130 ⟶ 220	14	2
5 PF + P**	130 ↘ 230	5 ↙	5

PF: Profunda femoris restoration alone.
PF + P*: Synchronous restoration of profunda femoris and popliteal arteries.
PF + P**: Profunda femoris and secondary popliteal restoration.

Thus peroperative measurements in 16 cases have allowed us to complete at the same time the PF revascularization by a popliteal restoration with 14 good results. In five cases poor results correlated with low peroperative flow measurements made us proceed to a secondary repair. This gave a good flow increase (230 ml) with good clinical results in all cases. Lastly in order to appreciate the distal supplying of PF, we have added rheography and distal plethysmography.

To conclude, analysis of these observations confirms the hemodynamic value of PF in the surgical repair of combined aortoiliac and femoropopliteal arteritis disease. The popliteal repair alone should be made only when the PF could not be used. Lastly peroperative flow measurements and arteriography allowed us to appreciate more the hemodynamic value of the PF repair. Thus we limit the number of simultaneous restoration of both levels when peroperative flow measurements of PF is critical.

References

1. Andersen CA, Rich NM, Collins GJ, McDonnald PT (1978) Limb salvage by extended profunda femoris revascularization. Am Surg 44
2. Baird RJ, Feldman R, Milles JT (1977) Subsequent downstream repair after aorto iliac and aorto femoral bypass operations. Surgery 82:785
3. Benson JR, Whelen TJ, Cohen A, Spencer F (1966) Combined aorto iliac and femoropopliteal occlusive disease. Ann Surg 163:121
4. Collins GJ, Rich NM, Andersen CA, McDonnald PT (1978) Staged aorto-femoropopliteal revascularization. Arch Surg 113:149
5. Dardik H, Ibrahim IM, Jarrah M, Sussman B, Dardik I (1979) Synchronous aortofemoral or iliofemoral bypass with revascularization of the lower extremity. Surg Gynecol Obstet 149:676
6. Edwards WH, Wright RS (1978) A technique for combined aorto-femoral popliteal arterial reconstruction. Arch Surg 113:149
7. Garret WV, Slaymaker EE, Heintz SE, Barnes RW (1977) Intraoperative prediction of symptomatic result of aorto-femoral bypass from changes in ankle pressure index. Surgery 82:504
8. Gruss JD, Kawai J, Karabedos C (1979) Conception actuelle du traitement dans l'obstruction mixte des artères du bassin et de la cuisse. Chirurgie 105:575
9. Heyden B, Vollmar J, Voss EU (1979) Therapiekonzept bei Zweietagenverschlüssen (Aorto-iliakal und femoro-popliteal). Zentralbl Chir 104:519

10. Masson B, Quancard X, Catherine G, Janvier G (1978) La restauration ilio-fémoro-poplitée en un temps. Sa place dans le traitement de l'artèrite des membres inférieurs. Chirurgie 104:833
11. Mozersky DJ, Summer DS, Strandness DE (1972) Long-term results of reconstructive aorto-iliac surgery. Am Surg 123:503
12. Muclare RJ, Royster TS, Lynn RA, Conners RB (1978) Long-term results of operative therapy for aorto-iliac disease. Arch Surg 113:601
13. Nicaise H, Marconj M, Baehrel B (1978) Peroperative arteriography by ampliphotography and flow measurement as control methods in vascular surgery. 27th International Congress of the European Society of Cardiovascular Surgery, Lyon, 28 June - 1 July 1978, vol II, pp 99-103
14. Noer I, Tonnesen KH, Sager P (1978) Peroperative estimation of run-off in patients with multiple level arterial obstructions as a guide to partial reconstructive surgery. Ann Surg 188/5:663
15. O'Donnel TF, Lahey SJ, Kelly JJ, Ransil BJ, Millan VG, Korwin S, Calow AD (1979) A prospective study Doppler pressures and segmental plethysmography before and following aorto-femoral bypass — Implications for predicting success and for adopting a uniform method of classifying arterial disease. Surgery 86:120
16. O'Donnel TF, Raines JK, Darling C (1979) Relationship of muscle surface pH to noninvasive hemodynamic studies in arterial occlusive disease. Arch Surg 114:600
17. Sautot J (1969) La chirurgie des oblitérations aorto-iliaques. CMM 45:1303
18. Tingaud R, Serise JM, Le Heron D, Busquet J, Janvier G, Torrielli R (1979) La coexistence de lésions aorto-iliaques et de thrombose fémorale ou fémoro-poplitée. Le risque ischémique après chirurgie de restauration. Lyon Chir 75:299

Aorto-iliac Thrombo-endarterectomy

M. Goldstein, G. Vincent, J. P. Barroy, and J. P. Dereume*

Introduction

In the surgery of the aortic bifurcation, the controversy between supporters of bypass grafting and those of thromboendarterectomy is not yet settled (1, 2, 6, 11-14).

We wish to bring our personal contribution while stating that we are not definitively against the use of Dacron grafts, which we regularly use in the surgery of aortic aneurysm. Besides, one of the authors participated with our colleague J. van der Stricht in the first Dacron bypass procedure in Belgium in 1958. Since then, the use of this prosthetic material has been progressively developed in our department as much for the aortoiliac segment (level 1) as for the femoropopliteal one (level 2).

If the patency after 5 years has shown good results for the aorto-iliac segment, it is not very encouraging for the femoropopliteal segment.

That is one of the reasons why we have given up arterial reconstruction of the femoropopliteal segment in patients with grade two arteritis, with intermittent claudication; in those cases we prefer a lumbar sympathectomy giving a sufficient increase of the blood flow (10), or a medically controlled physical training (5). We have the same attitude in arterial disease with associated lesions of the aortoiliac segment and of the femoral segment; in those cases, we perform a reconstruction of the aortoiliac level and a lumbar sympathectomy; it is very exceptional to be obliged to add a femoropopliteal reconstruction.

Our choice for the thromboendarterectomy (TEA) in aortoiliac reconstruction is associated with the two major complications encountered with synthetic prostheses: infection and false aneurysm (1).

To avoid the above mentioned complications, we started again with TEA of aortoiliac level in 1964 and our first results have been presented in Moscow in 1971 (7). The main conclusions of this paper can be summarized as follows: an increase in the number of TEA since 1965, the continuing use of Dacron for aortic aneurysm, and a decrease of the number of Dacron prostheses for chronic arteriosclerotic disease of the aortic bifurcation. Since then, we have seen the specter of infection and false aneurysm vanishing in this type of surgery.

---

*Department of Vascular Surgery, Hôpital Saint-Pierre, Université Libre de Bruxelles, Belgium

Technique

At first, we classically made longitudinal incisions to realize the TEA; the closure was done with or without angioplasty (continuous suture with 4-0 silk). The subsequent development of cicatricial stenosis prompted us to change to transversal incisions and to close with interrupted 4-0 silk stitches. If the TEA is not realizable, we proceed to a Dacron bypass procedure.

For aortic and iliac lesions, we generally use the transperitoneal approach, which permits a bilateral lumbar sympathectomy. The extraperitoneal appraoch is used in unilateral iliac lesions and in high risk patients. To achieve the TEA on the common femoral artery, we actually frequently perform a profundoplasty.

Material

This study is based on a series of 289 patients which represents 423 operated limbs:

Men	251	Mean age	58.9 years	(31-86)
Women	38	Mean age	60.5 years	(38-86)

The severity of the arterial disease is estimated by the stage according to the classification of Fontaine.

	Male	Female
Stage II	150	20
Stage III	41	7
Stage IV	60	11

We already mentioned that, in case of associated lesions of the femoral and/or distal level, the arterial reconstruction of the femoropopliteal segment is rarely made. In our series of 289 patients, 159 had associated lesions on level 2 and/or level 3 (distal lesions). In the series of 423 reconstructed limbs (operated at the aortoiliac level) we have associated the following operations of the femoropopliteal level: ten TEA, eight venous grafts, and two Dacron bypass grafts. This means associated reconstruction of the femoropopliteal segment in less than 5% of the cases (9). Lumbar sympathectomy has been associated in 276 patients (95%).

Results

We have had early occlusion for seven out of 423 limbs at risk (1.5%) and 29 late failures (7%). Sixteen patients out of 289 died at the hospital, which gives a mortality of 5.5%: six of cardiac insufficiency or infarctus, four of pulmonary embolism, three of marasmus, two of shock, and one of sepsis.

We have had the following complications in the postoperative period: five deep venous thromboses (one pulmonary embolism), eight intestinal occlusions (5 laparotomies), four pneumopathies, three cerebrovascular accidents, four ventral incisional hernias, four lymphorrheas in the groin, and one acute renal failure. We have had to amputate five limbs because of failure of revascularization (three cases of isolated aortoiliac TEA and two cases of associated femorodistal reconstruction).

In our follow-up we have found 29 cases of reobliteration (7%), of which some have been reoperated and corrected. This reocclusion has led to 15 amputations (eight cases of isolated aortoiliac TEA and seven cases of associated femorodistal reconstruction). Altogether, we have had 4.7% of amputation (20/423) in our follow-up.

We have found two cases of false aneurysm and no case of sepsis in our series. This represents 0.4% out of 423 operated limbs.

Table 1 and Figure 1 show the cumulative patency rate of the aorto-iliac TEA calculated by the life-table method. The cumulative patency rate of our series is 86.99% with a standard error of patency of 2.17%.

Discussion

Our preference for TEA as a method for the treatment of atherosclerotic occlusive lesions in the aortoiliac segment has relieved us from the obsession of graft infection and of false aneurysm which are very rare after TEA.

Infection

In spite of all the precautions observed by the vascular surgeons, 2% to 5% of prosthesis infection is found in many statistics (1, 4). This very serious complication too often leads to limb amputation or even death. Wylie (14) mentions six deaths and four amputations in a series of 18 referred cases (3). The development of extra-anatomical bypass procedures has permitted us to save some of those patients.

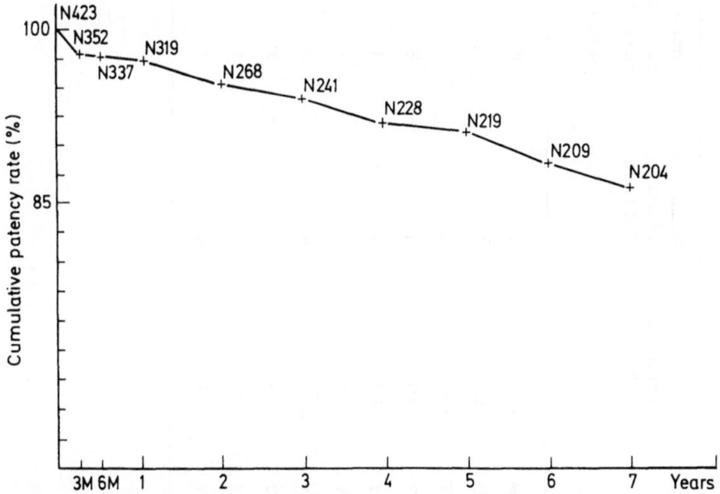

Fig. 1. Patency rate of aortoiliac TEA: life-table method

Table 1. Cumulative patency rate

A	B	C	D		E	F	G	H
Interval	Number of limbs at risk	Number of limbs failing	Number of reconstructions not observed throughout period due to		Interval failure	Interval patency rate	Accumulated patency rate	Standard error
			Death	Duration of follow-up	(%)	(%)	(%)	(%)
0 - 3 M	423	8	16	47	2.04	97.96	97.96	0.71
3 M - 6 M	352	1	0	14	0.29	99.71	97.67	1.11
6 M - 1 Y	337	3	1	14	0.91	99.09	96.78	1.23
1 Y - 2 Y	319	4	3	44	1.35	98.65	95.47	1.38
2 Y - 3 Y	268	4	4	19	1.55	98.45	93.99	1.55
3 Y - 4 Y	241	5	3	5	2.14	97.86	91.97	1.75
4 Y - 5 Y	228	4	3	2	1.77	98.23	90.34	1.90
5 Y - 6 Y	219	6	1	3	2.76	97.24	87.84	2.10
6 Y - 7 Y	209	2	1	2	0.96	99.04	86.99	2.17
7 Y - 8 Y	204	0	0	0	0	100	86.99	2.17

False aneurysm

False aneurysm remains a matter of controversy. In turn, the suture material, the infection, the type of anastomosis, the local endarterectomy, etc., have been incriminated. *This complication is found in 2% to 6% of most series.*

False Aneurysm in the Groin. This localization is the most common and its correction is usually possible by a new anastomosis, sometimes a more distal one with or without interposition of another graft material.

Aortic Localization of False Aneurysm. This localization often leads to an aortointestinal fistula with secondary infection of the aneurysmal sac. This complication is often fatal. Its only treatment is removal of the prosthesis and realization of extra-anatomical bypasses.

General Complications and Mortality

The general complications and operative mortality are also comparable to those found in bypass procedures. The 5-year patency rate seems to be as good as in Dacron bypass grafting (8, 14). Early and late failure of an aortoiliac TEA can always be corrected by a bypass procedure.

References

1. Agrifoglio G, Costantini S, Zanetta M, Castelli P (1979) Infections and anastomotic false aneurysms in reconstructive vascular surgery. J Cardiovasc Surg 20:25-32
2. Agrifoglio G, Costantini S, Castelli P, Lorenzi G, Gabrielli L, Agus GB (1979) Thromboendarterectomy for peripheral occlusive arterial disease. J Cardiovasc Surg 20:369-372
3. Baker MS, Baker BH, MacMillan JC (1976) In situ treatment of an infected vascular graft. Am Surg 42:308-310
4. Cormier JM, Ward AS, Lagneau P, Janneau D (1980) Infection complicating aortoiliac surgery. J Cardiovasc Surg 21:303-314
5. Dereume JP, Barroy JP, Azama M, Rondeux C, Goldstein M (to be published) Notre expérience du réentraînement physique ambulatoire. Méthode et résultats. Acta Belg
6. Descotes J, Barral X (1977) Fiabilité de l'endartériectomie dans le traitement du syndrome de Leriche. Résultats de 170 interventions réalisées de 1960 à 1970. Compte - Rendu de la Société de Chirurgie de Lyon, 1977, 114-119
7. Goldstein M, Flamand JP, Belenger J, Van der Stricht J (1972) Early and late results of aortic and iliac reconstructive operations. J Cardiovasc Surg 13: 454-458
8. Harbrecht PJ, Ahmad W, Fry DE (1978) Management of aortic bypass graft thrombosis: utility of thrombectomy. Am J Surg 136:363-368
9. Summer DS, Strandness DE (1978) Aortoiliac reconstruction in patients with combined iliac and superficial femoral arterial occlusion. Surgery 84:348-355
10. Terry HS, Allan JS, Taylor GW (1972) The relationship between blood-flow and failure of femoropopliteal reconstructive arterial surgery.
11. Traverso LW, Baker JD, Dainko EA, Machleder HI (1978) Infrarenal aortic occlusion. Ann Surg 187:397-401
12. Van Lent D, Kuijpers PJ, Skotnicki SH, Meyer I (1974) Aortoiliac surgery: a comparative study between thromboendarterectomy and bypass. J Cardiovasc Surg 15:352-355
13. Voss EU, Vollmar J, Heyden B, Rudolph F (1980) Chirurgische Therapie der chronischen aorto-iliacalen Arterienverschlüsse. Aktuel Probl Chir Orthop 15:77-94
14. Wylie EJ, Olcott C, String ST (1976) Endarterectomy versus bypass operation for aortoiliac occlusive disease. In: Varco RL, Delaney JP (eds) Controversy in surgery. Saunders, Philadelphia

Concomitant Revascularization of Aorto-iliac-Femoropopliteal Atherosclerotic Lesions

G. Agrifoglio, S. Costantini, G. B. Agus, and P. Castelli*

Introduction

The occurrence of combined atherosclerotic occlusive disease in both the aortoiliofemoral and femoropopliteal segments is a common clinical and angiographic entity, with an incidence reported between 45% and 82.5% (1). Generally the vascular reconstruction is limited to the proximal district, eventually associated to lumbar sympathectomy or to profundoplastic procedure; by this approach, according to previous reports, between 9% and 57% of patients obtain inadequate relief and many of these have required a subsequent more distal operation and in some case even major amputation.

Personal Series

In the Institute of Vascular Surgery of the University of Milan, from January 1971 to April 1980, we have performed 181 simultaneous revascularizations of both aortofemoral and femoropopliteal segments, that is 21.1% out of 855 procedures performed in the same period at proximal level (Table 1). One hundred and sixty-eight patients (92.8%) were men and only 13 (7.2%) women, aged between 38 and 73 years, with the highest frequency in the sixth decade (50%). Among these patients, there were myocardial diseases in nine, diabetes in six, respiratory failure in five, chronic renal failure in five, and systolic hypertension in two.

One hundred and sixty-one patients (88.9%) were operated on for disabling claudication and only 20 (11.1%) for rest pain or distal gangrene. At the proximal level, in 116 cases (64.0%) we performed a thromboendarterectomy (TEA) and in 65 cases (36.0%) a bypass graft, while at the distal level we always performed a femoropopliteal TEA, in 27 cases (14.9%) bilaterally. A lumbar sympathectomy was associated in 47 cases (25.9%).

Results

We have classified as a good result the complete relief from claudication or rest pain, with femoral pulse as well as one or more distal pulse palpable and healing of trophic lesions; poor results are the inadequate relief of ischemic symptoms (Table 2). We obtained 167

*Institute of Vascular Surgery, University of Milan, Italy

early good results (92.3%), four poor (2.2%); three amputations (1.6%) The operative mortality rate was 3.9%; five patients died of cardiac complications and two of acute renal failure. Postoperative thrombosis occurred in 10 cases (5.5%), all successfully treated by Fogarty's thrombectomy.

Table 1. Combined aortoiliofemoral and femoropopliteal reconstructions

Aortobipopliteal TEA	13
Aortobifemoral and unilateral femoropopliteal TEA	11
Aortoiliac and aortoilio-femoropopliteal TEA	9
Iliofemoropopliteal TEA	83
Aortobifemoral bypass and bilateral femoropopliteal TEA	14
Aortobifemoral bypass and unilateral femoropopliteal TEA	42
Iliofemoral bypass and femoropopliteal TEA	9
Total	181

Table 2. Combined aortoiliofemoral and femoropopliteal reconstructions: early and late results

	Early		Late	
	No.	%	No.	%
Good	167	92.3	101	82.1
Poor	4	2.2	14	11.4
Amputation	3	1.6	6	4.9
Death	7	3.9	2	1.6
Total	181	100.0	123	100.0

Follow-up ranging from 1 to 5 years on 123 cases (73.6%), shows a good result in 101 cases (82.1%), poor in 14 patients (11.4%); six patients (4.9%) were amputated and two other patients (1.6%) died after a major amputation.

We have successfully reoperated 8 out of 14 patients with poor results: in three we have performed a femoropopliteal re-TEA, while the other five were reoperated at the proximal level.

Discussion

In our series, indication to one-stage aortofemoropopliteal reconstruction is based on four criteria: clinical picture, angiographic pattern, hemodynamic study, and surgical procedure. According to Fontaine's stages, we think that the patients with a multilevel occlusive disease should be operated on at the second stage to obtain a complete relief of claudication.

Many authors agree with this point and recently Hill et al. (2) have pointed out that in patients who have undergone aortofemoral bypass with untreated superficial femoral artery, only 26% were relieved of claudication. Instead at the third and fourth Fontaine stages, where the surgical purpose is limb salvage, combined reconstruction is indicated when profundoplasty, eventually associated with lumbar sympathectomy, is believed insufficient to relieve rest pain and to heal trophic lesions.

The angiographic pattern indicates the need of femoropopliteal revascularization when there is: a poor collateral network from the profunda femoris artery, with ostial stenosis of the branches which recanalize the distal third of the superficial femoral artery; an early division of the profunda femoris artery with hipoplasic branches; diffuse atherosclerotic stenosing lesions of the profunda femoris artery; or occlusion of the above-knee segment of the popliteal artery.

Regarding hemodynamic study, according to Sumner and Strandness (7), we calculate an index of run-off resistance by dividing the difference between the thigh and ankle pressure by the brachial pressure, with the Doppler technique. We operate at the femoropopliteal level when the run-off index is greater than 30 mm Hg. In our series the average preoperative run-off index was 49 mm Hg and the postoperative 10 mm Hg. However, according to previous reports, we think either pressure gradient or increase in the ankle pressure after aortoiliac reconstruction is not of prognostic value.

From a technical point of view, we always prefer a femoropopliteal TEA by semiclosed or even closed technique with Vollmar's ring stripper, because it is easier to perform and less time consuming than reversed saphenous vein bypass graft. For aortofemoral lesions, when unilateral reconstruction is required, we always prefer to perform a TEA, via the retroperitoneal approach. We apply an alloplastic bypass graft when there are kinked or aneurismatic arteries or when TEA fails (9 cases out of 92). Also for bilateral revascularization we prefer the TEA procedure but in these cases bypass graft may be more suitable, especially in high risk patients, because the operation is technically easier and takes less time.

Conclusion

One-stage treatment of combined aortoiliofemoral and femoropopliteal lesions, when indicated, depends on the capital principle of vascular surgery that reconstruction must be as complete as possible. Furthermore, revascularization limited to the proximal district is often inadequate to obtain complete relief of claudication.

Many of these patients undergo a subsequent operation that generally requires greater technical care and increases the possibility of infective complication and proximal thrombosis. Performing a femoropopliteal TEA, associated to aortofemoral TEA or bypass graft, does not significantly increase operative time and risk, and allows a complete relief of ischemic symptoms, with a mortality rate and incidence of poor results similar to those obtained after aortoiliofemoral reconstruction alone.

References

1. Berguer R, Cotton LT, Higgins RF (1975) Analysis of deep femoral artery hemodynamics and the effect of reconstruction. J Cardiovasc Surg 16:148
2. Hill DA, McGrath MA, Lord RSA, Tracy GD (1980) The effect of superficial femoral artery occlusion on the outcome of aortofemoral bypass for intermittent claudication. Surgery 87:133
3. Myhre HO (1977) Surgical treatment of aortoiliac atherosclerosis. Acta Chir Scand 143:15
4. Royster TS, Lynn R, Mulcare RJ (1976) Combined aortoiliac and femoropopliteal occlusive disease. Surg Gynecol Obstet 143:949
5. Sumner DS, Strandness DE Jr (1978) Aortoiliac reconstruction in patients with combined iliac and superficial femoral arterial occlusion. Surgery 84:348
6. Viver Manresa E, Callejas Perez JM, Rodriguez Mori A, De Sobregrau RC (1979) Reconstruction simultanea de las lesiones obliterantes de los sectores aorto-iliaco y femoro-popliteo. Angiologia 31:163
7. Vollmar I (1968) Chirurgia ricostruttiva delle arterie. PEM, Rome

Value of Popliteal Artery TEA in Treatment of Combined Aorto-iliac-Femoropopliteal Disease

R. de Nunno, F. Prestipino, C. Ballarini, R. Ballabio, P. Insalaco, and A. Bertolini*

Treatment of combined atherosclerotic lesions of the aortofemoropopliteal axis by revascularization does not always yield rewarding results. In fact, persisting claudicatio intermittens, although reduced, occurred in some of our patients treated with aortobifemoral (AbF) bypass or aortoiliacfemoral (AIF) TEA either associated or not associated with profundoplasty.

In the hope of finding the reasons of some insufficient results, we began a critical review of clinical and radiological data regarding a group of revascularized patients. The angiographic picture, particularly in those cases in which profundoplasty was performed, often induced us to evaluate the importance of the extension of the collateral bed of the popliteal artery and, as a consequence, to consider femoropopliteal (FP) TEA or FP bypass whenever popliteal collaterals were scarce (Figs. 1-2). The first follow-up results obtained by associating direct popliteal revascularization with AbF bypass or TEA instead of profundoplasty in third and fourth Fontaine stage patients showed us the possible solution to the problem and encouraged us to persue the matter.

Materials and Methods

We considered a group of 130 of 186 patients revascularized between 1974 and 1979, showing combined atherosclerotic lesions of the aortofemoropopliteal axis. Of these (Table 1), 52 were treated by simple AbF bypass or TEA; 21 also underwent profundoplasty, and 57 had direct popliteal revascularization with lumbar gangliectomy.

Angiographically, the profundoplasty group (Table 2) presented, in seven cases, apart from AIF lesions, also an obliterated femoralis superficialis with a popliteal flow fed by a good collateral bed from the femoralis profunda, which showed some atherosclerotic lesion. Follow-ups on these patients have been satisfactory with disappearance of claudication; in one case only, due to closure of a bypass branch, did trophic lesions appear after 3 years. In another five patients, presumably because of obstruction or delayed flow due to proximal disease, the popliteal artery and its collaterals could not be visualized by means of preoperatory angiography.

After 1 year from operation, two of these patients (40%) still had claudication, while two patients (40%) presented the same problem after 2 years; one patient (also a diabetic) suffered from rest pain. After 3 years, all patients (100%) had claudication (the diabetic patient also presenting trophic lesions). In the remaining nine profundo-

*Ente Ospedaliero Fatebenefratelli e Oftalmico, 2nd Division of Surgery, Milan, Italy

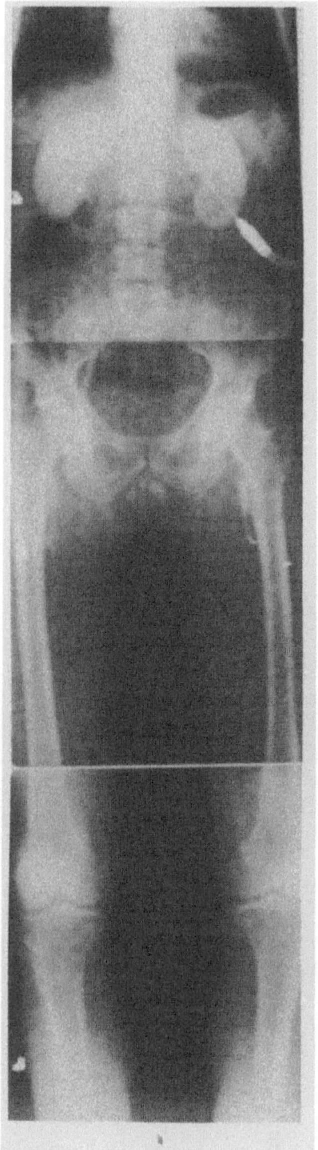

Fig. 1

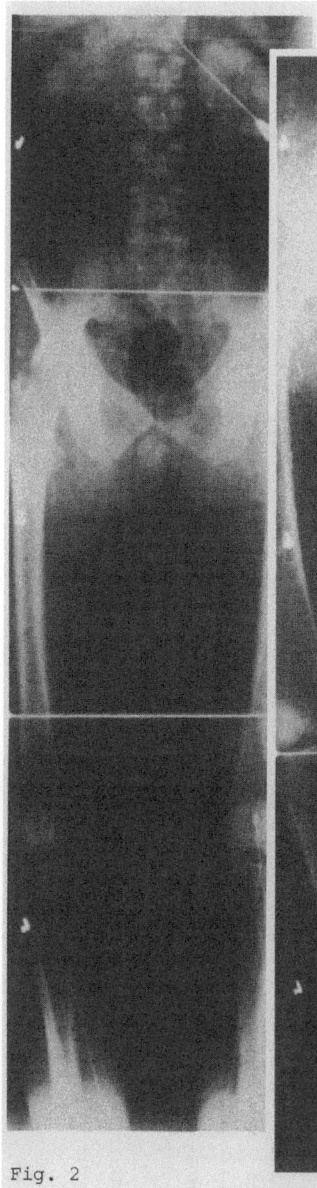

Fig. 2

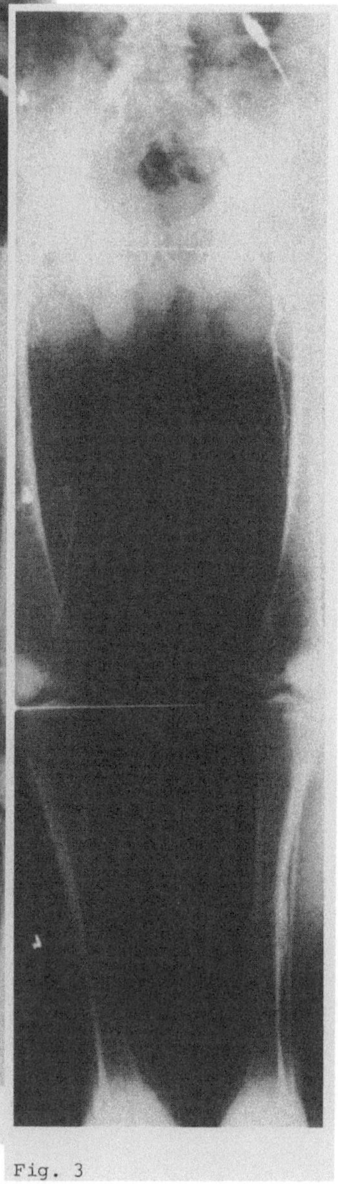

Fig. 3

Table 1. Combined aortoiliac-femoropopliteal disease

Surgical treatment	Preoperative angiographic picture		
	Nonvisualized popliteal and peripheric vessels	Patent popliteal artery with scarce collaterals	Patent popliteal artery with good collaterals
TEA AIF	4	6	28
AbF bypass	2	-	12
TEA or AbF bypass + TEA or FP bypass + gangliectomy	15	42	-
TEA or AbF bypass + profundoplasty	5	9	7
Totals	26	57	47

Table 2. Follow-ups in TEA-AIF or AbF bypasses with profundoplasty

Preoperative angiographic picture		Claudication						Rest pain or trophic lesions					
		At 1 year		At 2 years		At 3 years		At 1 year		At 2 years		At 3 years	
		Pres.	Abs.	Pres.	Abs.	Pres.	Abs.	Pres.	Abs.	Pres.	Abs.	Pres.	Abs.
Nonvisualized	No.	2	3	2	2	2	–	–	5	1	3	1	1
popliteal artery	%	40	60	50	50	100	–	–	100	25	75	50	50
Patent popliteal artery with scarce collaterals	No.	3	6	3	4	2	3	–	9	–	7	1	4
	%	33	67	43	57	40	60	–	100	–	100	20	80
Patent popliteal artery with good collaterals	No.	–	7	–	6	1	1	–	7	–	6	1	1
	%	–	100	–	100	50	50	–	100	–	100	50	50
Totals	No.	5	16	5	12	5	4	–	21	1	16	3	6

plasty patients, angiography showed an obstructed femoralis superficialis, a patent, if damaged, popliteal and poor collaterals. Follow-ups on this last group were reasonably good after 1 year; persistent, though slight, claudication returned in three cases (33%); such a percentage remained unvaried after 2 years; after 3 years, one patient (20%) was suffering from rest pain and trophic lesions requiring succesful femoropopliteal TEA.

After this, in other cases with similar angiographic situations (good or at least visible popliteal and poor collaterals), we performed revascularizations by associating AbF bypasses or TEA and lumbar gangliectomy with FP TEA or, if impossible, FP bypass. Results from this group (Table 3) of 57 patients have been, we would say, very good; of 15 of these patients in which angiography could not show the popliteal artery, a slight claudication persisted in only one case, appearing after 3 years in two out of eight of them (25%). One of the two had an obstruction of the femoralis superficialis and the other of a branch of the bypass. The latter who came to observation 20 days after the onset of obstruction in poor general condition, was treated medically and had to be amputated 1 year later. After 4 years, one of the two patients had an obstructed femoralis superficialis while the other was suffering from rest pain; therefore, after angiography showing a patent distal popliteal tract, we performed a successful FP bypass (patency is conserved after 1 year).

In the remaining 42 cases in which angiography showed a patent, if damaged, popliteal and poor collaterals, follow-ups at 2 years were excellent with absence of claudication in 100% of cases; at 3 years, slight claudication occurred in 2 out of 23 patients; at 4 years only 1 out of 14 patients had claudication leading to rest pain after 1 year. Pre- and intraoperatory angiographic study on this patient showed an obstruction of the previously disobliterated femoralis superficialis and no peripheric vascular bed.

As stated above, we wish to point out that all of the patients treated with TEA were given (some for 6 months and some indefinitely) coumadin drugs in order to maintain prothrombin activity around 30%.

Conclusions

Good long-term results and prolonged patency of disobliterated vessels in the 57 patients treated with AbF bypass or TEA associated with either FP TEA or bypass leads us to think that, whenever angiography reveals poor popliteal collaterals, in order to potentiate flow to the limb, the treatment of choice should be a direct revascularization by means of FP bypass or TEA with gangliectomy for reduction of peripheric resistance.

We perform profundoplasty only in patients of the older group and in third and fourth stages having an obstructed femoralis superficialis and a good proximal popliteal flow with efficient collaterals (Fig. 3). In fact, association of profundoplasty did not satisfy us because postoperatory angiography did not demonstrate the popliteal artery, even if patent, presumably because of poor collaterals that do not allow the peripheric bed to take advantage of flow increase. Some of the cases, purposely excluded from our study groups, help enforce our point of view.

In these, because of persisting claudication after bypass on the femoralis profunda and lumbar gangliectomy and in view of poor general conditions, we tried a simple disobliteration of the distal tract of the popliteal artery (from the channel of Hunter to the bifurcation)

Table 3. Follow-ups in TEA-AIF or AbF bypasses with TEA or FP bypass

Preoperative angiographic picture		At 1 year Pres.	At 1 year Abs.	At 2 years Pres.	At 2 years Abs.	At 3 years Pres.	At 3 years Abs.	At 4 years Pres.	At 4 years Abs.	At 5 years Pres.	At 5 years Abs.
Claudication											
Nonvisualized	No.	1	14	1	10	2	6	2	2	1	1
Popliteal artery	%	7	93	9	91	25	75	50	50	50	50
Patent popliteal artery with scarce collaterals	No.	-	42	-	32	2	21	1	13	1	4
	%	-	100	-	100	9	91	7	93	20	80
Totals	No.	1	56	1	42	4	27	3	15	2	5
Rest pain or trophic lesions											
Nonvisualized	No.	-	15	-	11	-	6	1	3	1	1
Popliteal artery	%	-	100	-	100	-	100	25	75	50	50
Patent popliteal artery with scarce collaterals	No.	-	42	-	32	-	23	-	14	1	4
	%	-	100	-	100	-	100	-	100	20	80
Totals	No.	-	57	-	43	-	29	1	17	2	6

obtaining, to our surprise, a great improvement of clinical symptoms, lasting, in one case, for 2 years.

We think that these cases, although lacking statistical meaning, lay emphasis on the importance of treatment of the popliteal in limb revascularization by means of the femoralis profunda. This brief operation, well tolerated by patients, feasible under local anaesthesia, could well be a solution for a lot of cases. This could be due to the fact that, with TEA of the distal popliteal, some of the collaterals become patent (as seen especially by intraoperatory angiography). These collaterals, being in relation with the femoralis profunda, improve its flow.

Summary

The study refers on 186 arteriopathic patients undergoing lower limb reconstructive vascular surgery from 1974 to 1979. Of these, 130 showed combined atherosclerotic lesions of the aortoiliac-femoropopliteal axis.

Results regarding patients treated by revascularization of the AIF axis associated to profundoplasty (21 cases) were not satisfactory, particularly when indication to such surgery was placed by rest pain or trophic lesions. The search for the causes of such results brought to revision of pre- and intraoperatory angiographies; this showed that in many cases a reduction of collateral circulation at the popliteal lèvél was to blame.

Therefore, whenever angiographic studies showed a poor collateral circulation of the popliteal bed, the A.a carried out a direct revascularization of the aortoiliac-femoropopliteal (AIFP) axis in 57 cases, with excellent results. In choosing between profundoplasty and femoropopliteal TEA, the A.a stress the importance of popliteal artery revascularization both in the effort of reestablishing a direct flow and in improving the vascular bed distal to the branches of the femoralis profunda, with simple TEA of the distal popliteal segment.

References

1. Darling RC, Linton RR (1972) Durability of femoropopliteal reconstructions; endarterectomy versus vein bypass grafts. Am J Surg 123:427
2. De Nunno R, Ballabio R (1976) Sulla rivascolarizzazine aortoiliaco femoropoplitea.
3. De Nunno R, Ballabio R, Bertolini A (1977) The problem of lower limb revascularization in III and IV stage arteriopathies. International Congress of Cardiovascular Surgery, Tokyo
4. Martin P, Eawley JE (1972) On the surgery of atherosclerotic lesions of the profunda femoris artery. Surgery 71:182
5. Morris-Jones CDP (1974) Profundoplasty in the treatment of femoropopliteal occlusion. Am J Surg 127:680
6. Royster TS, Lynn R, Mulcare RJ (1976) Combined aortoiliac and femoropopliteal occlusive disease. Surg Gynecol Obstet 143:949
7. Sumner DS, Strandness DE (1978) Aortoiliac reconstruction in patients with combined iliac and superficial femoral occlusion. Surgery 84:348

Evaluation of the Profundoplasty in Reconstructions of Combined Aorto-iliac and Femoro-popliteal Occlusive Disease

W. Simma, C. Gross, P. Hartl, F. Pressl, G. Sfetsos, H. Bassiouny, and P. Brücke*

Combined aortoiliac and femoropopliteal lesions are more commonly encountered and indicate in most of the cases an advanced stage of arterial occlusive disease (4, 8, 10). The majority of the involved cases are old and to a relatively high percentage, they present with rest pain and tissue necroses (10, 11). Total reconstructions in both regions with these patients carry a high operative risk. The purpose of this study is to demonstrate the possibility of resubstituting such major procedures with more simple ones.

Material and Methods

In a 6-year period (January 1, 1974 – December 31, 1979) in the Surgical Department I of the General Hospital Linz, 135 bifurcation prostheses were implanted for occlusive diseases of the distal abdominal aorta and the iliac arteries. The group included 123 men and 12 women, i.e., a ratio of 10:1. The average age of the patients was 64 years (Table 1).

In 36 cases only the aortoiliac region was affected (Table 2); in 99 patients there were additional occlusions in the femoropopliteal system. In the following presentation, the isolated aortoiliac lesions are excluded.

Out of 99 patients operated upon for combined aortoiliac and femoropopliteal occlusive disease (Fig. 1), there were 92 men and 7 women with an average age of 67.2 years (Table 3). Compared with those, the average age in the aortoiliac group was 56.3 years (10). Clinically 48 patients presented with stage II-III, 51 with stage III-IV, 15 had a past history of cerebral infarction, 5 of myocardial infarction, 6 had hypertension, 4 were diabetics, and all of them were smokers, some heavy. A transabdominal approach was used for the implantation of all the aortobifemoral prostheses except for one patient who had a retroperitoneal approach.

Table 1. Total number of bifurcation grafts

No.	135
Males	123
Females	12
Age range	37-80 years
Average age	64 years

Table 2. Aortoiliac reconstructions

No.	36
Males	31
Females	5
Age range	37-78 years
Average age	56.3 years

*Surgical Department I of the Allgemeines Krankenhaus Linz, Krankenhausstr. 9, A-4020 Linz

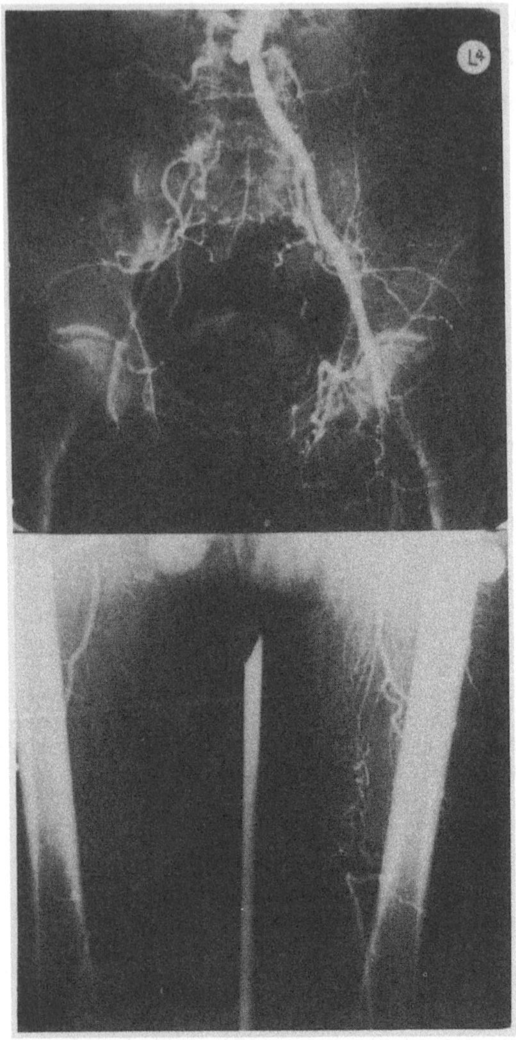

Fig. 1. Angiogram of a 76-year-old man with combined aortoiliac and femoropopliteal occlusion. Successful repair by means of an aortobifemoral Dacron graft and additional bilateral profundoplasty

Table 3. Combined aortoiliac and femoropopliteal lesions

No.	99
Males	92
Females	7
Age range	41-80 years
Average age	67.2 years

In 63 patients the limbs of the bifurcation prostheses were anastomosed to the profunda femoris with an associated profundoplasty, in 39 cases bilaterally, in 24 patients unilaterally. In two patients an additional bilateral lumbar sympathectomy was done, in one a femoropopliteal venous bypass grafting. In 36 patients the bifurcation implantation was done without profundoplasty. Three bilateral lumbar sympathectomies and two femoropopliteal bypass graftings were done simultaneously.

In the 63 patients with profundoplasties, 15 of them had secondary vascular procedures from 1 day to 2 years postoperatively (23.8%) (Table 4): these included 12 femoropopliteal bypass grafts and 3 profundoplasties. In the 36 patients without profundoplasties, 12 secondary vascular procedures became necessary from 1 day to 4 years postoperatively (33%): nine femoropopliteal bypass grafts, two profundoplasties, and one anastomosis reconstruction for stenosis. On observing Table 4 meticulously we can find that 6 out of the 15 delayed procedures in those patients who had previous profundoplasties became necessary on the opposite side of the unilaterally operated patients. This modifies remarkably the percentage of delayed procedures to 12.7% in the profunda group and to 42.8% in the nonprofundoplasty group.

Table 4. Delayed procedures n = 15 (23.8%)

Initial bif. + bil. prof. (39)		+ Unilat. prof. (24)	
No	6	No	9
T. of tr. fempopl. gr.		6 fempopl. 3 prof. pl. (6 of these operations became necessary on the opposite side)	

N.B. 15-6 = 9 (12.7%) of the delayed procedures were performed due to inefficiency of the primary treatment.

Results

Fourteen patients out of 99 died in the immediate postoperative (2 days to 3 weeks) period: four from myocardial infarction, two from bilateral pneumonia, two from cardiorespiratory insufficiency, two from colon necrosis, and one mortality each from sepsis after graft infection, shock, uremia, and paralytic ileus.

Ten patients died in the delayed postoperative period (7 weeks to 5 years): three from myocardial infarction and one mortality each from colon carcinoma, carcinosis peritonei, suppurative cholecystitis, sepsis, and three from unknown causes.

Eighty out of 85 patients submitted to postoperative control (80.9%). They all underwent Doppler examinations and a careful clinical examination. An excellent result was determined by unlimited activity, good result for a walking distance of 800-1000 m, and claudication for a distance not more than 150 m. Fifty-seven cases had an excellent result, five a good result, and eight patients complained of intermittent claudication.

Only two patients experienced an above-knee amputation 3-6 months postoperatively.

Discussion

The importance of the profunda femoris in the treatment of peripheral vascular occlusive disease of the lower limbs has been proved in numerous clinical and experimental studies (2, 5, 6, 9, 11). Due to the abundant anastomoses to the popliteal artery, it is thus the most important collateral of the lower limb. Also the profunda femoris is usually spared from extensive atherosclerosis and if involved this is localized at the take-off in most cases. This site of affection can be readily corrected by plasty (3, 8, 12).

Combined aortoiliac and femoropopliteal occlusions occur in 45%-69% of cases as reported in the literature – 73% in our patients (4, 8, 10). Reconstruction of these lesions by a profundoplasty after restoration of an adequate inflow provides a satisfactory outflow. Thus in the long-term results much fewer subsequent downstream repairs are needed (1-3, 7, 10, 12). Flow measurements showed that flow through the profunda femoris is equal to flow through aortofemoral grafts to the common femoral artery when both superficial and deep femoral vessels are patent (2).

We have to pay special attention to the surgical technique and to the selection of patients (3, 7, 9, 12). In all cases it is essential to extend the arteriotomy beyond the atheromatous stenosis. In some lesions the arteriotomy may extend to 10 cm and more. In these cases an autologous vein graft is more efficient than the tailored end of the prosthesis (7). However, the latter is used efficiently in limited lesions extending 1-2 cm beyond the take-off (Fig. 2).

If a short segment of the superficial femoral artery is occluded and is abundantly collateralized (Fig. 3), we tailor an additional tongue for the superficial femoral artery (Fig. 4). In some of these cases, a peripheral pulse can be palpated postoperatively. However, if the profunda femoral artery is extensively involved by atherosclerosis or is absent on angiography, then a femoropopliteal bypass grafting should be additionally performed in the same session.

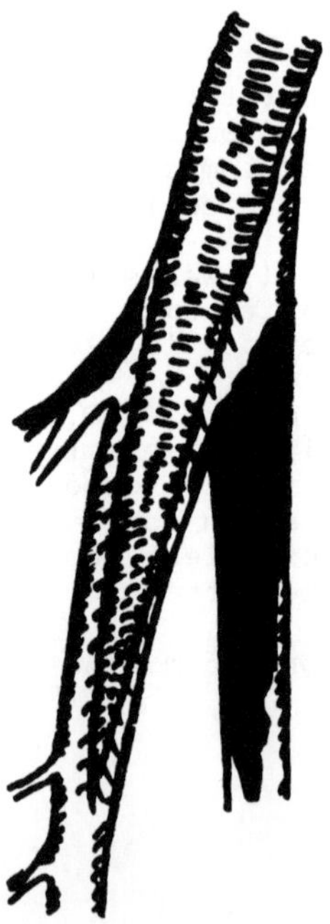

Fig. 2. Drawing of a tailored prosthesis limb serving as a profundoplasty

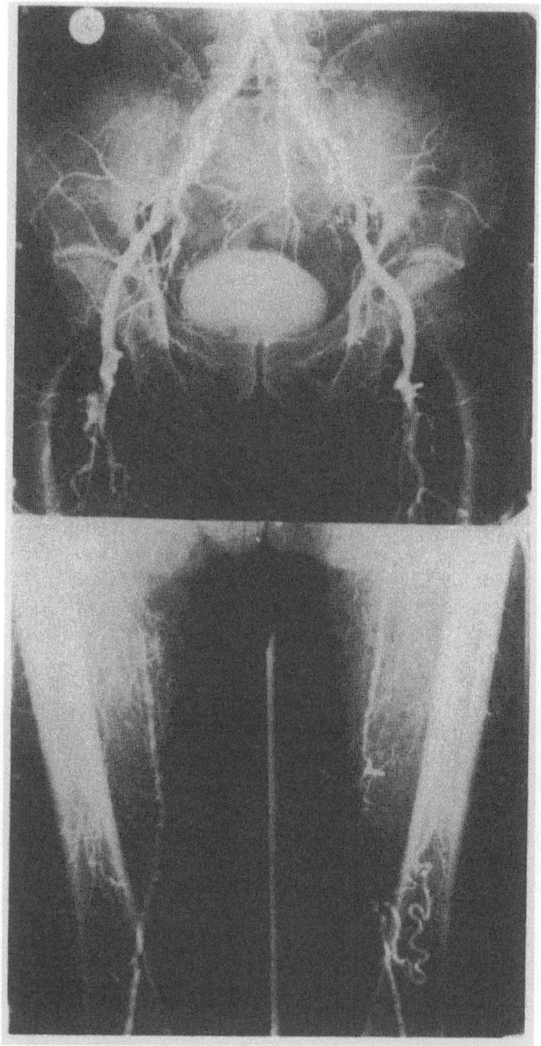

Fig. 3. Angiogram of a 65-year-old man with a combined aortoiliac and femoropopliteal occlusion with a good collateralization of the superficial femoral artery. Palpable pulses in the periphery after restoration of the iliac arterial inflow and after additional revascularization of the profundal arteries and a plasty at the origin of the superficial femoral arteries

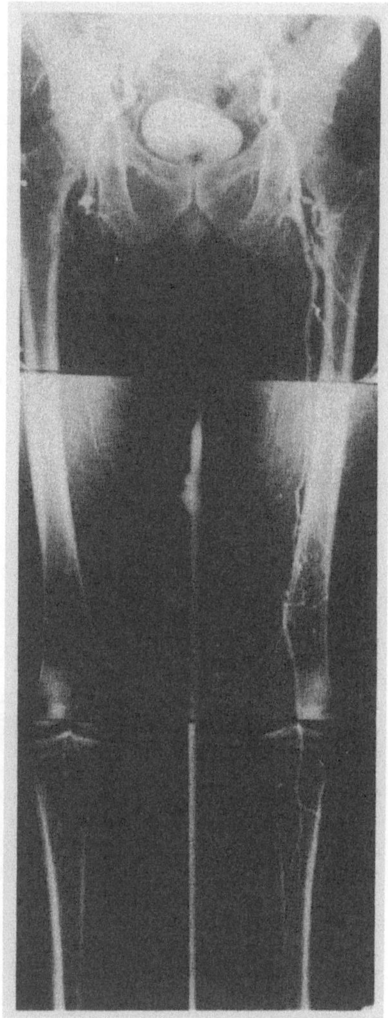

Fig. 4. Angiogram of a 74-year-old man showing subtotal stenoses of both common iliac arteries and a complete atherosclerotic occlusion of both superficial arteries. There is no profunda seen on the right side. In such cases, a femoropopliteal bypass graft has to be done as an additional procedure in the same session after restoration of the proximal inflow

Summary

The results in 135 patients undergoing aortoiliac and aortofemoral bypass grafts during 1974-1979 were examined. In most cases occlusive disease of the iliac arteries was combined with total atherosclerotic occlusions of the superficial femoral arteries and sometimes with additional alterations of the profundal artery.

In 42.8% subsequent vascular procedures became necessary in patients who had undergone aortoiliac or aortofemoral anastomic procedures without additional profundoplasties. In those cases where the primary reconstruction was combined with profundoplasty, the results very satisfying and in only 12.7% subsequent repairs became necessary.

The aortoprofunda bypass is now preferred for patients with combined aortoiliac and femoropopliteal occlusive disease. Results and technical details are discussed.

References

1. Baird RJ, Feldman P, Miles JT, Madras PM, Gurry JF (1977) Subsequent downstream repair after aortoiliac and aortofemoral bypass operations. Surgery 8:785-793
2. Bernhard M, Ray LJ, Militello JP (1976) The role of angioplasty of the profunda femoris artery in revascularization of the ischemic limb. Surg Gynecol Obstet 142:840-844
3. Bone GE (1979) Profundoplasty in the management of severe limb ischemia. American College of Surgeons, 56th Annual Clinical Congress, Chicago, Oct 21-26, 1979, Postgraduate Course 17: Peripheral vascular surgery, pp 9-12
4. Edwards WH, Wright RSA (1974) A technique for combined aorto-femoral-popliteal arterial reconstruction. Ann Surg 179:572
5. Lange J, Maurer PC, Liepsch D (1978) Strömungsdynamik der Arteria profunda femoris: Experimentalphysikalische Untersuchungen am naturgetreuen Modell vor und nach Profundaplastik. In: Wagner O, Kubiena K (eds) X. Jahrestagung der Österreichischen Gesellschaft für Gefäßchirurgie, Krems/Donau, Oct 19-22, 1978, pp 175-178
6. Martin P, Renwich S, Stephenson C (1968) On the surgery of the profunda femoris artery. Br J Surg 55:539
7. Malone JM, Goldstone J, Moore WS (1978) Autogenous profundoplasty; the key to long-term patency in secondary repair of aortofemoral graft occlusion. Ann Surg 188:817
8. McCombs PR (1979) The physiopathologic characteristics of superficial femoral artery occlusion. Surg Gynecol Obstet 148:775-784
9. Oberlinner R, Maurer PC (1976) Revaskularisation der Arteria profunda femoris: Typische Fallberichte und Ergebnisse. In: Denck H, Hagmüller GW (eds) IX. Jahrestagung der Österreichischen Gesellschaft für Gefäßchirurgie, Vienna, Nov 12-14, 1976, pp 261-268
10. Royster TS, Lynn R, Mulcare RJ (1976) Combined aorta iliac and femoro popliteal occlusive disease. Surg Gynecol Obstet 143:949-952
11. Vänttinen E, Inberg MV (1975) Aorto-ilico-femoral arterial reconstructive surgery; with special reference to profunda revascularization. Acta Chir Scand 141:600
12. Winegarner FG, Michl LG, Madura JA, Jesseph JE (1974) Revascularization of the severely ischemic lower extremity by aorta-profunda femoris bypass. Am J Surg 128:649-651

Long Grafts in the Treatment of Combined Iliac and Femoral Artery Disease

R.E.Horton, D.R.Bird, and P.C.Clifford*

The long graft is defined in this paper as from the common iliac artery or sometimes the aorta to the popliteal artery. The distal popliteal is preferred to the proximal part because in advanced atherosclerosis it is nearly always less diseased so that technical failure is rare. We have used the long graft in two circumstances. The first is when a femoropopliteal vein graft is indicated but no long saphenous vein is available. The second indication which is the subject of this presentation occurred in 21 patients (24 grafts) with combined iliac and femoral artery disease. All the patients were suffering from critical ischaemia and were subjects for early amputation if a reconstruction could not be carried out (Fig. 1).

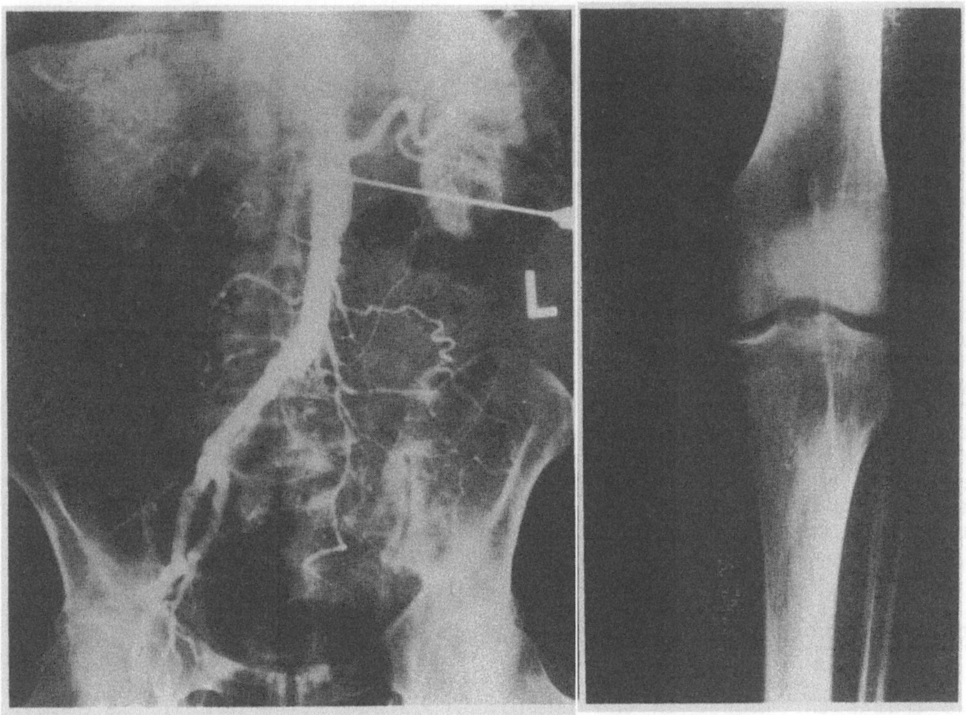

Fig. 1. Combined iliac and femoral artery occlusion treated by aortopopliteal graft

*Bristol Royal Infirmary, Bristol BS 2 8 HW, Great Britain

A number of different operative procedures have been described in the treatment of combined iliac and femoral disease but in the United Kingdom the most commonly used reconstruction is probably the ilioprofunda graft. The iliopopliteal graft gives a much more dramatic clinical result and pulse volume recordings which are much nearer to normal than is seen following the ilioprofunda graft.

There is no evidence that length is a significant cause of graft thrombosis but diameter should not be less than 10 mm which is adequate for iliac artery flow. Dacron grafts develop a 1-2 mm pseudointima of compressed fibrin and platelets and this results in a considerable reduction of flow. Strandness and Sumner (2) emphasise the importance of using a 10 mm graft because the deposition of a 1 mm pseudointima inside a 10 mm graft increases the haemodynamic resistance by 144% while the same depth of pseudointima in an 8 mm graft increases the resistance by 216%.

The Operation

The operation is simple and blood loss is usually minimal, transfusion needs rarely exceeding one unit. The patient is little disturbed because the approach to the iliac arteries is extraperitoneal.

The operation comprises three parts,

1. An extraperitoneal approach is made to the iliac arteries, using the incision described by Helsby and Moosa (1). This extends from the costal margin near the tip of the ninth costal cartilage and curves down and medially ending some 5 cm from the midline and 5 cm above the symphysis.
2. A short subinguinal incision is made and this is used to pull the graft through from the pelvis and also to tunnel down to join the popliteal incision. The opportunity is taken to divide the inguinal ligament which may contribute to kinking in the graft.
3. The popliteal artery is approached medially and the distal part exposed by dividing the medial head of gastrocnemius.

When the exposures have been completed the 10 mm woven graft is preclotted. The patient is heparinised intravenously and the graft placed in position and sutured with a continuous 5/0 prolene suture.

The long grafts have been studied and their continued patency judged by the pulse clinically felt in the graft and by ultrasonic studies using a 30-channel pulsed Doppler imaging system (MAVIS) manufactured by GEC (Medical) which gives an image of the moving stream of blood. In a prospective study it was found that no change in graft diameter occurred in the first 3 months following implantation of the graft but after this time there was a tapering in the distal third of the graft caused by an increase in depth of pseudointima. We believe that this is a haemodynamic effect resulting from the insertion of a 10 mm Dacron graft into the narrower popliteal artery.

Early Thrombosis

Two grafts thrombosed in the immediate postoperative period. In each case the graft was explored, opened transversely about its middle and thrombus removed with Fogarty catheters. These two grafts have remained patent for 8 and 36 months so far.

We believe this complication to be due to a combination of the thrombogenic characteristics of the graft and reduced cardiac output and graft flow following surgery. We were not, at this time, using the heparin irrigation technique to neutralize thrombin in the graft as described by Yates et al. (3).

Late Thrombosis

Late thrombosis occurred in two cases at 4 and 13 months following insertion of the graft. One has remained patent for a further 8 months following thrombectomy but in the second case flow could not be re-established and the leg was amputated. One patient had been working all day in a stooping position with acutely flexed knees and hips. At the end of the day his graft thrombosed. This raised the possibility that graft thrombosis might be caused by kinking of the graft with the knee or hip flexed. To investigate this, grafts have been studied with the Advanced Technology Laboratories' Duplex Ultrasound System which, by rapid automatic scanning, gives the impression of motion on the screen (real time). Graft or artery wall can be studied dynamically during joint flexion and when imaged the picture can be frozen for measurements to be taken. Sixteen out of 18 (78%) grafts kinked at the knee with 90° of flexion and the resulting occlusion was up to 54% in diameter (Fig. 2). Flexion of the hip to 60° only showed kinking in one of 21 cases studied.

Based on these studies we now advise patients with grafts sutured to the distal popliteal artery that prolonged knee flexion should be avoided and that the knee should never be flexed beyond 90°. Air and car travel is potentially hazardous to the graft and patients should be warned of the importance of not sitting in a cramped position for a long period of time. Kinking can be eliminated by using the proximal popliteal artery but technical difficulties caused by severe disease in the proximal popliteal artery generally outweigh this disadvantage.

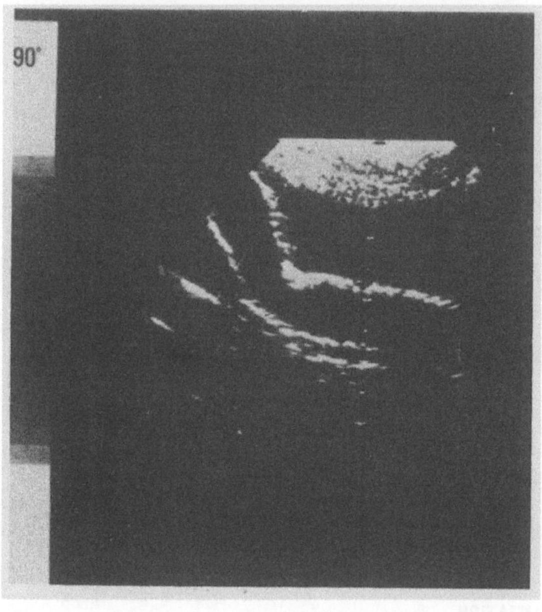

Fig. 2. Scan demonstrating kinking of Dacron graft with knee flexion to 90°

Mortality

One patient died on the fifth day from a coronary artery thombosis giving a mortality of 4%. Cardiovascular disease was the cause of six out of seven later deaths. Four patients died of myocardial infarcts, one from congestive heart failure and one from a massive stroke. The seventh patient died from carcinoma of the colon.

Graft Patency

The results have been studied by the life-table method (Fig. 3). The 4-year analysis shows a patency rate of 79%. The high patency rate is probably due to the high flow which results from taking the graft from the common iliac artery. Kinking of grafts sutured to the distal popliteal is not a cause of thrombosis unless the knee is kept in flexion for a long period of time.

At the time of this study, 14 patients were still alive and relieved from pain. They had retained their legs and were able to walk. As an alternative to amputation in combined iliac and femoral disease, the long graft patients generally remain mobile until death from some other manifestation of atherosclerosis.

Summary

Twenty-four 10 mm Dacron grafts have been used in 21 patients with combined iliac and femoral artery disease causing critical ischaemia. After 3 months, the grafts show tapering in the distal third. Kinking at the knee joint occurred in 78% of grafts but this did not have any obvious effect on long-term patency. Follow-up studies show 79% of grafts to be patent at the 3- to 4-year interval.

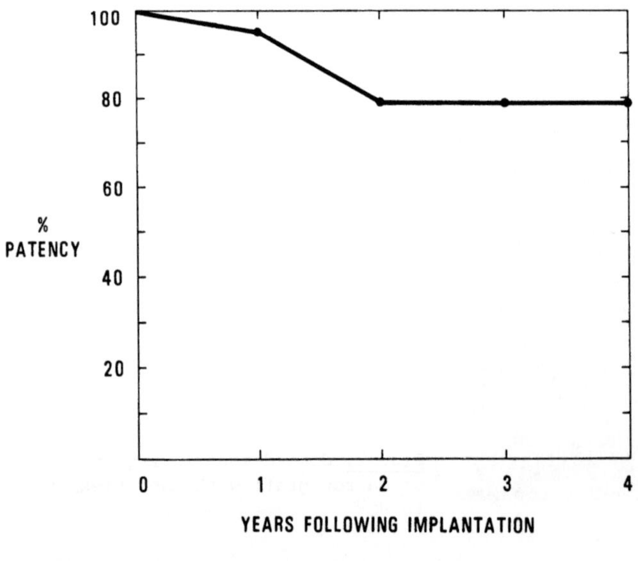

Fig. 3. Life-table analysis of the long-term patency of iliopopliteal Dacron grafts for limb salvage

References

1. Helsby CR, Moosa AR (1975) Br J Surg 62:596
2. Strandness DE, Sumner DS (1975) Hemodynamics for surgeons. Grune & Stratton, New York, p 343
3. Yates SG, Barros D'Sa AAB, Berger K, Fernandez LG, Wood SJ, Rittenhouse EA, Davis CC, Mansfield PB, Sauvage LR (1978) The preclotting of porous arterial prostheses. Ann Surg 188:5

Disease of the Aorto-iliac and Femoro-popliteal Arteries. Combined Surgical Repair in 48 Cases

E. Tovar and A. Tovar*

Forty-eight patients were submitted to direct aortoiliac and femoropopliteal surgery simultaneously, between January 1973 and December 1979. All sorts of technical combinations were carried out, and we emphasize the difficulty of finding a suitable method of performing superior and inferior anastomosis at the femoral level.

The clearest indications are the aortic aneurysms, with associated aneurysm and thrombosis at the femoral or popliteal level, and those cases with serious popliteal damage, and in which only one vessel is permeable, associating with aortoiliac surgery the femorotibial or fibula, in general, with femoral profunda atheromatosis.

The overall results are bad, with early femoropopliteal occlusion, because of difficulties at the level of the proximal anastomosis. In our experience, we consider that this simultaneous surgery is only indicated when no reasonable possibility of saving the extremity can be seen with the femoral profunda and with especially selected cases.

Mortality was one patient in the series, so it is the results and not the death rate which cause our attitude.

Material and Method

In the period between January 1973 and December 1979, we operated on 48 patients in the aortoiliac and femoropopliteal sectors simultaneously. Age ranged between 51 and 72, with an average of 66. The majority were male. The etiology of the illness was arteriosclerosis in 35 patients, 9 aneurysms, and 4 thromboembolias in both sectors.

Sixteen cases were treated with thromboendarterectomies in the aortoiliac sectors, four bilateral and twelve unilateral, by the extraperitoneal approach. Of these cases, three were treated with bilateral femoropopliteal thromboendarterectomies, one with a bypass in one site and thromboendarterectomies in the other, 12 unilateral, 10 with bypass, and two with thromboendarterectomies in the femoropopliteal sector.

Four with thromboembolic disease of both sectors were treated with thrombectomies by the femoral approach, in all cases bilateral.

Nine patients had aneurysm in the abdominal aorta, associated in two cases with bilateral femoral aneurysm and obliterations of the superficial femoral; three unilateral popliteal aneurysms and three femoropopliteal obliterations that were treated with a vein bypass, the three unilateral. One popliteal aneurysm was treated with excision and a bilateral bypass.

*Instituto Policlinico Sta. Teresa, La Coruña, Spain

Results

The operatory mortality among the 48 patients was one case, 6 days after being operated on, due to a heart attack. The patient, 70 years old, had no previous history of ischemic cardiopathy. Seven extremities were amputated as a result of femoropopliteal occlusion in the 3 months following the operation.

The occlusion was more frequent and earlier in the thromboendarterectomy than in the bypass at any level, although more marked in the femoropopliteal sector. Occlusion was not always followed by amputation. The fact that the majority of the patients systematically received lumbar sympathectomy uni- or bilaterally probably contributed to this. The value of the associated sympathectomy cannot be clearly defined objectively, but we think that the results improve and the ischemia is prevented when the inferior sector is occluded.

The majority of the patients operated on had the inferior sector occluded after 2 years; not all could be followed, and about 20% had some problem at the superior level: occlusion of one branch of the bypass, obliteration of the external iliac, etc. In general the results, except in 16 patients, were not better than if we had acted only at the superior level, for which reason, in our experience, this technique is restricted to cases in which it is really indicated.

Discussion

The simultaneous approach in lesions of both sectors seems to be the ideal solution, but practice shows that the results obtained are not satisfactory in more than half the patients, and that the results are not better than those obtained acting on the superior sector and lumbar sympathectomy.

The most important problem observed was technical at the level of the inferior and superior anastomosis of the two respective sectors. The use of the iliac as a terminal bed in the superior sector and the common femoral as origin or the femoropopliteal is the simplest and easiest, but the external iliac is quickly occluded. The most frequent solution was taking the inferior bypass at the level of the superficial femoral, in a terminal way and 4 to 6 cm from the common. The saphena vein, at the level of the bifurcation graft, gave very bad results and the same can be said of the compound grafts.

Conclusions

Simultaneous surgery of the aortoiliac and femoropopliteal sector did not give good results in the short term or long term. Mortality was very low, about 2%. We consider that it is only justified in carefully selected cases and that it is necessary to individualize.

Late Results in Surgery of Aorto-iliac-femoral Occlusive Disease

G. Walterbusch, R. Flade, A. Staufenbiel, and H. G. Borst*

Combined disease of the aortoiliac and femoropopliteal arteries generally results in more severe ischemia of the lower limb than isolated disease of either segment. Furthermore, two-segment disease often reflects generalized arteriosclerotic morbidity, most significantly involving the coronary and cerebral artery system. Therefore, in this group of patients an urgent therapy is required more often and the operative risk is markedly increased.

Fortunately, in most cases isolated repair of the proximal aortoiliac occlusive disease results in limb salvage and considerable reduction of claudication (1). Controversy remains in cases with completely occluded popliteal artery, i.e., the questions whether additional femorocrural repair is necessary and whether this should be performed at the same procedure or at a second stage (2). In this study our patient material with two-segment disease was reviewed with particular interest of long-term results in relation to preoperative angiographic findings.

Material and Methods

Two hundred and eighty-three patients underwent surgery of aortoiliacofemoral occlusive disease between March 1973 and December 1979. Among these patients, 475 limbs had two-segment disease. Male patients (n = 263) predominated with 93% vs 7% female patients (n = 20). Mean age at the time of operation was 61.5 ± 6 years. Twenty-three patients (8.1%) were lost to follow-up, 46 patients had died before reinvestigation. All the remaining patients were reexamined at our clinic within the past 12 months. The average follow-up duration of this group was 32 months. At the time of operation, 190 patients (67%) had ischemic rest pain or tissue necrosis. Ninety-three patients (33%) underwent surgery because of disabling claudication.

Primary operative procedures were planned on the basis of angiographic findings. In case of a patent profunda femoris artery and popliteal artery, only profunda revascularization was performed without attempt at two-segment repair. This condition was present in the vast majority of the patients. (n = 441, limbs = 92.8%) (see Fig. 1, right limb).

When the profunda femoris artery showed distal disease or occlusion, an additional femoropopliteal venous bypass was implanted in the same session. This condition was found in 12 limbs (2.5%) (see Fig. 1, left limb). In these cases, preoperative angiographic findings unequivocally

*Medizinische Hochschule, Abt. Thorax-, Herz- und Gefäßchirurgie, Karl-Wiechert-Allee 9, D-3000 Hannover 61

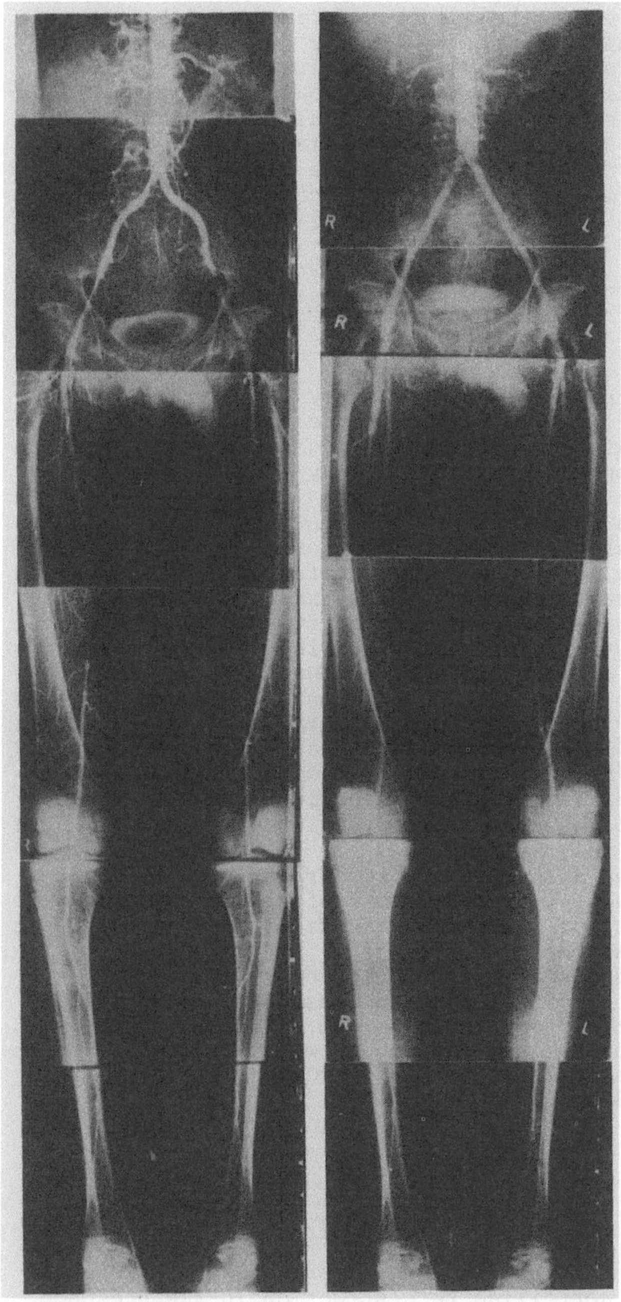

Fig. 1. Pre- and postoperative angiograms demonstrating the operative procedures in the femoropopliteal segment. Right limb: Profunda revascularization. Left limb: Additional venous bypass in presence of profunda artery disease

indicated the operative regime. In 22 limbs (4.6%) with popliteal artery occlusion, the operative procedure was a matter of debate in recent years since early results after proximal segment repair seemed to be unpredictable. Retrospective evaluation of preoperative angiograms identified only four patients (0.8%) with popliteal artery occlusion who had relief from ischemic symptoms following proximal repair only. Most interestingly, these patients showed patency of the superficial femoral artery up to the adductor foramen feeding the collaterals of the Rete articulare genus (see Fig. 2).

In a fourth group, characterized by total occlusion of the superficial femoral and popliteal artery, proximal repair alone always failed. In 13 patients with this condition, additional femorocrural grafting became necessary early after primary aortoiliac repair. Therefore, in this type of disease we now prefer a one-stage repair (aortoiliac and femorocrural) as performed in our last five cases (see Fig. 3, right limb).

Results

There were 13 hospital deaths among 265 patients with aortoiliac repair (4.9%). Hospital mortality was 6.2% after second stage femorocrural grafting and 11.7% after one-stage two-segment repair. Early death was attributed to respiratory insufficiency and myocardial infarction as a rule.

Nonlethal early and late complications are shown in Table 1. Aortoiliac graft failure was mostly related to improper profunda revascularization and at reoperation a more extensive profundoplasty was used. Thrombectomy of occluded grafts was successful except in three cases where extra-anatomic femorofemoral crossover grafts became necessary. In 11 cases of stenotic distal anastomosis, causing recurrent symptoms of ischemia, the same type of corrective repair was applied. In 16 patients, including the above-mentioned 13 patients with femoral superficial and popliteal artery occlusion, persistent or even aggravated ischemia was observed early after aortoiliac repair. Eighteen patients required late second-stage femoropopliteal or femorocrural bypass operation despite good profunda inflow. Late ischemic disease in these patients was related to progression of arteriosclerotic disease in the popliteal and trifurcation vessels.

No infection was observed after primary repair of aortoiliac segments. Three infections developed in the groin after late femoropopliteal segment grafting. One of these patients died after a subsequent extra-anatomic bypass operation.

Three patients developed distal anastomotic aneurysms and were reoperated. In one case, limb amputation was necessary for untractable embolic occlusion, originating from the aneurysm. The cumulative 7-year patency rate for aortoiliac segment repair was 84%, whereas patency rate for femoralpopliteal grafting was only 40%. Limb salvage rate for all limbs at risk was 87%.

Conclusion

Our experience with combined aortoiliac and femoropopliteal disease proves the value of single aortoiliac reconstruction in the presence of a patent proximal popliteal artery segment. It has been widely demonstrated that reconstruction of the aortoiliac segment and the profunda artery inflow is a very successful operation with excellent long-term results (3-5).

When the profunda femoris shows significant distal obstructive disease, simultaneous two-segment repair appears to be inevitable. In patients with popliteal artery occlusions. isolated aortoiliac repair may be successful in one condition: superficial femoral artery patency up to

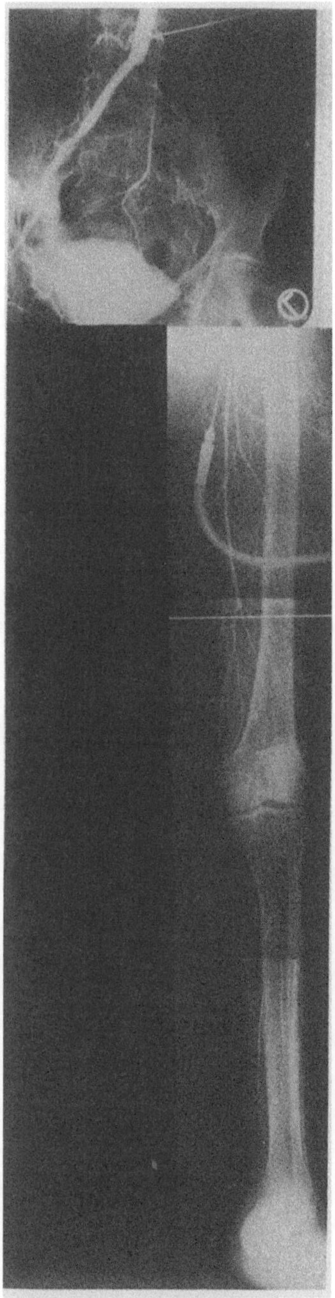

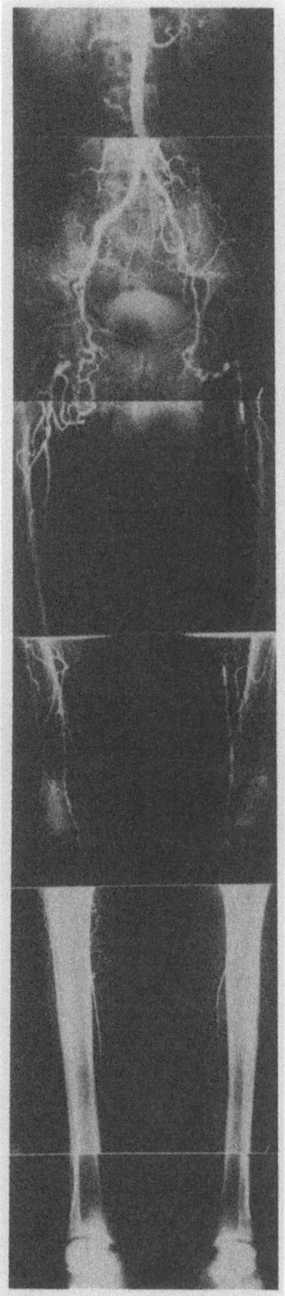

Fig. 3

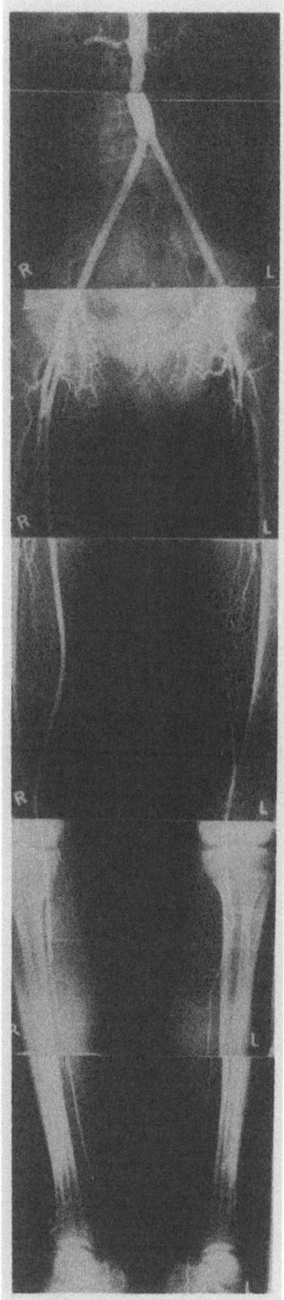

Fig. 2

Fig. 3

Fig. 2. In case of popliteal artery occlusion, proximal repair was sufficient when superficial femoral artery was patent

Fig. 3. In case of total occlusion of superficial femoral and popliteal artery, proximal repair failed. Additional femorocrural venous grafts became necessary

Table 1. Complications and secondary operations

Complications	Early		Late		Secondary operations: Profundo-plasty	Femoropoplital (crural) graft	Extra-anatomic graft	Resec-tion	Ampu-tation
	N	%	N	%	N	N	N	N	N
Graft failure	4	0.8	16	3.4	16	1	3	-	5
Stenosis	-	-	11	2.3	11	-	-	-	-
Ischemia despite intact aortoiliac inflow	16	3.3	18	3.8	-	31	-	-	16
Infection	-	-	3	1.0	-	-	3	-	-
Aneurysm	-	-	3	0.6	-	-	-	3	-

the adductor foramen, permitting direct connection with the large knee collaterals.

Except for this rare condition, popliteal artery occlusion appears to require two-segment repair. Since failure of one-segment repair under these circumstances seems to be predictable, one-stage two-segment repair is recommended.

References

1. Brewster DC, Darling RC (1978) Optimal methods of aorto-iliac reconstruction. Surgery 84:739-748
2. Van Dongen RJAM (1976) Operationstaktik bei Verschlüssen der Becken und Oberschenkelarterien. Angio 1/1:10-16
3. Morris GC, Edwards W, Cooley DA, Crawford ES, De Bakey ME (1961) Surgical importance of profunda femoris artery. Analysis of 102 cases with combined aorto-iliac and femoropopliteal occlusive disease treated by revascularization of deep femoral artery. Arch Surg 82:32
4. Vänttinen E, Tuberg MV (1975) Aorto-ilicofemoral arterial reconstructive surgery. With special reference to profunda revascularization. Acta Chir Scand 141:600-608
5. Malone JM, Moore WS, Goldstone J (1975) The natural history of bilateral aorto-femoral bypass grafts for ischemia of the lower extremities. Arch Surg 110: 1300-1306

Aorto-femoro-popliteal and Aorto-femoro-tibial Reconstructions: 10-Years Experience

A. Cavallaro, V. Sciacca, M. Garofalo, A. Alessandrini, and L. Di Marzo*

The very high incidence of cases in which significant lesions of the aortoiliac and of the femoropopliteal tracts coexist poses the problem of the surgical tactics to be used to achieve the best result.

While some authors (5) assert that a "total" reconstruction should be attempted almost routinely, according to the majority of others (7, 8), an aortofemoral procedure with profundoplasty, when necessary, is generally sufficient to obtain a satisfactory result. However, mainly in cases of heavy involvement of limb circulation with very low ankle pressure index and actual or impending gangrene, a double reconstructive procedure, even if charged by higher mortality and morbidity, may be desirable as the only means to achieve a significantly satisfactory result (4, 6). The double reconstruction could be a necessity and not a choice in a high percentage of reoperations for thrombosis of an aortofemoral graft (3). Baird et al. (1) assert that a distal extension of an aortofemoral reconstruction appears necessary in the early postoperative period in 10% of cases and within 8-9 months in 10% more.

From November 1969 to June 1980, on 280 patients consecutively submitted to aortofemoral reconstruction, the necessity or opportunity of extending distally the reconstruction itself was established in 40 (14.2%). Almost all 280 patients initially treated also presented occlusion of the superficial femoral artery. According to the type of actual circulatory involvement and of the operation therefore performed, we have divided the patients into five groups.

Group 1: One-Stage Aortofemoral + Distal Reconstruction by Necessity

One patient, in whom surgical reconstruction was planned on account of unilateral iliofemoral occlusion, a dissecting aneurysm of the femoral bifurcation was resected, including the proximal 5 cm of deep femoral; the Dacron prosthesis was anastomosed end-to-end to a branch of the deep femoral. An autologous vein femoropopliteal bypass was then established, putting the proximal anastomosis, side-to-end, on the branch of the deep femoral, 0.5 cm distal to the termination of the Dacron prosthesis. The result is very good (actual follow-up 60 months).

Group 2: One-Stage Aortofemoral + Distal Reconstruction, Elective

Six patients, aged 51-69 years (mean 59 years).

Associated diseases:	heart	3 (50%)
	diabetes	2 (33%)

*University of Rome, IV. Cattedra di Patologia Chirurgica, Rome, Italy

Operative indication was rest pain in three cases (50%) and gangrene in three (50%). Proximal reconstruction was bilateral in two patients, unilateral in four. In six limbs, on the basis of preoperative evaluation and intraoperative finding ("bad" profunda in four cases, involvement of popliteal and/or tibial vessels in two), the arterial reconstructive procedure was extended distally down to popliteal (five cases) or tibial (one case) vessels. The material used for the femorodistal bypass was autologous vein in four cases, Dacron in one, and PTFE in one. The results were not gratifying, consisting of one postoperative death, two early failures (with one major amputation), two late failures (6 and 36 months) without loss of the limb, and one extended patency with optimal functional result (follow-up 51 months).

Group 3: Two-Stage Aortofemoral + Distal Reconstruction for "Acute" Complications of the Former

Sixteen patients, aged 40-73 years (mean 57 years).

Associated diseases:	diabetes	3 (19%)
	lung	3 (19%)
	heart	2 (13%)
	hypertension	2 (13%)

Operative indication to the proximal reconstruction, which was bilateral in 14 cases, was: claudication four (25%), rest pain nine (56%), gangrene three (19%). In five cases an extra-anatomic reconstruction was performed (three femorofemoral, one axillofemoral, one axillobifemoral).

The complications which led to emergency reoperation were immediate or early in 17 limbs (13 thrombosis, 4 infection); the only late complication consisted of bilateral groin pseudoaneurysm in one patient. Twenty emergency operations were performed on 19 limbs of 16 patients, correcting the "acute" defect of the cranial reconstruction and extending this down to the popliteal artery (15 times) or to one of the tibial vessels (five times). The graft material was mainly autologous vein (nine times) but also PTFE and Dacron were used (six and five times, respectively).

The results were disappointing: five postoperative deaths (31%), eight early failures with five major amputations and only three saved limbs; persistent good result was achieved in five limbs of four patients (actual follow-up: 20, 28, 38, and 50 months) (Fig. 1).

Group 4: Two-Stage Aortofemoral + Distal Reconstruction for Progression of Disease

Six patients, aged 52-78 years (mean 65).

Associated diseases:	hypertension	3 (50%)
	heart	2 (34%)
	lung	2 (34%)
	Kidney	1 (17%)

The aortofemoral procedure, bilateral in three patients, was indicated by: claudication in one case (17%), rest pain in four (66%), and gangrene in one (17%). At an interval of 1-15 months (mean 5 months), a second operation was judged necessary on account of the worsening of patient conditions ameliorated after the first surgical treatment. The cause of deterioration of limb circulation is uncertain, consisting probably in a progressive failure of the cranial reconstruction; however, true progression of the basic disease or chronic damage of distal arterial tree by microembolism could play a significant role.

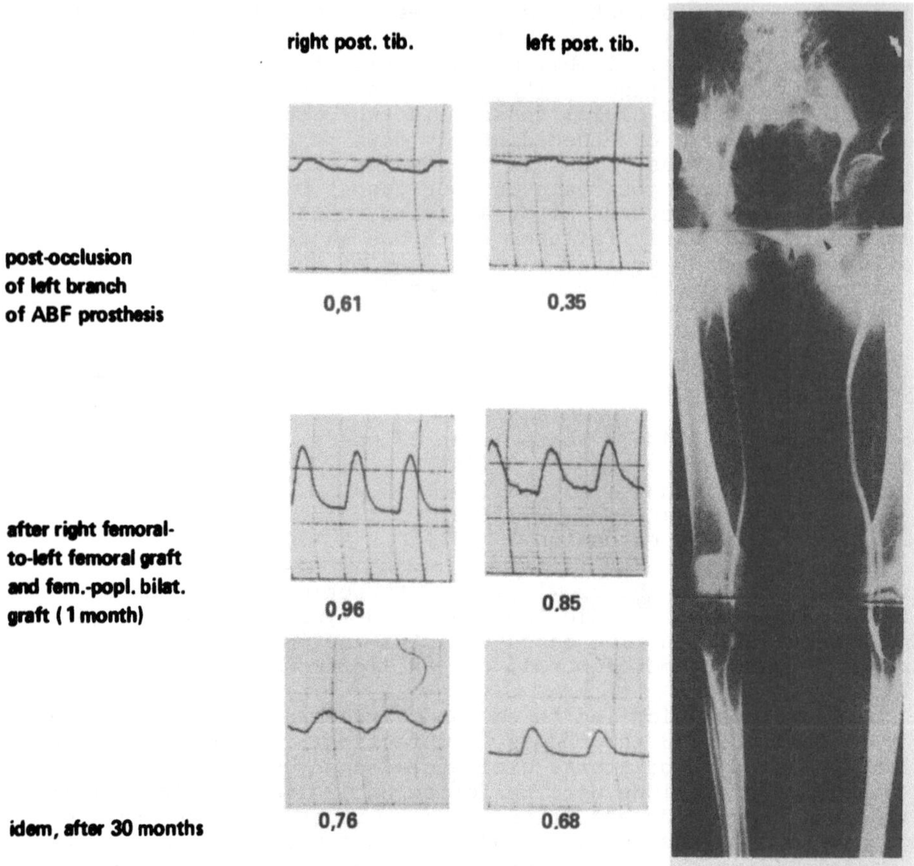

Fig. 1. In this patient of Group 3, occlusion of the left branch of an aortobifemoral prosthesis was treated unsuccessfully by thrombectomy; a right femoral-to-left femoral and popliteal artery bypass was performed; a femoropopliteal bypass was added on the right side to avoid excessive steal. Both distal reconstructions were performed by Dacron prostheses; angiography (on the right) shows a good function of the reconstruction (2 years postoperative) and Doppler flowmetry confirms continuing patency

The distal reconstruction was performed seven times on six limbs of six patients (four femoropopliteal bypasses, three femorotibial bypasses): the graft material was PTFE four times and autologous vein three times. Late patency was achieved in four patients (actual follow-up: 11, 26, 36, and 65 months); early failure and subsequent amputation affected two patients (Fig. 2).

Group 5: Two-Stage Aortofemoral + Distal Reconstruction for Persistence of Significant Symptoms after the Former (Fig. 3)

Eleven patients, aged 53-74 years (mean 62 years)

Associated diseases:	heart	4 (36%)
	lung	3 (27%)
	diabetes	2 (18%)
	hypertension	2 (18%)

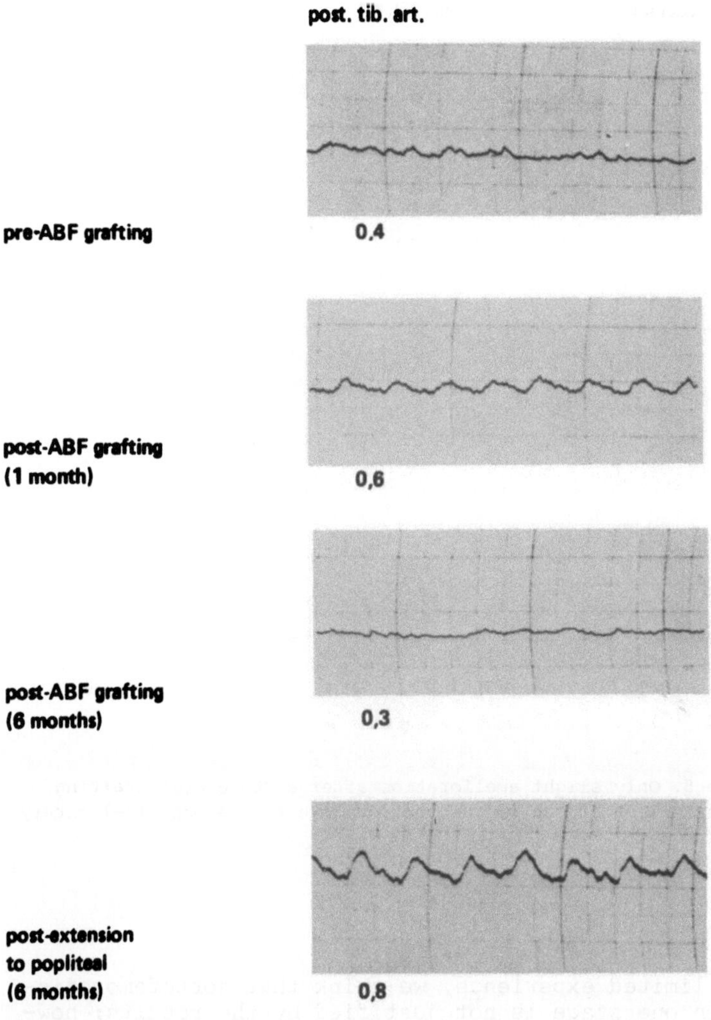

Fig. 2. In this patient of Group 4, the initial good result after aortobifemoral grafting was not maintained on the left limb, a progressive worsening of distal pressure index and of clinical conditions being apparent; good result after distal extension down to the popliteal artery

Aortofemoral reconstruction (bilateral in nine patients) was performed on the basis of: claudication, three (27%); rest pain, one (9%); gangrene, seven (64%). The probable cause of persistence of symptoms (unchanged or only slightly improved) after the first operation was identified in a "bad" profunda in five cases (46%) and in popliteal or tibial artery involvement in six cases (54%). The interval between the first and the second operation ranged from 15 days to 11 months (mean 3.5 months).

Seventeen reoperations were performed on 11 limbs of 11 patients, putting the end of the distal reconstruction 6 times on the popliteal and 11 times on the tibial arteries. Graft material was mainly PTFE (11 times); autologous vein was used in four operations and Dacron in two. Early failure affected the result in five cases, with unavoidable major amputation in four; late patency was achieved in six patients (actual follow-up: 3, 7, 8, 9, 60, and 62 months).

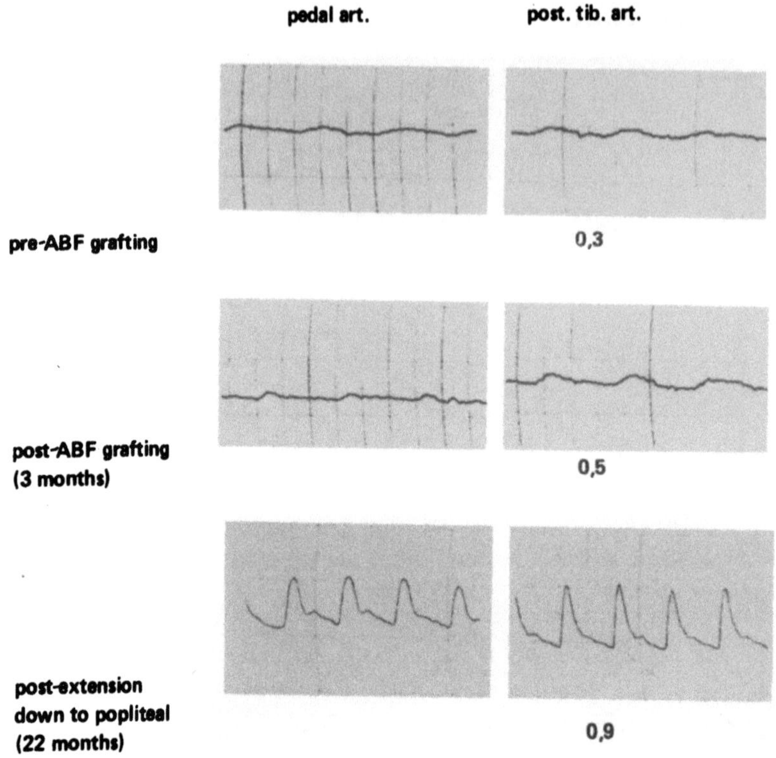

Fig. 3. Patient of Group 5. Only slight amelioration after aortofemoral grafting; very good result after extension of the reconstruction down to the popliteal artery

Conclusion

On the basis of our limited experience, we think that aortofemorodistal reconstruction in one stage is not justified by the results; however, an extension of an aortofemoral reconstruction, down to the leg vessels, may appear necessary after a shorter or longer period, to achieve a better rehabilitation of the patient: in such cases, long-term success was achieved in about 60% of cases. In emergeny conditions, as in reoperations for acute complications of an aortofemoral procedure, the attempt to save the limb is fully justified, but the results were very poor (only about 25% of permanent good results).

References

1. Baird RJ, Feldman P, Miles JT, Madias PM, Gurry JF (1977) Subsequent downstream repair after aorta-iliac and aorta-femoral bypass operation. Surgery 82:785
2. Cavallaro A, Sciacca V, Alessandrini A, Stipa S (1978) Le ricostruzioni aorto-femoro-poplitee: considerazioni su 20 casi. Policlin Sez Chir 85:543
3. Courbier R, Jausseran JM, Reggi M, Monin P, Chamant M (1978) Rôle de la perméabilité de la voie fémorale superficielle dans les thromboses des prothèses aorto-ilio-fémorales. Chirurgie 104:563

4. Dardik H, Ibrahim IM, Jarrah M, Sussman B, Dardik I (1979) Synchronous aorto-femoral or iliofemoral bypass with revascularization of the lower extremity. Surg Gynecol Obstet 149:676
5. Favi P, Marranci PL, Ponzalli M, Moretti R, Massimo C (1978) Cinquanta casi di ostruzione aorto-femoro-poplitea trattati con by-pass aorto-bifemorale e femoro-distale con innesto venoso. VI Congr Naz Soc It Chir Card Vasc, vol II, p 215
6. Masson B, Quancard X, Catherine G, Janvier G (1978) La restauration ilio-fêmoro-poplitêe en un temps. Sa place dans le traitment de l'artêrite des membres in-fêrieurs. Chirurgie 104:833
7. Provan JL, Patterson GA, Madras PN (1980) Is proximal reconstruction alone ad-equate treatment for combined aortoiliac and femoropopliteal disease? Can J Surg 23:81
8. Voss EU, Heyden B, Vollmar J (1979) Le traitement chirurgical des obstructions êtagêes aorto-iliaques et fêmoro-poplitêes. Angeiologie 31:3

Session V Cardiac Surgery

Infection in Cardiac Surgery

Chairman: R. Soyer, Rouen; Co-Chairman: P. Naumann, Düsseldorf

Positive Blood Culture: Germ Number and Distribution in 706 Patients After Open Heart Surgery

U. Mähner, A. Laczkovics, F. Wewelka, H. Benzer, and E. Wolner*

Positive blood cultures were obtained in 32 of 706 patients after open heart surgery with extracorporeal circulation.

Results:

	1978			I/79 - IX/79		
Valve replacement + anuloplasty or aortocor. bypass	22	4	18%	13	1	7.6%
Simple valve replacement	109	5	4.5%	87	5	5.7%
Aortocor. bypass	146	10	6.8%	103	2	1.9%
Congen. heart dis.	112	5	4.5%	77	0	0.0%
Total	409	24		297	8	

Concordant with the literature, infections occur more frequently in the older age groups and after longer lasting, complicated operations. Beside this, a reduction in germ number can be achieved by changing the antibiotic therapy plus observation of specific hygiene rules. Without frequent changes of different antibiotics, and without penicillin, a selection of dangerous gram-negative bacteria could be avoided.

*2nd Surgical Clinic, University Vienna, Austria

Antibiotic Concentration in Human Hearts

P. Satter and P. Eigel*

Early postoperative endocarditis is a major complication of open heart surgery particularly after valve replacement. By definition it is a clinical picture within 60 days after the initial operation due primary to staphylococcal infection. The incidence is approximately 1% with a high mortality of between 40% and 100% (1). Contamination occurs probably intraoperative. The clinical picture develops either as a primary sepsis and endocarditis or as secondary sepsis arising from an infected sternotomy with consequent infection of blood and valves. Since general resistance is reduced during and after ECC and because many patients are of advanced age, it is generally agreed that antibiotic prophylaxis is necessary particularly if an artificial valve is implanted (2, 3). In order to find the most suitable drug it is important to know not only the antibiotic potential against different strains of bacteria but also the concentration of the administered antibiotic at the site of its intended activity.

Technique

In this study the tissue concentration of different cephalosporins was measured in 50 noncalcified human heart valves (27 aortic and 23 mitral) in 40 specimens from the right atrium and in 7 resected papillary muscles.

The antibiotics in the test were: Cefamandole (Mandokef, Eli, Lilly), Cefoxitin (Mefoxitin, Merck, Sharp and Dome), Cefotaxim (Claforan, Hoechst, Glaxo), or Cefuroxime (Zinacef, Hoechst).

A dose of 1.5 g Cefuroxime or 2 g Cefamandole, Cefoxitin, or Cefotaxim was administered by intravenous infusion just before introduction of anesthesia. All specimens were taken at the same time approximately 10 min after starting ECC and 60 min after administration. They were cleaned of blood and immediately deep frozen at -24°C. The antibiotic concentration was analysed at the Department of Microbiology, University Frankfurt/Main, by the plate dilution test using bacterium subtilis as a test strain (4).

Results

Table 1 demonstrates the tissue concentration for the four antibiotics in the test and within the different structures. The tissue con-

*Clinic for Thoracic- and Cardiovascular Surgery, University Frankfurt/Main, Theodor-Stern-Kai, D-6000 Frankfurt/Main centration for Cefamandole and Cefoxitin are highest with mean values of 28 mcg/g and 23 mcg/g for the aorta, and 32 mcg/g and 53 mcg/g for the mitral valve respectively. The tissue concentration was somewhat lower with Cefuroxime, 7 mcg/g for the aorta and 12 mcg/g for the mitralis, while the lowest concentrations were found after the administration of Cefotaxim, 2.4 mcg/g for the aorta and 2.2 mcg/g for the mitral valve. The same tendency appears in the atrial wall and the papillary muscles.

Table 1. Tissue concentrations of different cephalosporins in mcg/g

		Atrium	Aortic v.	Mitral v.	Pap. musc.
Cefamandole	n	6	6	5	-
	$\bar{x}$	67.76	28.82	32.87	
	SD±	28.44	11.51	6.52	
Cefoxitin	n	8	7	6	2
	$\bar{x}$	38.17	23.59	53.74	21.62
	SD±	16.85	19.75	20.81	1.46
Cefuroxime	n	9	4	5	-
	$\bar{x}$	17.64	6.81	11.99	
	SD±	5.90	1.76	4.22	
Cefotaxim	n	17	10	11	5
	$\bar{x}$	1.92	2.40	2.22	1.37
	SD±	0.63	0.64	0.56	0.47

Discussion

The minimal effective concentration for penicillin sensible and resistant staphylococci lies for the tested cephalosporins around o.5 - 1 mcg/g (5). With concentrations well above this minimum level, the tissue concentration for Cefamandole, Cefoxitin, and Cefuroxime within the resected heart valve and heart muscles is certainly in a safe range against most strains of staphylococci which are known to cause early postoperative valve endocarditis. Significantly lower, however, was the tissue concentration for the fourth antibiotic in test, Cefotaxim. Whether this fact is due to a change in the molecule during the concentration test which distorted the results, or whether Cefotaxim has less permeability into the human heart muscle and valves, has as yet not been determined. Further studies are necessary and underway. Until such time as they are completed we cannot recommend Cefotaxim as a routine prophylaxis in open heart surgery particularly since the other three cephalosporins in test are, due to their pharmacokinetics, their tissue penetration and their antibacterial spectrum, optimally suited for this purpose.

Summary

In order to prevent early postoperative endocarditis, 50 human heart valves, 40 biopsies from the right atrium, and 7 papillary muscles were studied for concentration of different cephalosporins during ECC. With Cefamandole, Cefoxitin, and Cefuroxin the necessary bactericide tissue concentration could be found and they are therefore suitable for prophylaxis of this serious complication. The tissue concentration of Cefotaxim did not reach the necessary level in our test and is, at this time, not equally recommendable.

References

1. Wilson WR (1977) Prosthetic valve endocarditis: Incidence, anatomic location, cause, morbidity, and mortality. In: Duma RJ (ed) Infections of prosthetic heart valves and vascular grafts. University Park Press, Baltimore London Tokyo, p 3
2. Eigel P, Tschirkov A, Satter P, Knothe H (1978) Assays of cephalosporin antibiotics administered prophylactically in open heart surgery. Infection 6/1:3-8
3. Schaffner W (1977) Antibiotic prophylaxis in valvular replacement surgery. In: Duma RJ (ed) Infection of prosthetic heart valves and vascular grafts. University Park Press, Baltimore London Tokyo, p 313
4. Plaue R, Fabricius K, Wysocki S (1974) Cephalotinspiegelbestimmung in menschlichen Geweben. Chirurg 45:274-278
5. Simon C, Stille W (1979) Antibiotika-Therapie in Klinik und Praxis, 4th edn. Schattauer, Stuttgart New York

Gentamicin Pharmacokinetic During Open Heart Surgery: Serum and Tissue Concentrations in Valvular, Muscular and Subcutaneous Tissue

M. Schmuziger, E. Eschenbruch, E. Beyer, B. Metz, and F. Daschner*

Introduction

More than 15 years after clinical introduction, gentamicin is still one of the antibiotics of choice for the treatment of hospital infections due to pyocyanic pseudomonas, Klebsiella, and other coli. Until now, the pharmacokinetics of gentamicin in heart surgery with extracorporeal circulation (ECC) has been unknown. The aim of our investigations was to determine these pharmacokinetics as well as the concentrations of gentamicin in postinflammatorily changed scarred valvular tissue.

Material and Methods

In 38 candidates for valvular replacement with normal renal function, 1.5 mg/kg body weight of gentamicin was injected (within 5 min) intravenously between 7 and 0 h preoperatively. There were 22 men and 16 women with a mean age of 54.6 years and a mean weight of 65.4 kg (Table 1).

During the subsequent operations, valvular, muscular, and subcutaneous fat tissues were taken and their gentamicin concentrations were determined by the agar diffusion method. The operations were always performed by the same surgical team and were done with nonpulsatile flow, total hemodilution, moderate hypothermia with hypothermic cardiac arrest, and hyperpotassic cardioplegia as well as topical heart cooling. Mean extracorporeal circulation time was 129 min.

*Benedikt-Kreutz-Rehabilitationszentrum, Südring 15, D-7812 Bad Krozingen

Table 1. Gentamicin study

n = 38	♂	n = 22
	♀	n = 16
Mean age	♂	55 years
	♀	54 years
Mean weight	♂	70 kg
	♀	59 kg

Gentamicin 1.5 mg/kg slowly iv 7-0 h preop.

Blood, obtained from the venous line, subcutaneous fat, and muscle were taken simultaneously at various intervals following injection of the drug, while valvular tissue and blood were taken at the time of valve replacement. Specimens were immediately frozen at -72°C and assayed during the next 4 weeks by an agar diffusion method using Bacillus subtilis ATCC 6633 as test organism (Spore suspension: BBL; antibiotic medium No. 2, Oxoid). Tissue fluid in 1:3 dilution (wt/vol.) with 0.15 molar phosphate buffer, pH 8, was obtained by use of a Coleworth Stomacher No. 80.

Standards for plasma antibiotic assays were made in phosphate-buffered bovine serum albumin (1:1), for tissue fluid in phosphate buffer, pH 8. All determinations were done in triplicate and read by the same technician.

Results

Tissue and concomitant plasma antibiotic concentrations are shown in Table 2. Peak levels in plasma and tissue were reached within 1 h after administration which from thereon declined slowly to lower values. Subcutaneous and muscle concentrations varied between 0.51 µg/g and 2.1 µg/g. Gentamicin concentrations in cardiac valvular tissue were higher than those in subcutaneous tissue only during the first hour after administration. They reached between 58% and 65% of the corresponding plasma levels within 2 h and up to 93% from 2 to 5 h after application of the drug.

Histologic examination of the valves revealed either no or only few small capillaries, hyaline deposits, scars, and old inflammatory reactions.

Table 2. Plasma (µg/ml) and tissue (µg/g) concentrations of gentamicin in cardiac surgery patients after a single injection of 1.5 mg/kg body weight

	0 - 1 h	1 - 2 h	2 - 3 h	3 - 4 h	4 - 5 h	5 - 6 h	6 - 7 h
Plasma	5.5 ± 3.1/	2.7 ± 1.6	1.6 ± 1.2	1.5 ± 0.7	1.3 ± 0.6	1.3 ± 0.9	0.9
	(22)X	(21)	(21)	(11)	(11)	(9)	(1)
Heart valves	3.6 ± 3.3/	1.59 ± 0.9	1.5 ± 0.6	1.2 ± 0.48	1.2 ± 0.54	-	-
	(6)X	(5)	(13)	(4)	(4)		
Muscle	1.9 ± 1.7/	0.99	-	-	-	0.9	0.51
	(4)X	(2)				(2)	(1)
Subcutaneous tissue	2.1 ± 1.5/	1.8 ± 1.2	1.8 ± 2.4	1.2 ± 0.9	1.8 ± 1.2	1.2 ± 0.6	0.0
	(5)X	(10)	(5)	(5)	(4)	(9)	(2)

/ = ± Standard deviation

X = Number of specimens

- = No specimen assayed

Conclusions

Slow intravenous injection of 1.5 mg/kg body weight of gentamicin never reaches toxic serum levels of 10 µg/ml. ECC has an influence on serum levels due to its dilution effect. Tissue concentrations seem to depend on the degree of vascularization of the corresponding tissue during ECC.

In nonvascularized scarred valvular tissue, which is constantly in touch with the blood stream, gentamicin concentration ranges constantly between 58% and 93% of the actual serum level.

After iv administration of 1.5 mg/kg body weight of gentamicin in heart surgery with extracorporeal circulation, therapeutic gentamicin tissue concentrations for gentamicin-sensitive strains are observed in valvular tissues up to 3 h, in subcutaneous fat tissue for 3 h, in muscular tissue only during the first hour. Serum concentrations are within a therapeutic range for approximately 3 h.

Antibiotic Levels in the Human Serum, Pericardial Fluid and Heart Tissues

J. I. Kiss, E. Faragó. S. M. Békássy, and A. Gömöry*

One of the most frequently occurring complications following heart interventions is infection. This may have the form of wound infection, respiratory, or urinary infections; however, its most frequent form is postoperative endocarditis. According to Rapaport (9), it is an ironic situation that one of the therapeutic possibilities for bacterial endocarditis is just the prosthetic valve replacement. Antibiotics are essential tools in prevention and therapy of postoperative infections and bacterial endocarditis. Antibiotic therapy may be succesful if the bacteria involved in the disease are susceptible to the antibiotic applied. This basic principle has been known for several decades. Nevertheless, the therapeutic failures and the new results of clinical pharmacology revealed that apart from the principle cited above, we shall have success only if, apart from the serum, the antibiotics reach an efficient concentration even at the place of the disease, i.e., in the tissues. The tissue levels are sufficient if they reach or superate the minimal inhibitory concentration for the given bacteria. Therefore, the knowledge of the tissue levels is of even higher importance from a clinical point of view than that of the serum levels. The most effective antibiotic, the dosage, and mode of application can only be properly selected for a given infection if we know exactly the actual tissue levels. In order to meet these requirements, we studied the antibiotic levels in the serum, the pericaridal fluid, the auricle, and cardiac valves during heart operations.

Material and Methods

Patients

Antibiotic levels in the serum, pericardial fluid, the auricles, and the valves were determined 30-180 min subsequent to the preoperative application of the antibiotics. The patients were thoroughly checked before the operations; their hepatic and kidney functions were in the physiological ranges. For 3 days before the operations, the patients received no antibiotics. All the patients were adults. The operations (commissurotomy, valve implantation, patch closure) were carried out because of mitral and aortic valve defects as well as congenital defects.

---

*Second Department of Surgery, and Department of Pulmonology, University Medical School, Debrecen 4004, Hungary

Antibiotics used

Methicillin (Chinoin, Budapest, Hungary); flucloxacillin (Floxapen) (Brentford, Bencard, England); cephacetrile (Celospor) (CIBA-GEIGY); gentamicin (Pharmachim, Bulgaria); tobramycin (Brulamycin) (BIOGAL, Debrecen, Hungary); amikacin (Schering Co. and Bayer AG). The number of patients per group, the doses, and modes of application are summarized in Table 1.

Table 1. Antibiotics, patients, doses, route

Antibiotic	No. of cases	Dose/route
Methicillin	11	1 g /im
Flucloxacillin	19	500 mg /im
Cephacetrile	10	3 + 3 g /iv
Gentamicin	15	1 mg/kg/im
Tobramycin	15	1 mg/kg/im
Amikacin	14	500 mg /im

Method

Antibiotic levels of the serum, the pericardial fluid, and the heart tissues were determined by using an agar diffusion hole method (2, 4). The test strain was a spore suspension of Bacillus subtilis ATCC 6633.

Calculations

The semilogarithmic graphic method was used. The antibiotic levels of serum and the pericardial fluid was expressed in μg/ml, those of the tissues in μg/g units. Average values are given.

Results

The results obtained during 84 heart operations, using six different antibiotics are summarized in Table 2. Sixty to 180 min subsequent to an im application of 1 g methicillin, the average values were 14.7 and 1.8 μg/ml in the serum and pericardial fluid, respectively, whereas the auricle contained 8.2 μg/g.

The serum level reached 14 μg/ml 35-160 min after the im administration of 500 mg flucloxacillin. At the same time in most cases no flucloxacillin was detected in the pericardial fluid, in several cases 0.7 μg/ml was found. Levels of 2.6, 1.7, and 1.6 μg/g were found in the auricle, the mitral, and the aortic valves, respectively.

Cephacetrile was administered intravenously. Twice given 3 g doses resulted in 130-140 μg/ml serum level between 30-120 min. The pericardial fluid contained 20.2 μg/ml, whereas in the auricle, the mitral, and the aortic valves 12.5, 19.9, and 18.5 μg/g levels were detected, respectively.

Table 2. Serum, pericardial fluid, auricle, and valve level of antibiotics

Antibiotic	Time (min)	Serum level (μg/ml)	Pericardial fluid level (μg/ml)	Auricle level (μg/g)	Mitral valve level (μg/g)	Aortic valve level (μg/g)
Methicillin	60-180	14.7	1.8	8.2	-	-
Flucloxacillin	35-160	14.0	0.0-0.7	2.6	1.7	1.6
Cephacetrile	30-120	130-140	20.2	12.5	19.9	18.5
Gentamicin	30-155	5.2	1.1	1.8	2.5	2.0
Tobramycin	35-140	5.6	1.0	0.7	2.2	1.7
Amikacin	35-160	16.4	3.5	4.5	-	10.5

Gentamicin was applied intramuscularly in a dose of 1 mg/kg body weight. Thirty to 155 min subsequent to the application, the serum level reached 5.2 μg/ml, the pericardial fluid contained 1.1 μg/ml. At the same time, the auricle, the mitral, and the aortic valves displayed 1.8, 2.5, and 2.0 μg/g, respectively.

Similar doses of tobramycin (1 mg/kg body weight) resulted in 35-140 min subsequent to the application 5.6 and 1.0 μg/ml, as well as 0.7, 2.2, and 1.7 μg/g levels in the same order as given for gentamicin.

Intramuscular application of amikacin (500 mg) resulted in 16.4 μg/ml concentration in the serum after 35-160 min. The pericardial fluid contained 3.5 μg/ml, and in the tissues (auricle and aortic valve) showed 4.5 and 10.5 μg/g, respectively.

Discussion

Serum levels of antibiotics have been studied by numerous authors using different doses and modes of application as well as after different time intervals. Our results regarding the serum levels agree with the data in the literature. However, as regards the tissue levels of human organs, there are only very few data at our disposal. Such studies can only be carried out if the surgeons are interested and collaborate precisely with the laboratory specialists. Such a possibility was given in our laboratory during the last 10 years. It is especially important to know human tissue levels, since similar organs of different animals display quite different values (11).

According to our knowledge of the six antibiotics we studied, only the levels of cephacetrile have been studied in human pericardial fluid (10) and in the heart muscle (1). The published data on cephacetrile agree with ours. The other antibiotics were measured in human tissues only by us. The clinical significance of the numeric values obtained can only be judged if we compare the actual levels with the minimal inhibitory concentrations for the given bacteria.

The heart muscle level of methicillin reaches the minimal inhibitory concentration of the bacteria in its spectrum; however, that of the pericardial fluid does not. Therefore, one can treat the endocarditis by using 1 g methicillin im with success, if the bacterium is susceptible. Nevertheless, for the treatment of pericarditis one needs some other antibiotics or other modes of application (5).

The flucloxacillin levels of the pericardial fluid were insignificant after an im application of 500 mg. However, the tissue levels were multiples of the minimal inhibitory concentrations. This offers a great possibility in the therapy of endocarditis caused by flucloxacillin-sensitive bacteria (8).

High doses of cephacetrile assured suitable antibiotic concentrations in both the pericardial fluid and the heart tissues. The intravenous application of 3 + 3 g cephacetrile may be of vital importance in severe cases of pericarditis and endocarditis (7).

Among the antibiotics of the aminoglycoside type (gentamicin, tobramycin, amikacin), the first two display identical or very similar pharmacokinetics. One mg/kg body weight doses result in levels of pericardial fluid and heart tissues being efficient only against a part of the bacteria involved (6).

An im application of 500 mg amikacin resulted in effective concentrations in both the pericardial fluid and the heart tissues. This represents an extraordinary, sometimes the last therapeutic possibility in the infections caused by gentamicin-resistant, especially gram-negative bacteria (3).

According to our results, the pericarditis can be treated with usual doses of amikacin or high doses of cephacetrile, if applied im or iv. The endocarditis can be successfully treated by methicillin, flucloxacillin, amikacin, high doses of cephacetrile, and sometimes by gentamicin and tobramycin.

Summary

Methicillin, flucloxacillin, cephacetrile, gentamicin, tobramycin, and amikacin levels were studied in the serum, the pericardial fluid, the auricle, and the cardiac valves during 84 cardiac interventions, by using an agar diffusion method. On the basis of the results obtained, the therapeutic values of the antibiotics were judged in the therapy of pericarditis and endocarditis.

References

1. Adam D, Pätzold J, Reichardt B (1976) Konzentration von Cephacetril im Herzmuskelgewebe. Infection 4:215-216
2. Bennett JV, Brodie EJ, Benner EJ, Kirby WMM (1966) Simplified, accurate method for antibiotics assay of clinical specimens. Appl Microbiol 14:170-173
3. Faragó E, Kiss J, Gömöry A, Aranyosi J, Juhász I, Mihóczy L (1979) Amikacin: in vitro bacteriological studies, levels in human serum, lung and heart tissue, and clinical results. Int J Clin Pharmacol 17:421-428
4. Grove DC, Randall WA (1955) Assay methods of antibiotics, a laboratory manual. Med Encyclopedia, New York
5. Kiss J, Faragó E, Gömöry A, Czakó Z, Fábián E, Bacsa S (1975) Untersuchung der Methicillinkonzentration im Serum, in der perikardialen Flüssigkeit und im Myokard beim Menschen. Acta Chir Acad Sci Hung 16:351-357
6. Kiss J, Faragó E, Gömöry A, Homolay P, Kiss IS (1977) Gentamicin in cardiac surgery. Acta Chir Acad Sci Hung 18:133-139

7. Kiss J, Faragó E, Gömöry A, Kiss B, Várhelyi I (1978) Human pharmacokinetics of cephacetrile (Celospor). In: Siegenthaler W, Lüthy R (eds) Current chemotherapy, vol 1. Soc Microbiol, Washington DC, pp 392-395
8. Kiss J, Faragó E, Gömöry A, Szamaránszky J (1979) A flucloxacillin szérum, tüdöszövet, pericardiális folyadék és szivszövet szintjének vizsgálata emberben. Kisérletes Orvostudomány 31:578-585
9. Rapaport E (1978) The changing role of surgery in the management of infective endocarditis (Editorial). Circulation 58:598-599
10. Regamey CC, Vicquerat C, Suter PM, Waldvogel FA (1976) Cephacetril-Konzentrationen im Pericardexudat nach Herzoperation. Infection 4:209-214
11. Wahlig H, Metallinos A, Hameister W, Bergmann R (1974) Gentamycin-Konzentrationen in Geweben und Körperflüssigkeit von Versuchstieren. Int J Clin Pharmacol 10:212-229

Intraoperative Changes of Immunoglobulins and Complement Fractions During Open-heart Surgery Using Membrane Oxygenators

R. Lozano, M. Navarro, J. C. Salinas, J. Suárez, J. Revilla, C. Pastor, M. D. Abós, E. Tejero, and M. R. Casado*

The immunological changes that follow open-heart procedures have received, so far, scant attention, in spite of the well-known fact that pump oxygenation perfusion and blood transfusion are responsible for many haematological disturbances (11, 12, 24, 26, 27, 30, 31).

In 1969, Hairston et al. (12) found a significant decrease of complement activity and immunoglobulins (IGB) in the sera of patients after open-heart surgery performed using disc or bubble oxygenators. The authors concluded that a "depression of immunological surveillance" was to be expected after pump oxygenation perfusion with nonmembrane oxygenators, which lasted for 5 to 7 days. Parker et al. (24) observed strikingly similar changes in patients operated on after extracorporeal circulation (ECC) with bubble oxygenators. In both papers, it was speculated that protein denaturation, a consequence of the polarizing forces that occur at the blood-gas interface in nonmembrane oxygenators, could be responsible of the decrease observed in immunoprotein factors after ECC. Other less comprehensive studies have also reported direct or indirect evidence of IGB denaturation following open-heart surgery (26, 27).

In membrane oxygenators (MO), blood is not exposed to a direct interface with gas, as it is in bubble and disc oxygenators, and trauma to blood is consequently reduced (2, 3, 25, 33). The purpose of the present study was to assess whether the use of MO could avoid or at least minimize the immunological disturbances which had been reported.

Patients and Methods

Twenty-nine adult patients were included in the study group. There were 12 males and 17 females. Age ranged from 15 to 66 years (mean age: 46.6 years). All underwent open-heart surgery: 19 had uni- or multivalvular surgery, 7 had aorto-coronary vein grafts, 1 patient was operated on for a hydatid cyst, 1 for a ventricular aneurysm, and 1 for an ASD.

ECC was performed in all cases with a Travenol Teflo MO. Ringer's lactate solution, albumin and NA CO_3 was used for priming. Blood loss was minimal during sternotomy and cannulation except for one patient, and was not replaced. Moderate hypothermia (29-32°C) was routinely induced. Patients were on cardiopulmonary bypass (CPB) for times ranging from 23 to 130 min (mean: 72.2 min). Ten patients who underwent peripheral vascular or abdominal surgery for nonmalignant conditions lasting from 3 to 4 h were used as a control group.

---

*Services of Cardiovascular Surgery and General Surgery "A", University Hospital and Medical Faculty, University of Zaragoza, Zaragoza, Spain

In patients in the study group, arterial blood was drawn before the skin was incised, immediately before the onset of CPB, immediately after coming off CPB, and after skin closure. When the patient was on CPB for more than 1 h, another sample was drawn. In patients in the control group, arterial blood was drawn before incision and after skin closure. Blood was centrifugated at 4°C for 5 min. Serum was collected in sterile tubes with one microdrop of EDTA and was frozen at -23°C, once the tubes were hermetically closed, and stored for a maximum time of 15 days.

IgA, IgG, IgM, C3, C4, and C5 serum concentrations were measured by single radial immunodiffusion techniques, following Mancini et al. (21). IgE serum concentration was measured by radioimmunoassay, following Leonardy and Peacock (18).

The patients in the control group did not receive heparin routinely during surgery. In order to ascertain that heparinization did not interfere with our determinations, IgA, IgG, IgM, C3, C4, and C5 were measured in sera from six healthy volunteers. Two samples were drawn from each volunteer. In one of each, tests were performed as in the study and control groups. In the other sample, blood was incubated with heparin (4 mcg/ml) before the laboratory procedures were started. There were no significant differences in the results obtained with the two techniques.

Results

IgG, IgA, and IgM concentrations were reduced to 78.1% to 74.75% of preoperative values *before* the onset of CPB. The decreases were significant. During the first hour of CPB, concentrations of IgG, IgA, and IgM showed a further nonsignificant decrease. No further decrease was observed until the end of surgery. Changes in IgE concentration were not significant for any of the intervals (Table 1).

Changes in C3, C4, and C5 concentrations were very similar (Table 2): a decrease of 75.8% to 84.5% of preoperative values before the onset of CPB (significant), and no further significant changes during the whole procedure. Nevertheless, a decrease during the first hour of CPB from 67.5% to 71% of preoperative values can be observed.

There was no statistical correlation between changes in IGB and complement fractions (CF) and changes in haematocrit in the interval between incision and the completion of CPB, as measured by the correlation index r (Table 3). Changes in concentrations of IGB and CF were of much smaller amount and not significant in patients in the control group (Table 4).

Mean values of IgG were below normal limits during the whole procedure in patients in the study group. Other immunoproteins, though decreased, stayed within normal ranges.

Most patients had postoperative concentrations of IgG which were below normal limits. This was not the case for patients in the control group.

Discussion

The striking fact in our results is that the decrease in IGB and CF concentrations is observed *before* the onset of CPB, in a percentage very close to those reported by others (12, 24). These authors measured the concentrations of immunoproteins before and after surgery,

Table 1. Changes in immunoglobulins during open-heart surgery

	IgG mg/100 ml	Δ % IgG	IgM mg/100 ml	Δ % IgM	IgA mg/100 ml	Δ % IgA	IgE mg/100 ml	Δ % IgE
Range of normal values	800-1800		60-250		90-450		170	
Preop	1032 ± 81.3		152 ± 14.9		193 ± 21		58.8 ± 16	
Pre bypass	705 ± 64.9	-25.25 ± 5.9[a]	105 ± 10.63	-25.35 ± 5.8[a]	137 ± 17.4	-21.9 ± 6.4[a]	54.3 ± 14.8	2.7 ± 9.12
1H bypass	653 ± 62.5	-33.92 ± 4.63[b]	90 ± 6.4	-32.78 ± 4.8[b]	112 ± 9.8	-31.45 ± 5.4[b]	47.7 ± 10	22 ± 25.32[b]
End bypass	588 ± 45.5	-34.24 ± 5.43[b]	92 ± 10	-30.21 ± 6.9[b]	113 ± 11.4	-27.7 ± 9.4[b]	50.4 ± 9.39	46.38 ± 25.9[b]
End op	624 ± 46.5	-29.71 ± 6.19[b]	94 ± 7.4	-20.25 ± 8.9[b]	126 ± 12.18	-25.8 ± 8.9[b]	48.8 ± 11.7	61.28 ± 31.94[b]

[a] $P < 0.001$

[b] $P > 0.05$ (compared with pre bypass values)

Table 2. Changes in complement fractions during open-heart surgery

	C_3 mg/100 ml	Δ % C_3	C_4 mg/100 ml	Δ % C_4	C_5 mg/100 ml	Δ % C_5
Range of normal values	101-189		12-75		8.1-25	
Preop	96.4 ± 7.4		28.3 ± 3		11.2 ± 1.5	
Pre bypass	77.8 ± 7.2	-18.6 ± 4.3[a]	19.6 ± 2.3	-24.21 ± 6.2[a]	8.9 ± 1.3	-15.49 ± 4[a]
1H bypass	59.5 ± 11.2	-29.7 ± 4.3[b]	7.8 ± 1.6	-32.45 ± 7.4[b]	7.2 ± 0.8	-29 ± 3[b]
End bypass	59.4 ± 4.4	-34.59 ± 4.4[b]	15.6 ± 2	-34.9 ± 5.7[b]	7.6 ± 0.8	-22.6 ± 4.5[b]
End op	64.8 ± 5.8	-29.29 ± 5.5[b]	14.25±2	-40.5 ± 6.8[b]	8.3 ± 1.3	-25.8 ± 5[b]

[a] $P < 0.001$

[b] $P > 0.05$ (compared with pre bypass values)

Table 3. Correlation index (r) between changes in immunoglobulins and complement fractions and changes in haematocrit in the period between incision and the end of CPB

	Δ %	r	P	Δ % Haematocrit
IgG	-34.24	0.12	0.7	
IgA	-27.7	0.36	0.2	
IgM	-30.2	0.32	0.3	-31.5
C_3	-34.59	0.17	0.6	
C_4	-34.9	0.17	0.6	
C_5	-22.6	0.44	0.1	

Table 4. Changes in immunoglobulins and complement fractions during noncardiac surgery lasting 3 to 4 h

	Range of normal values	Preoperative	After operation	Δ %
IgG mg/100 ml	800 - 1800	1080 ± 98.3	993 ± 93.19	-7.8 ± 2.68
IgM mg/100 ml	60 - 250	117 ± 15.39	102.1 ± 13.14	-2.3 ± 7.1
IgA mg/100 ml	90 - 450	182.4±30.25	234.6 ± 43.67	+8.53 ± 11.65
IgE UI/ml	170	34.4±11.37	29 ± 9.22	-5.8 ± 4.74
C_3 mg/100 ml	101 - 189	68.6 ± 4.19	64.1 ± 3.51	-5.87 ± 3.6
C_4 mg/100 ml	12 - 72	34.5 ± 5.98	30 ± 5.17	-11.6 ± 49[a]
C_5 mg/100 ml	8.1 - 25	9.7 ± 0.29	9.34 ± 0.35	-0.36 ± 0.25

[a] $P < 0.05$

but not immediately before the onset of CPB, so that it can be assumed that the decrease of IGB and CF happened before the onset of CPB also in their cases.

The lack of statistical correlation between the decreases in IGB and CF and the decreases in haematocrit rules out the effect of haemodilution. As a matter of fact, significant changes in our study happened before the onset of CPB, and, consequently, before haemodilution could show its effect. But the nonsignificant decrease which we have observed during the first hour of CPB may be partly related to dilution which would add its effect to the depletion of IGB and CF which happens before CPB.

The cause of the decrease of IGB and CF during sternotomy and cannulation is not very clear. Several authors reported changes in IGB and CF after surgery, and both general anaesthesia and the effect of trauma and stress have been advocated as causative factors (5, 7, 9, 14, 20, 23, 34). In our study, similar anaesthetic techniques were used in both the study and the control group. On the other hand, sternotomy and cannulation do not involve greater tissue damage than a whole procedure of complex abdominal or vascular surgery. Since changes in IGB and CF were minimal and not significant in the control group, the depletion of IGB and CF in the study group must be related to the *specific* action of cardiotomy, and cannulation. A control group of "closed" cardiac operations should have been most useful in elucidating if these manoeuvres are able to induce a decrease of IGB and CF per se. Unfortunately, we did not have the opportunity of building up such a group, since "closed" cardiac surgery is very rare in our service.

Cardiotomy and cannulation may induce the formation of immune complexes (IC), which would consequently deplete IGB and CF from the serum. Several facts support this theory: First, IgE concentrations did not change significantly and it is known that IgE very rarely participates in circulating IC. Second, IgG is the IGB that shows the greater decrease, both in our study and in the results reported by others (12, 24, 26, 27), and IgG represents the main bulk of IGB in almost every circulating IC described up to now in human disease (16).

Furthermore, recent research indicates that the presence of circulating immune complexes or heart reacting antibodies (HRA) may be a secondary reaction to cellular heart damage (6, 19). Circulating IC or HRA (which preclude the existence of IC) have been repeatedly found after myocardial infarction (13, 15), in the postpericardiotomy syndrome (8, 19, 32), and even the presence of blood in the pericardium has been proved to be a precipitating factor for the production of IC (29). As it happens in extracardiac diseases, IgG represents the main bulk of IGB which is present in circulating IC in heart disease: Pretty et al. (25) described circulating anti-IgG antibodies after open-heart surgery. Goldman et al. (10) showed that IgG was antibody directed at heart antigens in a heart transplant model in dogs.

Moreover, the in vivo half-time of plasminogen activator activity is known to be prolonged after CPB in patients (31). This could be explained by the presence of circulating IC that would activate Hageman's factor, thus activating the fibrinolitic system (28). Lastly, the pattern of decrease of CF which we have observed further enhances the theory of IC being formed during the initial steps of cardiac surgery: Circulating IC formed during cardiotomy and cannulation would trigger complement activation, thus leading to a depletion of CF.

Concluding, we have found no evidence of immunoproteins being "denaturated" by membrane oxygenators and strongly believe that other kinds of oxygenators do not have that action either. Our results strongly suggest that cardiotomy and cannulation, by means of the trauma to the heart and of the presence of blood in the pericardium, induce the formation of circulating IC, which is responsible for the depletion in immunoproteins which has repeatedly been observed after open-heart surgery. IgG is very often below normal values at the end of open-heart surgery and this may play an important role in the increased susceptibility to infections of these patients. On the other hand, the consequences of circulating IC, such as the activation of the complement system and kinin liberation via activation of the Hageman factor, as has been described by Movat (22) and Ratnoff (28), may be a cause of some of the still obscurely understood complications of open-heart surgery, such as haemorrhagic phenomena, changes in capillary permeability, membrane damage, etc. (1, 17).

These considerations stress the importance of further studies concerning the pathogenesis of immunologic disturbances induced by open-heart surgery. Those studies should include the measurement of circulating IC at several sequential intervals during the cardiac procedure.

Summary

Immunoglobulins and complement fraction concentrations were measured at different times during open-heart surgery (OHS) performed with membrane oxygenators in 29 patients, and before and after surgery in a control group of 10 patients operated on without extracorporeal circulation. Significant decrease of all immunoproteins happened between the beginning of surgery and the onset of cardiopulmonary bypass (CPB). No further significant depletions of immunoproteins were found during CPB, but the initial decrease resulted in pathologically low values of IgG in almost every patient during the whole procedure and at the end of surgery. No correlation was found between these changes and changes in haematocrit. Patients in the control group did not show significant decreases of immunoproteins during surgery. Decrease of immunoproteins during OHS should not be related only to the trauma to blood by the heart-lung machine, as has been done up to now. Rather, further studies should try to detect circulating immune complexes which could be formed as a consequence of the pericardial and cardiac injury that ensues during the initial steps of OHS, i.e., during cannulation and intracardiac exploration.

References

1. Austen KF (1970) Inborn and acquired abnormalities of the complement system in man. Trans Assoc Am Physicians 83:49-61
2. Bramson ML, Osborn JJ, Gerbode F (1976) The membrane lung. In: Ionescu MI, Wooler GH (eds) Current techniques in extracorporeal circulation. Butterworths, London, pp 65-90
3. Byrick RJ, Noble WH (1978) Postperfusion lung syndrome. Comparison of Travenol bubble and membrane oxygenators. J Thorac Cardiovasc Surg 76:685-693
4. Clark RE, Beauchamp RA, Magrath RA, Brooks JD, Ferguson TB, Weldon CS (1979) Comparison of bubble and membrane oxygenators in short and long perfusions. J Thorac Cardiovasc Surg 78:655-666
5. Cohnen G (1972) Changes in immunoglobulin level after surgical trauma. J Trauma 12:249-257
6. Dass SK, Cassidy JT, Petty RE (1974) The significance of heart-reactive antibodies in heart disease. Chest 66:179-181
7. Dittrich A, Dittrich K (1975) Immunoglobuline nach Operationen. Gelbe Hefte 15: 198-227
8. Engle MA, McCabe J, Denham B (1970) Immunologic studies in postpericardiotomy syndrome. Pediatr Res 7:290-296
9. Gierhake FW, Plock-Kömnilk P, Torrau E, Heide G, Shaper G (1973) Postoperative Verminderung der Immunoglobuline und des Komplements und ihre mögliche Bedeutung für infektiöse Komplikationen. Langenbecks Arch Klin Chir [Suppl Chir Forum]:385-397
10. Goldman BS, Shumak KH, Silver MD (1971) Antibodies in the serum and the heart of dogs with cardiac allografts. Transplant Proc 3:515-518
11. Hairston P, Manos JP, Grober CD, Lee WH Jr (1968) Alteration of intrinsic bactericidal potential of blood by pump-oxygenation perfusion. Symposium: Organ perfusion and preservation. Appleton, New York, pp 911-928

12. Hairston P, Manos JP, Graber CD, Lee WH Jr (1969) Depression of immunologic surveillance by pump-oxygenation perfusion. J Surg Res 9:587-593
13. Heine WI, Friedman H, Mandell MS, Goldberg H (1966) Antibodies to cardiac tissue in acute ischemic heart disease. Am J Cardiol 17:798-803
14. Jubert AV, Lee ET, Hersch EM, McBride CM (1973) Effects of surgery, anaesthesia, and intraoperative blood loss on immunocompetence. J Surg Res 15:399-407
15. Kuch J (1973) Autoantibodies directed against heart antigens and endocrine reactivity in patients with recent myocardial infarction. Cardiovasc Res 7:649-654
16. Lambert PH, Zubler R (1977) La formation de complexes immuns: Role physiologique et manifestations pathologiques. In: Touraine JL, Traeger J, Triau R (eds) Transplantation et immunologie clinique. Simep, Villeurbaine, pp 10-15
17. Lee WH Jr, Krumhaar D, Konkalsrud EW, Scheide OA, Maloney JV Jr (1961) Denaturation of plasma proteins as a cause of morbidity and death after intracardiac operations. Surgery 50:29-35
18. Leonardy JG, Peacock LB (1972) An evaluation of quantitative serum immunoglobulin determinations in clinical practice. Ann Allergy 30:378-381
19. Lessof M (1978) Immunological reactions in heart disease. Br Heart J 40:211-214
20. Maeso J, Beneyto M, Montero R, Vicente JL (1977) Influencia del acto quirúrgico y de la fluidoterapia en el proceso inmunitario. Aspectos de la terapia con gammglobulina de acción inmediata por vía intravenosa. Rev Esp Anestesiol Reanim 24:2-9
21. Mancini G, Carbonara AC, Heremans JF (1965) Immunological quantitation of antigens by single radial immunodiffusion. Immunochemistry 2:235-241
22. Movat HZ (1968) Activation of the kinin system by antigen-antibody system complexes. In: Rocha e Silva M, Rotschild HA (eds) International symposium on vasoactive polypeptides: Bradikinin and related kinins. Brasil Livraria, Sao Paulo, p 177
23. Navarro M, Lozano R, Salinas JC, Cornudella R, Revilla JM, Gutièrrez M, Tres A (1977) A study of human immunological response to major surgery (Abstract). XXVII Congress of the *Societè Internationale de Chirurgie*, Kyoto, p 155
24. Parker DJ, Cantrell JW, Karp RB, Stroud RM, Digerness SB (1972) Changes in serum complement and immunoglobulins following cardiopulmonary bypass. Surgery 71: 824-827
25. Peirce E, Converse II, Corrigan JJ, Kent BB, Cate CL, Johnson RL, Dreves AE (1969) Comparative trauma to blood in the disc oxygenator and membrane lung. Trans Am Soc Artif Intern Organs 15:33-42
26. Pretty HM, Fudemberg HH, Perkins HA, Gerbode F (1968) Antigamma-globulin antibodies after open-heart surgery. Blood 32:205-209
27. Pruitt KM, Stroud RM, Scott JW (1971) Blood damage in the heart-lung machine. Proc Soc Exp Biol Med 137:714-719
28. Ratnoff OD (1969) Some relationships among haemostasis, fibrinolytic phenomena, immunity, and inflammatory response. Adv Immunol 10:145-149
29. Segal F, Tabaznik KB (1960) Postpericardiotomy syndrome following penetrating stab wounds of the chest: Comparison with the postcommisurotomy syndrome. Am Heart J 59:175-183
30. Subramanian V, McLeod J, Gans H (1968) Effect of extracorporeal circulation on reticuloendothelial function. I. Experimental evidence for impaired reticuloendothelial function following cardiopulmonary bypass in rats. Surgery 64: 775-784
31. Subramanian V, Lande AI, Gans H (1969) Depression of host-defense mechanism following extracorporeal circulation. Trans Am Soc Artif Intern Organs 15: 105-111
32. Versey JM, Gabriel R (1974) Soluble-complex formation after myocardial infarction. Lancet 2:493-494
33. Wright JS, Fisk GC, Torda TA, Stacey RB, Hicks RG (1975) Some advantages of membrane oxygenators for open-heart surgery. J Thorac Cardiovasc Surg 69: 844-890
34. Yoginder K, Chitakara A, Avertano BC, Norhonha LI (1977) Serum immunoglobulins after surgical operations. Int Surg 62:165-169

Serum C-reactive Protein Levels in Septicaemia and Endocarditis

A.T.M. Ghoneim, S.L. Haworth, and M.I. Ionescu*

Introduction

Post-operative infections, including prosthetic valve endocarditis (PVE), are among the most serious complications following cardiac surgery. Early diagnosis and treatment may be life saving. Recently, the detection and quantitation of circulating immune complexes (CIC) was used in the diagnosis of infective endocarditis (1), but these complexes appear in the circulation several days after the onset of septicaemia (1) and may persist for several months (2). Detection of circulating bacterial antigens may be a more sensitive test for bacteraemia. However, the polymicrobial nature of the disease and the antigenic variation between different members of the same species may complicate the test. C-reactive protein (CRP) is a protein normally present in human serum at a low concentration, ~5 mg/l (0-20 mg/l) (3), but rises rapidly after the onset of inflammatory or destructive processes in the body often reaching levels above 100 mg/l and decreases promptly during convalescence (4). The CRP levels can be measured accurately and its rapid rate of change was considered to make it a more sensitive immediate marker of infection when compared with other tests used at present. Although it is appreciated that such a rise is a nonspecific mechanism, its use in monitoring infective complications after surgery has been advocated (4). This paper describes the time course of CRP levels after open-heart surgery (OHS) and its behaviour in patients who developed septicaemia with and without endocarditis.

Materials and Methods

Patients with Cardiac Operations

The pattern of post-operative CRP response was studied in 100 consecutive patients who underwent various cardiac operations. Two ml of clotted blood were collected 1 day prior to and then twice weekly after surgery. From 40 patients, four to ten samples were collected, from 60 patients one to four.

Early Post-Operative Infective Complications (Onset <3 Months after Surgery). From all 600 patients subjected to open-heart surgery during the last 3 years, 9 have developed infective complications in the early post-operative period. Five had *Staphylococcus aureus* wound infection with

*Departments of Microbiology and Cancer Research, The University of Leeds, and the Cardio Thoracic Unit, The General Infirmary at Leeds, Leeds LS2 9JT, Great Britain

Table 2. Serum C-reactive protein levels in 11 patients with septicaemia and/or endocarditis

Infection	Organism	No.	CRP levels mg/l[a]
Septicaemia	*E. coli*	1	150
	P. aeruginosa	1	240
	K. aerogenes	1	165
	Not isolated	1	210
Endocarditis	S. "viridans"	2	106, 120
	Group C. strept.	2	66, 95
	S. aureus	1	134
Bacteraemia/	S. "viridans"	1	24
? endocarditis	*S. faecalis*	1	19

[a]The CRP levels given in the table represent the serum levels when first tested after the clinical diagnosis of infection had been made

difference in CRP levels between patients with late onset PVE and those with endocarditis. Patients with severe septicaemia were infected by virulent bacteria and produced high levels of CRP (150-210 mg/l). Two patients with bacteraemia who were suspected of having endocarditis showed persistent low levels of CRP (19-24 mg/l).

Figure 2 shows the changes in CRP levels in 11 patients with infections during antibacterial therapy. Patients who responded to treatment showed a rapid decline in serum CRP levels. Patients in whom CRP levels remained high or started to rise deteriorated.

When compared with body temperature, white blood cells (WBC) and erythrocyte sedimentation rate (ESR) (Fig. 3), the CRP levels were a much more sensitive test in showing changes in the inflammatory process in the body. The ESR in particular remained high for at least 4 weeks after recovery in nearly all cardiac patients with infections.

Discussion

Infection after cardiac surgery is a major hazard because it may lead to serious complications, i.e., septicaemia and PVE. Because of the use of prophylactic antibiotics immediately before and for a short period after surgery, it is unlikely that early signs of infection will be noticed. There is no simple laboratory test/method for the screening of infection in the latent period between seeding of bacteria and the full clinical picture of the disease. Any test which will draw attention to this group of infected patients will be of considerable value because it will call for extensive investigation and early diagnosis and treatment.

The demonstration of CRP in various biological fluids has been shown to be a sensitive indicator of active inflammatory or necrotic processes in the body (4, 6-8). In 1957, Rapport et al. (9) described the pattern of post-operative CRP responses in a group of patients who underwent various surgical procedures. Several reports followed

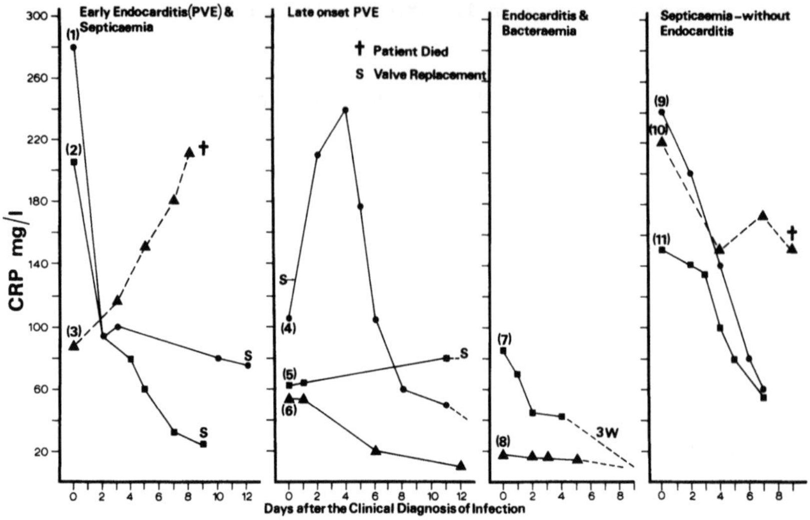

Fig. 2. Changes in serum C-reactive protein levels in 11 patients with infection during antimicrobial therapy. The infecting organisms were: *S. aureus (1, 2)*, *K. aerogenes (3)*, *S. epidermidis (4)*, streptococcus viridans *(5)*, *S. faecalis (6, 8)*, haemolytic streptococcus group C *(7)*, *P. aeruginosa (9)*, *E. coli (11)*. In patient *10*, blood cultures were sterile. The increase in CRP levels in patient *4* was due to surgery as he needed emergency valve replacement. Patients who responded to treatment showed rapid decline in CRP levels within 2 days of treatment. Patients in whom levels remained high or started to rise deteriorated and patients *3* and *10* died

this publication (4, 10, 11) and confirmed Rapport's observations. Our results in uncomplicated cardiac surgery patients showed a similar pattern. A level of 20 mg/l was achieved by the third post-operative week. High CRP levels during or after the third week were associated with clinical infection.

It can be speculated in the two patients with bacteraemia who had persistently low CRP levels that in the absence of bacterial invasion the CRP levels may remain low in contrast to septicaemia or endocarditis where high levels are usually achieved. The possible role of CRP in differentiating between endocarditis and bacteraemia in patients with valvular disease deserves further investigation.

We used the CRP levels as an aid to monitor the response to therapy. Within 24-48 h of successful therapy, the CRP levels showed a marked reduction and this was interpreted as an indication that the inflammation was subsiding (Fig. 2). Compared with the ESR, CRP levels were a much more sensitive test in showing such changes (Fig. 3).

We did not find any noticeable effect of antibiotics in variable concentrations on the natural course of CRP synthesis. Gentamicin, tobramycin, ampicillin, penicillin, lincomycin, clindamycin, metronidazole, and vancomycin were the antibiotics used. Transient changes in renal function, i.e., high blood urea or high creatinine levels, did not seem to affect the CRP levels. We did not investigate patients in acute renal or hepatic failure to find out the effect of these conditions on the CRP. However, changes in the liver function may influence both production and elimination of CRP from serum (12).

In conclusion, the serum CRP level in conjunction with blood cultures and other bacteriological investigations may be of value in the detection of early infective complications after cardiac surgery and it may be used as an aid in monitoring the response to chemotherapy.

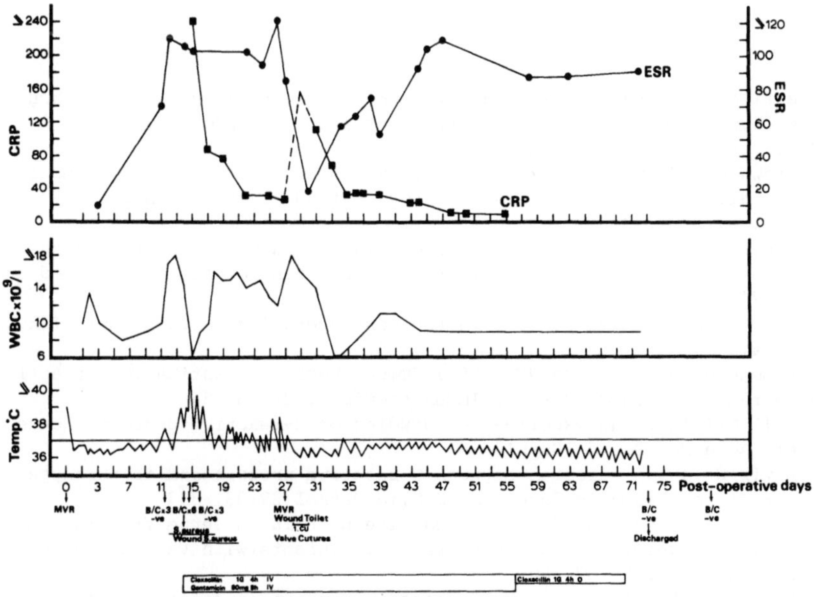

Fig. 3. Case No. 2 (Mrs. A.E.), *Staphylococcus aureus* wound infection, septicaemia and PVE 2 weeks after mitral valve replacement. Note that during the first days of treatment there was a marked decrease of CRP levels while the ESR remained elevated and only after 14 days started to show a decline. The WBC and temperature remained elevated. After the second valve replacement, the CRP levels, temperature, and WBC were within the normal range while the ESR remained elevated

Summary

Longitudinal studies of serum C-reactive protein (CRP) in 100 patients who underwent cardiac surgery and another 12 patients with early and late infections after cardiac surgery were performed to assess the value of CRP as an early "marker" of infection. Eleven patients with endocarditis and/or septicaemia, not related to cardiac surgery, were also investigated. The assay method used was radial immunodiffusion. Patients without post-operative complications showed a typical pattern. The pre-operative levels were all below 6 mg/l. These started to rise to reach a peak in 48 h, then gradually returned towards the baseline. The differences between the CRP levels in infected and non-infected patients were significant, $P < 0.01$. Patients with infection showed high CRP levels, with marked decrease following successful antibiotic treatment. Patients in whom CRP levels remained high or started to rise deteriorated.

Acknowledgements. We are grateful to Professor E.H. Cooper and to Professor E. Mary Cooke for advice in the preparation of this paper.

References

1. Bayer AS, Theofilopoulos AN, Tillman DB, Dixon FJ, Guze LB (1979) Use of circulating immune complex levels in the serodifferentiation of endocarditic and nonendocarditic septicemias. Am J Med 66:58-62
2. Harkiss GD, Brown DL, Evans DB (1979) Longitudinal study of circulating immune complexes in a patient with *Staphylococcus albus* – induced shunt nephritis. Clin Exp Immunol 37:228-238
3. Nilsson LA, Tibblin C (1968) C-reactive protein in a random sample of Swedish men aged fifty. Distribution and relation to clinical manifestation. Acta Med Scand 183:467-471
4. Matsushima Y (1967) C-reactive protein in the post-operative patient. Bull Tokyo Med Dent Univ 14:1-22
5. Mancini G, Carbonara AO, Heremans JF (1965) Immunochemical quantitation of antigens by single radial immunodiffusion. Immunochemistry 2:235-254
6. Hedlund P (1961) Clinical and experimental studies on C-reactive protein (acute phase protein). Acta Med Scand [Suppl] 361
7. Rozansky R, Davis E (1958) Relation between C-reactive protein and erythrocyte sedimentation rate in rheumatic fever. Am J Clin Pathol 29:331-333
8. Saxtad J, Nilsson LA, Hanson LA (1970) C-reactive protein in serum from infants as determined with immunodiffusion techniques. II. Infants with various infections. Acta Paediat Scand 59:676-680
9. Rapport MM, Schwartz AE, Graf L (1957) C-reactive protein in patients following operation. Ann Surg 145:321-325
10. Elster SK, Wood HF (1954) Studies of the C-reactive protein in the "post commissurotomy" syndrome. J Clin Invest 33:931
11. Fischer CL, Gill C, Forrester MG, Nakamura R (1976) Quantitation of "acute-phase proteins" post-operatively. Value in detection and monitoring of complications. Am J Clin Pathol 66:840-846
12. Hurliman J, Thorbecke GJ, Hochwald GM (1966) The liver as the site of C-reactive protein formation. J Exp Med 123:365-378

Perioperative Antibiotic Prophylaxis in Cadiac Surgery With Cephalosporins

B. Reichart*, B. Rothenfußer**, and D. Adam**

Though antibiotics are generally inappropriate prophylactic agents presumably one-fourth to one-half of all used in hospitals are for prevention. Side effects of this widespread practice are change of hospital flora, change of antibiotic susceptibility, and, last but not least, increasing medical costs (1, 7, 10). Yet, perioperative antibiotic short-term prophylaxis in cardiac surgery is recommended worldwide especially since consequences of infection following valve replacement are serious (8, 9, 11).

Besides the antimicrobial spectrum, the selection of the compound depends on the concentration of antibiotics in tissues and organs within the thorax. So, diffusibility of cephalosporins into the myocardium is an important in vivo parameter (2-5).

Method

The study was carried out with seven different cephalosporins: cephalothin, cephradine (Sefril^R), sephacetrile (Celopspore^R), cefapirin (Bristocef^R), cefamandole (Mandocef^R), cefacedone (Refosporin^R), cefoxitin (Mefoxitin^R). The serum and tissue levels of these antibiotics were determined by biological assay using the agar diffusion method and Bacillus subtilis as the test organism (6). Heart muscle samples were collected during mitral valve replacement taking papillary muscles 55 to 65 min after administration of 100 mg/kg body weight of cephalothin, cephradine, cephacetrile, cefapirin, or cefacedone iv, respectively. A dose of cefamandole and cefoxitin was administered at 50 mg/kg body weight.

Results

Approximately 60 min after the iv bolus injection the following concentrations in papillary muscle were assessed: cephalothin 1.4 µg/g, cefapirin 4.7 µg/g, cephacetrile 11.2 µg/g, cephradine 15.4 µg/g; serum levels varied from 51 to 92 µg/ml. The values for cefacedone, cefamandole, and cefoxitin were 26.9, 40.3, and 43 µg/g in heart muscle tissue; the serum levels ranged from 78 to 130 µg/ml.

*Herzchirurgische Klinik der Universität München, Klinikum Großhadern, Marchionistr. 15

**Kinderklinik der Universität München, D-8000 München 70

Table 1. Serum and tissue levels of seven cephalosporins, 60 min after iv bolus

	Cephalothin	Cefapirin	Cephacetrile	Cephradine	Cefacedone	Cefamandole	Cefoxitin
Serum (S) (µg/ml)	51 ± 21	59.4 ± 21	73 ± 37	92 ± 39	129.9 ± 12	123.8 ± 39	78 ± 32
Pap. muscle (T) (µg/g)	1.4 ± 0.4	4.7 ± 2	11.2 ± 4	15.4 ± 4	26.9 ± 17	40.3 ± 14	43 ± 27
T/S Ratio	0.03	0.08	0.15	0.17	0.21	0.33	0.55

Table 1 summarizes the just mentioned results (mean ± standard deviation). Additionally tissue/serum ratios are depicted: ratios were highest for cephamandole and cefoxitin.

In the mean time same datas are available for 50 mg/kg iv cefotaxim (Claforan[R]; trade name in Germany). Investigations were performed by Adam and Struck from Munich (personal communication 1980). After 60 min heart muscle concentration was 25 µg/g, tissue/serum ratio 0.11. According to our ranking, cefotaxim would be between cephradine and cefacedone, though half of the dose was administered.

Conclusion

If properly timed all investigated cephalosporins, except cephalothin, revealed heart muscle concentrations which exceeded minimal antimicrobial concentrations of the most pathogen microorganisms. Cefamandole and cefoxitin had the highest tissue and serum levels.

References

1. Adam D (1979) Der Stellenwert der Antibiotika-Prophylaxe. Hyg Med 4:224-230
2. Adam D, Hofstetter AG, Jacoby W, Reichart B (1976) Studies on the diffusion of Cephradine and Cephalotin into human tissue. Infection [Suppl 2] 4:105-107
3. Adam D, Pätzold J, Reichart B (1976) Konzentration von Cephacetril im Herzmuskelgewebe. Infection [Suppl 3] 4:215-216
4. Adam D, Reichart B, Feist W (1978) Diffusion von Cefamandol in das Herzmuskelgewebe. Infection [Suppl 2] 6:245-246
5. Adam D, Hofstetter AG, Reichart B, Schneider C, Wolff H, Koch E (1979) Zur Diffusion von Cefazedon in das Herzmuskel-, Prostata- und Hautgewebe sowie in die Gallenflüssigkeit. Arzneim Forsch 29/2:1901-1906
6. Bennett J, Brodie JL, Benner EJ, Kirby WMM (1966) Simplified accurate method for antibiotic assay for clinical specimens. Appl Microbiol 14:170
7. Brumfitt W, Hamilton-Miller JMT (1975) The place of antibiotic prophylaxis in medicine. J Antimicrob Chemother 1:163-169
8. Goldmann DA, Hopkins CC, Karchner AW, Abel RM, McEnany MT, Akins C, Bucklex MJ, Moellering RC (1977) Cephalotin prophylaxis in cardiac valve surgery. J Thorac Cardiovasc Surg 73:470-479
9. Goodman JS, Schaffner W, Collins HA, Battersby EJ, Koenig MG (1968) Infection after cardiovascular surgery. N Engl J Med 18:117-123
10. Hirschmann JV, Inui TS (1980) Antimicrobial prophylaxis. A critique of recent trials. Rev Infect Dis 2:1-23
11. Slaughter L, Morris JE, Starr A (1973) Prosthetic valvular endocarditis. Circulation 47:1319-1326

Cephalosporins Versus Penicillins in Open-Heart Surgery: A Prospective Randomized Clinical Trial

O. Søreide, H. Engedal, L. Segadal, S. Gullestad, and A. Digranes*

Antimicrobial prophylaxis is well established in open-heart surgery owing to the catastrophic nature of prosthetic endocarditis. Some authors do not recommend prophylactic use of antimicrobial agents in non-prosthetic cardiac surgery (2), but recent surveys have shown that the majority of surgeons use prophylaxis even in this type of surgery (9). The benefit of prophylaxis has also been established for coronary bypass operations (3).

The antibiotics selected should have an antibacterial spectrum that covers the microorganisms most likely to be encountered during and after operation, and an effective concentration of the drug must be present in the operative site at the time when bacterial contamination occurs. We have performed a prospective randomized clinical trial comparing two prophylactic antibiotic regimes in order to investigate their safety.

Material and Methods

Part I: Clinical Prospective Study

One hundred and eleven patients above the age of 16 undergoing cardiac surgery involving the use of cardiopulmonary bypass were randomized in two prophylactic antibiotic treatment groups (Table 1). Three patients were excluded from the penicillin group (I) (active bacterial endocarditis two patients, allergy to penicillin one patient), and five patients from the cephalosporin group (II) (active bacterial endocarditis three patients, wrong randomization two patients). The results were thus obtained in 53 patients in Group I and in 50 patients in Group II.

The chest, abdomen, and lower limbs were routinely draped (Steridrape) after scrubbing with chlorhexidine. Cardiopulmonary bypass was performed with Bentley BOS 10 bubble oxygenator involving hemodilution and hypothermia in nearly all cases. During and after the operative procedure, specimens for bacteriological cultures were collected at fixed intervals from sites given in Figure 1. Specimens from the sternal wound area were taken intraoperatively by the use of a cotton swab and transported in a modified Stuart's medium. The same technique was used to obtain specimens postoperatively from wounds with secretion. All specimens were processed in the microbiological laboratory with standard methods.

Wound infection was characterized by drainage and clinical signs of inflammation plus isolation of bacteria. Urinary tract infection

*Departments of Surgery, Anaesthesiology, and Microbiology, University of Bergen, Haukeland Hospital, Norway

Table 1. Antibiotic regimes in the two treatment groups

Group	Drug	Dose	Method	Time
Penicillin	Penicillin G	5×10^6 IU	iv	1 h before operation
	Penicillin G	5×10^6 IU	Prime	Operation
	Ampicillin	2 g	iv	Every 8 h day 1-3
	Cloxacillin	2 g	iv	Every 8 h day 1-3
	Amoxycillin	1 g	Oral	Every 6 h day 4-7
Cephalosporin	Cephalothin	2 g	iv	1 h before operation
	Cephalothin	2 g	Prime	Operation
	Cephalothin	2 g	iv	Every 8 h day 1-3
	Cephalexin	0.5 g	Oral	Every 6 h day 4-7

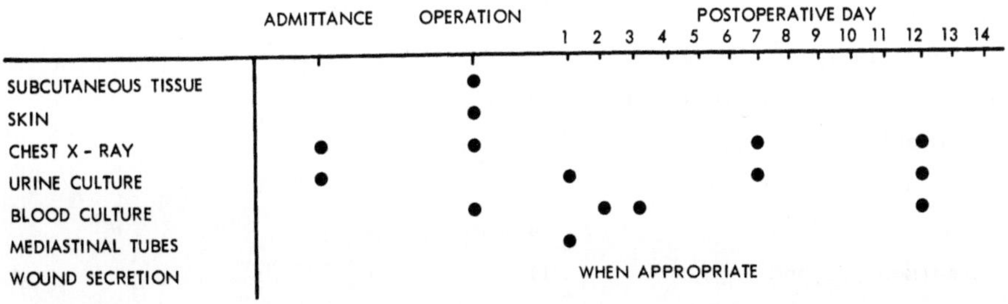

Fig. 1. The surveillance regime for bacteriological sampling and for identification of infections

was considered present when 10^5 organisms or more per milliliter urine could be cultured. Respiratory tract infection was defined by clinical and radiological signs in addition to a temperature exceeding 37.5°C. Bacteriemia was defined as growth of bacteria from one blood culture irrespective of other clinical signs of infection. Valve endocarditis was identified by bacteriemia, clinical septicimia, and dehiscence of the valve.

Part II: Intraoperative Serum Concentration Levels

Serum concentrations of the respective antibiotics were determined in 27 consecutive patients, 14 in Group I and 13 in Group II before, during, and immediately after cardiopulmonary bypass. During bypass, samples were obtained 10 and 30 min after initiating bypass, and then every 1/2 h throughout the bypass period.

The antibiotic concentrations in patient sera were determined by an agar well diffusion method (1). *Staphylococcus aureus 209* was used as the test organism and PDM antibiotic sensitivity medium (AB Biodisk) as the test medium. Each determination was made in duplicate, and the mean was calculated.

Results

Comparison of groups

No significant differences could be found in the variables under study (Table 2).

Table 2. Comparison of groups

	Penicillin group	Cephalosporin group
No. of patients	53	50
Mean age (years)	55	57
Preoperative hospitalization (days)	2.9	3.1
Type of operations (No.)		
Aortocoronary bypass	28	36
Single valve replacement	17	10
Double valve replacement	2	1
Others (congenital, aneurysm, etc.)	6	3
Duration of operation (min ± SD)	210 ± 45	210 ± 40
X-corporeal bypass time (min ± SD)	94 ± 33	96 ± 28
Reoperation due to bleeding	4	3
Antibiotic treatment beyond 7 days	11	5
Prophylaxis discontinued before day 7	4	1
Days in hospital (mean)	19.3	18.4

Infection Rates

Septicemia was not encountered in any patient. Two patients, one in each group, developed a superficial sternal wound infection. No other incisional wound infections were registered. Respiratory tract infection rate recorded at 5-7 days and 12-14 days postoperatively was 30% and 2%, respectively, in the penicillin group, compared with 24% and 4% in the cephalosporin group. Urinary tract infection rate recorded at 7 days and at 12 days postoperatively was 8% and 11%, respectively, in the penicillin group compared to 2% and 8% in the cephalosporin group (P >0.10). One patient (cephalosporin group) developed prosthetic endocarditis 2 months after aortic valve replacement (*Staphylococcus aureus* isolated from blood cultures. No bacteria were isolated from this patient intra- or postoperatively).

Bacteriological Surveillance

Table 3 gives the isolates from the samples taken from the sternal wound incision intraoperatively. Bacteria were found in the subcutaneous tissue in 13% of the patients, and from the skin margin in 29% of the patients (no significant differences between the groups). In the majority of cases (29/42), coagulase negative staphylococci were cul-

Table 3. Bacteriological findings in samples collected peroperatively from 103 patients given prophylactic antibiotics. Figures in parentheses indicate the number of patients

Antibiotic given	Subcutaneous tissue only	Bacteria isolated from skin only	Subcutaneous tissue plus skin
Penicillin group	Coagulase-negative staphylococci (1)	Coagulase-negative staphylococci (9)	Coagulase-negative staphylococci (5)
	Micrococci (1)	Diphteroids (4)	
		Anaerobic Gram-positive cocci (2)	
		α-hemolytic streptococci (1)	
Cephalosporin group	Coagulase-negative staphylococci (1)	Coagulase-negative staphylococci (11)	Coagulase-negative staphylococci (3)
		Escherichia coli (1)	Diphteroids (3)
		Diphteroids (1)	
		α-hemolytic streptococci (1)	
		Propionibacterium acnes (1)	
		Lactobacilli (1)	
		Yeast (2)	

tured. In the penicillin group, bacteria were isolated from the blood in three patients on the day of operation (anaerobic streptococci, 1; Propionibacterium acnes, 2), and in one patient day 12 postoperatively (coagulase negative staphylococci). In the cephalosporin group, coagulase negative staphylococci were isolated from the blood in one patient on day 3 and one patient day 12 postoperatively. The isolates from patients with urinary tract infection are given in Table 4. Significant drainage from incisional wounds was found in 28 patients in the penicillin group, compared to 32 patients in the cephalosporin group. Coagulase negative staphylococci could be isolated in seven of these patients, six in the penicillin group and one in the cephalosporin group. This difference is statistically significant ($0.02 < p < 0.05$). Bacteria were not isolated from the mediastinal tubes except in one patient (probably contamination due to broken sample vial).

Side Effects

In four patients (penicillin group) and one patient (cephalosporin group), the prophylactic regime was terminated before schedule. In two patients, one in each group, this was due to an allergic reaction.

Table 4. Bacteriological findings in urine specimens from 103 patients given prophylactic antibiotics. Figures in parentheses indicate the number of patients

Antibiotic given	Specimens collected on Day 1	Day 7	Day 12
Penicillin group	Klebsiella (1)	Escherichia coli (1)	Klebsiella (1)
		Klebsiella (2)	Enterococci (1)
		Micrococci (1)	Micrococci (1)
			Candida albicans (1)
			Mixed flora (2)
Cephalosporin group		Enterococci (1)	Escherichia coli (2)
			Staph. epidermidis (1)
			Mixed flora (1)

Serum Concentration Levels

The serum concentrations of penicillin G and cephalothin before, during, and after cardiopulmonary bypass are given in Table 5.

Discussion

Both antibiotic regimes used in this study seem to be safe as the infection rates in both groups of patients are low compared to those reported in recently published series (3, 4, 6). On the basis of the clinical results, we cannot establish whether cephalosporins or penicillins are to be preferred as prophylactic agents. With our current low infection rates, the size of the study groups must be very large (i.e., thousands of patients) to discover significant differences, if such exist.

However, bacteria were found in specimens collected peroperatively from about 40% of the patients. This is a minimum figure as bacteria would probably have been isolated from a greater number of patients with a better sampling technique (7). The dominating organisms in the specimens collected both per- and postoperatively were coagulase negative staphylococci, bacteria which are potentially pathogenic in this type of surgery (4, 8). The bacteria isolated from the blood are probably of no significance. None of the patients with positive blood cultures developed endocarditis or had other signs of systemic infection.

The blood and tissue concentrations of the prophylactic drugs should be adequate at the time of maximum contamination, i.e, during operation. The serum concentration levels of penicillin G and cephalothin found during the bypass period were all well above recommended values. Furthermore, the antibiotics chosen for prophylaxis should be effective against the majority of possible pathogens identified. Because of the decreasing sensitivity of coagulase negative staphylococci to penicillins, and the nearly uniform sensitivity to cephalothin at our hospital, cephalothin appears to be the preferable alternative. The penicillin regime used in this study lacks the theoretical

Table 5. Serum concentrations (mg/l ± SD) before, at different time intervals during, and immediately after terminating cardiopulmonary bypass (No. of observations in parentheses)

	Penicillin G	Cephalothin
Before bypass	110 ± 245[a] (n = 13)	23 ± 31 (n = 13)
10 min bypass	156 ± 55 (n = 14)	117 ± 11 (n = 13)
30 min bypass	130 ± 41 (n = 14)	84 ± 10 (n = 13)
60 min bypass	93 ± 28 (n = 13)	61 ± 19 (n = 12)
90 min bypass	59 ± 27 (n = 7)	35 ± 17 (n = 10)
120 min bypass	55 ± 15 (n = 3)	37 (n = 1)
After bypass	39 ± 16 (n = 14)	26 ± 14 (n = 12)

[a]The high SD is caused by a single value

advantage of an effective protection during the operation since penicillin G was the only drug given peroperatively. The low infection rate in the penicillin group may indicate that our operative technique and performance is acceptable.

The prophylactic antibiotic used should furthermore be selected on the basis of low toxicity, ease of administration, and minimum cost. Whether cephalosporins are substantially better than penicillins with respect to these considerations is a matter of discussion. From a nursing point of view, a one-drug regime is more easy to handle than a two-drug regime.

In this study, prophylactic antibiotics were probably given for too long a period (2) as the risk of bacterial contamination is reduced after closure of the wound(s). However, in prosthetic surgery it is of major importance that the antibiotic is incorporated into clots and fibrin material. New clots are continually formed in the course of the first day, and fibrin is incorporated at the base of the prosthetic device. The antibiotic should therefore be continued for some days postoperatively (5). However, we cannot find any evidence for extending the prophylaxis beyond 3 days.

Based on this study, we now advocate cephalothin prophylaxis for 3 days. If such a regime is followed, the risk of allergic reactions, alteration in the normal bacterial flora, and development of resistant strains will be minimized. We also recommend that bacteriological surveillance should be performed periodically in each hospital in order to determine the sensitivity of potential pathogens to the antimicrobials used.

References

1. Bennett JV, Brodie LJ, Benner EJ, Kirby WMM (1966) Simplified, accurate method for antibiotic assay of clinical specimens. Appl Microbiol 14:170-177
2. Flynn NM, Lawrence RM (1979) Antimicrobial prophylaxis. Med Clin North Am 63: 1225-1245
3. Fong IW, Baker CB, McKee DC (1980) The value of prophylactic antibiotics in aorto-coronary bypass operations. J Thorac Cardiovasc Surg 78:908-913

4. Myerowitz PD, Caswell K, Lindsay WG, Nicoloff DM (1977) Prophylactic use of antibiotics. Open heart surgery. South Med J 70:61-64
5. Neu HC (1977) Clinical pharmacokinetics in preventive antimicrobial therapy. South Med J 70:14-24
6. Pien FD, Michale NL, Mamiya R, Tavaki H, Slavish S, Bruce A, Moreno-Cabral RJ (1979) Comparative study of prophylactic antibiotics in cardiac surgery. Clindamycin versus cephalothin. J Thorac Cardiovasc Surg 77:908-913
7. Raahave D (1975) New technique of quantitative bacteriological sampling of wounds by velvet pads: clinical sampling trial. J Clin Microbiol 2:277-280
8. Speller DC, Mitchell RG (1973) Coagulase-negative staphylococci causing endocarditis after cardiac surgery. J Clin Pathol 26:517-521
9. Weiner JP, Gibson G, Munster AM (1980) Use of prophylactic antibiotics in surgical procedures: peer review guideline as a method for quality assurance. Am J Surg 139:348-351

Prospective Randomized Comparative Study of Cefamandole Versus Ampicillin-Cloxacillin Antibiotic Prophylaxis in Extra-corporeal Cardiovascular Surgery

A. Nevelsteen, P. Lauwers, R. Demeyere, R. Suy, W. Daenen, H. van Ermen, and G. Stalpaert*

Introduction

In most forms of clean surgery, no antibiotic cover is necessary. On the other hand, cover is advisable in open-heart surgery when some contamination is inevitable or when prostheses are inserted, especially because of the disastrous consequences when prosthetic valve endocarditis develops (1, 2). For this reason and because the efficacy of prophylactic antimicrobial therapy has been emphasized (3), prophylactic administration of antibiotics is common for patients undergoing cardiac surgery. Although it has been proved that the prophylactic therapy should be directed both against *Staphylococcus aureus*, *Staphylococcus epidermidis*, and gram-negative bacilli (4-6), the choice of the suitable agent and the duration of the therapy are still controversial. Cefamandole, a new cefalosporin antibiotic, has an excellent antibacterial activity against these offending organisms and provides fast rising and dose-dependent serum and tissue concentrations (7-9). For these reasons we selected it as a suitable agent for prophylaxis in cardiovascular surgery. We decided to set up a prospective randomized comparative trial using our previous antibiotic regimen (ampicillin-cloxacillin) as the control versus cefamandole.

Clinical Material and Methods

Selected for this clinical trial were all adult patients undergoing extracorporeal cardiac surgery between July and November of 1978. Excluded were only patients with seriously reduced renal function or patients with known hypersensitivity to the penicillins or to the cefalosporins. During this period we operated on 170 patients. They were randomly divided into two groups of 85 patients each.

Group 1 consisted of 63 men and 22 women with a mean age of 53.5 years (range 25 to 72 years). Forty-eight patients underwent a coronary bypass operation. Valvular replacement was performed in 22 patients. Eleven patients underwent a coronary bypass in combination with valvular replacement (Table 1). All these patients received cefamandole intravenously, diluted in 150 cc of dextrose and infused over a period of 30 min. The dosage was 2 g every 6 h on the day of operation (first dose at the time of anesthesia induction) and 2 g every

*Department of Cardiovascular Surgery and Department of Anesthesiology, AZ St. Rafaël, Kapucijnenvoer 33, 3000 Leuven, Belgium

8 h for 2 days postoperatively or 4 days in patients with valvular replacement.

Group 2 consisted of 62 men and 23 women with a mean age of 51.5 years (range 25 to 70 years). Forty-three patients underwent a coronary bypass operation. Valvular replacement was performed in 33 patients. Seven patients underwent a coronary bypass in combination with valvular replacement or an aortobifemoral graft (Table 1). These patients received the combination ampicillin-cloxacillin, intravenously during the first 2 or 3 days and perorally after discharge from the intensive care unit. The dosage was 500 mg of each every 6 h during 8 days started also at the time of anesthesia induction. The patients in this group with valvular replacement received cloxacillin 500 mg every 6 h for another 3 weeks.

Blood cultures were routinely taken in all patients with fever exceeding 39°C. In any patient, who developed clinical signs of sepsis, a blood culture was taken and the prophylaxis was immediately stopped and converted to gentamicin or tobramycin without knowledge of the result of the haemoculture. With regard to the occurrence of late onset endocarditis, all patients were followed for at least 1 year.

Table 1. Surgical procedures in the studied group of patients

Group 1	63 men			Group 2	62 men		
	22 women				23 women		
Mean age	53.5 years			Mean age	51.5 years		
Coronary bypass			48	Coronary bypass			43
Valvular replacement			22	Valvular replacement			33
	MVR	8			MVR	8	
	AVR	4			AVR	11	
	AVR + MVR	8			AVR + MVR	11	
	MVR + TVR	1			MVR + TVR	1	
	AVR + MVR + TVR	1			MVR + AVR + TVR	2	
Commissurotomy			2	ASD II			1
Aneurysm LV			2	Aneurysm LV			1
Coronary bypass comb. with			11	Coronary bypass comb. with			7
	Valvular repl.	8			Valvular repl.	4	
	Aneurysm LV	3			Aneurysm LV	1	
					AF graft	2	

Results

Four patients in group 1 died within 30 days of the operation, for an operative mortality of 4.7%. One patient died of myocardial infarction and two because of low cardiac output. The last patient died of infection, namely pneumonia caused by *Pseudomonas aeruginosa*. With one operative death in group 2, the mortality here was 1.1%. After a mediastinal infection with *Escherichia coli*, successfully treated with local measures and gentamicin, this patient died of septic shock due to cholecystitis.

Blood cultures had to be taken in 21 patients of group 1, in 15 patients because of fever exceeding 39°C (Table 2). Two of these haemocultures were positive, namely for *Klebsiella oxytoca* and *viridans streptococci*. The prophylaxis in these two patients remained unchanged and they recovered without problems. In six patients of group 1, haemocultures were taken because of clinical signs of sepsis. All cultures were negative. Nevertheless, as stated in the conditions of the trial, the antimicrobial prophylaxis was converted to gentamicin or tobramycin and all patients recovered without problems. In group 2, haemocultures were taken in 16 patients, in nine because of fever exceeding 39°C and in seven because of clinical signs of sepsis. All cultures were negative and all patients recovered without problems.

Table 2. Early results

Haemocultures
- Group 1: 21 patients
  - 15 patients fever >39°C
    - 13 negative
    - 2 positive
      - *Klebsiella oxytoca*
      - *viridans streptococci*
  - 6 patients signs of sepsis
    - 6 negative
- Group 2: 16 patients
  - 9 patients fever >39°C
    - 9 negative
  - 7 patients signs of sepsis
    - 7 negative

Postoperative morbidity included a postperfusion syndrome and a myocardial infarction in two patients of group 1. There were no complications related to the prophylaxis itself and no patient showed a wound infection or an early onset prosthetic valve endocarditis. A self-limiting Cytomegalovirus infection and a deep venous thrombosis were seen in two patients of group 2. A chronic fistula at the sternotomy wound, caused by *Candida albicans*, was successfully treated by local measures in a third patient. In one patient of this group, the prophylaxis was stopped because of hypersensitivity to the penicillins. There were no patients with postoperative endocarditis.

All patients were followed for at least 1 year and in both groups there were two late deaths. In group 1, there was one death due to pulmonary embolism. The cause of death of the second patient is unknown, but certainly not infection. In group 2, the two late deaths were due to pulmonary embolism and myocardial infarction. Neither in group 1 nor in group 2 was there any patient with a late infection or a late onset prosthetic valve endocarditis.

Comments

As for any operative procedure, it is generally agreed that the best prevention of postoperative infection and/or prosthetic valve endocarditis in extracorporeal cardiac surgery remains a meticulous surgical technique to prevent bacterial contamination during operation. Nevertheless, the great morbidity and mortality associated with these complications justifies completely the prophylactic use of antibiotics in this kind of surgery. With our combinative ampicillin-cloxacillin regimen, the incidence of postoperative endocarditis in our department decreased from 8% to 0.8% (10). Although we felt that the patient should be covered during the ingrowth of tissue into the teflon ring of the prosthesis, it has been proved that the prolonged use of antibiotics is associated with several theoretical and practical disadvantages (11). Since the prophylaxis must be directed not only against *Staphylococcus aureus* and *Staphylococcus epidermidis*, but also against a wide range of gram-negative bacilli, cefamandole was chosen as an alternative for our previous regimen because of its more favourable MIC figures on gram-positive and its extended spectrum against likely offending gram-negative bacilli (12). It provides fast arising and dose-dependent serum concentrations (13) and shows a good penetration into cardiac tissue (14). Furthermore, used as indicated in this study, there are practically no associated complications.

As for the results, the only difference between the two groups consisted of the two positive blood cultures in group 1 (*Klebsiella oxytoca and viridans streptococci*). Viewing the fact that the prophylaxis remained unchanged and that these patients recovered without further problems, these positive cultures have to be considered as the result of a transient bacteraemia and not as a failure of the prophylactic therapy. Besides, after χ^2 relating of the results there were no statistically significant differences between the two groups ($\chi^2 = 2.6303$, $P = 0.268$). So it appears from this study that a 3-day cefamandole regimen (or 5 days in valvular surgery) constitutes a safe and an effective prophylaxis in cardiac surgery. The fact, however, that in six patients the prophylaxis had to be converted to gentamicin or tobramycin demonstrates that cefamandole, as is true for other prophylactic regimens, is not suitable for all-purpose use. Although on a theoretical basis, gentamicin or tobramycin is the best prophylaxis against the offending gram-negative bacilli, we cannot recommend them as the first choice for prophylaxis in cardiac surgery. Because the incidence of prosthetic valve endocarditis is low, the potential iatrogenic complications (15-17) reported with these antimicrobials may exceed the risk of infection. For these reasons, we constrict their use to patients who fail to respond to more convenient antibiotics.

References

1. Sandusky WR (1980) Use of prophylactic antibiotics in surgical patients. Surg Clin North Am 60:83
2. Tyers GFO, Williams EH, Pierce WS, Waldhausen JA (1977) Present status of cardiac valve replacement. Curr Probl Surg 115:10
3. Myerowitz PD, Caswell K, Lindsay WG, et al. (1977) Antibiotic prophylaxis for open-heart surgery. J Thorac Cardiovasc Surg 73:625
4. Wilson WR, Jaumin PM, Danielson GK, et al. (1975) Prosthetic valve endocarditis. Ann Intern Med 82:751
5. Block PC, De Sanctis RW, Weinberg AN, et al. (1970) Prosthetic valve endocarditis. J Thorac Cardiovasc Surg 60:540
6. Slaughter L, Morris JE, Stan A (1973) Prosthetic valvular endocarditis: a 12 year review. Circulation 47:1319
7. Ernst EC, Berger S, Barza M, et al. (1976) Activity of cefamandole and other cephalosporins against aerobic and anaerobic bacteria. Antimicrob Agents Chemother 9:852

8. Jones RN, Fuchs PC (1976) Comparison of in vitro antimicrobial activity of cefamandole and cefazolin with cephalothin against over 8000 clinical bacterial isolates. Antimicrob Agents Chemother 9:1066
9. Waterman NG, Eickenberg UG, Scharfenberger L (1976) Concentration of cefamandole in serum interstitial fluid, bile, and urine. Antimicrob Agents Chemother 10:733
10. Daenen W, Stalpaert G (1976) Experience with the Björk-Shiley prosthesis (365 cases). In: Late results of valvular replacements and coronary surgery; European Press, Ghent, p 47
11. Bernard HR (1975) Dangers of indiscriminate antibiotic therapy. Surg Clin North Am 55:1303
12. Shemonsky NK, Carrizosa J, Levison ME (1975) In vitro activity and pharmacokinetics in patients of cefamandole, a new cephalosporin antibiotic. Antimicrob Agents Chemother 8:679
13. Myers BR, Ribner B, Yancovitz S, et al. (1976) Pharmacological studies with cefamandole in human volunteers. Antimicrob Agents Chemother 9:140
14. Archer GL, Polk RE, Duma RJ, et al. (1978) Comparison of cephalothin and cefamandole prophylaxis during insertion of prosthetic heart valves. Antimicrob Agents Chemother 13:924
15. Argov Z, Mastaglia FL (1979) Disorders of neuromuscular transmission caused by drugs. N Engl J Med 301:409
16. Appel GB, Neu HC (1978) Gentamicin in 1978. Ann Intern Med 89:528
17. Neu HC (1976) Tobramycin: an overview. J Infect Dis [Suppl] 134:S3

An Investigation of the Influence of Perioperative Antibiotic Treatment on the Resistancy-Characteristics of Bacteria Isolated from Patients Undergoing Cardiac Surgery

B. G. Hansen*

On account of actual cases of postoperative valvular endocarditis due to multiresistant strains of Staph. epidermidis (epid.), a two-step prospective investigation was made concerning changes in resistancy properties of bacteria isolated in the pre- and postoperative phase from patients undergoing open-heart surgery.

In phase 1, all were given streptomycin and methicillin for 7 days starting 12 h before the operation. None of the patients were colonized with multiresistant strains before or immediately after the operation. Two days after the operation (while situated in the intensive care unit), 79% of the patients carried multiresistant Staph. epid. in the nose and 59% had multiresistant enterobacteria in the urine. No strains isolated from the air of the operating room were multiresistant while 34% of strains isolated from the intensive care unit were so.

In phase 2, all were given methicillin for only 3 days. The cleaning routine was changed. A new investigation showed a reduction of 20% of the prevalence of multiresistant strains. Days of bacteriuria were reduced. The frequency of wound infections was unaltered; endocarditis did not occur.

The investigation concludes that administration of methicillin for 3 days gives sufficient protection in cardiac surgery against postoperative infections, that reduced use of antibiotics will reduce the risk of selecting multiresistant strains and that improved cleaning reduces the risk of early colonization with resistant strains. A halving of the antibiotic expense is an essential economic gain.

*Department of Thoracic Surgery, Odense University Hospital and the State Serum Institute Regional lab. Odense, Denmark

Treatment of Infective Endocarditis. An Analysis of 68 Surgically Treated Patients

A. Brunet, G. Cohen, M. Redonnet, C. Hubscher, B. Letac, and R. Soyer*

As emphasized by Rapaport (3), striking changes have recently occurred in the clinical picture and in the management of infective endocarditis (1, 4-6). In the present study, we have tried to better appreciate the modern surgical aspects of native valve endocarditis by reviewing our experience of 68 cases.

Clinical Material

All patients presenting with infectious valvular lesions and operated between 1973 and 1978 are inlcuded in these series. These 68 cases represent 12% of the total of valvular replacement done in our department during the same period. There were 58 males and 10 females between 19 and 73 years of age (mean 49 years). Only 28 patients had a history of valvular disease preexistent to infective endocarditis.

Our series are to be divided into two groups. In group A, nonactive endocarditis, 52 patients, operation was performed after complete cure of infectious process. In group B, active endocarditis, 16 patients, operation was performed in the primary course of antibiotherapy. Duration of antimicrobial therapy prior to surgery ranged from 15 to 60 days. Clinical control of infection was obtained preoperatively in seven patients. Nine patients had to be operated in spite of a still rampant infection.

An infectious organism was identified in 38 patients. The offending bacteria was a streptococcus in 27 cases, a staphylococcus in six cases, and various types of gram-negative organisms in five cases. The infection site was the aortic valve in 49 patients, the mitral valve in ten, both aortic and mitral valves in eight, and aortic and tricuspid valve in one.

Primary indication for all patients was cardiac decompensation. Most severe hemodynamic impairment were seen in group B. No patient was operated on for sepsis alone and major preoperative embolism occurred in only three patients.

Results

In group A (nonactive endocarditis), there was no hospital mortality. Follow-up analysis has been possible in 47 of 52 patients operated on. The follow-up period has been 2 to 81 months (mean 22.2 months). Three late deaths were from progressive heart failure. Three patients have

*Department of cardiac surgery, Centre hospitalo-universitaire, Rouen, France

been successfully reoperated: two for periprosthetic leak, one for postcannulation coronary stenosis. A mild diastolic murmur is present in 13 patients with no hemodynamically significant incompetence. At the present time, all the 44 middle-term survivors are functional class I or II.

In group B (active endocarditis), five patients died at surgery and hospital mortality is 31%. These deaths are related to annular rupture (one) and low cardiac output (four). One patient, a tramp, has been lost to follow-up. As to the ten other patients surviving operation, follow-up ranges from 2 to 36 months (mean 16 months). During this period, one patient died suddenly of unexplained cause and one patient had to be reoperated for periprosthetic leak. There was no recurrence of infection. Three patients present a mild diastolic murmur. The nine middle-term survivors are functional class I or II.

Discussion

Our patients are all from the same geographic area (French Normandy) and have been referred to us by the same cardiologist team. Clinical aspects of infective endocarditis, as encountered in our patients, can therefore be considered as representative of this pathology in a Western European country.

The role of infection in valvular pathology is important and more than 10% of our valvular replacements are done for infectious lesions. Classic patterns of subacute endocarditis are infrequently seen. Many patients have no known previous cardiac abnormality. Hyperacute as well as torpid clinical pictures can be encountered. The most common site of infection is the aortic orifice and mitral involvement appears usually secondary to aortic infection in case of mitroaortic disease.

On such aspects, North American series (1, 4-6) compare with ours but they differ in some respects: no isolated tricuspid insufficiency and no fungal infections have been encountered by us. That is probably explained by the infrequency of drug addiction in our area (4). More surprising is the lasting preeminence of streptococcus infections in our and other European series (2). Even in patients operated on for active endocarditis, this germ is identified in more than half of the cases.

Anyway, surgical treatment of active endocarditis remains a real surgical challenge. Our series confirm the usual findings: more severe heart failure, more frequent multivalvular lesions, and annular abscess. Six patients/16 had multivalvular lesions in group B vs 3/52 in group A; five patients/16 had annular and myocardial abscess in group B vs 2/52 in group A.

Hospital mortality is high and related to the importance of anatomic destructions and degree of preoperative hemodynamic impairment. Three of our six patients presenting with multivalvular lesions died in the postoperative period.

Early operation, whether infection is controlled or not, is the only way to lower hospital mortality. In our series, operative risk is similar if infection is preoperatively controlled (two deaths in seven patients) or not (three deaths in nine patients). Mortality is less important if the patients are operated in the first month of antimicrobial therapy (two deaths in ten patients). On the whole, our experience supports current concepts of an aggressive surgical approach to infective endocarditis (1, 2, 4-6).

References

1. Boyd AD, Spencer FC, Isom OW, Cunningham JN, Reed GE, Acinapura AJ, Tice DA (1977) Infective endocarditis. An analysis of 54 surgically treated patients. J Thorac Cardiovasc Surg 73:23-30
2. Piwnica A, Soyer R, Eisenmann B, Diamant-Berger F, Haas C, Menasche P (1974) Remplacements valvulaires en urgence au cours de l'endocardite bactérienne aigue. Coeur [Suppl: Journées internationales de Deauville]:839-854
3. Rapaport E (1978) The changing role of surgery in the management of infective endocarditis. Circulation 58:598-599
4. Richardson JV, Karp RB, Kirklin JW, Dismukes WE (1978) Treatment of infective endocarditis: a 10-year comparative analysis. Circulation 58:589-597
5. Wilson WR, Danielson GK, Giuliani ER, Washington JA II, Jaumin PM, Geraci JE (1978) Valve replacement in patients with active infective endocarditis. Circulation 58:585-588
6. Young JB, Welton DE, Raizner AE, Ishimori T, Montero A, Guinn GA, Mattox K, Gentry LO, Alexander JK, Miller RR (1979) Surgery in active infective endocarditis. Circulation [Suppl 1] 60:77-81

Airborne Contamination Hazard in Open-Heart Surgery. Efficiency of Air Filtration and Laminar Flow

G. Soots, H. Leclerc, A. Pol, and C. Savage*

The purpose of this study is to evaluate the role of airborne contamination in open-heart surgery. In 1975, after an episode of postoperative infection, classical prophylactic measures were reinforced and they were maintained all through this study. Results were, however, disappointing. We recognized that we had excessive activity in an old and overcrowded hospital (12). But we found it necessary to investigate the mechanism of contamination. Since 1968, our attention had been focused on possible airborne contamination, as we found contaminated bacterial plates when they were exposed below ventilation ports.

Material and Methods

During the study (from September 1, 1975, to March 31, 1979), 824 open-heart operations were performed. Patients were distributed in four groups corresponding (Table 1) to operating room ventilation. In group I, ventilation was old, turbulent, and not filtrated. In group II, ventilation was "rebuilt" in 1976 but again with turbulence and no filtration. In group III, operations were performed in the same operating room as in Group I, but with a blowing unit equipped with high efficiency particulate air (HEPA) filters, determining an area of laminar flow where patient and operating personell were concentrated (partial horizontal laminar flow). In group IV, patients were operated on in a new hospital where the operating room was equipped with HEPA filters and laminar flow between a blowing unit on one wall and an aspirating unit on the opposite (total horizontal flow).

Table 1. Patient grouping according to operating room ventilation (N = 824)

	Group I (N = 274)	Group II (N = 166)	Group III (N = 233)	Group IV (N = 151)
Ventilation	Built 1965;	Rebuilt 1976;	Horizontal;	Horizontal;
	turbulent;	turbulent;	part. lam. flow;	total lam. flow;
	no filters	no filters	HEPA filters	HEPA filters

*Hôpital Cardiologique, Boulevard du Professeur J. Leclercq, 59037 Lille Cedex, France

Table 2 shows patient distribution in each group in regard to operations performed. Air sampling as close as possible to the operative field was performed during a number of operations in each group at different times during the operative procedure. We used a Casella air sampler collecting 1 m^3 of air which is projected on bacterial plates for cultures. Bacterial colonies are counted and results expressed in terms of "colony forming units" (CFU) as described by Blakemore (1).

Table 2. Surgery performed

	Group I (N = 274) %	Group II (N = 166) %	Group III (N = 233) %	Group IV (N = 151) %
Valve repl.	34.3	38.5	42.4	43.04
C.A.B.P.	24.8	31.9	32.6	35.09
Congenital	33.5	27.7	20.1	13.2
Misc.	7	1.8	4.7	9.2
Total	274	166	233	151

Patient study was established using the following parameters: wound infection, mediastinitis, temperature equal to or over 38.5°C, and blood cultures. Late prosthetic valve endocarditis was not investigated.

The antibiotics policy was as follows: all patients received prophylactic penicillin G only, starting the day before surgery. Blood cultures were performed on the basis of 10 in 24 h when temperature was ⩾38.5°C. No antibiotic change was made before results of blood cultures were obtained. However, in cases of severe hyperthermia associated with alarming symptoms (such as shivering), antibiotic therapy was altered (only after blood cultures sampling) by giving cephalosporin and gentamycin in group I and pristinamycin alone in all other groups. Antibiotic therapy was eventually modified according to the results of blood cultures and antibiograms.

Results

Figure 1 shows four examples of the usual findings in the four groups. In group I with turbulent air and old, nonfiltrated ventilation, maximum CFU per cubic meter was as high as 1400/m^3; "peaks" of CFU were demonstrated at the time of patient preparation and at removal of drapes. CFU counts remained at lower levels during bypass. In group II, similar peaks were also present but maximum CFU count was below 300. In group III with HEPA filters and partial horizontal laminar flow, CFU was as low as 50 to 100, with no peaks, and in group IV it was always below 10 CFU.

Clinical results are indicated in Table 3. A statistically significant difference was demonstrated between total percentage of clinical sepsis from group I to all other groups, but no significant difference was found between groups II, III, and IV.

Postoperative hyperthermia is shown in Table 4. By considering temperature curves of patients, we could separate them into two catego-

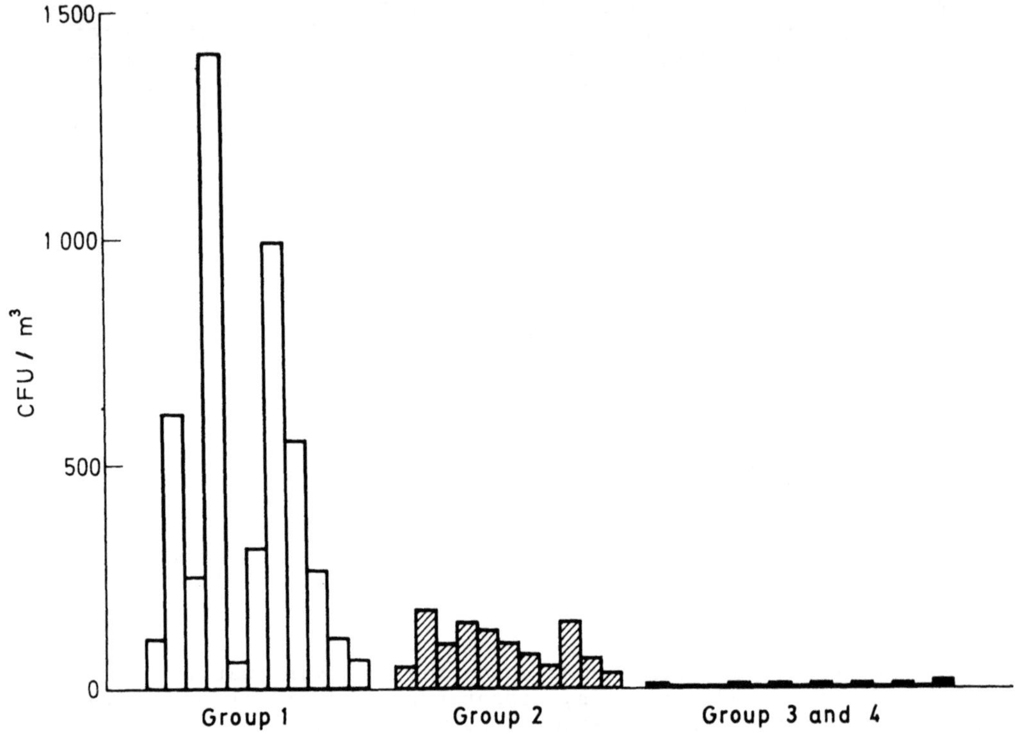

Fig. 1. Results of air sampling

ries. 1) In some subjects, temperature increased above 38.5°C the first day and returned to normal after 2 to 3 days. 2) In others, after initial rise the first day, temperature went down slowly or persisted more than 5 days. Patients who developed mediastinitis were all in the second category.

Considering hyperthermia of any type (Table 4), significant differences were demonstrated only between groups I and III ($p = 0.0004$) as well as groups I and IV ($p = 0.003$), showing better results by use of laminar flow of both designs than with the old turbulent and not filtrated ventilation. No improvement was found between groups I and II ($X^2 = 2.3$) from old to "rebuilt" ventilation. But no significant difference was shown between groups II, III, and IV ($X^2 < 2.6$), so the benefit from laminar flow against a recently rebuilt ventilation was questionable. But if one looks at hyperthermia lasting more than 5 days (Table 4), there are significant differences between each group from I to IV, showing that each modification in ventilation resulted in progress.

Percentage of positive blood cultures (BC) fell significantly between groups I and II ($p = 0.001$) and between group I and all others (Table 5). No difference was seen between groups II and III ($X^2 = 0.002$) ("rebuilt" ventilation versus partial laminar flow). But a significant improvement was demonstrated between groups II and IV ($p = 0.04$) and groups III and IV ($p = 0.03$), showing greater improvement from total laminar flow than partial.

If one considers cases associating positive blood cultures and hyperthermia over 38.5°C and lasting more than 5 days (Table 5), percentages falling from 21.1% in group I to 9.6% in group II, to 6% in group III, and to 1.9% in group IV are impressive; however, the number of cases is too small for statistical evaluation.

The study represented in Table 6 shows the predominance of gram + microorganism and especially *staphylococcus albus*. Total gram - organisms (7.6%) in group I fell to 3.2% in group IV. The high level of contamination with enterobacter in groups II and III (3.6% and 2.6%) in a group of patients operated on in the same period was related to accidental contamination of scrub water.

Table 3. Clinical sepsis

	Group I (N = 274) %	Group II (N = 166) %	Group III (N = 233) %	Group IV (N = 151) %
Wound inf.	12	2.4	5.1	5.3
Mediast. inf.	3.6	1.8	0.4	1.3
Total[a]	15.6	4.2	5.5	6.6

[a]Group I/II $p = 0.0002$, significant
Group I/III $p = 0.0002$, significant
Group I/IV $p = 0.006$, significant
Group II/III/IV $X^2 = 0.8$, nonsignificant

Table 4. Postoperative hyperthermia ≥38.5°C

	Group I (N = 274) %	Group II (N = 166) %	Group III (N = 233) %	Group IV (N = 151) %
Hyperth. (all types)[a]	77	70.4	62.6	63.5
Hyperth. (lasting ≥5 days)[b]	35.7	26.5	18.2	5.9

[a]Group I/III $p = 0.0004$, significant
Group I/IV $p = 0.003$, significant
Group I/II $X^2 = 2.3$, nonsignificant
Group II/III/IV $X^2 < 2.6$, nonsignificant

[b]Group I/II $p = 0.04$, significant
Group II/III $p = 0.04$, significant
Group III/IV $p = 0.0006$, significant

Table 5. Results of blood cultures

	Group I (N = 274) %	Group II (N = 166) %	Group III (N = 233) %	Group IV (N = 151) %
BC + [a]	35.7	21.6	21.8	13.2
BC + and hyp. ⩽5D	14.59	12	15.8	11.2
BC + and hyp. ⩾5D[b]	21.1	9.6	6	1.9

[a]Group I/II $p = 0.001$, significant
Group II/III $\chi^2 = 0.002$, nonsignificant
Group II/IV $p = 0.04$, significant
Group III/IV $p = 0.03$, significant

Table 6. Bacteria found in blood cultures

	Group I (N = 274) %	Group II (N = 166) %	Group III (N = 233) %	Group IV (N = 151) %
Positive blood cult. patients	35.7	21.6	21.8	13.2
Staph. albus	23	12.6	14	9.2
Staph. aureus	0.7	1.2	1.7	0.6
Strepto non hem.	0.7	-	-	-
Enterocc.	3	-	0.4	0.6
Escher. coli	1	1.2	0.4	-
Enterobacter	0.7	3.6	2.6	-
Klebsiella	2.1	0.6	0.4	1.3
Pseudom. aerog.	-	0.6	0.8	-
B 5 W	-	0.6	0.4	-
Micrococcus	1.8	-	1.7	1.3
Serratia mar.	1.4	1.2	-	-
Clostrid perf.	0.3	0.6	-	-
Bacillus	0.3	0.6	-	-
Citrobacter freun.	-	-	0.4	-

Discussion

Patient distribution in regard to surgery performed has been different between groups, with an increasing percentage of coronary and valve surgery. As shown by Engelmann et al. (6), these patients are more susceptible than others to postoperative infection.

Results of air sampling expressed in CFU per cubic meter showed that operating-room air was highly contaminated in group I with old not filtrated and turbulent air distribution. The number of CFU in air samples was especially high during preparation of the patient for monitoring and anesthesia, and at the end of the procedure. The CFU number was high when a large number of operating-room personnel were active. Bypass time was consistent with a low CFU count. This reproduces the findings of Blakemore et al. (1).

Better results were obtained in group II after the ventilation was "rebuilt" but the absence of filtration would probably result in the same situation as in group I with elapsing time.

HEPA filters are recognized (1, 3, 9, 12) as being able to retain particulates over 0.3 μm diameter and to deliver practically bacteria-free air. Laminar flow has been advocated particularly by orthopedic surgeons (2) to avoid turbulence and spread of bacteria which are produced by shedding from operating-room personnel. Partial laminar flow and even more total laminar flow were able to deliver almost "sterile" air in the operating room in our experience.

While a significant improvement was found from group I to all other groups, it was impossible to show a difference in clinical results between groups II, III, and IV. This finding is similar to that of Szilagyi et al. (14) in vascular surgery, pointing out the difficulty in demonstrating the benefit of prophylactic measures against infection on a clinical basis only.

Such a study should involve a considerable number of patients, requiring a long time and the consequences of modifications of many parameters during the study. Clark et al. (3) obtained a significant lowering of rate of deep wound infection but their program did not concern only ventilation modifications, making it difficult to isolate the role of air filtration in their work.

Postoperative hyperthermia is often considered as noninfection-related after open-heart surgery and due to the use of cooling and rewarming, affecting the thermal regulation of the patient. In our experience, significant reduction of postoperative hyperthermia lasting 5 days or more has been parallel to improvement of bacterial content of air in the operating room. The high frequency of positive blood cultures in these patients allows one to suspect the role of contamination in postoperative hyperthermia.

The high level of positive blood cultures may be surprising and even alarming. In fact, results would have been different if one had performed a smaller number of blood cultures in hyperthermic patients. Our practice to realize systematically 10 blood cultures over a 24-h period on every patient experiencing hyperthermia equal to or above 38.5°C, was certainly responsible for the high number of positive results.

As sampling was by necessity done via the jugular venous catheter and not by needle venous puncture, one may think that some accidental contamination of blood samples could have induced false positive results. The chances to alter results seems low, however, since at a given period of time only 4.9% positive cultures were obtained among 1130 blood cultures performed. Kotin (11) showed the frequency of positive blood cultures on many occasions, even in healthy patients. Positive transient blood cultures should be considered as transient bacteremia which do not always lead to clinical complications, depending on host response and quantity of contamination. Probably our antibiotic policy, using only penicillin G and no wide-spectrum prophylactic antibiotics, allowed cultures to grow more frequently. But we found it an advantage to be able to determine the choice of antibiotics on the basis of cultures and antibiograms.

The frequency of *Staphylococcus albus* coagulase negative (Table 6) is a surprising fact. This bacterium has for a long time been considered as nonpathogenic or a blood culture contaminant. Some recent studies, however, demonstrated its responsibility in postoperative septicemia (8) and bacterial prosthetic heart valve endocarditis (1o).

The parallelism found in this study between bacterial quality of operating-room air, postoperative hyperthermia lasting more than 5 days, and positive blood cultures is an argument to suspect the role of airborne contamination in open-heart surgery.

The mechanism of contamination has been investigated by Blakemore et al. (1). They made the remark that the extracorporeal blood is exposed to the air which is constantly drawn through the coronary suction lines. Identical organisms were isolated from the air and the blood of the heart-lung machine. *Staphylococcus albus* was the most frequent organism. He stated that 1200 CFU could be introduced into the blood per hour of bypass.

Dankert and Eijgelaar (5) demonstrated the contamination of disposable oxygenators after open-heart surgery and the disappearance of this contamination with laminar flow. Contamination by this route in open-heart surgery is hematogenic and this could explain the frequency of hyperthermia on the first day, related to plus or minus transient and severe bacteremia.

Clark et al. (3) stated that postoperative soft tissue infections are the results of a break in the observance of Halsted's principles but that architectural, engineering, and functional improvements affected the deep infection rate. As the efficiency of HEPA filtration has been demonstrated by the studies of Blakemore et al. (1), Clark et al. (3), Dankert and Eijgelaar (5), and our own, further investigation should be necessary to assess an additional benefit from laminar distribution of flow (12).

Conclusions

This study shows that airborne contamination hazard should be considered in open-heart surgery as well as the efficiency of HEPA filtration in reducing the risk of contamination for the patient. This is, however, not the only way of infection for open-heart surgery patients and the use of HEPA filters and laminar flow units should not induce heart surgeons to neglect the principles of good aseptic surgery.

References

1. Blakemore WS, McCarrity GJ, Thurer RJ, Wallace HW, MacVaugh H III, Corriel LL (1971) Infection by airborne bacteria with cardiopulmonary bypass. Surgery 6:830
2. Charnley J, Eftekhar N (1969) Postoperative infection in total prosthetic replacement arthroplasty of the hip-joint. With special reference to the bacterial content of the air of the operating room. Br J Surg 56 9:641-649
3. Clark RE, Amos WC, Higgins V, Bemberg KF, Weldon CS (1976) Infection control in cardiac surgery. Surgery 79:89-96

4. Corriel LL, McGarrity GJ, Blakemore WS (1968) Studies on HEPA filtered vertical flow air in the microbiological laboratory and operating room. J Am Assoc Contamin Control 1:48
5. Homan van der Heide JN, Dankert J, Eijgelaar A (1978) A crossflow unit, to prevent airborne infections during open-heart surgery. 27th International Congress of the European Society of Cardiovascular Surgery, Lyon, 28 June - 1 July, 1978, Tome I. 225, 228
6. Engelman RM, Williams D, Gouge TH, Chase RM, Falk EA, Boyd AD, Reed GE (1973) Mediatinitis following open-heart surgery. Arch Surg 107:772-778
7. Firor WB (1967) Infection following open-heart surgery, with special reference to the control of prophylactic antibiotics. J Thorac Cardiovasc Surg 53/3: 371-378
8. Force RA, Dixon C, Bernard RNK, Martinez L, McLean APH, Meakins JI (1979) Staphylococcus epidermidis: An important pathogen. Surgery 86/3:507-514
9. Hoet T (1979) La prévention en matière d'aérobiocontamination en site opératoire. Symbiose - Nouv Rev Santé [Suppl April]
10. Hornick RB (1977) Sources of contamination in open heart surgery. In: Duma RJ (ed) Infections of prosthetic heart valves and vascular grafts. University Park Press, Baltimore London Tokyo, pp 81-99
11. Kotin P (1952) Techniques and interpretation of routine blood cultures. Observations in five thousand consecutive patients. JAMA 149/14:1273-1276
12. Laufman H (1976) Is laminar airflow necessary for prophylaxis against wound infection? Med Instrum 10/6:269
13. Maillard JN, Flusin JL, Rodary M, Elman A (1976) Un nouveau critère de gestion hospitalière. Le seuil de sécurité. Mém Acad Chir 102/4:229
14. Szilagyi DE, Smith RF, Elliott JF, Vrandecic MP (1972) Infection in arterial reconstruction with synthetic grafts. Ann Surg 176/3:321-333

Session VI Cardiac Surgery

Heart Disease in Infancy and Childhood

Chairman: A. Senning, Zurich; Co-Chairman: E. Bos, Rotterdam

Surgery of the Interrupted Aortic Arch

V. Jelesijević, R. Achatzy, E. Anyanwu, D. Knoll, F. Klinke, and H. Dittrich*

The interruption of the aortic arch is a rare vascular anomaly which is most often combined with congenital heart diseases. The first pathological description of this entity dates back to the 18th century. Eighty per cent of the neonates with this anomaly die in the first month of life.

But before we give a detailed description of the interrupted aortic arch, we would like to say a few words about its normal development. Proceeding from the hypothesis of Edwards (2), the double anlage of the aortic arch is the embryonic starting point. The normal left aortic arch arises as the result of the interruption of the dorsal segment of the embryonic right arch between the right subclavian artery and the descending aorta, under the disappearance of the right ductus arteriosus. But the development can take a different course altogether, leading to other anomalies of the aortic arch. One of these presents as the right aortic arch, with possibilities of interruption in four different locations.

The double aortic arch (Fig. 1) which also shows interruptions, is a further anomaly which stands out against the interruption of the aortic arch. Two types are distinguished according to whether or not a functioning lumen is present.

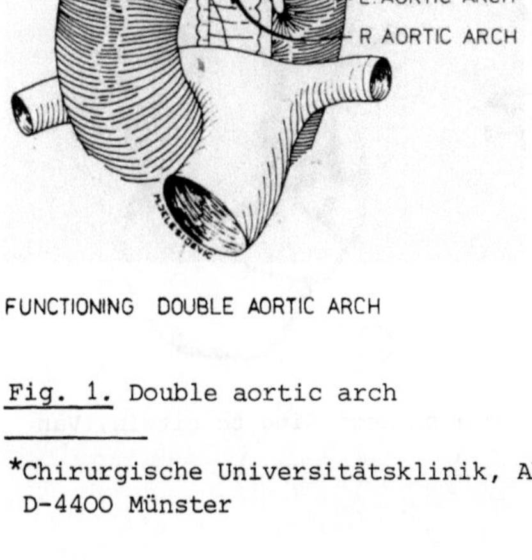

FUNCTIONING DOUBLE AORTIC ARCH

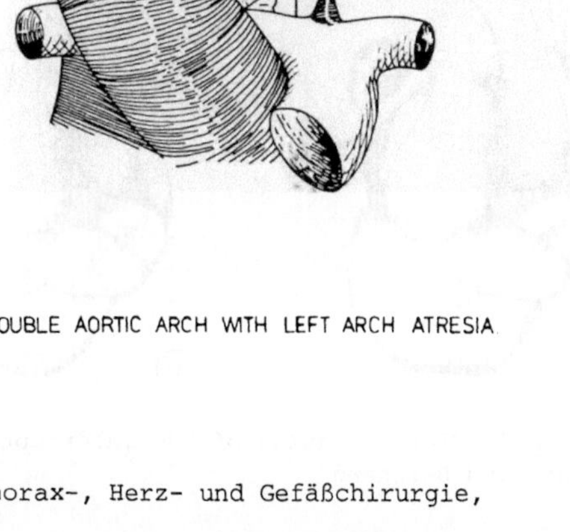

DOUBLE AORTIC ARCH WITH LEFT ARCH ATRESIA

Fig. 1. Double aortic arch

*Chirurgische Universitätsklinik, Abt. Thorax-, Herz- und Gefäßchirurgie, D-4400 Münster

In type I, both arches are open and functioning. This anomaly is more common than type II. These functioning two aortic arches may lead to the constriction of the trachea and the esophagus, and eventually to their obstruction. Among the anomalies of the arch which build a vascular ring around the trachea and the esophagus, the double aortic arch is the most important. This vascular ring can be without symptoms. On the other hand, it can be a reason for respiratory difficulties right from birth.

In type II, the continuity of the arch remains, but a segment of it is atretic and presents as a fibrous cord without a lumen. The second arch is open and functions well. Theoretically, the atresia or aplasia can be on either of the sides, although to date, not a single case of an atretic right arch has been described. However, on the left side they have different localizations.

Now, to the interruption of the single aortic arch of which there are two forms. The one form shows a complete interruption, the other an interruption with a bridging fibrous cord between the proximal arch and the descending aorta. This last form is known as atresia of the aortic arch.

With reference to our cases, we would like to restrict ourselves to the complete interruption of the aortic arch. Almost always an open ductus arteriosus maintaining a connection with the descending aorta is present. Several anatomic variations are possible, depending on the position of the brachiocephalic vessels. The interruption of the aortic arch is a result of the complete cessation of the integration of the embryonic arches into the doubled aortic arch system.

Litwin's (3) classification of the interrupted aortic arch (Fig. 2) shows three variations. The commonest interruption (type A) is located distal to the left subclavian artery, that is, the embryonic left arch is interrupted between the left subclavian artery and the ductus arteriosus. In the case of an embryonic right arch, the interruption lies between the right subclavian artery and the descending aorta. In this variation, the brachiocephalic vessels arise from the proximal aorta. Approximately half of all the cases presenting with interrupted aortic arch shows this variation.

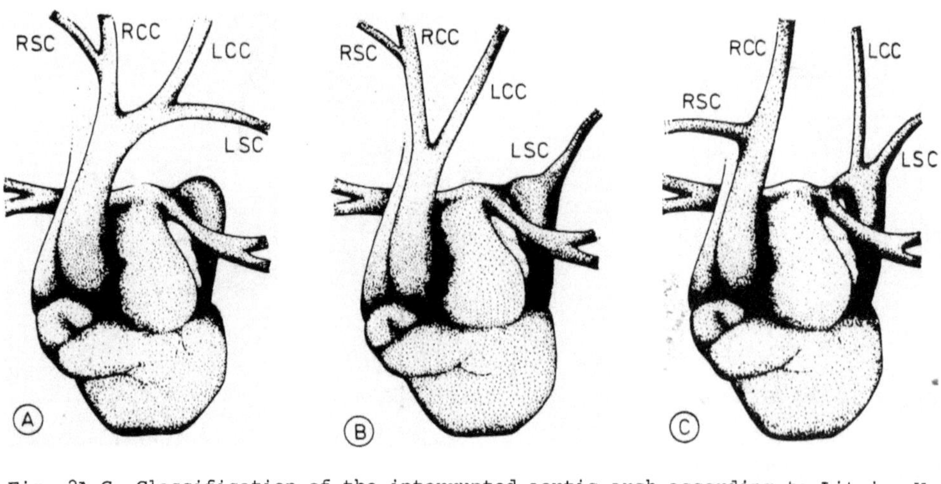

Fig. 2A-C. Classification of the interrupted aortic arch according to Litwin, Van Praagh, and Bernhard

Type B is characterised by a discontinuity between the left common carotid and the left subclavian artery in the case of the left embryonic arch, alternatively between the right subclavian artery and the descending aorta, in the case of the right embryonic arch. In this variation, the left subclavian artery arises from the descending aorta and the left common carotid, from the proximal aorta. Approximately, one third of the cases of interrupted aortic arch present with this variation of the vascular anomaly.

A further variation is seen in type C, where the aortic arch is interrupted between the brachiocephalic trunk and the left common carotid artery. This form represents 10% of all the cases. Aside from these, there is a subgroup which is assigned to the B type. Here, both carotids arise from the ascending aorta and both subclavian arteries, from the descending aorta.

A connecting fibrous cord distinguishes the atresia from the completely interrupted aortic arch. A patent ductus arteriosus is present. The ascending aorta is supplied by the left ventricle and the descending aorta by the right ventricle via the patent ductus.

From January 1, 1974, to date, we have operated five patients with interrupted aortic arch and thereby performed aortic arch replacement. All the operated cases belonged to the group of people that survived early childhood. We have not operated a newborn with this anomaly. Four of the operated patients belonged to type B of Litwin's classification and one to type C. We preferred a left lateral thoracotomy through the fourth intercostal space. Having dissected the descending aorta, the pericardium is incised over the pulmonary artery following which the ascending aorta is dissected (Fig. 3).

After exteriorising part of the aorta with a clamp, a woven Dacron prosthesis of 16-22 mm is sutured to it and pulled through the left side of the mediastinum, passed from the front backwards, and thence pulled on to the descending aorta with which it is anastomosed. In all patients, the same blood pressure was registered postoperatively both at the arms and at the legs. Because of the hypoplasia of the subclavian artery, two patients had a difference of 10-15 mm Hg in the blood pressure measurements. During the follow-up of these patients for 6 years, no late complication was observed.

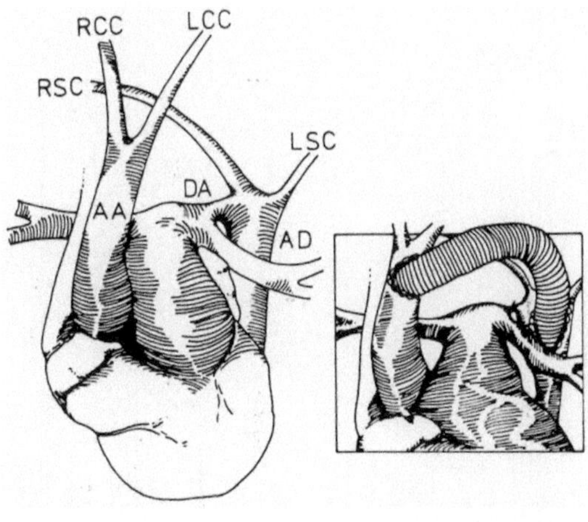

Fig. 3. Interrupted aortic arch type B (Litwin), operative correction, prosthetic replacement

Summary

During the last 6 years, we operated five patients with interrupted aortic arch in the Department of Thoracic and Cardiovascular Surgery in Münster. In each case, we reconstructed the aortic arch with a pro-prosthesis. These patients belonged to the group of people that survived early childhood. There was no intra- or postoperative death and late complications were not observed.

References

1. Barrat-Boyes GB, Nicholls TT, Brandt WTP, Neutze MJ (1972) Aortic arch interruption associated with patent ductus arteriosus, ventricular septal defect, and total anomalous pulmonary venous connection. J Thorac Cardiovasc Surg 63: 367-373
2. Edwards JE (1948) Anomalies of the derivatives of the aortic arch system. Med Clin North Am 32:925
3. Litwin SB, Van Praagh R, Bernhard FW (1972) A palliative operation for certain infants with aortic arch interruption. Ann Thorac Surg 14:369-375
4. Shuford HW, Sybers GR (1974) The aortic arch and its malformations. Thomas, Springfield, p 264
5. Ventemiglia R, Oglietti J, Wukasch CD, Hallman LG, Cooley AD (1976) Interruption of the aortic arch. J Thorac Cardiovasc Surg 72:235-242

The Mitral Valve in Atrioventricular Canal Defect (A.V.C.D.)

S.P. Allwork*

Introduction

Mitral valve stenosis and regurgitation are inimical to successful surgical treatment of AVCD whether they are present initially or are iatrogenically produced.

Nineteen hearts were studied with respect to the anatomy of the mitral component of the atrioventricular valve or valves. Eight hearts had "partial" AVCD (i.e., without ventricular septal defect) and eleven had complete AVCD with interventricular communication.

Results

Partial AVCD

In each case the mitral valve consisted of three leaflets, anterior (aortic), septal, and lateral (mural) (Fig. 1a). The lateral edge of the aortic leaflet had a variable number of chordae tendinae (often thick and short) which inserted into the anterior papillary muscle group. This muscle was normally positioned fairly high on the ventricular wall, and also received some chordae from the septal and mural leaflets. The posterior papillary muscle group received the chordae from the remainder of the septal and lateral leaflets. This muscle group also tended to be placed quite high in the left ventricle.

With respect to the aortic region of the anterior leaflet, this inserted sheet-like directly into the outlet septum, below the aortic valve (Fig. 1b). In most of the specimens, thickened, rolled edges to the mitral leaflets indicated that they had been regurgitant during life.

Five of the eight hearts had been operated upon. One of these (an adult) survived for 3 years, but with increasing mitral dysfunction. The "cleft" had been closed by direct suture, producing a tunnel-like mitral valve (Fig. 2a). The anterior leaflet had torn away from its tenuous insertion into the inlet septum, creating a hole, 1 cm in diameter, in the anterior leaflet. The margins of this hole were quite markedly calcified (Fig. 2b). Valvar pulmonary stenosis had also been present at the time of operation and was surgically released.

*Department of Surgery, Royal Postgraduate Medical School, Hammersmith Hospital, Ducane Road, London, W12 OHS, Great Britain

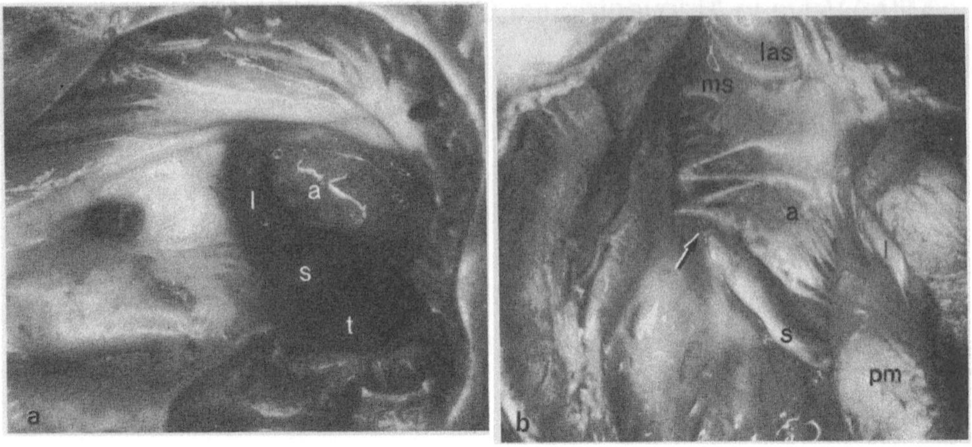

Fig. 1. a Atrioventricular defect seen from the right atrium. The left atrioventricular valve has three distinct leaflets, anterior *(a)*, septal *(s)*, and lateral *(l)*. The architecture of the atrial septum is normal – all the morphological features are present. *t*, "posterior" tricuspid leaflet. b The left ventricular outflow tract and left atrioventricular valve in partial AVCD. The anterior leaftlet *(a)* is intact and is inserted into the narrow outlet septum. There is a small gap ("cleft" – arrowed) between the anterior and septal leaflet *(s)*. The latter has a thickened, rolled edge. Note the abnormal plane of the atrioventricular valve, and the short distance between the annulus and the apex. This makes the papillary muscles *(pm)* appear "high up" on the ventricular wall. *ms*, membranous septum; *las*, left aortic sinus

Complete AVCD

Of the 11 specimens, three were of the Rastelli type C, but the septal and lateral leaflets were recognised. All three hearts had double outlet right ventricle and marked pulmonary outflow tract obstruction. The remaining eight specimens were equally divided between type A and type B. In every case, septal and lateral components of the posterior leaflet were recognised, and these inserted, by way of usually deficient short, thick chordae tendinae, into two groups of papillary muscles. The anterior group was abnormally robust but the posterior was small. In type B hearts the anterior aortic leaflet had chordal attachment to the concave ventricular septum. These chordae were, like those of the other leaflets, short and rather thick. Only secondary chordae (i.e., not attached to the free edge) were represented.

With respect to the interventricular communication (VSD), it was in every case situated in the inflow (posterior) ventricular septum, so that the atrioventricular valve leaflets formed its "roof". The septum was concave posteriorly, but the outflow septum was intact in all but two hearts. In these two, there was also a perimembranous VSD (Fig. 3).

The left ventricular outflow tract was narrow and tunnel-like in all the hearts, due to the muscular insertion of the aortic leaflet, but neither fibrous nor muscular obstruction was observed in this series. One heart, however, had a rather small, bicuspid aortic valve.

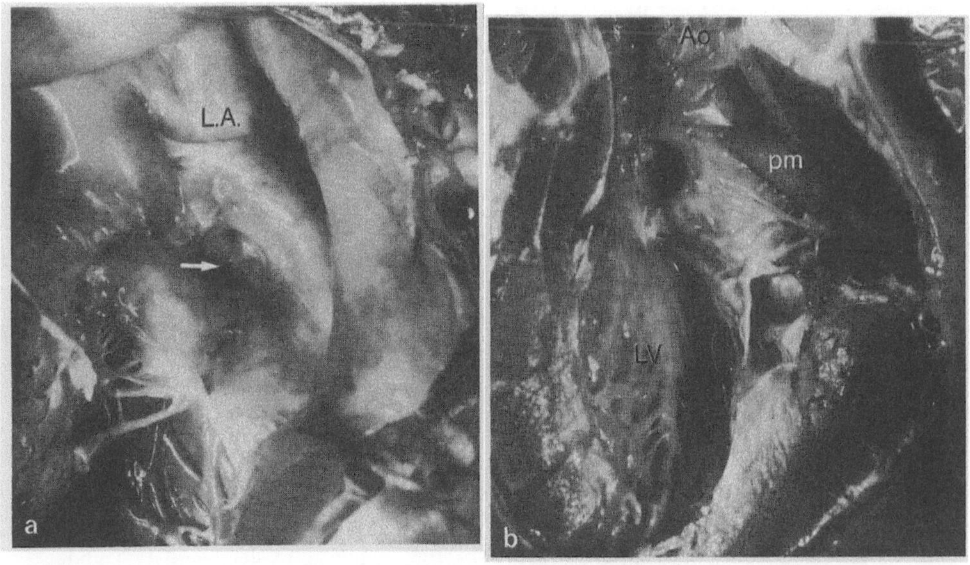

Fig. 2. a Inflow view of partial AVCD with direct suture of the "cleft" which has produced a tunnel-like deformity of the anterior and septal leaflets. The subaortic attachment of the valve has torn (arrowed). *LA*, left atrium. b Left ventricular *(LV)* view of the same heart. The tunnel-like stenosis and hole in the leaflet are obvious. Note the "high", thick anterolateral papillary muscle *(pm)*. *Ao*, aortic valve

Discussion

The observations in this small *post mortem* series accord with the finding of Carpentier (2) that the left component of the atrioventricular valve in AVCD has three leaflets, not two. The "cleft" is in fact a commissure between the anterior and septal leaflets. The competence of the commissure is reflected in the presence or absence of mitral regurgitation during life: it may be assessed anatomically by the presence and degree of thickening and rolling of the free edge of the leaflet, and by the increase in wall thickness of the atria. The presence of a cleft between two atrioventricular valve leaflets does not, of itself, cause regurgitation in AVCD (7). Furthermore, clefts between the inferior and septal tricuspid leaflets tend to develop in normal hearts as age advances (1) and these are not necessarily associated with regurgitation. It seems possible, therefore, that the left septal commissure in AVDC may become incompetent as life advances, consequent, perhaps, upon ventricular dilatation.

The finding of multiple chordal attachment to the outflow septum was noted by Edwards (3) who observed that closure of the "cleft" in such hearts could produce both stenosis and regurgitation. This was well exemplified by one heart in this series (Figs. 2a,b) in which severe mitral dysfunction developed after operation and was progressive.

With respect to the nature of the interventricular communication in complete AVCD, in every case the VSD was posterior. According to Wakai and Edwards (8), VSD is membranous in nature, but the above findings and those of Piccoli et al. (5, 6) do not support this observation. Instead, the membranous part of the (outlet) septum was

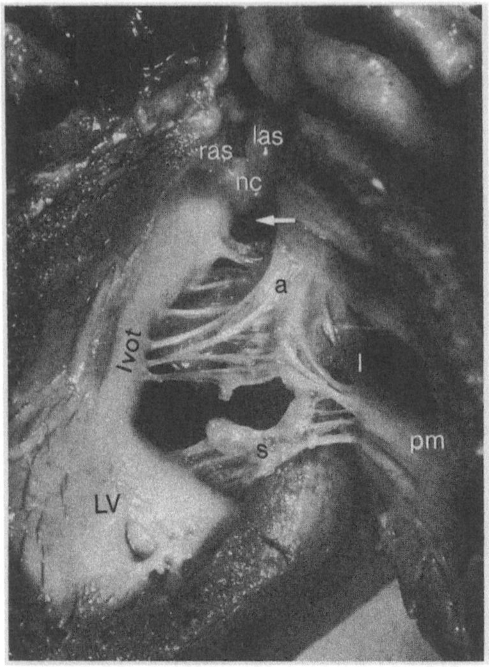

Fig. 3. Complete AVCD, left ventricular *(LV)* view. Most of the posterior (inlet) septum is missing, so that the septal summit is deeply concave. The anterior leaflet is attached by short chordae to the slender outlet septum *(lvot)*, causing a long narrow outflow tract. In left ventriculograms, the very dense opacification of the outflow tract is sometimes likened to the curve of a goose's back. Above this leaflet, immediately below the aortic valve, is a small membranous VSD (arrowed). *nc*, non-coronary aortic sinus; *ras*, right aortic sinus

intact in all but two hearts. In these two, subaortic VSD was additional to the major inlet septum defect. The outlet septum is abnormally orientated (5, 6, 9) but usually imperforate in AVCD.

Concerning the nature of AVCD, the primary anomaly is maldevelopment of the inlet part of the ventricular septum.

The abnormalities of the atrioventricular valves are of supreme functional and surgical importance, but they are secondary to the septal maldevelopment. The author has also observed, with Goor et al. (4), that in the normal heart the distance from the mitral annulus to the apex of the left ventricle is almost equal to that from the apex to the aortic root, whereas in AVCD the former is always considerably shorter. This deficiency is reflected in the relatively "high" position of the papillary muscles in the left ventricle.

In AVCD, the atrial septum is usually present and is usually morphologically normal, although patency of the foramen ovale is quite common. Common atrium occurred once in this series in a situs solitus patient: it is, of course, much commoner in heterotaxy. What is abnormal in AVCD is the inflow ventricular septum. When the valve apparatus is attached to the deficient inflow septum, its plane is distorted. Its morphology may be distorted by abnormal alignment between the remnant of the posterior septum and the anterior septum. Thus both "complete" and "partial" AVCD are essentially malformations of the ventricular, not the atrial septum (10).

Conclusion

The left atrioventricular valve has been described and illustrated in 19 hearts with AVCD. This structure has three leaflets, not two; nor is its morphology remotely like that of a bishop's mitre! The nature of the anomaly has been outlined briefly.

References

1. Allwork SP, Anderson RH (1979) The developmental anatomy of the membranous part of the ventricular septum in the human heart. Br Heart J 41:275-280
2. Carpentier R (1978) Surgical anatomy and management of the mitral component of atrioventricular defects. In: Anderson RH, Shinebourne EA (eds) Paediatric cardiology 1977. Churchill-Livingstone, Edinburgh London New York, pp 477-490
3. Edwards JE (1960) The problem of mitral insufficiency caused by accessory chordae tendinae in persistent common atrioventricular canal. Proc Staff Meet Mayo Clin 35:299-305
4. Goor D, Lillehei CW, Edwards JE (1968) Further observations on the pathology of the atrioventricular canal malformation. Arch Surg 97:954-962
5. Piccoli GP, Gerlis LM, Wilkinson JL, Lozsadi K, Macartney FJ, Anderson RH (1979) Morphology and classification of atrioventricular defects. Br Heart J 42:621-632
6. Piccoli GP, Wilkinson JL, Macartney FJ, Gerlis LM, Anderson RH (1979) Morphology and classification of atrioventricular defects. Br Heart J 42:633-639
7. Somerville J (1966) Clinical assessment of the function of the mitral valve in atrioventricular defects related to the anatomy. Am Heart J 71:701-711
8. Wakai CS, Edwards JE (1958) Pathologic study of persistent common atrioventricular canal. Am Heart J 56:779-794
9. Wenink ACG (1980) The ventricular septum in atrioventricular defects (Abstract). In: The ventricular septum. Boerhaave Committee for Postgraduate Medical Education, pp 53-55
10. Wenink ACG (1980) Multifocal origin of the ventricular septum (Abstract). In: The ventricular septum. Boerhaave Committee for Postgraduate Medical Education, pp 9-15

Complete Atrioventricular Canal. Long Term Results With Special Reference to Block and Mitral Valve Function

K. Böök, V. O. Björk, C. Thorén, and P. Zetterqvist*

The complete atrioventricular (AV) canal is a complicated congenital malformation posing several difficulties in its surgical correction. The early results reported carried a high rate of complications mainly due to valve dysfunction and atrioventricular block. Scott et al. (4) reported a mortality of 75%. A detailed description of the anatomy of the complete AV canal by Rastelli et al. (2) greatly contributed to the understanding of this malformation and made possible a description of a method of surgical repair by Rastelli et al. (3). This technique of repair is now uniformly accepted and with slight modification adopted by most surgeons. This paper will present our experience with surgical correction for complete AV canal, the early as well as long-term results with special reference to mitral valve function and conduction disturbances.

Material

During the period 1969 to February 1980, 52 patients underwent surgical repair for complete AV canal defects. The age at operation ranged from 3 months to 15 years and 19 patients (37%) were below 2 years of age. Equilibrated intraventricular pressures were present in 39 cases (75%). Other malformations co-existed with the AV canal in 12 patients ASD secundum seven, Fallot three, patent ductus one, and partial abnormal pulmonary venous return one. Thirty-four patients (65%) had Down's syndrome. Previous pulmonary artery banding had been performed in 16 patients (31%).

Operative Procedure

The operation was performed on the non-beating heart from the incised right atrium. A single Dacron patch was utilized for closure of the common ventricular and atrial defect. The patch was first sutured to the right side of the ventricular septal ridge with isolated mattress sutures buffered by small teflon pearls. When approaching the bundle of His, the sutures were placed in the base of the mitral valve, thus effectively avoiding the conduction system (Fig. 1). The common anterior and posterior valve leaflets were divided, always giving priority to the mitral valve side in order to ensure competence in this valve. A valve cleft was approximated with fine isolated sutures. The divided

*Thoracic Surgical Clinic, Karolinska Hospital, the Departments of Pediatric Cardiology at Karolinska Hospital and St. Görans Hospital, Stockholm, Sweden

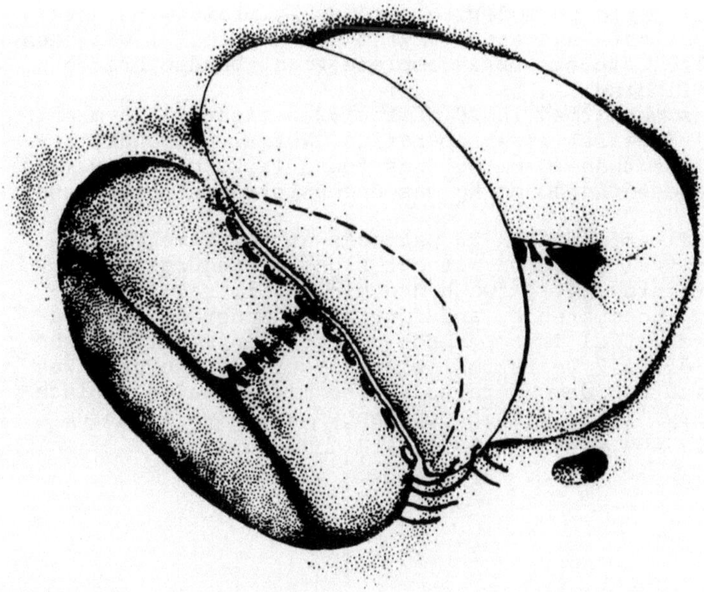

Fig. 1. Technique of avoiding the conduction system in repair of atrioventricular canal. The sutures are placed in the base of the mitral valve and then continued on the atrial septal ridge

valves were then sutured to both sides of the patch and the atrial portion of the patch was attached to the septal rim with a running suture. In the patients who had a pulmonary band, the band was removed and usually a plastic procedure had to be performed on the pulmonary artery because of the stricture caused by the band.

Mortality

Total mortality was nine patients (17%) where six died early (within 1 month of operation) and three late. All patients in the early mortality group had low output in the postoperative period and succumbed to myocardial failure. At autopsy, good local results were seen in all cases and no patch detachment or other technical detail could be regarded as responsible for the failure. In one patient, an AV block III may have been present – the patient was continuously paced in the postoperative period. Fibroelastosis was seen in two patients and one had a gravely misformed tricuspid valve. Two of the late deaths were caused by myocardial failure and one of liver failure (reaction to antibiotics).

Long-Term Follow-up

The first 34 consecutive survivors have now been followed for 1-8 years with a mean of 3.9 years. Two of these patients were lost to follow-up (living abroad). Twenty-five (78%) were leading a normal asymptomatic life while mild to moderate cardiac symptoms were noted in seven (22%). All patients had sinus rhythm and AV block I was seen in five patients (16%). Complete or incomplete right bundle branch block was a frequent finding.

Catheterization was performed in 28 of the 32 patients at a mean of 2.8 years (range 1-8 years) after operation. Normal pulmonary artery mean pressure (less than 20 mm Hg) was found in 20 patients (71%) and a mean pressure exceeding 40 mm Hg was encountered in three cases (11%) (Fig. 2).

Cineangiograms were performed in 26 patients at the time of reevaluation and good mitral function without signs of regurgitation was present in 14 patients (54%), two had a minimal mitral incompetence, six had a mild incompetence, and four had a moderate incompetence. The most marked mitral incompetence was seen in a patient who got bacterial endocarditis 2 years following surgery. In no case was severe mitral regurgitation demonstrated and no mitral valve replacement has been necessary. Tricuspid incompetence was shown in three patients, mild in one, and moderate in two.

Discussion

Surgical repair of complete AV canal can be performed with a reasonable risk. In our experience, the presence of Down's syndrome does not increase the risk. The success of the repair is very dependent on the surgical technique and the aim must be to avoid the two most important complications, namely total AV block and mitral dysfunction. This may be achieved with the Rastelli method of repair which we have modified slightly. The division and attachment of the valve tissue must be done with utmost care to ensure the best possible mitral valve function. Pulmonary artery banding as a palliative operation should

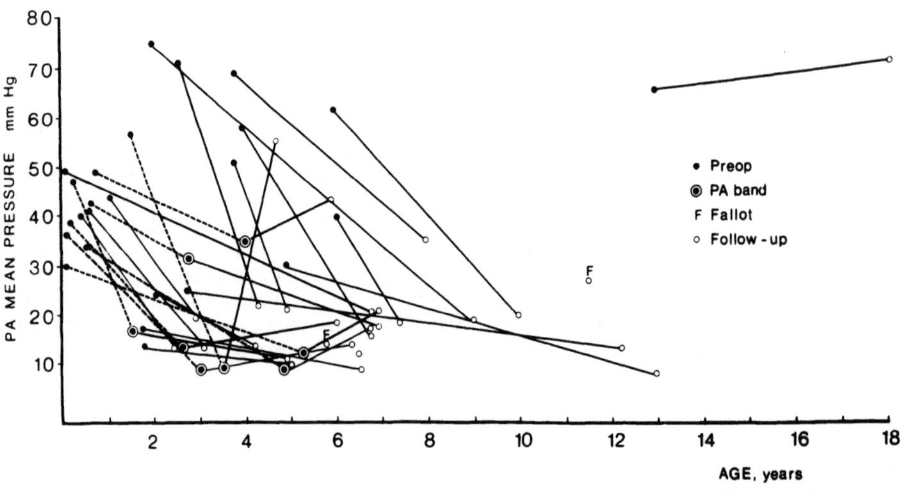

Fig. 2. Mean pressure in the pulmonary artery before and at follow-up after repair of atrioventricular canal in 26 patients. Dashed lines denote patients with pulmonary banding

be avoided since this operation in itself carries a certain risk and the pulmonary artery is sometimes difficult to restore at the following repair and pulmonary artery branch stenosis may result from a band that slips peripherally on the main stem. Two of the three patients with remaining severe pulmonary hypertension were previously banded. Early complete repair on infants in failure is the method of choice and this is in accordance with the editorial presented by Kirklin and Blackstone (1).

Marked reduction in pulmonary arterial pressure and pulmonary vascular resistance may be expected after surgical correction. Even up to the age of 6 years at surgery, severe pulmonary hypertension was shown to be reduced to normal levels in the long-term follow-up study presented. Good mitral valve function may also be expected in most cases and so far mitral valve replacement has not been necessary but further follow-up is necessary to see how the valve will function in the long run. Some patients will undoubtedly need valve surgery but hopefully not until adult age.

References

1. Kirklin JW, Blackstone EH (1979) Management of the infant with complete atrioventricular canal. J Thorac Cardiovasc Surg 78:32
2. Rastelli GC, Kirklin JW, Titus JL (1966) Anatomic observations on complete form of persistent common atrioventricular canal with special reference to atrioventricular valves. Mayo Clin Proc 41:296
3. Rastelli GC, Ongley PA, McGoon DC (1969) Surgical repair of complete atrioventricular canal with anterior common leaflet undivided and unattached to ventricular septum. Mayo Clin Proc 44:335
4. Scott LP, Hanck AS, Nodas AS, Gross RE (1962) Endocardial cusion defect. Preoperative and postoperative survey. Circulation 26:218

Total Anomalous Pulmonary Venous Drainage (TAPVD) in Infancy. Results of Corrective Surgery

I. Louhimo and E. L. Lindfors*

Before 1970, the results of surgical correction of total anomalous pulmonary venous drainage (TAPVD) in infancy were usually quite poor (see, e.g., 1, 2, 8). During the last 10 years, however, the operative mortality has in many centres dropped below 20% (7, 9, 10). Due to the rarity of the disease, the experience of individual surgeons remains limited and this may be one factor why some controversial points in the treatment of TAPVD still exist. These include the operative approach, the question of left atrial enlargement, whether to close the systemic communication and ASD primarily or not, and perhaps also the best timing of the operation (7). For further evaluation of these problems, the Finnish experience is analysed in this paper.

Material

In 1972 to 1979, 11 infants with TAPVD were operated on at the Children's Hospital, University of Helsinki. Before that time, three older children had had corrective operation using conventional bypass, with one death.

The main features of the present series are seen in Table 1. There were four females and seven males. Five of the patients were under 2 months of age, the youngest 1 week old. The weight varied between 3.2 and 6.6 kg. The defect was supracardiac in six cases, cardiac in four, and mixed in one. There were no patients with infracardiac anomaly in this series. The drainage of the supracardiac defect was to the left innominate vein in four and to the right superior vena cava in two cases. In the cardiac types, one patient had four separate openings into the right atrium, the other three had drainage to the coronary sinus. The mixed type had the main drainage also to the coronary sinus but the left upper lobe vein went to the superior vena cava. In addition to TAPVD, one patient had also a patent ductus and one patient common atrium and univentricular heart. Extracardiac anomalies in the series include one rectovaginal fistula and one palatoschisis.

Preoperatively, eight of the 11 patients were in cardiac failure and pulmonary congestion was so severe in six of them that respirator treatment was needed before the operation. Patient No. 2 had four cardiac arrests before the operation, three during attempted angiography and one in the intensive care unit. The diagnosis was confirmed only during the operation. Patient No. 4 had renal and liver failure before the operation and had a severe bleeding tendency. The prothrombin value was only 22%, P + P 3.6%, Factor V 19%, and Factor VII 65% of normal.

---

*Children's Hospital, University of Helsinki, Stenbäckinkatu 11, 00290 Helsinki 29, Finland

Table 1. TAPVD in infancy

Case	Year of operation	Age (months)	Weight (kg)	Type	Cardiac failure	Result
1	1972	5.5	5.0	Mixed	+	Good
2	1972	3.5	3.5	Cardiac	+	Good
3	1973	4	4.7	Cardiac	+	Good
4	1975	2.5	5.0	Suprac.	+	Death
5	1975	1	3.8	Cardiac	-	Good
6	1976	7	6.6	Suprac.	+	Single ventricle
7	1977	1.5	4.0	Suprac.	+	Good
8	1978	5	5.7	Suprac.	+	Good
9	1978	1.5	3.7	Cardiac	-	Good
10	1979	0.75	3.8	Suprac.	-	Good
11	1979	0.25	3.2	Suprac.	+	Good

On the other hand, three patients were in good condition when operated on and were not in cardiac failure.

At cardiac catheterization, the pulmonary artery pressure was at systemic or suprasystemic level in nine of the 11 patients. In case No. 5, it was 20/10 while the RV pressure was 43/0. In case No. 9, the pulmonary artery pressure was 63% of the systemic pressure.

Surgical Technique

All patients were operated on by using deep hypothermia and total circulatory arrest. Hypothermia was started with surface cooling, and perfusion was used to get the temperature further down to 18-20°C. In addition to general hypothermia, cold cardioplegia was used in the last three patients. The time of circulatory arrest varied between 25 and 50 min.

In the first three cases, the right anterior thoracotomy was used but in the last eight patients the approach was through median sternotomy. In supracardiac types, the anastomosis between the left atrium and the common pulmonary vein was performed in one patient through the right-sided approach (8) while in five others the approach was from below, lifting the ventricles up. This latter approach was found easier, especially when the incision into the common pulmonary vein was extended to one of its branches on the left side. No kinking occurred. When the drainage was to the coronary sinus, this was widely opened to the left atrium and connected to the foramen ovale. In the last two cases, the patch was then placed so that the coronary vein drainage was to the right side while the pulmonary vein drainage went to the left side. The left atrium was enlarged only in the patient with individual pulmonary veins draining to the right atrium. The connecting vein to the systemic circulation was always closed primarily, and so was the ASD except in the case of common atrium. This patient was operated on for pulmonary venous obstruction. In the patient with mixed anomaly, the left upper pulmonary vein was left untouched.

In the three youngest patients, the left atrium and the left ventricle enlarged so much after the anastomosis that it was difficult or impossible to close the sternum. Therefore, in each case the posterior pericardium was opened vertically to give more room for the heart. Catecholamines were needed immediately after the perfusion in eight patients but in three of them for a very short time only. Patient No. 2 with previous cardiac arrests had transient atrioventricular dissociation and needed pace-maker assistance for the first postoperative day. He had one cardiac arrest also after the operation and developed tension pneumothorax necessitating a re-thoracotomy but survived all these incidents without obvious neurological damage.

Results

Ten of the 11 patients survived the operation and are alive. Patient No. 4 with severe liver failure died of anuria and hyperkalemia on the first postoperative day.

The ten surviving patients have been followed-up for 1-8 years with a mean follow-up time of 4 years. The patient with univentricular heart, single atrium, and pulmonary hypertension is obviously suffering from her inoperable main cardiac lesion but is alive 4 years after TAPVD correction. The other nine are doing well from the cardiac point of view. So far, there has been no evidence of anastomotic strictures or other types of pulmonary venous obstruction. No re-catheterizations have been performed, however. Patient No. 3 has some problems with fecal continence because of her anorectal malformation and patient No. 10 is still waiting for her palatoschisis operation. She has also muscular hypotony and slow growth but no cardiac symptoms and needs no drugs. The first three patients have had a thorough neurological examination which revealed some "minimal brain disease" in case No. 2 with five cardiac arrests in his previous history.

Discussion

The present material differs from many others in the respect that there were no cases of infracardiac anomalies. This reflects the fact that the diagnosis of TAPVD is not easy and many patients die before reaching hospital or operating table. According to the report of the New England Regional Infant Cardiac Program (5), in 1969 to 1974 only 42 of the 63 TAPVD patients ever came to surgery and only 33 underwent reparative operation with correct preoperative diagnosis. Our autopsy reports in 1972 to 1979 revealed five undiagnosed TAPVD infants, three with supracardiac, two with infracardiac lesions.

Ten survivors among 11 TAPVD infants with operative repair reveals that the good results recently reported from many centres can be repeated and stresses the importance of early diagnosis. The one operative death in this series was not caused by the age or type of the defect but was due to the poor preoperative condition. Therefore, it seems justified to operate on these patients when the diagnosis is confirmed, without any postponement (3, 11). This is at least true for the patients with pulmonary hypertension, and by far the majority of TAPVD patients diagnosed in infancy belong to this group.

Although in one of the best reported series of TAPVD (no deaths among ten infants) the ASD was sometimes left open (9), this does not seem to be necessary. The systemic connection can also be closed primarily although there is a possibility that this is not necessary or even safe in infracardiac types of lesion (7). The left atrium is already enlarged by anastomosing the common pulmonary vein into it, and further means to increase the left atrial size do not seem to be needed. The thin-walled atrium is rapidly enlarged, anyway, by the pulmonary blood when correction is performed. The posterior common vein can be approached from the right side, from the transversal sinus, or from the left side (3) but the simplest way to do it is from below, and the danger of causing kinking (1, 8) is perhaps overestimated, when the possibility is kept in mind. The most important factor, after all, is to achieve as large an anastomosis as possible. Thin polypropylene seems to be a good suturing material and was used also in the present series.

The follow-up time on our patients is not long enough to make any conclusions about the final results. However, the patients with 7-8 years follow-up are in good condition, and so far no case of secondary obstruction of pulmonary veins has occurred in this series. This is a definite possibility, however, and in addition to a stenosis at the anastomotic level also a fibrotic stenosis of the ostia of the pulmonary veins has been reported (4, 12). This condition has been seen in our unit in three patients without TAPVD, and if diagnosed, is amenable to surgical correction. In the majority, the late results are good (3, 6).

Summary and Conclusions

Eleven infants with TAPVD were operated on during 8 years with one death (Table 1). It seems that on the basis of the present and several other recent series the following conclusions can be made. Early diagnosis is important, because surgery should be performed before irreversible deterioration of the patient. With modern intensive care even infants with severe cardiac failure can be safely operated on. Deep hypothermia with total circulatory arrest gives good operative conditions. The communication to systemic vein as well as the ASD can be closed primarily. Enlargement of the left atrium is not needed. The late results at least in the majority of the patients are good.

References

1. Barrat-Boyes BG (1973) Primary definitive intracardiac operations in infants: Total anomalous pulmonary venous connection. In: Kirklin JW (ed) Advances in cardiovascular surgery. Grune & Stratton, New York London, pp 127-139
2. Clarce DR, Stark J, De Leval M, Pincott JR, Taylor JFN (1977) Total anomalous pulmonary venous drainage in infancy. Br Heart J 39:436-444
3. Di Eusanio G, Sandrasagra FA, Donnelly RJ, Hamilton DI (1978) Total anomalous pulmonary venous connection (surgical technique, early and late results). Thorax 33:275-282
4. Fleming WH, Clark EB, Dooley KJ, Hofschire PJ, Ruckman RN, Hopeman AR, Sarafian LMN, Mooring PK (1979) Late complications following surgical repair of total anomalous pulmonary venous return below the diaphragm. Ann Thorac Surg 27: 435-439

5. Fyler DC, Buckley LP, Hellenbrand WE, Cohn HE (1980) Report of the New England regional infant cardiac program. Pediatrics 65:377-461
6. Gomes MMR, Feldt RH, McGoon DC, Danielson GK (1971) Long-term results following correction of total anomalous pulmonary venous connection. J Thorac Cardiovasc Surg 61:253-257
7. Katz NM, Kirklin JW, Pacifico AD (1978) Concepts and practices in surgery for total anomalous pulmonary venous connection. Ann Thorac Surg 25:479-487
8. Kirklin JW (1973) Surgical treatment for total anomalous pulmonary venous connection in infancy. In: Barratt-Boyes BG, Neutze JM, Harris EA (eds) Heart disease in infancy. Diagnosis and surgical treatment. Churchill Livingstone, Edinburgh London, pp 89-100
9. Mansfield PB, Hall DG, Rittenhouse EA, Sauvage LR, Stamm SJ, Herndon PS, Furman EC (1979) Cardiac surgery under age two years. J Thorac Cardiovasc Surg 77: 816-825
10. Mathew R, Thilenius OG, Replogle RL, Arcilla RA (1977) Cardiac function in total anomalous pulmonary venous return before and after surgery. Circulation 55: 361-370
11. Sade RM, Castaneda A (1976) Recent advances in cardiac surgery in the young infant. Surg Clin North Am 56:451-465
12. Whight CM, Barrat-Boyes BG, Calder AL, Neutze JM, Brandt PWT (1978) Total anomalous pulmonary venous connection. Long-term results following repair in infancy. J Thorac Cardiovasc Surg 75:52-63

Hemodynamic Results After Reconstruction of the Right Ventricular Outflow Tract in Severe Tetralogy of Fallot With Monocusp Patch

D. Regensburger, H. H. Sievers, P. Lange, and A. Bernhard*

Insertion of a patch across the pulmonary valve ring in patients with tetralogy of Fallot will always cause a pulmonary insufficiency, the degree of which being dependent on the hypoplasia of the outflow tract which in turn determines the size of the patch. The clinical and hemodynamic significance of this pulmonary insufficiency is usually judged to be of minimal importance. The often dramatic clinical improvement of the preoperatively cyanotic, dyspneic, and disabled patients after the corrective surgery is dominating.

The preoperatively pressure loaded right ventricle is involved in most of the so-called corrective surgical procedures like ventriculotomy, valvotomy, infundibulectomy with or without patch insertion as well as the closure of the VSD with a patch. This will practically always result in a large dyskinetic area of the outflow tract. An additional volume overload caused by the pulmonary insufficiency could have deleterious effects on long-term right ventricular function. Furose et al. concluded that such a pulmonary insufficiency which is due to a patch insertion across the pulmonary ring will cause an increase of the end-diastolic pressure. A regurgitant fraction of 30% of the right ventricular stroke volume was found to cause an increase of the pressure gradient across the pulmonary valve ring by 100%. Follow-up studies up to 19 years postcorrection revealed an enlarged right ventricle. The patients, however, were asymptomatic at that time. The final fate of these patients with a corrected tetralogy of Fallot remains to be determined. Little is known about the long-term results of corrective surgery utilizing an outflow patch. A homologous or heterologous valve, inserted into the outflow tract at the level of the pulmonary valve ring together with an outflow patch, could prevent a postoperative pulmonary insufficiency. As a technically simple procedure, the use of homologous aortic segments with only one cusp or the Ionesco "monocusp patch" made out of xenogen glutaraldehyde stabilized pericard was proposed. It enlarges the outflow tract and is inserted like a simple patch. The semilunar cusp is supposed to adapt during diastole to the rudimentary damaged posterior pulmonary cusp or the posterior pulmonary wall.

Figure 1 depicts schematically the correct as well as the incorrect position of the monocusp valve. In the upper part of Figure 1 is demonstrated the adaption of the monocusp with the posterior pulmonary wall, in the lower part the adaption with the rudimentary pulmonary cusp. We have utilized so far a monocusp patch in ten patients at ages 1/2 to 55 years with severe tetralogy of Fallot. We would like to discuss critically here our early experiences with these monocusp valves which consisted of five homologous aortas and five Ionesco xenologous pericard patches.

---

*Department of Cardiovascular Surgery and Department of Pediatric Cardiology, University Kiel, Hospitalstr. 40, D-2300 Kiel 1

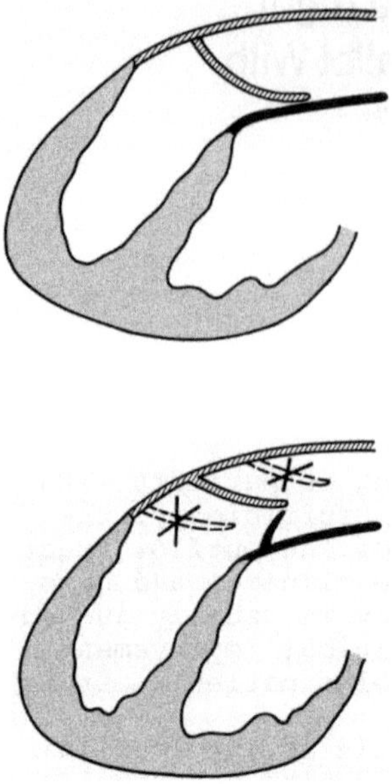

Fig. 1. Correct and incorrect positions of the monocusp valve

Out of these ten patients, we have restudied nine by left and right heart catheterization including oximetry, pressure measurements as well as biplane angiocardiography, and videodensitometry. The degree of the pulmonary insufficiency was quantified densitometrically by determining the blood volume regurgitating through the incompetent pulmonary valve during diastole. It is expressed as regurgitant fraction in percent of the total stroke volume of the right ventricle. Intraoperatively, the adequacy of the corrective surgery was judged by the maximal pressure ratio of right ventricle/left ventricle. We compared hemodynamic results of ten patients with monocusp patch, eight patients after pulmonary valve commissurotomy and infundibulectomy, and nine patients after enlargement of the outflow tract with a conventional patch (Table 1). The hemodynamic situation of all the ten patients with monocusp patch enlargement of the right ventricular outflow tract was excellent in terms of PRV/PLV ratio which was 0.44 ± 0.05 (0.25-0.58). The PRV/PLV ratio was similar in the two other groups of patients. Although the monocusp appeared to adapt satisfactorily during the operation, videodensitometry showed, however, in all patients a pulmonary regurgitation ranging from 8% to 50% with a mean value of 25.5% ± 4.5%. In the other two patient groups, we found regurgitation fractions of 22.0% ± 3.0 and 10.1% ± 2.9. The cause of this unexpected high degree of pulmonary valve incompetence in spite of monocusp insertion has to be analysed.

In the first five patients, we inserted monocusp patches from homologous aorta. Implanting these aortic monocusps, we had some technical difficulties and sometimes we found them too small. The regurgitant fraction in this patient group was 30%. Utilizing the Ionesco bovine pericardial monocusp patch in a second series of five patients, we were able to reduce the regurgitant fraction to a mean of 20.5% (Table 2). The different sizes of the Ionesco monocusp permit the implantation in infants as well as in adults.

Figure 2 shows a diastolic angiocardiographic frame of such a monocusp valve in a correct position closing sufficiently. The monocusp valve must have a sufficient size to adapt satisfactorily to the remnants of the posterior cusps of the pulmonary valve.

Table 1. Hemodynamic results of ten patients with monocusp patch, eight patients after pulmonary valve commissurotomy together with infundibulectomy, and nine patients with conventional pericardial patch

	n	Age (years)	PRV/ PLV	Gradient (mm Hg)	Regurgitation (%)
Infundibulectomy + commissurotomy	8	9.3 ± 0.8	0.44 ± 0.03	18.9 ± 4.5	10.1 ± 2.9
Patch insertion	9	7.3 ± 1.2	0.49 ± 0.04	12.2 ± 2.5	22.0 ± 3.0
Monocusp patch	10	13.4 ± 7.6	0.44 ± 0.05	9.1 ± 2.3	25.3 ± 4.5

Table 2. Hemodynamic results of five patients with Ionesco monocusp patch and five patients with homologue aortic monocusp patch

	Homologue aorta (n = 5)	Pericard (Ionesco) (n = 5)
Gradient (mm Hg)	8.2	9.5
PRV/PLV	0.41	0.46
Regurgitation (%)	30%	20.5%

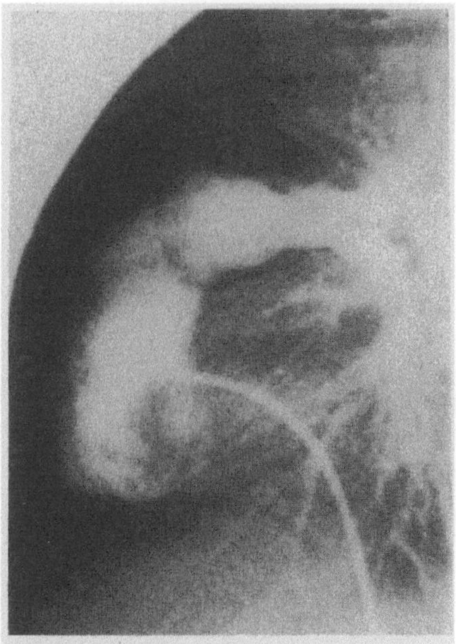

Fig. 2

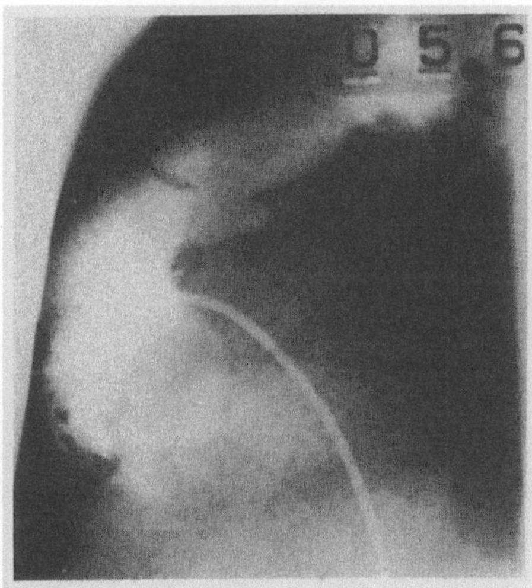

Fig. 3

Fig. 2. Diastolic angiocardiographic frame of an Ionesco monocusp in a correct position closing sufficiently

Fig. 3. Diastolic angiocardiographic frame of a homologue aortic monocusp closing insufficiently

Figure 3 demonstrates the diastolic angiocardiographic frame of a homologous aortic monocusp valve in a 55-year-old woman. This monocusp does not adapt sufficiently with the posterior cusp of the pulmonary valve. In this patient, we found a postoperative regurgitation of 27%.

On the basis of our early experiences, the implantation of the Ionesco monocusp seems to be superior to the use of homologous aortic monocusp patches and allogen and xenogen valves in the pulmonary position. In addition, insertion of this cusp is technically easier. In our last two patients – a 1-year-old infant and a 33-year-old woman – in whom we implanted the Ionesco monocusp, we found a postoperative regurgitant fraction of less than 10%.

References

1. Macartney FJ, Tandon AP, Ionescu MJ (1979) Right ventricular outflow tract reconstruction with pericardial monocusp patch and valved conduit. In: Tissue heart valves. Butterworths, London Boston
2. Marchand P (1967) The use of a cusp-bearing homograft patch to the outflow tract and pulmonary artery in Fallot's tetralogy and pulmonary valvular stenosis. Thorax 22:497-509
3. Sievers HH, Fischer K, Konertz W, Papachrysanthou C, Bernhard A (1977) Hämodynamische Resultate nach Rekonstruktion der Ausflußbahn bei Fallot'scher Tetralogie. Infundibulectomie, Erweiterungsplastik oder Umgehungsoperation. Thoraxchirurgie 25:368-373
4. Zavanella C, Miyamoto K, Subramanian S (1978) Reconstruction of the right ventricular outflow tract with a posterior monocusp valve. Cardiovasc Dis 2:128-131

Surgical Treatment of Fallot's Tetralogy in Children Under Four Years of Age

H. Oelert, G. Frank, Th. Stegmann, I. Luhmer, H. C. Kallfelz, and H. G. Borst*

Recently, Calder et al. (5), Radley-Smith et al. (11), and others (2, 8, 12) have shown that in children with tetralogy of Fallot (TOF) operated under the age of 2 years, primary total correction can give good long-term clinical and hemodynamic results. In accordance with Kirklin et al. (9), Sunderland et al. (13), Castaneda et al. (6), and others (1, 3, 12), the limiting factor for early correction appears to be not the degree of right ventricular outflow obstruction but the anatomy of the pulmonary vessels beyond the level of the pulmonary valve ring. In agreement with the clinical experience and the measurements of Tucker et al. (14) and others (4, 7, 10), primary intracardiac repair can be advocated when the diameter of the right pulmonary artery is more than one-third of the diameter of the ascending aorta.

Our choice between palliation and correction has been based primarily on the pulmonary artery anatomy defined by means of angiocardiography. In the past 4 years, patients with TOF, except newborns, were considered for intracardiac correction when the pulmonary artery appeared large enough to accommodate postrepair blood flow. In cases where the pulmonary arteries were small, pallation has been performed by enlarging the right ventricular outflow tract (RVOT), leaving the ventricular septal defect (VSD) open. In this presentation, we describe our experience with primary correction of tetralogy of Fallot in children under the age of 4 years. Patients who underwent partial relief of infundibular stenosis with or without subsequent VSD closure are not included in this series.

Clinical Material

Fourty-two patients with TOF were operated at the Hannover Medical School since 1976. There were 23 males and 19 females ranging in age from 5 months to 4 years with a mean age of 2.0 years. Indications for operation consisted in hypoxic episodes (mainly infants), polycytemia (hemoglobin above 17 g/100 ml), or both. Thirteen were infants under the age of 1 year. All patients underwent complete correction as the first and immediate operation after diagnosis because the pulmonary artery anatomy was judged favorable. By comparison, during the same period in 12 infants, all under the age of 6 months, the pulmonary arteries were not of satisfactory caliber and partial relief of right ventricular outflow obstruction was undertaken as a preliminary palliative measure.

*Medizinische Hochschule Hannover, Department of Surgery and Paediatric Cardiology, Karl-Wiechert-Allee 9, D-3000 Hannover 61

Operative Methods

The technique for intracardiac correction involved cardiopulmonary bypass[1] with moderate general body hypothermia and cold cardioplegic arrest. A vertical right ventriculotomy was used in all but one patient in whom an anomalous left anterior descending coronary artery required an incision into the inflow portion of the right ventricle. The ventricular septal defect was closed with a Dacron patch anchored by interrupted mattress sutures. Right ventricular outflow obstruction (Table 1) was treated by resection of muscle bands with or without patch enlargement, limited to the infundibulum in 13 patients. In 19 patients, the patch was carried across the pulmonary anulus.

Table 1. Incidence and site of right ventricular outflow tract patch plasty

	None	RV only	Transanular	Total
Correction under 1 year	3	3	7	13
Correction 1-4 years	7	10	12	29
Total	10	13	19	42

Transanular reconstruction was determined through intraoperative measurement of the pulmonary valve ring according to Pacifico's criteria (10). In cases with additional valvular stenosis, measurement was performed following pulmonary valvotomy. As a general rule, the pulmonary valve ring was transsected in infants when the anulus diameter was 11 mm or less. The same decision was made in older children with 1 mm per patient year added to the minimum anulus size for infants.

Outflow tract plasty originally was performed with a pericardial patch but later was abandoned because of a high incidence of aneurysmatic dilatation and calcification. In the cases operated on since 1978, a polytetrafluoroethylene (PTFE) (Gore-Tex) gusset was inserted and the pulmonary valve resuspended laterally. The width of the prosthetic patch again was chosen in accordance with the minimum acceptable pulmonary valve ring diameter.

Results

In the 42 patients (Table 2) who underwent complete intracardiac correction, there were two deaths. The causes were low cardiac output in an infant in whom the right pulmonary artery diameter was overestimated on the preoperative angiogram and in whom the postoperative right ventricular pressure did not fall below systemic values, and refractory nodal tachycardia in a 3 1/2-year-old child. Each of the deceased children had required transanular outflow patch reconstruction. No

[1]BOS 5 Oxygenator Bentley, Düsseldorf

Table 2. Operative results

	N	Early death	Percent
Correction under 1 year	13	1[a]	7.7
Correction 1-4 years	29	1[b]	3.4
Total	42	2	4.8

[a]Low cardiac output syndrome

[b]Refractory nodal tachycardia

late death occurred within a mean observation time of 2 1/2 years. The overall mortality amounted to 4.8%, being 7.7% for the infants and 3.4% for the older age group.

In most patients, ventricular and right pulmonary artery pressures (Table 3) were obtained at the end of the operation. In 11 infants, postrepair right ventricular systolic pressure showed an average decrease to 54% of systemic pressure. The right ventricle to pulmonary artery gradient dropped to a mean value of 15 mm Hg. Nearly the same early results were achieved in children between 1 and 4 years of age.

Late postoperative hemodynamic studies of survivors showed a progressive decrease of right ventricular pressure both in infants and children, demonstrated by the $P_{RV/LV}$ ratio. Similarly the RVOT gradient was further reduced, bringing the right ventricular pressure to normal or near normal values. Pulmonary insufficiency of varying degrees occurred in most patients following valvotomy or enlargement of the pulmonary anulus, but did not produce symptoms except in two patients. They both suffered from sinus bradycardia and had elevated pulmonary artery pressures.

Table 3. Mean values and SD of intra- and late postoperative pressure measurements (mm Hg)

	Early postop.			Late postop.		
	N	$P_{RV/LV}$	ΔP_{RVOT}*	N	$P_{RV/LV}$	ΔP_{RVOT}*
Correction under 1 year	11	0.54 ± 0.11	15.4 ± 7.9	4	0.39 ± 0.05	12.2 ± 4.5
Correction 1-4 years	17	0.56 ± 0.15	20.0 ± 10.6	11	0.46 ± 0.14	17.6 ± 15.4

* ΔP_{RVOT} = Right ventricular outflow tract gradient

Postoperative complications are summarized in Table 4. Early after the operation, complete heart block required permanent pacemaker implantation in two older children. Postoperative bleeding and detachment of the VSD patch demanded emergency reintervention on one patient each. In three instances, low cardiac output necessitated prolonged ventilation and positive inotropic support.

Five patients developed aneurysms of the right ventricular outflow tract. In all cases, pericardium had been used, three times transanular and twice limited to the right ventricular infundibulum. At reinvestigation, a narrow pulmonary valve anulus or stenosis at the pulmonary artery bifurcation was observed and confirmed at reoperation. No correlation was found to the residual right ventricular pressure ($P_{RV/LV}$ ranging from 0.34 to 0.57) nor the severity of pulmonary valve incompetence. In three cases, the aneurysm was resected and a new patch placed across the area of distal obstruction. So far, no aneurysmatic dilatation has followed Gore-Tex patch plasty.

Table 4. Early and late postoperative complications

Early	N	Treatment
Total AV block	2	Pacemaker impl.
Postoperative bleeding	1	Re-thoracotomy
Recurrent VSD	1	Re-closure (6th p.o. day)
Low cardiac output	3	Prolonged ventilation
Late		
RVOT — aneurysm	5	Resection in 3 (so far)
Pulm. hypertension[a]	1	-
Sick sinus syndrome	1	Pacemaker impl.

[a]Following PDA

Discussion

Our policy in the management of symptomic tetralogy of Fallot in infants and young children has been to undertake complete repair when the pulmonary arteries appear large enough to accommodate postoperative blood flow regardless of age. One of the determinant factors of operative success is the postrepair pressure ratio between the right and left ventricle. Unfavorable high residual RV pressure may result from hypoplasia or segmental stenosis within right or left pulmonary arteries (1, 3, 7). Also an inadequate postrepair diameter of the narrowest part of the right ventricular outflow tract may be incriminated. Accordingly, in cases considered for complete correction, the decision whether enlargement of the outflow tract must be transanular or can be limited to the infundibulum only, mainly depends on the size of the pulmonary valve ring as determined before and during operation. Based on our results and the experience of others (4, 7, 10), this should be at least 11 mm in infants; 1 mm per patient year is added in older children. If a transanular patch appears indicated Gore-Tex seems preferable to pericardium in order to prevent late aneurysmatic dilatation.

In summary, apart from children with underdeveloped pulmonary arteries, primary intracardiac correction in symptomatic children with tetralogy of Fallot can be performed with low operative risk and excellent hemodynamic late results. The majority of complications encountered in the presented series are believed to be avoidable by using proper pre- and intraoperative measurements as well as refined techniques of repair.

Summary

Based on the assumption that primary correction of tetralogy of Fallot can be undertaken when the diameter of the right pulmonary artery measures at least 30% of the diameter of the ascending aorta, 42 consecutive children, ranging in age from 5 weeks to 4 years, underwent intracardiac repair of their congenital heart lesion. Thirteen were infants under the age of 1 year. Thirty-two required patch enlargement of the right ventricular outflow tract; in 19, the patch extended across the pulmonary valve ring. All had patch closure of the ventricular septal defect (VSD).

One infant and one older child died early after the operation (4.8% mortality rate). There was no late death during a mean follow-up period of 2 1/2 years. Early and late complications consisted of complete heart block (two), recurrent VSD (one), postoperative bleeding (one), and aneurysms of the right ventricular outflow tract (five), all requiring reoperation. Since the use of Gore-Tex instead of pericardium for right ventricular outflow tract plasty, no further aneurysmal formation has been observed. Catheterization studies 1 or more years after the operation showed good hemodynamic late results with a right ventricular pressure approaching normal values. Pulmonary valve incompetence was insignificant except in two children with sinus bradycardia and elevated pulmonary artery pressures. It is concluded that our results justify primary repair of TOF (tetralogy of Fallot) in symptomatic children, regardless of age.

References

1. Alfieri O, Blackstone EH, Kirklin JW, Pacifico AD, Bargeron LM Jr (1978) Surgical treatment of tetralogy of Fallot with pulmonary atresia. J Thorac Cardiovasc Surg 76:321-335
2. Barrat-Boyes BG, Neutze JM (1973) Primary repair of tetralogy of Fallot in infancy using profound hypothermia with circulatory arrest and limited cardiopulmonary bypass. A comparison with conventional two-stage management. Ann Surg 178:406-411
3. Blackstone EH, Kirklin JW, Bertranou EG, Labrosse CJ, Soto B, Bargeron LM Jr (1979) Preoperative prediction from cineangiograms of postrepair right ventricular pressure in tetralogy of Fallot. J Thorac Cardiovasc Surg 78:542-552
4. Blackstone EH, Kirklin JW, Pacifico AD (1979) Decision-making in repair of tetralogy of Fallot based on intraoperative measurements of pulmonary arterial outflow tract. J Thorac Cardiovasc Surg 77:526-532
5. Calder AL, Barrat-Boyes BG, Brandt PWT, Neutze JM (1979) Postoperative evaluation of patients with tetralogy of Fallot repaired in infancy. J Thorac Cardiovasc Surg 77:704-720
6. Castaneda AR, Freed MD, Williams RG, Norwood WI (1977) Repair of tetralogy of Fallot in infancy. Early and late results. J Thorac Cardiovasc Surg 74:372-381

7. Daily PO, Stinson EB, Griepp RB, Shumway NE (1978) Tetralogy of Fallot choice of surgical procedure. J Thorac Cardiovasc Surg 75:338-345
8. Hirschfeld S, Tuboku-Metzger AJ, Borkat G, Ankeney J, Clayman J, Liebman J (1978) Comparison of exercise and catherization results following total surgical correction of tetralogy of Fallot. J Thorac Cardiovasc Surg 75:446-451
9. Kirklin JW, Blackstone EH, Pacifico AD, Brown RN, Bargeron LM (1979) Routine primary repair vs two-stage repair of tetralogy of Fallot. Circulation 60: 373-386
10. Pacifico AD, Kirklin JW, Blackstone EH (1977) Surgical management of pulmonary stenosis in tetralogy of Fallot. J Thorac Cardiovasc Surg 74:382-395
11. Radley-Smith R, Ilsley C, Reid C, Jacoub M (1980) Late clinical and hemodynamic results after primary correction of tetralogy of Fallot in the first 2 years of life. World Congress of Paediatric Cardiology, London, June 2-6, 1980, Abstract 038
12. Starr A, Bonchek LI, Sunderland CO (1973) Total correction of tetralogy of Fallot in infancy. J Thorac Cardiovasc Surg 65:45-57
13. Sunderland C, Nichols M, Feucht K, Ho L, Menashe V, Starr A, Lees M (1980) Primary total correction of tetralogy of Fallot in infancy – postoperative evaluation. World Congress of Paediatric Cardiology, London, June 2-6, 1980, Abstract 037
14. Tucker W, Turley K, Ullyot DJ, Ebert PA (1979) Management of symptomatic tetralogy of Fallot in the first year of life. J Thorac Cardiovasc Surg 78:494-501

Invited Lecture

Early and Late Results of Corrective Cardiac Surgery During the First Year of Life

A.R.Castañeda*

Introduction

The purpose of this paper is to present some of our early and late results following corrective cardiac surgery in neonates and infants. Therefore, I will forego details of surgical technique but will instead emphasize early and late hemodynamic results.

The mortality from congenital heart disease during the 1st year of life as identified by the New England Regional Infant Program (NERICP) in close to 3000 patients occurs principally during the first few months of life (Fig. 1). Clearly, to achieve a therapeutic impact in this group of critically ill infants, our surgical efforts must be directed at this early age group. The experience accumulated in our own department parallels this trend toward earlier operations in infancy, including neonates (Fig. 2).

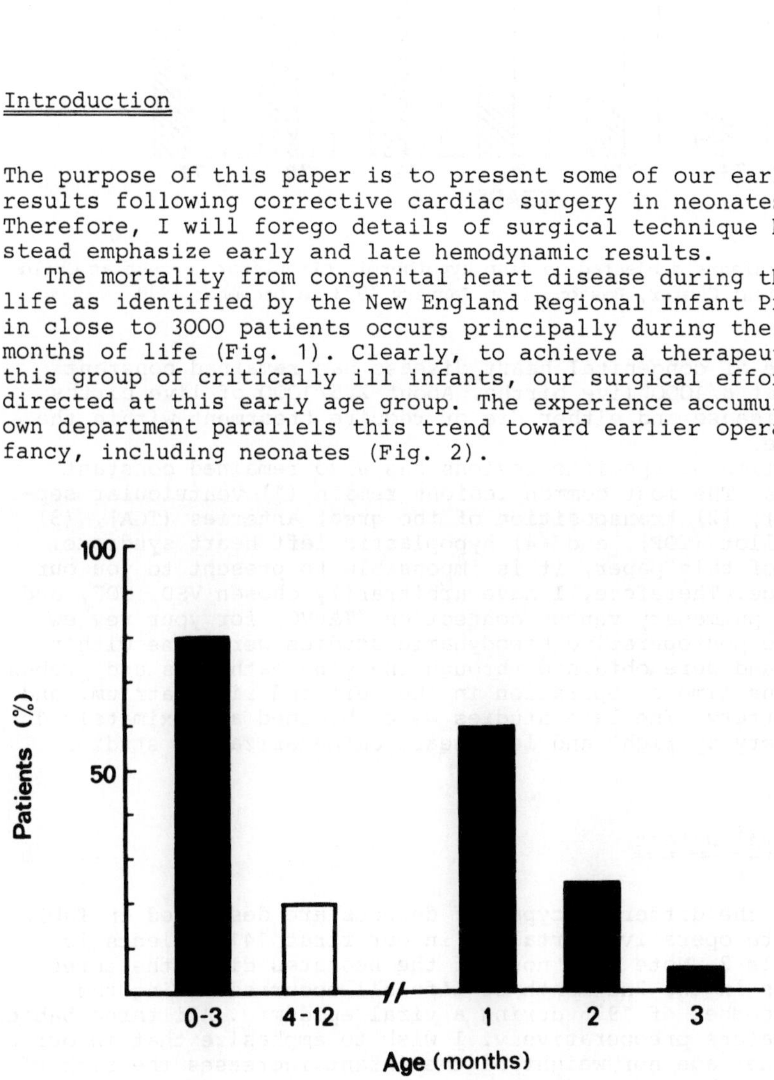

Fig. 1. Mortality from congenital heart disease during the 1st year of life. Data collected by the New England Regional Infant Cardiac Program (1037/2736 patients)

*Department of Cardiovascular Surgery, Children's Hospital Medical Center, Harvard Medical School, Boston, Massachusetts 02115, USA

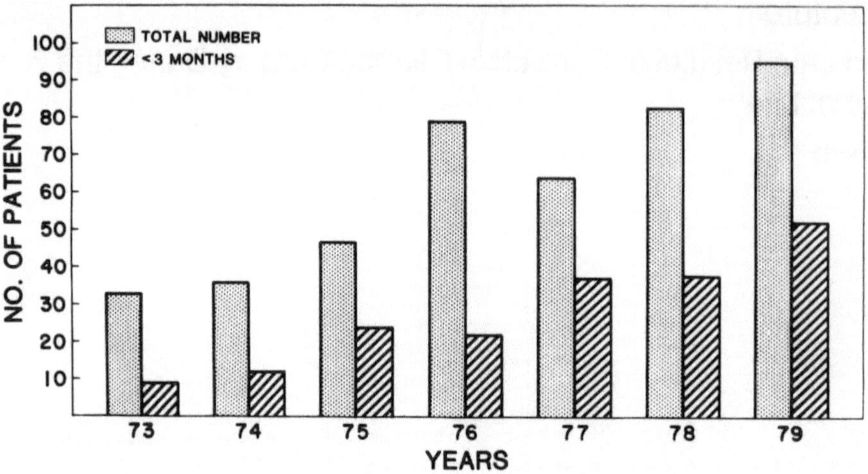

Fig. 2. Number of infants subjected to deep hypothermic circulatory arrest at Children's Hospital Medical Center, Boston, from January 1973 to December 1979

The incidence of congenital heart disease has remained constant over the years at 8/1000 live births. About 2.5/1000 of live births have critical disease and either die or require treatment within the 1st year of life.

The distribution of specific lesions has also remained constant over these years. The most common lesions remain (1) ventricular septal defect (VSD), (2) transposition of the great arteries (TGA), (3) tetralogy of Fallot (TOF), and (4) hypoplastic left heart syndrome. In the context of this paper, it is impossible to present to you our entire experience. Therefore, I have arbitrarily chosen VSD, TOF, and total anomalous pulmonary venous connection (TAPVC) for your review.

All immediate postoperative hemodynamic studies were done within the first 24 h and were obtained through in-lying catheters and probes positioned at the time of operation in the left and right atrium, and the pulmonary artery. The late studies were obtained approximately 1 year after surgery by right and left heart catheterization studies.

Ventricular Septal Defect

The location of the different types of defects are described in Table 1. Early and late operative mortality in our first 141 patients is outlined in Table 2. Note that none of the neonates died; the three deaths in babies in the 2nd month of life all occurred during the same week in December of 1976 during a viral epidemic. All three babies required respirators preoperatively. I wish to emphasize that in our experience neither age nor weight of the infant increases the risk of operation; rather the operative risk is mostly determined either by the preoperative metabolic condition of the child, the complexity of the cardiac defect, or the presence of important extracardiac defects.

We are concerned about the 6.4% incidence of right bundle branch block and left anterior hemiblock. This postoperative complication represents a technical problem during VSD closure which should be avoidable. Only one child after VSD closure remained in permanent com-

Table 1. Location of ventricular septal defects

Type of VSD	No. of Patients[a]
Infundibuloventricular	116 (82.5)
Multiple	10 (7.2)
Muscular	7 (4.9)
A-V canal type	6 (4.2)
Subpulmonary	2 (1.4)
Total	141

[a]Percentages are given in parentheses

Table 2. Age and outcome of VSD closure in infancy

Age (months)	No. of patients	Deaths Hospital[a]	Deaths Late
0 < 1	13	0	0
1 < 3	43	3 (7.5)	0
3 < 6	59	0	1
6 < 12	26	1 (3.3)	0
Total	141	4 (2.8)	1 (0.7)

[a]Percentages are given in parentheses

plete heart block; this child actually had the first episode of complete heart block preoperatively induced at the time of heart catheterization.

Changes in pulmonary artery pressure and in pulmonary vascular resistance are shown in Figures 3 and 4. Note that all patients had normal pulmonary artery pressure and pulmonary vascular resistance 1 year after surgery.

Interesting are the results of morphometric grading of pulmonary arteriolar changes as studied from pulmonary biopsy material. This classification focuses on changes which occur in the pulmonary arterioles prior to the development of the more advanced pulmonary vascular lesions as previously described by Heath and Edwards. Normally, at 1 year of age, a perivascular muscle layer progresses along the pulmonary arterioles up to the level of the alveolar duct arteries. The thickness of this muscle layer is about 10% of lumen size. At this age, there are also about six arterioles per 100 alveoli. In children with pulmonary hypertension, such as occurs with VSD, changes seen microscopically include (1) progression of the muscular layer up to and including the alveolar wall arterioles (type A lesion); (2) increase in the thickness of the muscular coat of the pulmonary arterioles (type B lesion); and (3) decrease in the number of arterioles per 100 alveoli (type C lesion). Comparing differences in pulmonary vascu-

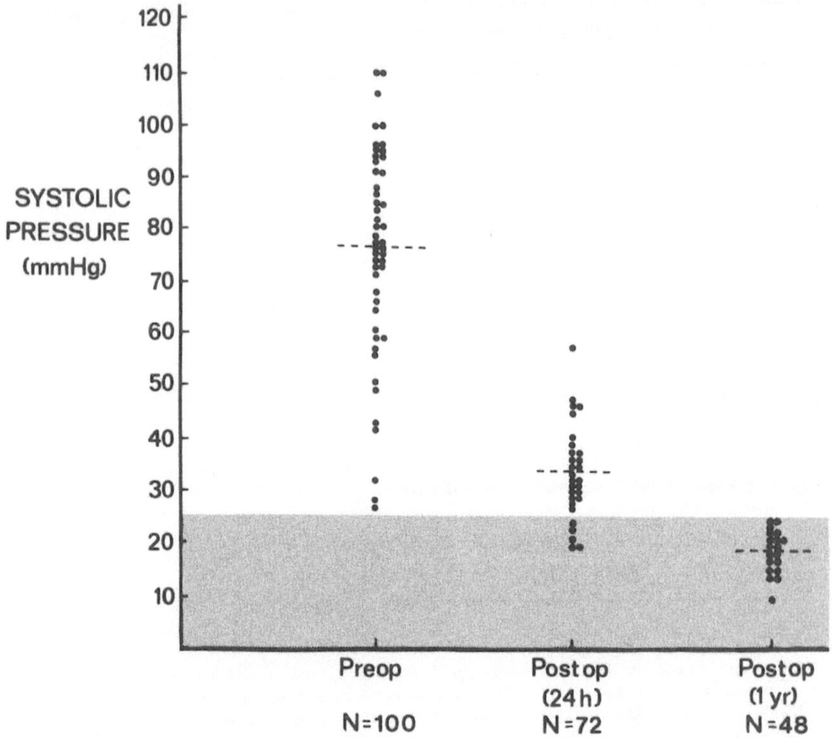

Fig. 3. Postoperative changes in pulmonary artery pressure after closure of VSD

lar lesions between children with VSD operated on during the 1st and 2nd year of life, we learned that the first group of patients had mostly type B lesions, none had Heath-Edwards stage 3 or 4 lesions; while in the 2nd year of life the majority had type B and C lesions, and three of the 20 patients had already stage 3 Heath-Edwards changes.

Left ventricular enddiastolic volume and ejection fractions are essentially normal 1 year after surgery (Fig. 5).

Left ventricular work function curves, relating LV minute work index to LV enddiastolic pressure in combination with methoxamine, a selective α pressor to increase afterload, were normal when compared to a group of controls.

In summary, closure of VSD during the 1st year of life in symptomatic infants can be performed at low operative risk and yielding normal late hemodynamic results. We recommend that all symptomatic infants have the VSD closed within the 1st year of life. Asymptomatic children with a hemodynamically significant VSD should have the defect(s) closed within the first 2 years of life.

Tetralogy of Fallot

Of a total of 166 patients with TOF seen at the RICP, 113 (60%) required admission during the first 3 months of life and over 50% required operation during the 1st year of life. A significantly smaller

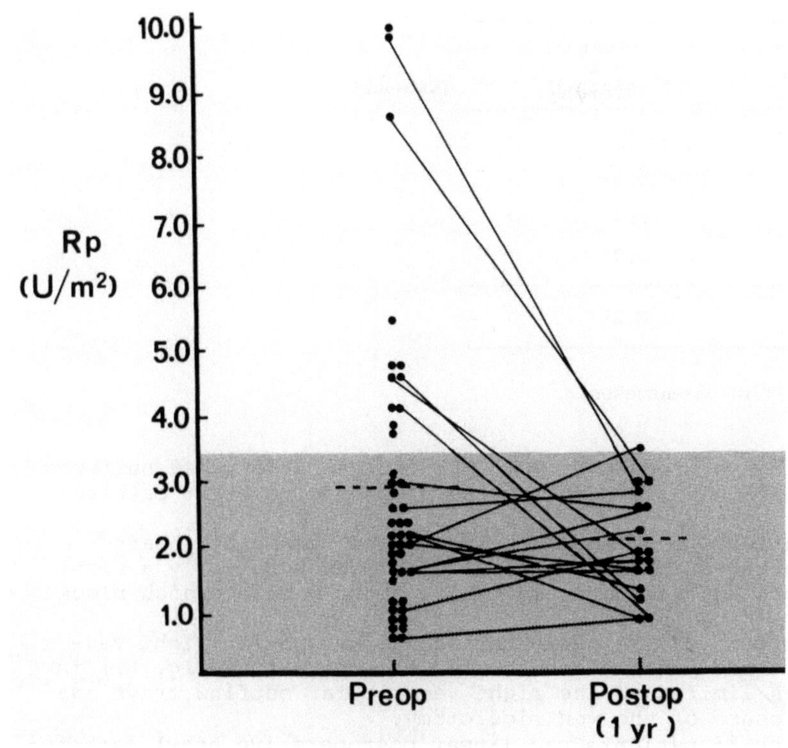

Fig. 4. Postoperative changes of pulmonary vascular resistance after closure of VSD

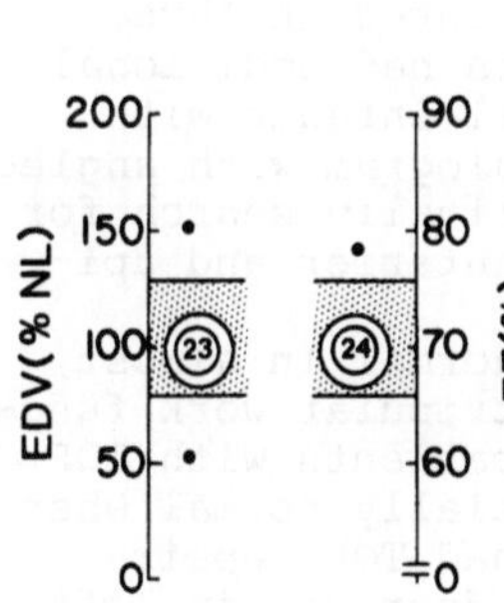

Fig. 5. Postoperative LV function after closure of VSD. EDV, enddiastolic volume; EF, ejection fraction

percentage required operations within the 1st week of life. Of our own group of 85 patients operated on between January 1973 and June 1980, 25 (30%) were operated on within the first 3 months of life (Table 3). Seven of the 85 patients died during or after surgery; however, four of these seven deaths were not directly related to the repair of TOF. Two patients had absent pulmonary valve syndrome with enormously dilated pulmonary arteries which extended into the pulmonary parenchyma, causing widespread compression of terminal bronchi and alveoli. The third patient had associated severe left-sided obstruction caused by idiopathic hypotrophic subaortic stenosis which was not adequately

Table 3. Age and outcome of TOF repair in infancy

Age (months)	No. of patients	Deaths Hospital[a]	Deaths Late
0 < 1	9	1 (11.0)	0
1 < 3	20	2 (10.0)	0
3 < 6	31	2 (6.4)	0
6 < 12	25	2 (8.0)	0
Total	85	7 (8.2)	0

[a]Percentages are given in parentheses

relieved at the time of repair of TOF. The fourth patient had suffered a severe myocardial infarction during the preoperative heart catheterization.

None of the patients had temporary or permanent complete heart block. Seventy-three patients (85%) developed postoperatively a right bundle branch block and six patients (7%) a right bundle branch block with a left anterior hemiblock.

Eighty-five percent of all patients had a transannular right ventricular outflow tract patch placed during the operation (Fig. 6); in 11%, the patch was limited to the right ventricular outflow tract and 4% had primary closure of the ventriculotomy.

Fifty-six of the 85 patients had 1-year postoperative heart catheterization studies. Of the patients with a transannular outflow tract patch, none had RV-PA gradients greater than 40 mm Hg (Fig. 7). Two of the patients with no outflow patches developed gradients of 70 and 90 mm Hg across a hypoplastic pulmonary valve annulus. These two have been successfully reoperated on for removal of right ventricular outflow tract aneurysms and placement of transannular patches.

A residual left to right shunt (>1.5 : 1.0) was measured in three patients. Curiously, at reoperation all three patients had additional anterior muscular VSD. To avoid this complication, all infants with TOF are now subjected to a preoperative left ventriculogram with angled-oblique views. Also during the operation, we systematically search for additional ventricular septal defects, particularly anterior and apical muscular defects.

Enddiastolic volumes and ejection fractions were normal in almost all patients 1 year after surgery (Fig. 8). Left ventricular work function curves following methoxamine administration in patients with TOF operated upon during the 1st year of life were essentially normal when compared to controls, while a group of patients who had TOF repair after 4 years of age showed a significant ($p < 0.001$) decrease in left ventricular function. The difference in the response to methoxamine between the older and younger patients was not related to preoperative resting hemodynamics or to the degree of hypoxemia before repair nor to the magnitude of pulmonary regurgitation after correction. The cause of left ventricular function abnormalities after TOF repair is not entirely clear. Diffuse and focal cardiac sclerosis in young children with TOF has been reported and such changes could conceivably be the anatomic substrate for compliance or contractile abnormalities in the left ventricle. Early repair may well prevent the development of these histologic changes.

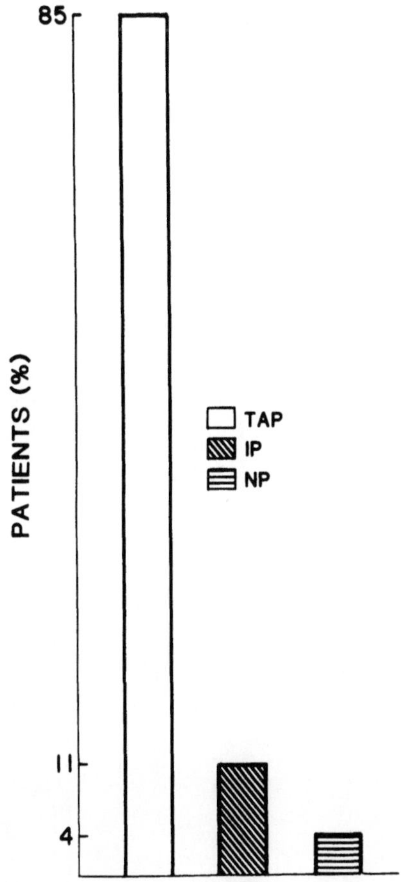

Fig. 6. Repair of TOF. Management of RV outflow tract. TAP, transannular patch; IP, infundibular patch; NP, no patch

Total Anomalous Pulmonary Venous Connection

Thirty-eight infants aged 16 h to 12 months had complete repair of TAPVC (Table 4). The supracardiac type was the most common form of TAPVC (Table 5). As mentioned earlier by Professors Borst and Oehlert, TAPVC is a disease mostly of neonates and very young infants. Note that seven of our patients were less than 1 week of age and that 23 of the 38 patients were less than 3 months of age. Similar to the Hanover experience, we also encountered a relatively high proportion of infracardiac type connections during early infancy (12/38). When comparing cardiac output (measured by thermodilution technique) in patients 2 and 24 h after VSD, TOF, and TAPVC repair, cardiac index was found to be consistently lower in the TAPVC group of patients. One year after surgery, the cardiac index was essentially the same among the three patient groups. Despite this initially low cardiac index, these patients were not symptomatic nor were they in a clinically recognizable state of low output.

Two patients, both with infracardiac type connections, had residual pulmonary hypertension measured 1 year after surgery. One of these patients had a residual stenosis at the anastomosis while the other patient had stenosis of individual pulmonary veins. This patient died at 10 months following the initial repair. One patient

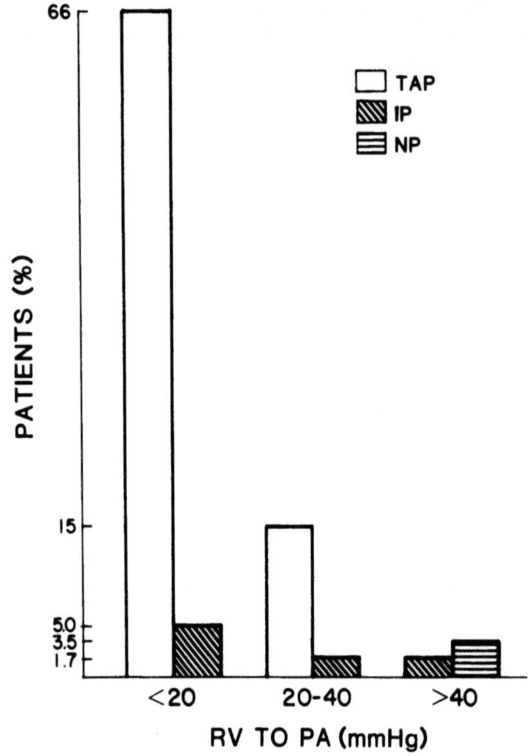

Fig. 7. Repair of TOF. Postoperative RV to PA gradients

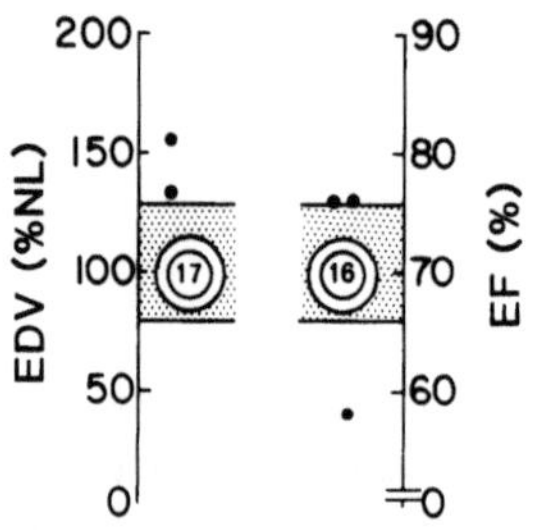

Fig. 8. Repair of TOF. Postoperative LV functions. EDV, enddiastolic volume; EF, ejection fraction

with infracardiac type drainage who underwent repair at the age of 4 months has pulmonary vascular obstructive disease despite an unobstructed anastomosis.

The residual stenosis in the one patient with infracardiac type of TAPVC was due to a technical error. The pulmonary venous anatomy resembled a tree with a dominant vertical rather than horizontal component. Instead of making a vertically oriented anastomosis, the incisions in the common vein and in the left atrium were horizontal. To avoid this complication, we have modified the technique for the repair of the infracardiac type of TAPVC. We now divide the descending vein almost at the level of the diaphragm. The vein is then incised vertically and a wide anastomosis is made to a vertical opening in the left atrium. The atrial septal defect is always closed.

Table 4. Age and outcome of TAPVC repair

Age (days)	No. of patients	Hospital mortality[a]
0 < 8	7	0
8 < 30	13	2 (15.3)
30 < 60	6	0
(months)		
2 < 6	9	1 (11.1)
6 < 12	3	0
Total	38	3 (7.9)

[a]Percentages are given in parentheses

Table 5. Type of connection of TAPVC and outcome of repair

Type of connection	No. of patients	Hospital mortality[a]
Supracardiac	21	2 (9.5)
Cardiac	5	0
Infracardiac	12	1 (8.3)
Total	38	3 (7.9)

[a]Percentages are given in parentheses

In summary, the use of deep hypothermic circulatory arrest has greatly facilitated repair of even the most complex cardiac defects in neonates and infants. We are encouraged by the immediate and late results of early repair for most lesions. Although I have not presented our entire experience, it suffices to say that neither age nor weight of the infant are significant risk factors. The significant risk factors are (1) the metabolic condition of the infant before surgery, (2) the type of cardiac lesion, and (3) the associated non-cardiac malformations. The need for early and complete hemodynamic and anatomic evaluation and prompt reparative surgical intervention (whenever feasible) has become established for the ill infant with complex congenital heart disease.

Cardiac Forum

Chairman: F. Sebening, Munich; Co-Chairman: H. Huysmans, Leiden

Surgical Treatment of Superior Vena Caval Obstruction

A. Forsyth, V. Ketharanathan, and S. Lennox*

Most surgeons are pessimistic about the surgical treatment of superior vena caval (SVC) obstruction. From our institution in 1958 Barrett (1) said: "Surgical operations have proved to be almost uniformly unsuccessful". Now, 22 years later, a recent publication by Morgans et al. (2), describing a case of SVC obstruction due to sarcoidosis wrote: "In benign S.V.C. obstruction conservative management is indicated, the obstruction being well tolerated and likely to improve with time. Successful surgical relief of S.V.C. obstruction awaits the development of a non-thrombogenic graft". Whilst we agree on the importance of a non-thrombogenic graft, we hope to demonstrate that there are other important factors concerned.

By far the majority of cases with obstruction to venous return from the head and neck and upper limbs are caused by carcinoma of the lung, and the diagnosis is usually obvious. We have seen, however, another group of patients presenting with SVC obstruction in whom the underlying pathology is not certain. Routine examination and blood tests give no clue to the diagnosis and a chest X-ray can show mediastinal widening or even be normal. Biopsies obtained by mediastinoscopy or anterior mediastinotomy may reveal carcinoma, but in our experience such cases commonly show fibrous tissue only. We believe that a mediastinotomy with full dissection of the great veins and the obstructing lesion must be done and that regardless of the diagnosis at this stage, bypass grafting is beneficial. Slow growing carcinomas are usually resistant to radiotherapy and the patient has many months to live with SVC obstruction that can be immediately relieved by grafting.

The main limiting factor in effecting surgical relief in the past has been the absence of a satisfactory venous conduit. Since 1969, we have placed a total of 20 grafts in 12 patients. Initially there were three saphenous veins used in two patients, then from 1971 to 1977, ten siliconised rubber conduits were used in seven patients. Since then, three patients have had ovine xenografts. Of the 12 patients operated on, ten were referred to us with the diagnosis of mediastinal fibrosis, and in only six was this diagnosis confirmed after full exploration.

Table 1 shows the six cases with venous obstruction due to malignant disease. There are two points to bring out:

1. Only one of the patients had carcinoma of the lung – the third patient. Of the others, the last man had a malignant thymoma, and the rest had a mediastinal carcinoma, commonly scirrhous in nature, with no primary site evident.
2. At least four of these people died within 1 year of operation but all were comfortable with no evidence of SVC obstruction leading up to their death.

*Brompton Hospital, Fulham Road, London SW3 6HP, Great Britain

Table 1. SVC bypass — malignant conditions

		Diagnosis	Graft	Result
1969	M 55	Large cell ca.	Saphenous vein	Died 5 m; no obst.
1971	M 57	Adeno ca.	Silicone rubber	Died 4 m; no obst.
1973	F 62	Ca. lung	Silicone rubber	Died 2 m; no obst.
1974	F 53	Adeno ca.	Silicone rubber	Died 1 yr; no obst.
1976	M 47	Adeno ca.	Silicone rubber	Lost to follow-up
1980	M 54	Malig. thymoma	1. Ovine Xenograft 2. Gore-tex	3 m; no obst.

The six patients with mediastinal fibrosis were young. Their ages ranged from 35 to 49 years, with a mean age of 39 years. There were five males and one female. It has been agreed that these people develop venous collaterals over the years that eventually relieve their symptoms. However, in our experience, this has not been so, particularly if the azygos vein is also obstructed, and we think it is unacceptable that young people who do not die of their disease should be denied the opportunity to have complete relief of their symptoms.

An example is in the first patient in Table 2. He was 49 years old in 1971 when he had two saphenous veins used to bypass SVC obstruction by decompressing the left innominate vein to the right atrium. At that time, we were not bold enough to attack the right side which remained obstructed. He continued to have symptoms on exertion and could not bend over because of a throbbing head. He recently pressed us into operating on his right side, which we did in June 1980, and he is now symptom-free. He had clearly not developed sufficient collateral flow over the past 8 years.

Table 2. SVC bypass — benign conditions

		Graft	Result
1971 1980	M 49	Saphenous veins x 2 — l. side Ovine xenograft — r. side	Venogram 1973 & 1976; l. side o.k.; no clinical obst.
1973	M 35	Silicone rubber x 2	Venogram 1974 — both narrow; no signs SVC obst.
1973	F 36	Silicone rubber x 2	Venogram 1974 — both patent; Venogram 1975 — l. blocked, r. patent; minimal signs SVC obst.
1974	M 45	Silicone rubber x 2	No obst. (Febr. 1978)
1977	M 34	Ovine xenografts x 2	No SVC obst.
1980	M 42	Ovine xenografts x 2	2 m. no SVC obst.

Table 2 shows the six patients with mediastinal fibrosis who were grafted. The first man we have just described. The next three patients had both sides decompressed with silicone rubber conduits, and all have good symptomatic relief. Follow-up venograms in these patients show that there appears to be narrowing at the distal anastomosis, although in some cases this can be explained by streaming from the internal jugular vein – as the studies were all done from the arms. The subclavian veins were not enlarged which suggests that there is no functional obstruction. In one case, the smooth lining of the rubber graft became irregular suggesting intramural thrombus formation which was thought to be the result of stasis in the graft consequent on stenosis at the anastomosis into the right atrium. We feel sure that the graft must be as large as possible (hopefully 15 mm diameter) and should be into the non-trabeculated wall of the right atrium.

It was partly as a result of problems such as these, and partly because of experimental work that one uf us (V. Ketharanathan) has done in the animal laboratory, that we changed to a newer biosynthetic graft. Produced in Melbourne, Australia, it is a composite vascular prosthesis of processed sheep collagen completely encasing a polyester skeleton and it fulfills many of the criteria we believe a low pressure venous graft should have:

1. Non-thrombogenic
2. Able to resist invasion by host tissue
3. Non-compressible
4. Easy to suture
5. Readily available

We feel that the third point is fundamental to low-pressure grafting. The graft should be pliable enough to change position slightly when the chest is closed, while at the same time be sufficiently rigid to resist compression by surrounding tissues or haematoma. Although the graft properties are important, we place equal importance on the aspects of surgical technique listed below:

1. A "bed" should be established for the conduit. This usually requires removal of most of the obstructing tissue.
2. The graft should be sutured under slight tension with the chest open – to allow for shortening when the chest is closed.
3. The suture lines should be everted and enlarged obliquely as for coronary artery grafting, and a continuous stitch of monofilament suture used.
4. An oval piece of non-trabeculated RA should be excised for the lower anastomosis in an effort to splint this end of the graft open.
5. Finally, the gradient across the graft should be measured with the sternum partly closed, and in a successful procedure, there should be no gradient.

We remain convinced that surgical relief of long standing SVC obstruction is worthwhile and hope to show in the future that our new biosynthetic graft is an "ideal" conduit.

References

1. Barrett NR (1958) Idiopathic mediastinal fibrosis. Br J Surg 46:207
2. Morgans WE, Al-Jilahawi AN, Mbatha PB (1980) Superior vena caval obstruction caused by sarcoidosis. Thorax 35:397-398

Surgery in Intensive Care Unit

M. Turina, J. Kugelmeier, L. Egloff, and Å. Senning*

Urgent reintervention is sometimes necessary after open-heart surgery. Massive exsanguinating bleeding can occur in the first hours or days after operation; surgical reexploration might be necessary in a patient too unstable to be moved into the operating room (OR), and in some cases, the primary closure of sternotomy will not be tolerated after prolonged open-heart procedures. A concept of surgery in intensive care unit (ICU) was developed to deal with such emergencies; the following communication relates our experience with this extreme and rare group of patients since 1977.

Definition

The term of surgery in ICU was applied to a heterologous group of patients subjected to operative interventions in their beds in ICU without transferring them to the OR facilities. The operations performed included reexploration for bleeding, implantation and removal of intraaortic balloon pump (IABP), and paracorporeal artificial heart, diagnostic or therapeutic pericardial decompression and delayed closure of sternotomy which had to be left open after intracardiac corrections.

Indications

Rethoracotomy for bleeding was performed in ICU in two groups of patients. The first group had a sudden massive exsanguination with consecutive rapid hemodynamic deterioration and tamponade mandating immediate intervention. The second group comprised the patients with postoperative low output, multiple infusions of pharmacologic agents, and IABP which exhibited postoperative blood loss warranting reexploration. Transportation to the OR was considered too risky and surgery was performed in ICU without interrupting the monitoring.

Delayed chest closure (leaving median sternotomy open at the end of operation) was practiced in patients with marked postoperative myocardial edema occurring either after prolonged or repeated periods of aortic cross-clamping or in the hearts with an extreme myocardial hypertrophy sometimes encountered in neglected congenital malformations. The indication to leave the chest open was based on diffuse postoperative bleeding after prolonged procedures and on hemodynamic deterioration or persistent ventricular arrhythmias after attempted closure of sternotomy.

---

*Kantonspital, Chirurg. Universitätsklinik A, Rämistraße, Zürich, Schweiz

The indications for use of the IABP have been widened in recent years. Only a brief trial of catecholamines and afterload reducing agents is attempted: if the cardiac output remains low and left ventricular filling pressure is adequate, the IABP is implanted in ICU without any delay. A paracorporeal artificial heart (1) was utilized in 1977/1978 in patients with terminal postoperative low output not responding to volume, catecholamines, and IABP treatment. Both implantation and removal of the artificial heart were performed in ICU without detaching the patient from the monitoring equipment.

Pericardial decompression by the subxyphoid approach is performed in ICU in patients with hemodynamic deterioration (increase in right atrial pressure, reduction in blood pressure, and cardiac output) where a tamponade cannot be ruled out. This small operation has been very useful as a diagnostic measure, allowing the differentiation between late onset of pericardial tamponade and right ventricular failure.

Surgical Technique

The operations in ICU are performed under standard aseptic conditions. A sterile set of instruments is placed on a trolley which also contains necessary suture material and electrocautery; a transportable surgical lamp provides an adequate light source. Two surgical nurses are available on short notice and the operation can be started within minutes. An additional small set of instruments (knife and wire-cutting scissors) is kept in the ICU to open the chest before the nurses arrive and the instrument tray is set up. In patients with delayed chest closure, the dressing is changed frequently (three to four times daily) to evacuate the hematoma and observe the condition of the heart. A gentamycin chain is used behind and in front of the sternum after closure of the incision.

IABP is implanted under local anesthesia through a small vertical inguinal incision which exposes the common femoral artery at its bifurcation. A standard implantation technique with a short segment of a 10 mm Gore-Tex graft is used.

Subxyphoid decompression is performed under either local or general anesthesia: the lowest part of the sternotomy incision is opened and the retrosternal space is explored digitally. Clots can be removed and the heart decompressed by this approach; when the bleeding persists, the whole length of incision is reopened to provide adequate vision for hemostasis. In "late" tamponade (days after operation), the evacuation of clot and fluid is usually sufficient to restore the normal hemodynamics; the sternal sutures stay intact.

Patient Material and Results

Emergency thoracotomy for massive exsanguinating bleeding was performed in seven patients with four long-term survivors (Table 1). The bleeding originated from the aortic cannulation site in two, aortic suture line in three, and proximal saphenous bypass graft anastomosis in two patients. Delayed chest closure was practiced in 16 patients and gave best results in patients with postperfusion myocardial edema: all four cases with acquired lesions (valvular and coronary) have survived and there were five long-term survivors among eight children in whom the primary closure of sternotomy was impossible after correction

Table 1. Surgery in ICU 1977-1980: Survival

		Patients	Survivors
Sudden massive bleeding		7	4
Delayed chest closure			
a) Prolonged perfusion + bleeding		4	2
b) Postperfus. myocardial edema	congenitals	8	5
	acquired	4	4
c) Paracorporeal artificial heart		5	2
Intraaortic balloon pumping		37	27

of complex congenital anomalies. When the chest had been left open after prolonged perfusions with diffuse bleeding from multiple anastomoses and pericardial adhesions, there were only two long-term survivors. IABP was utilized in 37 patients with 27 long-term survivors; in 11 cases, the implantation had to be performed in ICU and the device was removed in bed in 33 patients (Table 2). A paracorporeal artificial heart was utilized in six patients with profound postoperative heart failure: two implants were performed in ICU. The stabilization of circulation was achieved in four cases with a successful removal in bed; two patients were long-term survivors. The infection was encountered in one out of 21 patients with delayed chest closure; incidentally this was the only case in whom the gentamycin chain was not utilized during secondary closure. Long-term results in the group of patients with delayed chest closure have been very gratifying: there has been only late death due to arrhythmia 4 months after surgery in a patient with a paracorporeal artificial heart.

Table 2. Surgery in ICU 1977-1980: Mechanical circulatory assistance

	Implantation in ICU	Removal in ICU
Intraaortic balloon pump (37 patients)	11	33
Paracorporeal artificial heart (6 patients)	2	4

Discussion

Surgery in ICU has been practiced by many cardiovascular surgeons in extreme emergencies when the time does not permit the transfer to the OR. This method should by no means replace a planned reexploration after cardiovascular procedures and there are obvious disadvantages in performing surgery in bed in ICU: the lights are insufficient, the height of the operative field cannot be adjusted, and surgery is difficult in crowded conditions of ICU. Nevertheless, the concept of surgery in ICU is attractive because it avoids many logistic problems when transporting a critically ill patient to the OR. Monitoring and drainage are not interrupted, the infusions are continued in the controlled fashion, the patient is left on the respirator, and laborious detachment and reattachment of the monitoring lines with possibility of accidental removal of catheters is avoided.

From 1977 until July 1980, open-heart surgery was performed in approximately 2000 cases. Therefore, the policy of delayed chest closure (21 patients) was applied in approximately 1% of all cases. The incidence of postoperative myocardial edema and low output syndrome seems to be on the decline. The main reasons are to be found in more widespread use of hypothermia and potassium cardioplegia (2). Nevertheless, postoperative myocardial edema still can occur (3), especially in grossly hypertrophied ventricles which do not tolerate the primary closure of sternotomy. Our results show that the policy of delayed sternal closure, as advocated by other authors, too (4), does not expose the patient to any additional risks and indeed allows the heart to recover without subjecting it to the compression by the adaptation of sternum. A few general rules have emerged from the experience in delayed chest closure and surgery in ICU:

1. Sudden hemodynamic deterioration with high venous pressure can occur in the first hours or days after open-heart surgery: the distinction between tamponade and right ventricular failure is impossible and subxyphoid pericardial decompression mandatory. When blood and clots are found, the hemodynamic improvement is immediate; in right ventricular failure, no harm has been done and appropriate treatment can be instituted. In this situation, the old rule still holds: when in doubt, explore!

2. Sudden massive bleeding is possible in patients with friable vessels and multiple anastomoses; basic instruments for rapid opening of sternum by the first surgeon in the vicinity must be kept in ICU at all times. The evacuation of blood and digital compression can usually control the situation until the complete set of instruments arrives and the leak is repaired.

3. The transportation to the operating room is risky in patients with a low cardiac output or major arrhythmias; reexplorations should be carried in ICU without interruption of monitoring. Almost all postoperative bleedings can be controlled in ICU and we encountered only one complication which could not be repaired on the spot: the case of posterior wall rupture of the left ventricle after mitral valve replacement had to be taken to the OR and repaired in cardiopulmonary bypass.

Summary

Necessity for a rapid thoracotomy and logistic difficulties in transporting a desperately ill, heavily instrumented patient have prompted us to perform an increasing number of emergency procedures directly in intensive care unit. Following operations were done:

1. Rethoracotomy for bleeding in high-risk patients (implanted IABP, multiple infusions, and monitored pressures) and sudden tamponade with rapid hemodynamic deterioration: seven patients with four long-term survivors.

2. Delayed chest closure (median sternotomy left open for several hours or days) was utilized in patients with prolonged cardiopulmonary bypass

in diffuse bleeding (four cases with two survivors) and in patients with massive postperfusion myocardial edema precluding immediate closure of sternotomy (12 cases with nine survivors).

3. Implantation (11 patients) and removal (33 patients) of IABP; there were 27 long-term survivors out of 37 patients pumped.

4. Implantation (two cases) and removal (four cases) of the paracorporeal artificial heart: six patients pumped, two long-term survivors.

5. Pericardial decompression by subxyphoidal approach, both as a diagnostic measure (myocardial failure or tamponade) and therapeutic action (removal of subacute intrapericardial hematoma).

Surgery can be performed in intensive care unit with minimal equipment (sterile set of instruments, surgical light source, electrocautery, and suction). It is lifesaving in some patients and greatly simplifies the management of complicated cases; only one infection was encountered.

References

1. Turina M, Bosio R, Senning Å (1978) Clinical application of paracorporeal uni- and biventricular artificial heart. Trans Am Soc Artif Intern Organs 24:625-631
2. Kirklin JW, Conti VR, Blackstone EH (1979) Prevention of myocardial damage during cardiac operations. N engl J Med 301:135-141
3. Foglia RP, Steed DL, et al. (1979) Iatrogenic myocardial oedema with potassium cardioplegia. J Thorac Cardiovasc Surg 78:217-222
4. Ott DA, Cooley DA, et al. (1978) Delayed sternal closure: a useful technique to prevent tamponade a compression of the heart. Cardiovasc Dis 5:15-18

Is an Increase in Myocardial Perfusion in the Thallium Scintigram to be Expected After Left Ventricular Aneurysmectomy?

H. Eichstädt, U. Feine, K. Kochsiek, H. Schmutzler, and R. Felix*

Abstract

In 31 patients, thallium myocardial scanning was performed after aneurysm resection of the left ventricle. The aim of this study was to try an assertion about the completeness of adaptation of the marginal zones of aneurysm and about the postoperative reduction of left ventricular size. After standardization of picture focus distance and size of the cardiac scans, we suggested quantification of the dimensions of the left ventricle by counting picture points using a computer matrix. For that purpose, the left ventricle had to be delimitated exceptionally distinctly from the background. That intention was realized by an interpolating background subtraction, using a seven-pinhole collimator. Postoperatively an evident reduction of heart size, especially of ventricle cavity (ventricle/cavity ratio) could be proved, particularly when additional bypass grafting was applied. Thallium myocardial scanning therefore seems to be suitable for postoperative supervision after aneurysm resection as a follow-up measure.

Introduction

Thallium myocardial scanning has become part of the routine diagnostic program for coronary heart disease at a number of centers in recent years (1, 2, 5, 7, 11, 17, 19, 20, 29). There is as yet a great deal of unexplored territory in establishing the utility of the technique, especially in preoperative and postoperative evaluation in cases of coronary heart disease. We tested the applicability of the procedure in evaluating bypass patency several years ago (6-9). Aneurysm resection is becoming a more common procedure, too (3, 13, 14, 18, 23), so we have tested the applicability of thallium scanning to postoperative follow-up in these cases (10).

Our basic considerations were the following: Demonstration of the left ventricle in the thallium scan following anterior infarction results in an apical defect in the RAO view. The aim of aneurysm resection following anterior infarction is restoration of left ventricular pump function through a relative increase in functional myocardium on the circumference of the ventricle.

Left ventricular dilatation is a quantifiable parameter, especially in the tomoscintigrams of patients with aneurysm. In 45° LAO projection, the left ventricle can be demonstrated as an annulus area with a distinct core. High-quality scintigrams, especially tomoscintigrams, with a high degree of background subtraction allow determinations of the

*Universitätsklinikum Charlottenburg, Department Cardiology, D-1000 Berlin 19

relation of total ventricular area to the area of the ventricular cavity (ventricle/cavity ratio), as can be seen in Figures 1 and 2.

The purpose of our study was to determine whether thallium scans are adequate for postoperative evaluation of myocardial viability and of the degree of adaptation at the borders of the aneurysm. We did not intend to evaluate the results of individual surgical interventions or to judge the utility of aneurysmectomy per se. Other detailed studies which address these points are available (13. 16, 18, 23-25, 30).

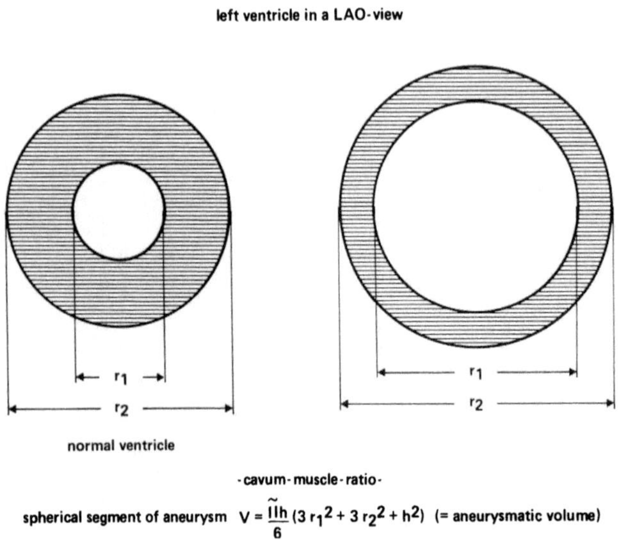

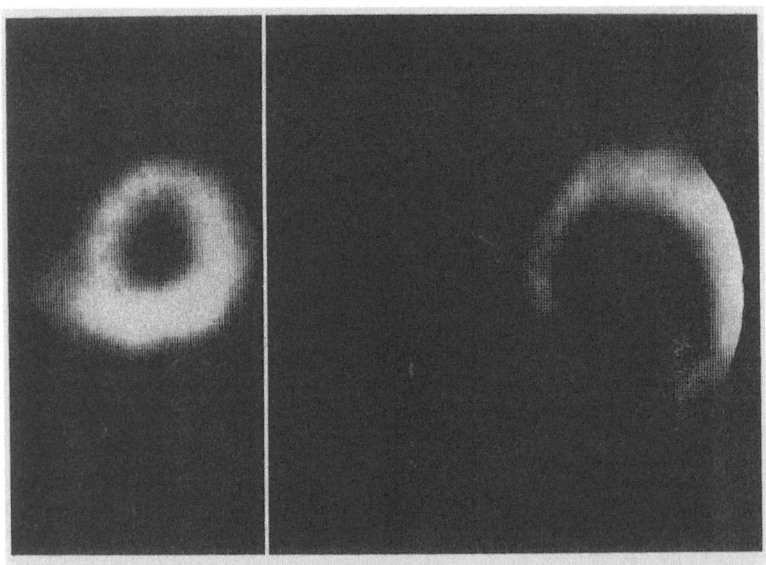

Figs. 1, 2. "Ventricle/cavity ratio" in a normal ventricle (left) and in an enlarged ventricle (right) in schematic representation (Fig. 1) and in the original scan (Fig. 2)

Material and Methods

Aneurysm resection was performed in 36 patients after transmural infarction in the University Hospital Tübingen between 1973 and 1978. Two patients died at operation (5.5%) and one other died after 1 month following surgery (2.7%). Twenty-eight of these patients were included in the current study and three other patients treated surgically at a later date completed the collective. Some of the cardiological findings in these 31 patients are summarized in Table 1.

Table 1. 31 patients with anterior wall aneurysm; preoperative data

ECG					
Anterior infarction		Posterior infarction			
n = 31		n = 1			
Angiogram					
1-vessel disease		2-vessel disease		3-vessel disease	
total	>75%	total	>75%	total	>75%
n = 16	3	6	3	-	3

Selection for aneurysmectomy was made according to the following criteria: Thirteen patients had intractable angina at rest, and 19 others had chest pain at low load levels. Seven patients had clinical evidence of congestive heart failure at rest (rales, or evidence of congestive failure in chest films), and two others had tibial edema or hepatic enlargement. Fourteen patients suffered severe dyspnea under light loads during bicycle exercise. Intractable arrhythmias secondary to infarction were observed in 12 cases, and an additional patient had recurrent emboli. Table 2 contains a summary of some relevant findings at operation.

Table 2. Intraoperative data

Localization of aneurysm		
ant.-lat. wall	+ apex	+ septum
n = 10	18	1
Area of resection (cm^2)		
10-19	20-29	30-50
n = 12	7	10
Additional bypass grafting		
LAD + diag. br.	cx + marg. sin.	RCA + branches
n = 4	4	7

Myocardial scanning was performed at rest and during exercise using standard procedures in all patients (7). Both Picker Dyna 4/15 and Ohio Nuclear Sigma 410 cameras were used. All patients had studies with a parallel hole collimator and additional views were made with a seven-pinhole collimator (27) in a number of cases; for that purpose, we used a Scintislice tomography system from CMS with pinhole diameters of 5.5 mm and 12.7 cm distance between collimator and crystal. We received at least three planes of the apex, the base and the middle portion of the left ventricle in each patient. Count rate analysis was performed on the circumference of the ventricle.

All the scans were smoothed down twice with a nine-point planing program. We employed modified interpolating background subtraction (12). The matrix contained 128 x 128 picture points. Matrix-cells were established for the entire area of the left ventricle (see Fig. 1, measure r_2) and for the area of the ventricular cavity (see Fig. 1, measure r_1). We have found that the ratio between total ventricular area and the area of the cavity is of diagnostic significance and we propose the "ventricle/cavity ratio" as a diagnostic parameter in heart failure of any genesis.

In addition, the circumference of the ventricle was divided into a number of "irregular regions" so that we were able to define the defect corresponding to the aneurysm and to express this area as a percentage of the total circumference of the left ventricle. Results were analyzed with a Gamma-11 system on a DEC computer. Space requirements do not allow us to go into details of the analytic program.

Results

Figure 3 presents the results of the quantitative valuation of matrix areas described above. Preoperative scintigrams in patients with aneurysm demonstrated a mean ventricular area of 727 matrix points and mean cavity area of 254 points, so mean ventricle/cavity ratio was 1 : 0.35. Total ventricular area was significantly less in a group of healthy controls, with a mean of 365 matrix points, about half as large as in patients with aneurysm ($p < 0.025$). Area of the cavity averaged 88 matrix points in this group, with a mean ventricle/cavity ratio of 1 : 0.24.

In healthy controls we obtained 76.5 counts in one single matrix cell, whereas the mean count rate in aneurysmatic segments was entirely 16.5 counts per matrix cell. Ventricular area was reduced in all patients following aneurysm resection, though the mean ventricular area of 597 matrix points was still 40% larger than in the group of healthy controls. Area of the ventricular cavity was reduced to 199 matrix points following aneurysmectomy, but the ventricle/cavity ratio remained essentially unchanged at 1 : 0.33. There was considerable variance in the reduction of ventricular area following surgery. Some patients demonstrated virtually identical relations after operation, while others showed a considerable reduction in ventricular area (Figs. 4 and 5).

Five patients experienced no relief of their anginal pain at rest, and 12 others still suffered chest pain during mild bicycle exercise (up to 50 watts). Signs of congestive heart failure at rest were evident in two patients, while ten patients suffered considerable dyspnea during exercise (Table 3). Subjective clinical improvement and a 100% increase in exercise tolerance were found postoperatively in the remaining 11 patients who had also received bypass grafts (see Fig. 6).

Left ventricular size measured in matrix-points

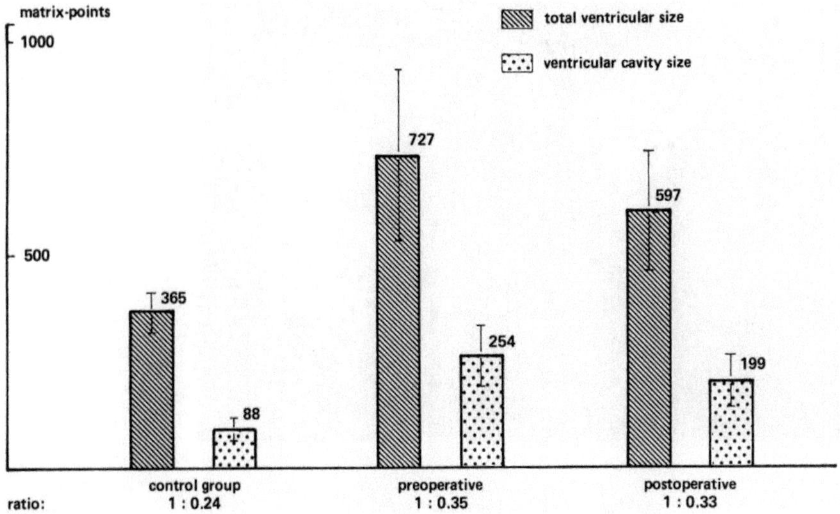

Fig. 3. Matrix area of the entire ventricle (striped column) as compared to the ventricular cavity (dotted column). On the left: healthy controls; in the middle: preoperative findings; on the right: following aneurysm resection

We were surprised to find no significant increase in functioning myocardial mass in the 20 patients with aneurysm resection but without bypass grafts. Figure 6 shows that the addition of bypass grafts is associated with a decrease in ventricle size and a clear increase in exercise tolerance (n = 11).

Table 3. Postoperative data

Angina pectoris		Congestive heart failure	
Rest	Exercise	Rest	Exercise
5	12	2/1	10

Discussion

Demonstration of myocardial scar tissue and diagnosis of load-related ischemia have found increasing importance as cardiological screening methods since 1975 (1, 2, 5, 7, 11, 19, 20, 22, 29). The questions at hand are whether a left ventricular aneurysm results in a circumscribed or diffuse reduction in thallium uptake, whether thallium is taken up at all and whether a defect in the thallium scan is reduced in size or eliminated completely after aneurysm resection. The problem is of particular interest when one considers that QS complexes usually remain unchanged in the ECG following aneurysmectomy (4, 18, 25, 26) which implies that the ECG is an unsuitable tool for postoperative

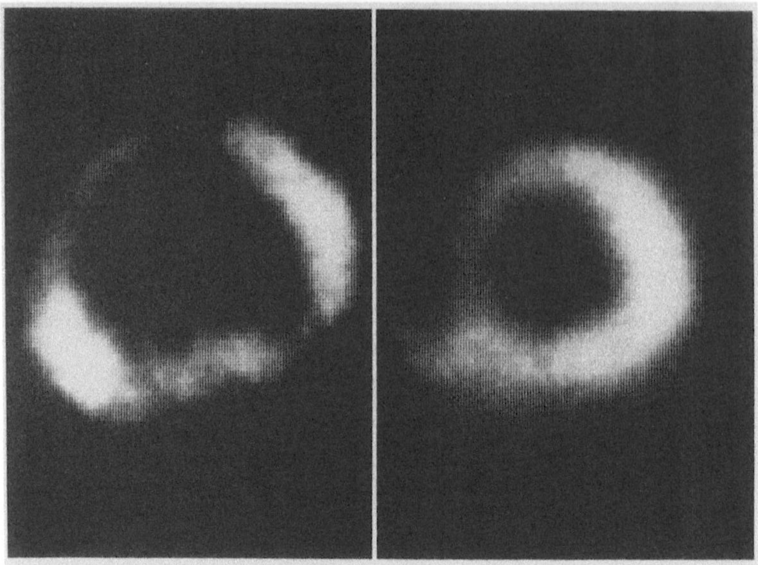

Fig. 4

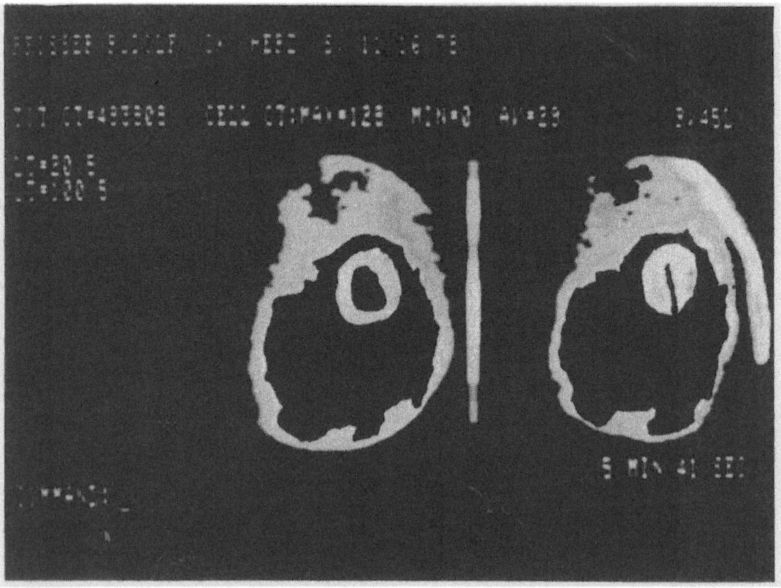

Fig. 5

Figs. 4, 5. Original scans in a patient before (left) and after (right) aneurysm resection. Tomoscintigraphic views made with a seven-pinhole collimator (4) and conventional scans with the parallel-hole collimator (5).

follow-up. It was our purpose to quantify postoperative reduction in ventricle size in the LAO view. This may be achieved by counting matrix cells over the entire ventricle in the LAO view and by relating this area to the area of the ventricle cavity (ventricle/cavity ratio). We believe that a relative increase in myocardial mass may be interpreted as an indirect sign of improved pump function.

Only invasive methods are capable of providing direct evidence of improved ventricular function. Postoperative improvement in hemodynamic parameters such as LVEDP, cardiac index, and left ventricular stroke volume index are the only objective diagnostic criteria of improved pump function (24). It was our intention to develop a noninvasive method that would allow indirect conclusions on improved function supplementary to radionuclide ventriculography.

We found that the cavity occupied more than a third of the total area of the ventricle in patients with aneurysm (ventricle/cavity ratio 1 : 0.35), in contrast to somewhat less than a quarter of total ventricular area in a group of healthy controls (1 : 0.24). This agrees with our angiographic results which demonstrate consistent increases in LVEDP as well as decreases in the ejection fraction in patients with aneurysm. Quantitative analysis in a number of studies has brought similar results (15, 16, 21, 30).

In postoperative studies, we found decreases in total ventricle size but found that there was no significant change in the relation between total ventricular area and area of the cavity (ventricle/cavity ratio 1 : 0.33). These findings lead us to the conclusions that aneurysm resection is followed by reduction in absolute size of the ventricle, but that end-diastolic volume remains large and ventricular function does not improve. However, patients who received bypass grafts in addition to aneurysm resection did experience a postoperative improvement in exercise tolerance (n = 11), a finding reported by other authors as well (23). But we were not able to demonstrate an unambi-

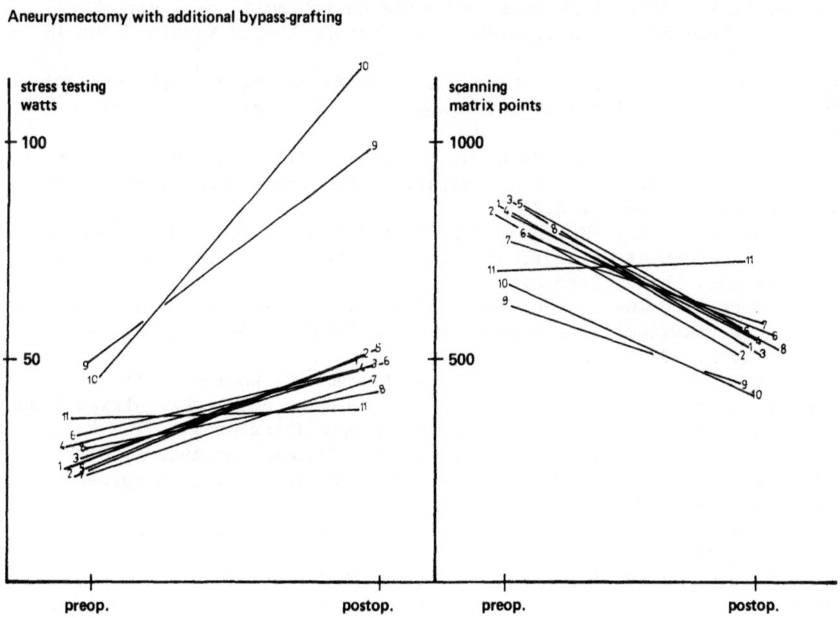

Fig. 6. Decrease in ventricular size associated with an increase in exercise tolerance in patients with additional bypass grafting

guous increase in the relation between perfused myocardial mass and the area of the ventricular cavity (ventricle/cavity ratio) in the relatively small number of patients in our collective.

Aneurysm resection of the type described here does not result in a significant decrease in the size of a myocardial scar which often extends more widely into the myocardial wall than is apparent on the surface. The proportion of functional myocardium does not increase after aneurysmectomy. These findings correlate well with the clinical state. In contrast, patients with additional bypass grafts demonstrate significant reductions in ventricle size and conspicuous improvement in exercise tolerance in the case of multi-vessel-disease.

Thallium myocardial scanning is a feasible diagnostic technique for follow-up studies after aneurysmectomy, given adequate picture quality which allows full development of the necessary data. As a result of our own studies, we propose the "ventricle/cavity ratio" as the most significant parameter in this regard.

References

1. Adam WE, De Jong R, Knapp WH, Stauch M, Tillmanns H (1978) Nuklearmedizinische Methoden in der Kardiologie. Z Kardiol 67:428
2. Aldor E, Blazek G, Gaul G, Heeger H, Kahn P (1978) Sensibilität des 201-Thallium-Szintigramms des Herzens unter Belastungsbedingungen. ROEFO 129:23
3. Cheng TO (1971) Incidence of ventricular aneurysm in coronary artery disease, an angiographic appraisal. Am J Med 50:340
4. Cokkinos DV, Hallmann GL, Cooley A, Zamalloa O, Leachmann RD (1971) Left ventricular aneurysm. Analysis of electrocardiographic features and postresection changes. Am Heart J 82:149
5. Cook DJ, Bailey J, Strauss HW, Rouleau J, Wagner HN, Pitt B (1976) Thallium-201 for myocardial imaging: Appearance of the normal heart. J Nucl Med 17:583
6. Eichstädt H, Gauss A (1978) Nichtinvasive Perfusionskontrolle nach aortokoronarer Bypass-Operation durch Thallium-Myokardszintigraphie. Z Kardiol [Suppl] 5:154
7. Eichstädt H, Schumacher M, Feine U, Kochsiek K (1978) Rechnerunterstützte 201-Tl-Myokardszintigraphie in der Routinediagnostik der koronaren Herzerkrankung. Nuklearmedizin 17:233
8. Eichstädt H, Gauss A, Andrasch R, Feine U, Kochsiek K (1979) Noninvasive perfusion control by Thallium-201 myocardial scintigraphy after coronary artery bypass surgery. Cardiovasc Radiol 2:243
9. Eichstädt H, Gauss A, Seybold-Epting W (1979) Thallium-201 myocardial imaging for non-invasive assessment of regional myocardial perfusion after aortocoronary bypass-grafting. Thorac Cardiovasc Surg 27:32
10. Eichstädt H, Gröber L, Feine U, Kochsiek K (1980) Verlaufskontrolle nach linksventrikulärer Aneurysmektomie durch die Thallium-201-Myokardszintigraphie. Fortschr. Röntgenstr. 133/3:245
11. Felix R, Thurn P, Pensky W, Wagner J, Simon H, Neumann G, Wahlen A, Winkler C (1975) Normales und pathologisches Perfusionsszintigramm des linksventrikulären Myokards und erste Ergebnisse des Thallium-201-Myokardszintigramms. In: Holtmeier HJ, Siegenthaler W (eds) Koronarinsuffizienz. Thieme, Stuttgart, p 72
12. Goris ML, Daspit SG, McLaughlin P, Kriss JP (1976) Interpolative background subtraction. J Nucl Med 17:744
13. Heberer G, Schramm G (1970) Resektion von Ventrikelaneurysmen. Verh Dtsch Ges Kreislaufforsch 36:167
14. Kluge TH, Ullal SR, Hill JD, Kerth WJ, Gerbode F (1971) Dyskinesia and aneurysm of the left ventricle. Surgical experience in 36 patients. J Cardiovasc Surg 12:273
15. Leighton RF, Wilt SM, Lewis RP (1974) Detection of hypokinesis by a quantitative analysis of left ventricular cineangiograms. Circulation 50:121

16. Letac B, Leroux C, Cribier A (1978) Large ventricular aneurysm occurring after myocardial infarction. Br Heart J 40:516
17. Lichte H (1977) Myokardszintigraphie mit 201-Thallium. Fortschr Med 95:899
18. Loop FD, Effler DB, Navia JA, Sheldon WC, Groves LK (1973) Aneurysm of the left ventricle: Survival and results of a ten-year surgical experience. Ann Surg 178:399
19. Mathey D, Montz R, Hanrath P, Kröger E, Knop J, Bleifeld W (1978) Reversible Myokardischämie oder irreversible Myokardfibrose. Dtsch Med Wochenschr 44:1736
20. Pachinger O, Probst P, Ogris E, Kaindl F (1977) Quantitative 201-Thallium-Myokardszintigraphie bei koronarer Herzkrankheit. Herz/Kreislauf 9:310
21. Parmley W, Chuck L, Kivowitz C (1973) In vitro length tension relations of human ventricular aneurysm. Relation of stiffness to mechanical disadvantage. Am J Cardiol 32:889
22. Ritchie JL, Zaret BL, Strauss HW, Pitt B, Berman DS, Schelbert HR, Ashburn WL, Berger HJ, Hamilton GW (1978) Myocardial imaging with Thallium-201: A multicenter study in patients with angina pectoris or acute myocardial infarction. Am J Cardiol 42:345
23. Rivera R, Delcau JL (1979) Factors influencing results in surgery of postinfarction ventricular aneurysms. In: Roskamm H, Schmuziger M (eds) Coronary heart surgery. Springer, Berlin Heidelberg New York
24. Rödiger W, Darup J, Rodewald G (1979) Die Funktion des linken Ventrikels nach Aneurysmektomie. In: Westermann KW (ed) Herzwandaneurysmen. Witzstrock, Baden-Baden
25. Shaw RC, Ferguson TB, Weldon CL, Connors JP (1978) Left ventricular aneurysm resection. Indications and long-term follow-up. Ann Thorac Surg 25:336
26. Tesler UF, Fernandez D, Morse D (1975) Combined revascularization and aneurysmectomy — rationale and results. In: Norman JC (ed) Coronary artery medicine and surgery — concepts and controversies. Appleton-Century Crofts, New York
27. Vogel RA, Kirch D, Le Free M, Steele P (1978) A new method of multiplanar emission tomography using a seven-pinhole collimator and an Anger scintillation camera. J Nucl Med 19:648
28. Vogel RA, Kirch DL, Le Free MT, Rainwater JO, Jensen DP, Steele P (1979) Thallium-201 myocardial perfusion scintigraphy: results of standard and multi-pinhole tomographic techniques. Am J Cardiol 43:787
29. Wackers FJT, Schoot JB, Sohole EB, Samson G, Niftrik GJC, Lie KJ, Durrer D, Wellems HJJ (1975) Noninvasive visualization of acute myocardial infarction in men with Thallium-201. Br Heart J 37:741
30. Watson LE, Dickhaus DW, Martin RH (1975) Left ventricular aneurysm. Preoperative hemodynamics, chamber volume, and results of aneurysmectomy. Circulation 52:868

The Effect of Left Ventricular Aneurysmectomy on Left Ventricular Function at Rest and During Exercise. A Retrospective Study of 350 Patients

G. Trieb, H. Mannebach, D. Faßbender, A. Müller, H. M. Mertens, and U. Gleichmann*

Introduction

The indications for left ventricular aneurysmectomy are still open for discussion. In contrast to many reports describing subjective improvement after aneurysmectomy in many patients, we are not able to demonstrate in a small group an improvement by means of objective parameters (1, 2, 4, 6-9). It is the purpose of this report to analyse the pre- and postoperative hemodynamic data at rest and with exercise in a greater group of patients and to reevaluate the indications for surgery using more quantitative parameters.

Methods

Between 1974 and 1979, out of a total group of 350 patients with left ventricular aneurysm, 75 patients were treated by left ventricular aneurysmectomy, 275 patients were treated medically. In all patients, left heart catheterization including quantitative analysis of left ventricular volumes were performed. This report deals with the data of the 75 patients treated surgically.
The indications for left ventricular aneurysmectomy were: dyspnea of NYHA class III-IV, large left ventricular aneurysm of 150-200 ml, concomitant bypass surgery, recurrent embolism, or life threatening tachycardia.

After operation, a complete hemodynamic and angiographic study at rest and with exercise including an ergospirometric test was carried out in 34 patients. In the remaining group of 41 patients, ergospirometry in combination with pulmonary pressure measurements at rest and with exercise was performed. Biplane cineangiocardiography was analysed for volume calculations according to the formula of Dodge et al. (3, 5).

Left ventricular anterior wall aneurysm was diagnosed when firstly there was a paradoxal outward movement of the anterior wall and secondly the absolute volume of the aneurysm was more than 50 ml/m^2 body surface area. The volume of the so-called rest ventricle was calculated in absolute values with determination of its ejection fraction.

*Gollwitzer-Meier Institute, D-4970 Bad Oeynhausen

Results

Fifty-two of the 75 patients reported an improvement in dyspnea; this was not confirmed by the results of the ergospirometry which show only in 8% a considerable enhancement of cardiac pump function. As shown by Figure 1, there were no significant changes between preoperative and postoperative values for heart rate, cardiac index, stroke volume index, and left ventricular end-diastolic pressure. There was a significant decrease in left ventricular volume indexes and a significant increase of total ejection fraction after surgery. Only in a few cases could a decrease of the left ventricular end-diastolic pressure at rest and with exercise be observed, especially in patients with isolated stenosis of left anterior descending artery or in patients with two- or three-vessel disease with an additional aortocoronary bypass graft. The stroke volume index, however, remained unchanged or decreased.

Looking for the best predictive preoperative parameter for an improvement in cardiac pump function after surgery, we found only a correlation between the ejection fraction of the rest ventricle measured during exercise and the left ventricular end-diastolic pressure measured after surgery. A good ejection fraction of the rest ventricle at exercise was followed by a marked decrease of the left ventricular end-diastolic pressure after surgery (Fig. 2).

Discussion

The report of subjective improvement of dyspnea contrasts markedly with the results of the objective measurements, therefore, the complaint of dyspnea seems not to be a good predictive parameter for the

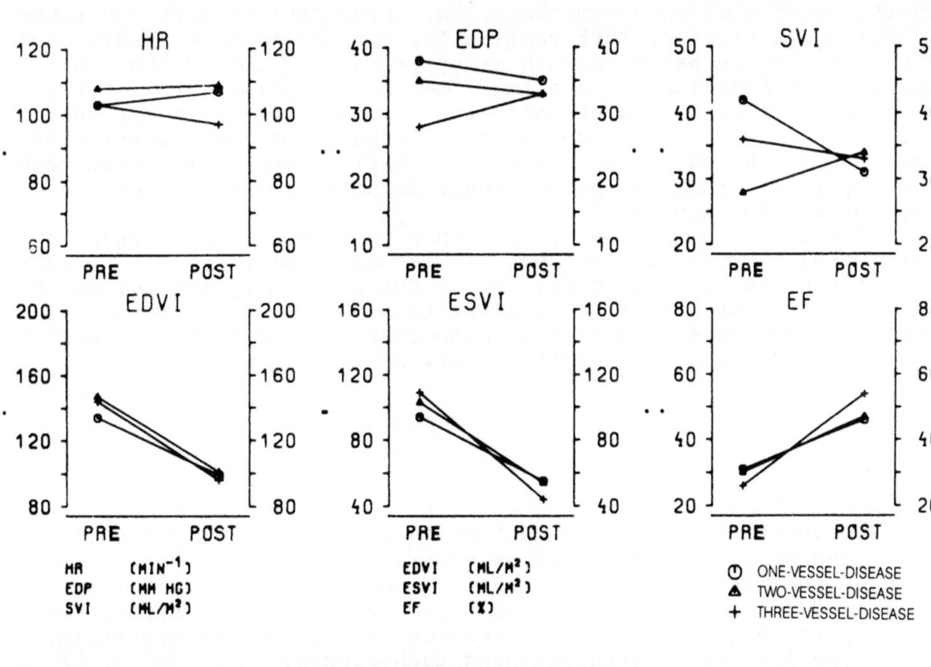

Fig. 1. Pre- and postoperative hemodynamics in patients with aneurysmectomy

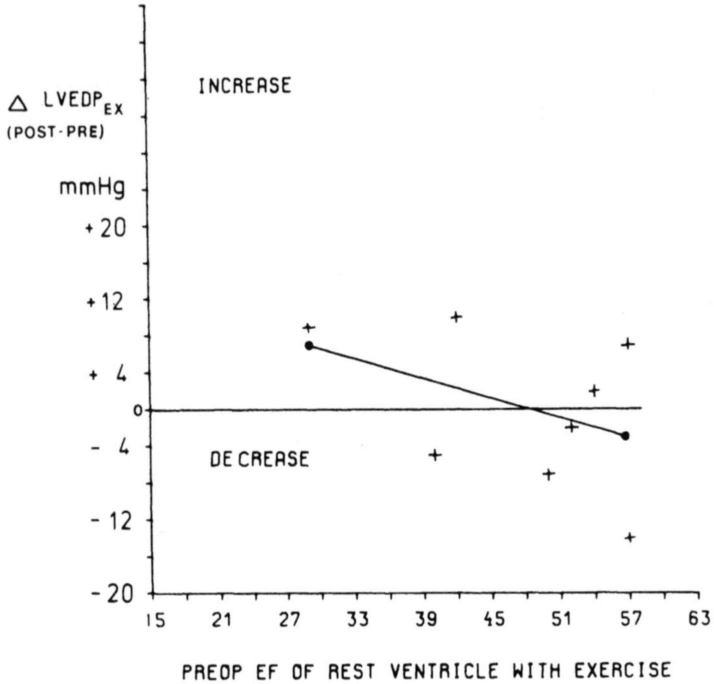

Fig. 2. Relation between preoperative ejection fraction of the rest ventricle with exercise (abscissa) and the decrease in left ventricular end-diastolic pressure after aneurysmectomy

potential benefit of aneurysmectomy. An improvement of left ventricular function in terms of left ventricular end-diastolic pressure could only be expected in patients with an ejection fraction of the rest ventricle with exercise of more than 50%. Not only the ejection fraction of the rest ventricle but also the absolute volume of the rest ventricle has an important impact on the results of left ventricular aneurysmectomy. As shown by Figure 3, a small volume of the rest ventricle may result in a low-output syndrome after surgery despite a nearly normal ejection fraction.

Our data show clearly that in patients with one-vessel disease and congestive heart failure, left ventricular aneurysmectomy has no benefit; in these cases, cardiac failure is not removed by the correction of left ventricular geometry. In patients with two- or three-vessel disease, an improvement in cardiac pump function could only be expected when concomitant bypass graft surgery is performed.

Conclusions

The first essential for aneurysmectomy is a good pump function of a normal-sized rest ventricle with an ejection fraction of more than 50% and an end-diastolic volume index of more than 60 ml/m^2. This kept in mind, aneurysmectomy is indicated in concomitant bypass surgery, very large aneurysm in the presence of a good rest ventricle, arterial embolism or life-threatening tachycardia.

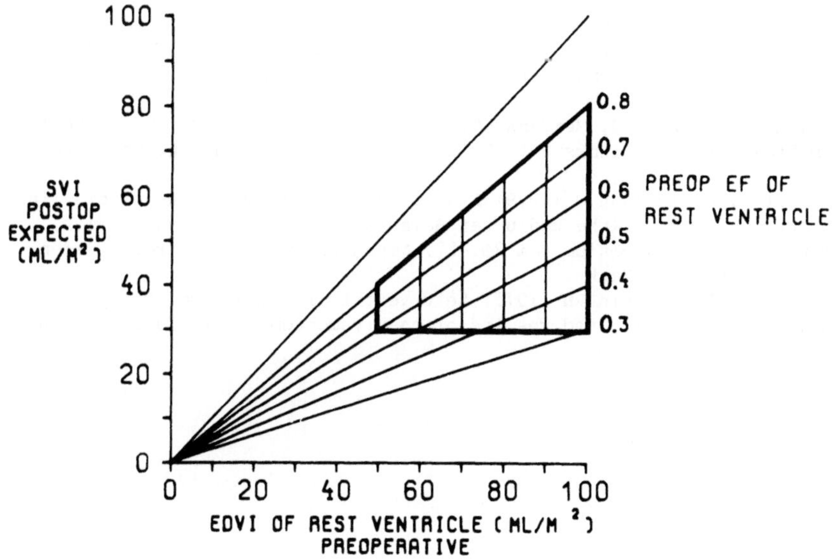

Fig. 3. The relation between expected postoperative stroke volume index and the preoperative end-diastolic volume index of the rest ventricle at different states of contractility of the rest ventricle (rest EF)

Summary

The results of left ventricular aneurysmectomy in 75 patients out of a total group of 350 patients with left ventricular aneurysm were reported. As demonstrated by hemodynamic and angiographic measurements, an improvement of left ventricular pump function could only be expected in patients with an ejection fraction of the rest ventricle with exercise of more than 50% and rest end-diastolic volume index of more than 60 ml/m^2.

References

1. Arthur A, Basta L, Kioschos M (1972) Factors influencing prognosis in left ventricular aneurysmectomy. Circulation [Suppl 2] 45:127
2. Björk VO, Henze A (1976) Left ventricular function at rest and during exercise before and after surgical treatment of ischemic heart disease, left ventricular aneurysm, aortic stenosis, and aortic incompetence. In: Roskamm H, Hahn C (eds) Ventricular function at rest and during exercise. Springer, Berlin Heidelberg New York, p 149
3. Dodge HT, Sandler H, Ballew DW, Cord JD (1960) The use of biplane angiocardiography for measurement of left ventricular volume in man. Am Heart J 60:762
4. Hazan E, Bloch G, Rioux C, Louville Y, et al. (1973) Surgical treatment of aneurysm and segmental dyskinesia of the left ventricular wall after myocardial infarction. Am J Cardiol 31:708
5. Sigwart U, Schmidt H, Bonzel T, Mertens HM, Gleichmann U (1975) Biplane LV cineangiographic evaluation of LV contraction at rest and during bicycle exercise. Circulation [Suppl II/4] 52:37

6. Swan HJ, Chattergee K, Kaushik VS, Matloff J (1976) Functional and clinical effects of surgical treatment of ventricular aneurysm. In: Roskamm H, Hahn C (eds) Ventricular function at rest and during exercise. Springer, Berlin Heidelberg New York, p 149
7. Trieb G, Schmidt H, Sigwart U, Mertens HM, Gleichmann U, Borst HG (1977) Einfluß der Aneurysmektomie auf die linksventrikuläre Belastungshämodynamik. Herz Kreislauf 511-514
8. Trieb G, Sigwart U, Gleichmann U (1979) Einfluß der Aneurysmektomie auf die linksventrikuläre Hämodynamik in Ruhe und unter Belastung. In: Herzwandaneurysmen, Rotenburger Diskussion, Symposium vom 20.-22. November 1978. Witzstrock, Baden-Baden Brussels Cologne New York
9. Watson LE, Dickhaus DW, Martin RH (1975) Left ventricular aneurysm. Preoperative hemodynamics, chamber volume, and results of aneurysmectomy. Circulation 52:868

Treatment of Sternal Dehiscence After Open Cardiac Surgery

G. Frank, M. Dziuba, and H. G. Borst*

Median sternotomy has become the approach of choice in open cardiac surgery (1, 6). However, postoperative sternal dehiscence can become a life-threatening complication. Incidence of sternal infection – as reported in the literature – ranges between 0.4% and 7.0% (1, 4, 5, 8). Regarding the treatment of sternal dehiscence, various recommendations were made (2, 3, 5, 7-9). This paper describes the evolution of our policy in the surgical management of sternal dehiscence and reports upon the results obtained by the various procedures employed.

Material

Eighty-three patients with sternal dehiscence were seen from October 1968 to June 1980, i.e., 1.8% of 4615 patients after open heart surgery (Fig. 1). There were 67 men and 16 women with an average age of 48 years (range 16 to 69 years). Forty-nine cases were primarily operated upon for valve disease, 25 for coronary heart disease, and nine cases for congenital lesions. Sternal dehiscence was twice as frequent in valve surgery as compared to operations for coronary and congenital lesions.

In 68 patients (82%), bacterial organisms could be cultured, in 15 patients (18%), no organism was found. In 13 individuals (16%), more than one organism could be detected (Fig. 2). The most frequent offending organisms were *Staphylococcus* with four deaths in the *S. aureus* group. Interestingly three deaths occurred in the *S. epidermidis* group. Infection with *Pseudomonas* and *Klebsiella aerobacter* had also a rather high mortality rate.

Method

While in our initial experience open treatment was preferred, we have used reclosure exclusively since 1972. Reclosure was performed as soon as sternal dehiscence became apparent: The wound was totally opened, the retrosternal and – if necessary – the pericardial space were cleaned of pus and debris and irrigated generously. The sternal edges were debrided with a curette and reapproximated with wires or steel bands for further stabilization. Skin and subcutaneous tissue were closed by interrupted sutures.

*Klinik für Thorax-, Herz- und Gefäßchirurgie, Medizinische Hochschule Hannover, Karl-Wiechert-Allee 9, D-3000 Hannover 61

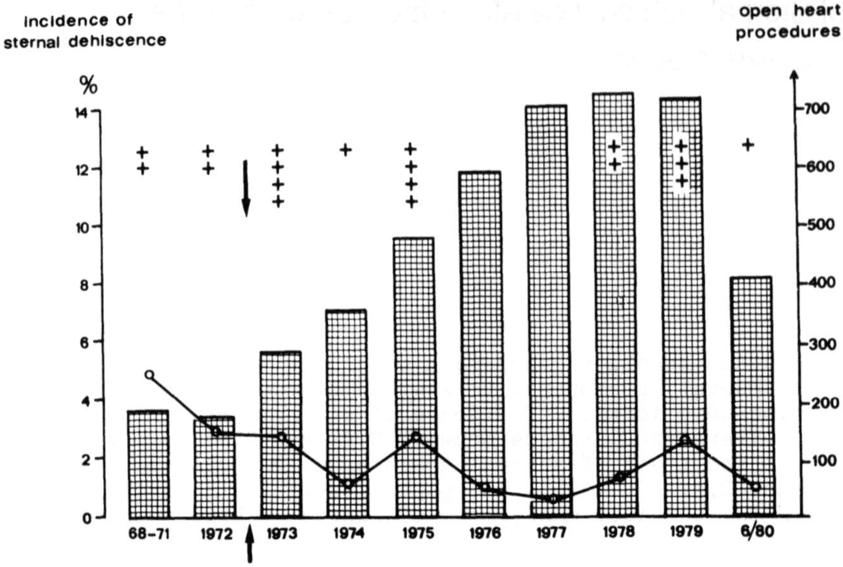

Fig. 1. Annual incidence and mortality (crosses) of sternal dehiscence

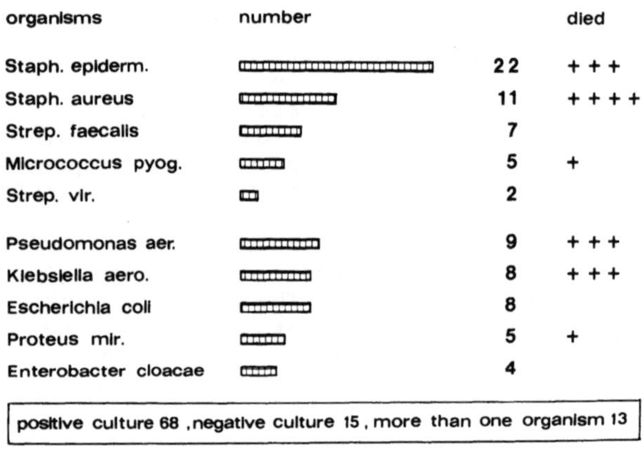

Fig. 2. Confirmed organisms in sternal infection

Two irrigation tubes were inserted from above and two drainage tubes from below for continuous irrigation using Ringer's lactate (50-100 ml/h) with antiseptic iodine solution (Polyvidon).

Irrigation was maintained for at least 3 days or was continued until bacterial controls were definitely negative. Thereafter the chest tubes were removed step by step under continuous suction to avoid open retrosternal spaces. In case of recurrent infection or dehiscence, the same procedure was repeated. Only if osteomyelitis and mediastinitis persisted was the sternum ultimately left open. Of course, proper antibiotic systemic therapy was administered intravenously at the time of reoperation and controlled by bacterial cultures.

Results (Fig. 3)

Of 23 patients in whom open treatment only was used and those in whom repeated reclosure finally ended in open therapy, nine (39%) were lost because of septic complications. The hospital stay of this group was 20 to 144 days (mean 75 days).

Of 60 patients in whom a consequent therapy of reclosure and irrigation was successful, eight (13%) died of various septic complications. Three of these patients died of bleeding from anastomoses of coronary bypass grafts or ascending aortic prosthesis. Hospitalization of this group was 14-58 days (mean 32 days).

	n	died	%		hospitalisation (d)		
open	7	4	(57)		20 – 144	(87)	
revision + open	11	4	(36)	39	34 – 120	(71)	75
revision + revision + open	5	1	(20)		42 – 90	(66)	
closed	51	5	(9,8)		14 – 58	(29)	
revision + revision	8	3	(37)	13	36 – 57	(52)	32
revision + revision + revision	1	–	–		240		

Fig. 3. Mortality (%) and period of hospitalization (days) after various treatments of sternal dehiscence

Discussion

The results of this study show a highly significant difference in mortality and period of hospitalization after sternal dehiscence depending upon the success of sternal reclosure. Thus, mortality rate was approximately three times as high in open as compared to successful closed treatment of sternal dehiscence. Likewise the period of hospitalization in the former group was twice as long as in the latter. This was true irrespective of the presence or absence of infection and of the organisms cultured.

In our mind, the first and most important aim of surgical therapy is prompt stabilization of the chest as soon as dehiscence becomes apparent. In this way, respiratory insufficiency and pain are avoided and the patient again is able to cough (3, 4, 7). From the experience in osteosynthetic surgery it may be assumed that stabilization of the sternum also counteracts spreading osteomyelitis (2). Even if this aim cannot be achieved ultimately repeated reclosure should be attempted in order to gain time so that granulation tissue piling up behind the sternum will wall off the infected space and limit the excursions of the sternal edges.

The role of continuous retrosternal irrigation is seen in its continuous mechanical washing effect preventing accumulation of debris and pus. The antiseptic effect of iodine or other additives remains conjectural and probably is of secondary importance to systemic antibiotic therapy (2, 4, 8, 9). In proven mediastinal infection, irrigation should be maintained until repeated cultures of the effluent have become negative after discontinuation of iodine (4, 9). Thereafter the chest tubes are removed only after proving – if necessary by contrast medium – that any retrosternal dead space has disappeared which may involve prolonged drainage.

Further arguments in favour of this aggressive management of sternal dehiscence is the psychological gain of the patient with his wounds closed and the avoidance of contamination of other patients in a cardiovascular unit.

Conclusions

1. In case of sternal dehiscence, infected or not, early reoperation should be performed with surgical debridement, rewiring, primary closure, and substernal irrigation.

2. Open treatment seems only indicated as an ultimate therapeutic step in cases of repeated dehiscence due to resistant sepsis with mediastinitis or osteomyelitis.

3. By performing a consequent closed treatment of sternal dehiscence, mortality rate and period of hospitalization can be reduced significantly.

Summary

On the basis of our experience in 83 cases of sternal dehiscence after median sternotomy, the treatment of choice was found to be early reclosure and irrigation. In comparison to open treatment, the mortality rate and the period of hospitalization could be significantly reduced.

References

1. Brown AH et al. (1969) The complication of median sternotomy. J Thorac Cardiovasc Surg 58:189
2. Bryant LR et al. (1969) Treatment of median sternotomy infection by mediastinal irrigation with an antibiotic solution. Ann Surg 169:914
3. Cheanvechai C et al. (1972) Treatment of infected sternal wounds. Cleve Clin Q 39:43
4. Engelmann RM et al. (1973) Mediastinitis following open heart surgery. Arch Surg 107:772
5. Grmoljez PF et al. (1975) Major complications of median sternotomy. Am J Surg 130:679
6. Julian OC et al. (1957) The median sternal incision in intracardiac surgery with extracorporeal circulation: A general evaluation of its use in heart surgery. Surgery 42:753
7. Ochsner JL et al. (1972) Disruption and infection of median sternotomy incision. J Cardiovasc Surg 13:394
8. Ott DA et al. (1980) Wound complications after median sternotomy: A study of 61 patients from a consecutive series of 9,279. Cardiovasc Dis 7/1:104
9. Thurer RC et al. (1974) The management of mediastinal infection following cardiac surgery. J Thorac Cardiovasc Surg 68:962

Sterno-mediastinitis Following Open-heart Surgery. Review of Five Years Experience

D. Duveau, M. Train, J. L. Michaud, and H. Dupon*

Median sternotomy incision is widely used for cardiac surgery. Post-operative sterno-mediastinitis is a redoubtable complication with a high morbidity and mortality. Experience of 37 infected patients among 2000 patients operated on for bypass is reported here and some problems such as predisposing factors, clinical data, and therapy are discussed.

Clinical Material

Distribution of Cases

Between January 1975 and May 1980, 1985 patients were subjected to heart surgery with bypass and underwent median sternotomy incision. Thirty-seven patients (1.9%) developed sterno-mediastinitis. There were 32 adults and five children less than 10 years old. The predominance of this complication in men (34 males and three females) suggests that pilosity is a predisposing factor. Figure 1 shows a homogeneous assessment by year, except in 1977 owing to a failure of the sterilizer.

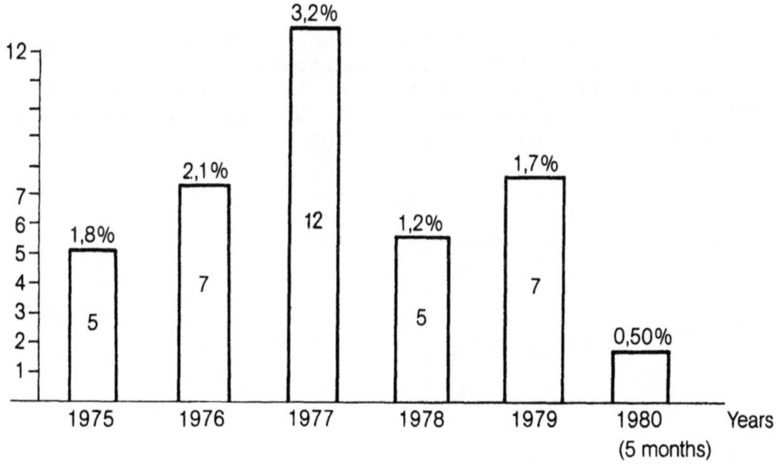

Fig. 1. Incidence of failure of the sterilizer

*Hôpital Laënnec - 35, rue Paul Bert, 44 100 Nantes, France

Standard median sternotomy incisions were made; the sternum was divided with an electric oscillating saw. Bleeding from the bone marrow was controlled by application of bone wax. Following correction of cardiac disease, the edges of the divided sternum were approximated by six or eight gauge steel wires. Soft tissues were approximated with interrupted nylon sutures and, for 2 years, by interrupted "resorbable" sutures.

Infecting Organisms

As shown in Table 1, *Staphylococcus aureus* or *albus* are the most common germs. But gram-negative germs are nonidentified with an incidence of 50%. Besides, isolation of multiple organisms is not exceptional.

Table 1. Bacteriological data (26 cases)

	No. of cases
Staphylo	9
Serratia	6
Enterobacter	3
Klebsiella	2
Strepto	2
Pyocyanic	1
Pneumocoq	1
Several germs	3
No germ	4

Operative Procedures

The incidence of sepsis connected with operation procedure is reported in Table 2. A high frequency of infective complication is observed in cardiac diseases requiring emergency operation, like surgery of complicated myocardial infarction, pulmonary embolism, aortic dissection, or surgery for thoracic and cardiovascular traumata.

Table 2. Operative procedure

Valvular replacement	18/856 = 2.1%
Congenital cardiovascular diseases	9/614 = 1.5%
Coronary bypasses	5/380 = 1.3%
Surgery of complicated myocardial infarction	3/ 79 = 3.8%
Miscellaneous	2/ 56 = 3.6%

Results

We used the method of treatment described by Bryant and Spencer with mediastinal irrigation. After a careful debridement of sternum and mediastinal tissues, the chest is closed on an irrigation-drainage system. Sternum soft tissues and skin are reapproximated in a single layer with 10 or 12 nylon sutures which are unstitched 3 weeks later. Thus no foreign bodies are left in the sterno-mediastinal space. The mediastinal space is washed by a povidone-iodine solution during 2 or 3 weeks; then, when liquid drainage is clean, washing is performed by a specific antibiotic solution during 15 days. Bacteriological controls are made in the drainage solution. Mediastinal tubes are gradually removed. Recovery is obtained in 2 or 3 months.

Sometimes sternal dehiscence reappears and the wound must be widely opened. Gauze packs irrigated with povidone-iodine, then smeared with vaseline, are inserted to attend granulations when mediastinal space and sternum edges are clean. The sternum can be reapproximated on a mediastinal drainage in order to reduce the length of recovery.

Our results are reported in Table 3. Death of 12 of the 14 patients was caused by septicopyemia complications in a period of less than 30 days (mean, 10 days). In two cases, late death was due to chronical sternal osteomyelitis. Among 23 healed cases, eight required iterative operations, the sternum could not be reapproximated and the chest wound was treated by gauze packing. In these cases, chronic cartilaginous infection or sinus tracts are very frequent (3/4 cases).

Table 3. Results

- 37 cases
- 14 deaths (38%)
  - 12 <1 month
  - 2 late (8-12 months)
- 27 good results
  - 15 by one-time surgery
  - 8 by two-time or multiple surgery
  - 4 cases of recurrent sternitis

Discussion

Predisposing Factors

Table 4 shows the different predisposing factors noted in our patients. It is very difficult to assert these factors have a significative incidence (8, 11). Nevertheless, we suggest there are particular circumstances or a particular atmosphere. We can recapitulate these circumstances in two groups. First of all, some patients are previously infected or very predisposed to infection, some have endocarditis or abdominal sepsis, or patients stay a long time in intensive care units with many catheters and a very succinct corporeal hygiene. Moreover, some patients have variations in their resistance to infection: patients with severely impaired myocardial function, defects in phagocytic function, and depression of host-defense mechanism due to bypass as was demonstrated by Silva et al. (10) and Kaplan et al. (7).

Table 4. Prejudicing factors

	No. of cases
Infective context	6 (16%)
Acute endocarditis = 3	
Septicaemia = 1	
Abdominal sepsis = 2	
Emergency surgery	9 (24%)
Weakened patients	19 (51%)
Long time of bypass (120')	8 (22%)
Long stay in intensive care unit	10 (27%)

Clinical Features

Sterno-mediastinal infection is clinically well known. Leukocytosis and fever are obvious signs of infection (3) but sometimes these symptoms are lacking (1, 3, 4, 6). Drainage from the sternal wound and some palpable movement of the sternal halves are late symptoms (6, 11) We shall emphasize some premonitory signs which are constant in our experience, such as abnormal cough and thoracic pain increased by moving arms. Bacteriological studies of drains and catheters are often unsuccessful or discordant.

Treatment and Prophylaxis

An early diagnosis is necessary. Intensive surgical therapy should be made. We would like to emphasize that the successful resolution of sepsis rests upon the surgeon's willingness to have an aggressive approach toward infection. Mediastinal irrigation as described by Bryant et al. (2), using povidone-iodine solution as reported by Thurer et al. (12), is the most common way of therapy. Sternal osteomyelitis is a very serious complication (two deaths in our series) as noted by Hehrlein et al. (5) and Wray et al. (14). In these cases, total excision of the sternum and transposition of the greater omentum may be a good stratagem in managing these cases (9).

We also would like to insist on prophylaxis [Vilde (13)]. Particular preparation of the skin, severe asepsis in operating room and especially in intensive care unit are very important. Prophylactic antibiotherapy is very useful. Antibiotics should be used before, during, and just a few days after operation, up to removal of drains and catheters.

For 1 year, we have applied these rules: skin is prepared the day before the operation with povidone-iodine solution; antibiotic used is cefamandole; 1.50 g of this solution are injected 3 h before induction; the same dose is reinjected at induction and repeated every 6 h until the time when chest tubes and catheters are removed. During this period, we observed only two cases of sterno-mediastinitis among 404 bypasses, an incidence of 0.5%.

Summary

Thirty-seven patients among 1985 bypasses had sterno-mediastinitis infection (1.9%). All of them are treated by mediastinal irrigation-drainage system using povidone-iodine solution. Fourteen patients (38%) died; 23 patients healed, eight of them required iterative operation. A better prophylaxis found on skin prepared by povidone-iodine and prophylactic antibiotherapy with cefamandole decreased infective complication incidence from 2% to 0.5%.

References

1. Brown AH, Braimbridge MV, Panagopoulos P, Sabar EF (1969) The complications of median sternotomy. J Thorac Cardiovasc Surg 58/2:189-197
2. Bryant LR, Spencer FC, Trinkle JL (1969) Treatment of median sternotomy infection by mediastinal irrigation with an antibiotic solution. Ann Surg 169/6: 914-920
3. Engelman RM, Williams CD, Gouge TH, Chase RM, Falk EA, Boyd AD, Reed GE (1973) Mediastinitis following open-heart surgery. Arch Surg 107/5:772-778
4. Fabiani JN, Lemerle JP, Beres J, Aubert M, Vilain R (1976) Traitement des sternites et sterno-chondrites après chirurgie cardiaque. A propos de 50 observations. Ann Chir Thorac Cardiovasc 15/4:297-304
5. Hehrlein F, Herrmann H, Kraus J (1972) Complications of median sternotomy in cardiovascular surgery. J Cardiovasc Surg 13/5:390-393
6. Jimenez-Martinez M, Arguero-Sanchez R, Perez-Alvarez JJ, Mina-Castaneda P (1970) Anterior mediastinitis as a complication of median sternotomy incisions: diagnostic and surgical considerations. Surgery 67/6:929-934
7. Kaplan EL, Castaneda AR, Ayoub EM (1968) Effects of cardiopulmonary bypass on the phagocytic and bacteriological capacities of poly-morphonuclear leukocytes. Circulation [Suppl 2] 37:158
8. Lecompte Y, Gilbert C, Hemmer C, Manuel C, Bure A, Hazan E (1975) Les complications infectieuses de la chirurgie cardiaque: facteurs de risque, définition et classification des manifestations cliniques. In: L'infection en réanimation, actualités et perspectives. Arnette (Problèmes actuels de réanimation, p 131-151)
9. Lee AB, Schimert G, Shatkin S (1976) Total excision of the sternum and thoracic pedicle transposition of the greater omentum; useful strategems in managing severe mediastinal infection following open-heart surgery. Surgery 80/4:433-436
10. Silva J, Hoeksema H, Fekety FR (1974) Transient defects in phagocytic functions during cardiopulmonary bypass. J Thorac Cardiovasc Surg 67/2:175-183
11. Soyer R, Brunet A, Menasche P (1977) L'infection en chirurgie cardiaque. Coeur 8/2:177-198
12. Thurer RJ, Bognolo D, Vargas A, Isch JH, Kaiser A (1974) The management of mediastinal infection following cardiac surgery, an experience utilizing continuous irrigation with povidone-iodine. J Thorac Cardiovasc Surg 68:962
13. Vilde JL, Baudet M (1977) La prophylaxie de l'infection en chirurgie cardiovasculaire. Coeur 8/2:199-204
14. Wray TM, Bryant RE, Killen DA (1973) Sternal osteo-myelitis and costochondritis after median sternotomy. J Thorac Cardiovasc Surg 65/2:227-233

Aneurysm of Ascending Aorta and Aortic Valve Insufficiency: Surgical Treatment

N. Spampinato, E. Covino, P. Oliviero, P. Stassano, and L. B. Tecchia*

Ascending aorta aneurysms with aortic valvular insufficiency is a severe and invaliding disease. Prognosis is very poor and natural history extremely short. Cardiac decompensation, dissection, and rupture are the most common complications (1). Surgical therapy consists in replacing the aortic valve and in treating the aortic dilatation by various techniques. Results have been satisfactory with acceptable hospital mortality and good long-term follow-up (2-4).

Controversies have been raised over the more suitable surgical technique in treating the aneurysm: resection followed by aortoplasty, external grafting, entire replacement of the ascending aorta, saving the coronary ostia, or using a valvulated conduit with coronary reimplantation or grafting have been advocated. We present our experience in the treatment of ascending aorta aneurysm and valvular regurgitation analyzing the various techniques employed and the results obtained.

Materials and Methods

Between 1976 and 1979, 215 aortic valve replacements have been performed in our department. In 16 cases (7.4%), an aneurysmatic dilatation of the ascending aorta was present, requiring appropriate treatment. There were 14 males and two females, ranging in age from 37 to 67 years (mean age 46.7 years). In the majority of the cases, the etiology was arteriosclerotic (14 cases) with one luetic patient and one with Marfan-like lesions. All underwent aortic valve replacement, seven receiving mechanical valves and 9 (more recently) bioprosthesis. In five cases, resection of saccular aneurysm was performed, followed by aortoplasty with low-porosity Dacron cloth (Fig. 1c); in eight cases, the entire ascending aorta was replaced by a woven Dacron graft (Fig. 1d). In three cases, a fusiform aneurysm was partially resected and an external grafting was performed, wrapping the ascending aorta with teflon fabric or felt (Fig. 1a,b). A valvulated conduit was never used. To limit the amount of diseased wall left in situ, the proximal suture line was shaped in such a way as to leave only two tongues of aortic wall corresponding to the coronary ostia. The functional and anatomical result of this technique can be compared to the coronary reimplantation technique using an aortic cuff.

Cardiopulmonary bypass was instituted through a femoral arterial line and a single right atrial cannula. In four cases, due to the limited distal extension of the aneurysm, aortic cannulation was performed. In nine cases of extremely large aneurysm with suspicion of ster-

*Department of Cardiac Surgery, 2nd Policlinico, Via S. Pansini, 5 Naples 80131, Italy

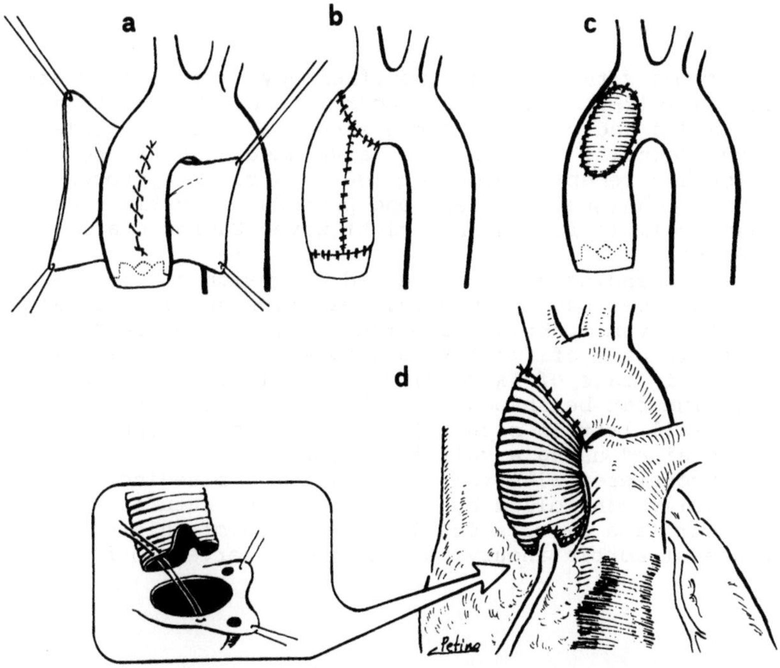

Fig. 1a-d. Operative techniques. a,b External grafting. c Aortoplasty after resection of saccular aneurysm. d Replacement of the ascending aorta by a woven Dacron graft. A small rim of aortic wall circumscribing the coronary ostia is preserved

nal erosion, a different technique of perfusion was employed: cardiopulmonary bypass was instituted by means of femorofemoral cannulation, full flow was obtained, and the patient was cooled to 25°C; then, after circulatory arrest and exsanguination, the median sternotomy was made with the aneurysm collapsed. The opening of the sternum and the surgical dissection under these conditions appeared safe.

Myocardial protection was achieved by direct injection into the coronary arteries of cold hyperkalemic cardioplegic solution: aorta cross-clamping time ranged between 40 and 117 min (mean 71 min). In the early cases (five), only moderate general hypothermia was used and the operation was carried out under anoxic arrest.

Results

There was one hospital death (6.25%) due to low cardiac output; this patient was not protected by cardioplegia. Postoperative bleeding was contained and no reoperations were needed.

Follow-up extended from 2 to 45 months (mean 13.5 months). There were three late deaths: one related to the operation (prosthetic endocarditis) and two unrelated (one patient died of carcinoma of the prostata and one of chronic respiratory failure). All the surviving patients are doing well, being in functional class I or II. No signs of recurrent aneurysm has been noted.

Discussion

Ascending aorta aneurysms with valvular insufficiency have been treated by various techniques (2-6). Danger of recurrence of the aneurysm has been emphasized and a radical approach has been advocated. Replacement of the entire ascending aorta with a valvulated conduit and coronary reimplantation has recently been considered a safer approach (4, 7). However, this technique requires long periods of aortic cross-clamping and coronary reimplantation in a tight woven Dacron graft can be cumbersome (4, 8, 9).

In our experience, depending on the size and extension of the aneurysm, different techniques have been used: resection and aortoplasty in case of saccular aneurysm, partial resection followed by wrapping with prosthetic cloth in case of fusiform aneurysm, entire replacement of the ascending aorta in case of large dilatation. In this last event, the proxymal suture line can be shaped in such a way as to minimize the amount of aortic wall left in situ (1). The functional result is comparable to that obtained using a valvulated conduit. No technical problems have been encountered with this procedure and bleeding from the suture line is easily controlled by reinforcing the sutures with teflon felt strips. Our late results confirm the value of this approach: no recurrence of aortic aneurysms has been observed so far.

Summary

Between 1976 and 1979, in the Department of Cardiac Surgery, University of Naples, 2nd Medical School, 16 cases of aneurysm of ascending aorta and aortic valve insufficiency were operated upon, out of 215 aortic valve replacements (7.4%). Fourteen male and two female patients ranging in age from 37 to 67 years (mean age 46.7 years) underwent aortic valve replacement associated with: external grafting of the ascending aorta in three cases, aortoplasty in five, and replacement of the ascending aorta with a tubular graft in eight.

Cardiopulmonary bypass was instituted by routine atrial and aortic, or femoral cannulation in seven cases, and by femorofemoral cannulation in nine. This peripheral route was preferred when a large aneurysm was suspected; the cardiopulmonary bypass in these cases was instituted before the sternotomy, general hypothermia was induced, and surgical dissection performed under circulatory arrest.

There was one hospital death, related to the operation, and three late deaths, two of which for causes not related to the operation. At the follow-up which extended from 2 to 45 months (mean 13.5 months), the surviving patients were doing well.

Resection of a saccular aneurysm and aortoplasty was done in the earlier cases; more recently, replacement of the ascending aorta with a tubular graft is preferred. If the aortic dilatation is not severe but the aortic wall is thin, external grafting with a teflon fabric is employed. A valvular conduit with coronary reimplantation has not been used. In fact, the proximal end of the tubular graft was shaped in such a way as to leave only two small segments of aortic wall corresponding to the coronary ostia, realizing thus a sort of partial reimplantation. No evidence of recurrent aneurysm has been found so far. This approach has been considered satisfactory.

References

1. Cooley DA, De Bakey ME (1952) Surgical considerations of intrathoracic aneurysms of the aorta and great vessels. Ann Surg 135:660-680
2. Miller CD, Stinson EB, Oyer PE, Moreno-Cabral RJ, Reitz BA, Rossiten SJ, Shumway NE (1980) Concomitant resection of ascending aortic aneurysm and replacement of the aortic valve. J Thorac Cardiovasc Surg 79:338-401
3. Singh MP, Bentall HH (1972) Complete replacement of the ascending aorta and the aortic valve for the treatment of aortic aneurysm. J Thorac Cardiovasc Surg 63: 218-225
4. Kouchoukos NT, Karp RB, Lell WA (1977) Replacement of the ascending aorta and aortic valve with a composite graft. Results in 25 patients. Ann Thorac Surg 24: 140-148
5. Nasrallah AT, Cooley DA, Goussous Y, Hallman GL, Lufschanowski R, Leachman RD (1975) Surgical experience in patients with Marfan syndrome, ascending aortic aneurysm, and aortic regurgitation. Am J Cardiol 36:338-341
6. Liddicoat JE, Bekassy SM, Rubio PA, Noon GP, De Bakey ME (1975) Ascending aortic aneurysms. Review of 100 consecutive cases. Circulation [Suppl 1] 51,52:202-209
7. Helseth HK, Haglin JJ, Stenlund RR, Peterson CR (1974) Evaluation of composite graft replacement of the aortic root and ascending aorta. Ann Thorac Surg 18: 138-141
8. McReady RA, Pluth JR (1979) Surgical treatment of ascending aortic aneurysms associated with aortic valve insufficiency. Ann Thorac Surg 28:307-316
9. Mayer JE, Lindsay WG, Wang Y, Jorgensen CR, Nicoloff DM (1978) Composite replacement of the aortic valve and ascending aorta. J Thorac Cardiovasc Surg 76:816-823

Stimulation of Myocardial Alpha-Adrenoceptors Mediating Positive Inotropic Effect in Human Atrial Preparations by Adrenaline and Dopamine

J. Wagner*, H. J. Schümann*, A. Knorr*, N. Rohm**, and J. Chr. Reidemeister**

Introduction

There is no longer any doubt about the presence of α-adrenoceptors in the heart of most mammalian species (10). In contrast to stimulation of β-adrenoceptors, that of α-adrenoceptors causes a positive inotropic but no chronotropic effect (10). Also in the anaesthetized intact cat, cardiac α-adrenoceptors have been demonstrated, stimulation of which also caused a positive inotropic effect – expressed as increase of left ventricular dp/dt_{max} – without increase in heart rate (12). The mechanism underlying stimulation of cardiac α-adrenoceptors is different from that of stimulation of β-adrenoceptors. Whereas stimulation of β-adrenoceptors is closely related to activation of myocardial adenylate cyclase (9) yielding to an elevation of cyclic AMP, that of α-adrenoceptors is not (2, 6, 7). Moreover, there is evidence that the positive inotropic effect induced by stimulation of α-adrenoceptors is strongly dependent on measures which influence the transsarcolemmal influx of Ca^{2+} as for instance organic calcium antagonists (3) as well as alteration of the extracellular calcium content or carbachol, for example (11). In isolated rabbit papillary muscle, these α-adrenoceptors have been found to be stimulated by the hormone adrenaline but not by the transmitter noradrenaline (4). This observation already has been obtained in the anaesthetized cat (12). Recently, myocardial α-adrenoceptors have been found also in human atrial preparations (8). Since these adrenoceptors were detected by use of phenylephrine, it was the aim of the present investigation to decide whether or not the endogenous catecholamines stimulate myocardial α-adrenoceptors also in the human heart.

Materials and Methods

From patients who underwent open-heart surgery (defects of atrial or ventricular septum, valvular pulmonary stenosis, Fallot's tetralogy, subvalvular aortic stenosis, atrioventricular canal, coronary artery disease; mean age of the patients: 17.2 ± 2.0 years; N = 38), right atrial appendage muscle strips were obtained. None of the patients had been treated with cardiac glycosides at least 3 weeks before operation. The premedication consisted of atropine, promethazine, diazepam, and droperidol. During the operation, the body temperature was kept between 28 and 30°C.

*Pharmakologisches Institut, Universitätsklinikum Essen, Hufelandstr. 55, D-4300 Essen 1
**Pharmakologisches Institut, Abt. für Thorax- und Kardiovaskuläre Chirurgie, Hufelandstr. 55, D-4300 Essen 1

The preparations immediately were transferred to oxygenated Krebs-Henseleit solution at room temperature. Thereafter, strips of a length of about 3 mm and a maximal diameter of 1 mm were cut. The preparations were suspended at a preload of 0.5 g at 37°C in Krebs-Henseleit solution. The force of contraction – expressed as g/g dry weight – was recorded isometrically by strain gauges. The stimulation frequency was kept at 1 beat/s, 3-30 ms duration and a voltage of 20% above threshold (8.8 ± 0.9 V, N = 80). For the experimental procedure, see Schümann et al. (8). Drugs used: (-)-noradrenaline base, (-)-adrenaline base, dopamine HCl, (±)-pindolol base, phentolamine HCl.

Results

The concentration-response curve of noradrenaline under control conditions is shown in Figure 1. The corresponding -log EC_{50} calculated from this curve amounts to 6.55 (Table 1). The β-adrenolytic drug pindolol shifts the concentration-response curve to the right, thus significantly reducing the -log EC_{50} by about 1 log unit to 5.59 (Table 1). When in addition the α-adrenoceptors are blocked by phentolamine no further shift of the concentration-response curve to the right occurs. The -log EC_{50} of 5.53 is not significantly different from that after block of the β-adrenoceptors, indicating that noradrenaline does not stimulate α-adrenoceptors (Table 1). In contrast, the concentration-response curve of adrenaline is displaced to the right not only by pindolol but in addition by phentolamine (Fig. 2). The corresponding -log EC_{50} of 7.39 is significantly decreased by phentolamine to 5.82 (Table 1). The third amine, dopamine, is influenced by both adrenolytic drugs in a comparable manner (Fig. 3): both pindolol and phentolamine decrease significantly the -log EC_{50} from 5.26 to 4.70 and to 4.17, respectively (Table 1).

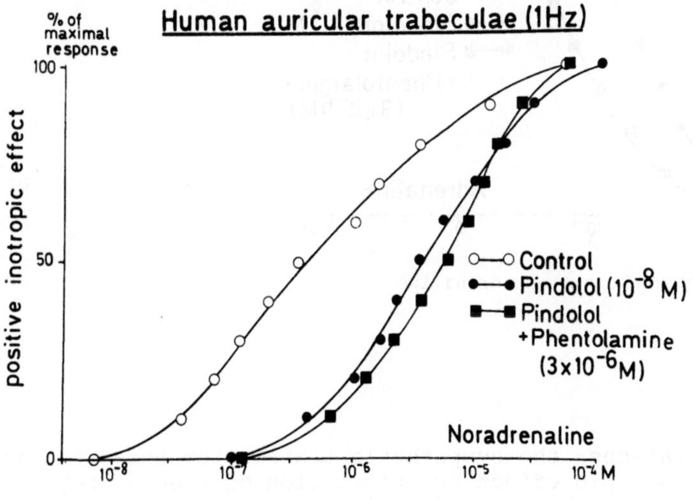

Fig. 1. Concentration-response curve of noradrenaline

Table 1. Human atrial strip preparations. Negative log EC_{50} values ($-\log EC_{50}$) for the positive inotropic effects of noradrenaline (NA), adrenaline (A), and dopamine (DA). (Given are means ± S.E.M., number of experiments in parentheses)

	None	Pindolol 10^{-8}M	Pindolol + phentolamine, 3×10^{-6}M
NA	6.55 ± 0.08 (7)	5.59 ± 0.19[a] (6)	5.53 ± 0.19[c] (9)
A	7.39 ± 0.1 (9)	6.29 ± 0.08[a] (9)	5.82 ± 0.11[b] (8)
DA	5.26 ± 0.04 (4)	4.70 ± 0.06[a] (6)	4.17 ± 0.21[b] (5)

[a] $p < 0.005$ compared with the control = none

[b] $p < 0.005$ vs pindolol

[c] Not significantly different from the value in the presence of pindolol

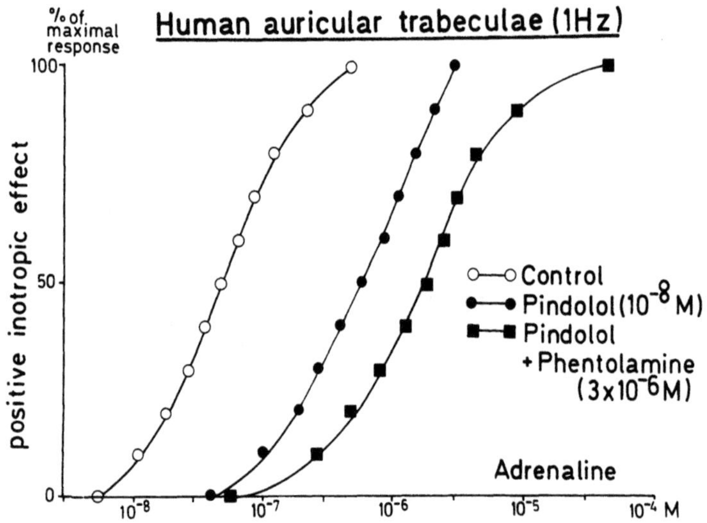

Fig. 2. Concentration-response curve of adrenaline

Discussion

In human atrial preparations, the sympathetic transmitter noradrenaline causes its positive inotropic effect by stimulation of β-adrenoceptors only. On the other hand, the hormone adrenaline acts by stimulating both β- as well as α-adrenoceptors. This observation is in accordance with those obtained from the papillary muscle of the rabbit (5) and from the heart of the anaesthetized cat (12). From these observations, speculations about the function of α-adrenoceptors can be made. The transmitter, secreted from nerve endings, is responsible for maintain-

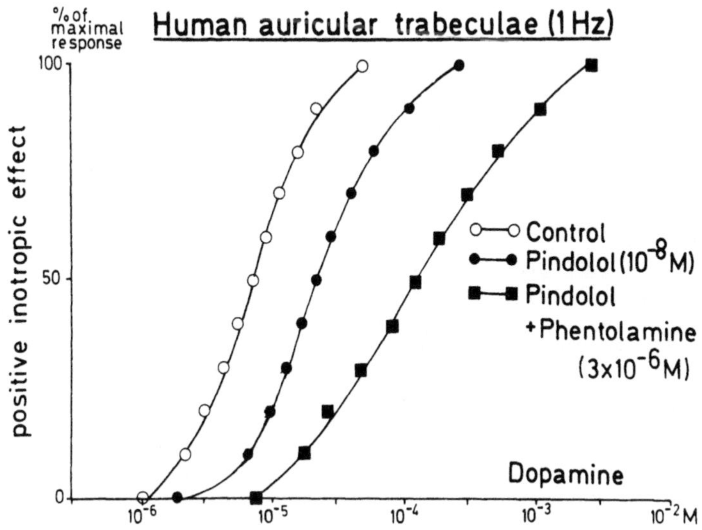

Fig. 3. Concentration-response curve of dopamine

ing the sympathetic drive of the heart by stimulating β-adrenoceptors. In situations of shock when the stores of energy-rich phosphates have been exhausted, α-adrenoceptors might get functional importance in maintaining a rest of contractility without consuming a lot of energy. In this case, the hormone adrenaline is liberated to a reasonable extent which is able to stimulate α-adrenoceptors. Recently, Baumann et al. (1) presented experiments which show a strong decrease of the susceptibility of β-adrenoceptors in non-ischaemic regions of the guinea pig heart after experimental infarction. Since under these conditions either the number of β-adrenoceptors or their sensitivity has been found to be diminished, it is very likely that α-adrenoceptors as mediators of a positive inotropic effect prevail. These results are in favour of a life-saving function of cardiac α-adrenoceptors.

Dopamine stimulated both β- as well as α-adrenoceptors to a comparable degree which can be derived from the -log EC_{50} values: Block of β-adrenoceptors lowered the -log EC_{50} by 0.56 log units, additional block of the α-adrenoceptors by further 0.53 log units. Therefore, the beneficial effect of dopamine in man in the treatment of shock might be attributed to its ability to stimulate cardiac α-adrenoceptors. It is worthwhile to mention that dopamine may exert a positive inotropic effect in those patients who have been treated beforehand with β-adrenolytic agents.

Summary

In human isolated right atrial appendage strip preparations, the cardiostimulating effect exerted by endogenous catecholamines noradrenaline, adrenaline, and dopamine was characterized.

1. Noradrenaline caused its positive inotropic effect by stimulation of β-adrenoceptors only.
2. Adrenaline and dopamine stimulate both adrenoceptors, β- as well as α-adrenoceptors.

References

1. Baumann G, Rieß G, Erhard W-D, Felix SB, Blömer H (1980) Reduzierte β-adrenerge Ansprechbarkeit im nicht ischämischen Myokard nach experimentellem Herzinfarkt. Z Kardiol [Suppl 124] 69
2. Benfey BG (1971) Lack of relationship between myocardial cyclic AMP concentrations and inotropic effect of sympathomimetic amines. Br J Pharmacol 43:757-763
3. Endoh M, Wagner J, Schümann HJ (1975) Influence of temperature on the positive inotropic effects mediated by α- and β-adrenoceptors in the isolated rabbit papillary muscle. Naunyn Schmiedebergs Arch Pharmacol 287:61-72
4. Endoh M, Schümann HJ, Krappitz N, Hillen B (1976) α-adrenoceptors mediating positive inotropic effects on the ventricular myocardium: Some aspects of structure-activity relationship of sympathomimetic amines. Jpn J Pharmacol 26:179-190
5. Schümann HJ, Endoh M, Wagner J (1974) Positive inotropic effect of phenylephrine in the isolated rabbit papillary muscle mediated both by α- and β-adrenoceptors. Naunyn Schmiedebergs Arch Pharmacol 284:133-148
6. Schümann HJ, Endoh M, Brodde O-E (1975) The time course of the effects of β- and α-adrenoceptor stimulation by isoprenaline and methoxamine on the contractile force and cAMP-level of the isolated rabbit papillary muscle. Naunyn Schmiedebergs Arch Pharmacol 289:291-302
7. Schümann HJ, Motomura S, Endoh M, Brodde O-E (1977) Comparison of the mechanisms underlying the positive inotropic actions of dopamine, adrenaline, and isoprenaline on the isolated rabbit papillary muscle. Naunyn Schmiedebergs Arch Pharmacol 297:257-267
8. Schümann HJ, Wagner J, Knorr A, Reidemeister JC, Sadony V, Schramm G (1978) Demonstration in human atrial preparations of α-adrenoceptors mediating positive inotropic effects. Naunyn Schmiedebergs Arch Pharmacol 302:333-336
9. Sutherland GW, Robinson GA, Butcher RW (1968) Some aspects of the biological role of adenosine 3', 5'-monophosphate (cyclic AMP). Circulation 37:279-306
10. Wagner J, Brodde O-E (1978) On the presence and distribution of α-adrenoceptors in the heart of various mammalian species. Naunyn Schmiedebergs Arch Pharmacol 302:239-254
11. Wagner J, Schümann HJ (1979) Different mechanism underlying the stimulation of myocardial α- and β-adrenoceptors. Life Sci 24:2045-2052
12. Wagner J, Rodrigues-Pereira E, Schümann HJ (1975) Alpha-Adrenozeptoren im Ventrikelmyokard der Katze. Verh Dtsch Ges Kreislaufforsch 41:226-229

Session VII Cardiovascular Surgery

Aortic Dissections

Chairman: Ph. Blondeau, Paris; Co-Chairman: A. Senn, Berne

Computed Tomographic Evaluation of Aortic Dissections

J.C.Couffinhal, R.A.Parienty, F.Michel, O.Nussaume, and B.Andreassian*

Aortic dissection continues to pose a real diagnostic problem as well as a therapeutic challenge; this condition being characterised by a high mortality rate at each step of its process. Often the surgeon forgets that he sees only patients already diagnosed.

To increase the survival rate, three kinds of measures are necessary:

1. Effective diagnosis at the emergency state must be considerably improved.
2. A review of therapeutic techniques and indications must be done.
4. Lastly, we must find a reliable and convenient monitoring procedure.

In our experience, computed tomography (CT) is perhaps an answer to at least two of these questions (1 and 3). Our goal was to identify the CT semeiological basis of the disease and to establish the most efficient use of the machine.

Material and Methods

In our department over the last 12 months, we have dealt with 11 aortic dissections (AD) of all sorts. Nine of them were investigated by using aortography together with CT. Two underwent aortographic screening only because of the urgent and precarious state of the patient. CT was carried out with a third-generation CT scanner. Scan time was 4 to 10 s. The shortest interval between two consecutive scans was 50 s.

CT techniques must always include slices of all of the aorta before and after the injection of contrast. In our earlier experience, contrast injection was performed by iv drip. For our last patient, we used dynamic scan: sequential scans are performed at the same anatomic level selected on a first series without contrast.

Results

Taking nine cases, our results are the following: In eight cases, CT diagnosis was positive; in the ninth, CT showed an abnormal aorta. On two occasions, arteriography was negative despite an obvious clinical finding; in these instances, CT confirmed the diagnosis without doubt.

*Department of Thoracic and Cardio-vascular Surgery. Hôpital Universitaire Beaujon 92110 Clichy, France

In all our cases of AD, we never found a normal aorta at CT examination. In eight cases, the false lumen appears whether patent or not; the intimal flap was visible on three occasions.

Discussion

In typical and evocative cases, aortography still remains the first and best procedure. With questionable cases there is room for preliminary noninvasive examinations which may lead to aortography. This is the same problem with typical cases with negative aortography. These methods are ultrasound and CT.

Ultrasound has been used in this disease since 1972 and is without substitute for the study of pericardium and aortic valve, but still, even in the M-mode or bidimensional, there currently exist too many false positive and negative cases to be able to determine with certitude the diagnosis of AD. Even though it is easily performed, its major inconvenience is that it only shows the aortic root.

CT – when enhanced by angio and dynamic scan techniques – exposes the whole of the aorta and this allows diagnosis of all forms of AD; it also shows pleura and mediastinum illustrating the eventual extent of the disease (hemopericardium).

The principal CT signs are the following: Visualization of parietal flap and visualization of a false lumen whether patent or not (CT numbers can indicate gain in density revealing a not obviously patent lumen). Finally, the modification of the size and form of the aorta may be an encouraging sign.

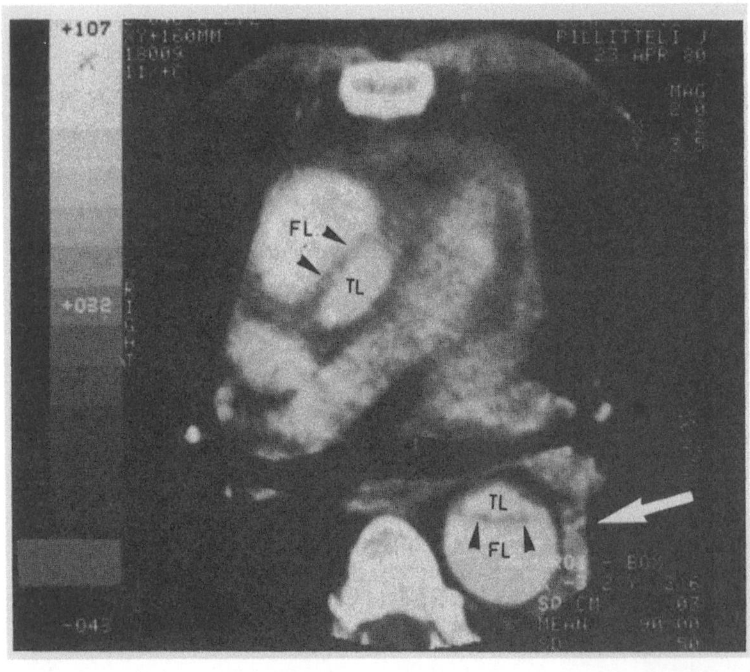

Fig. 1. Acute aortic dissection; angioscan. *FL*, false lumen; *TL*, true lumen

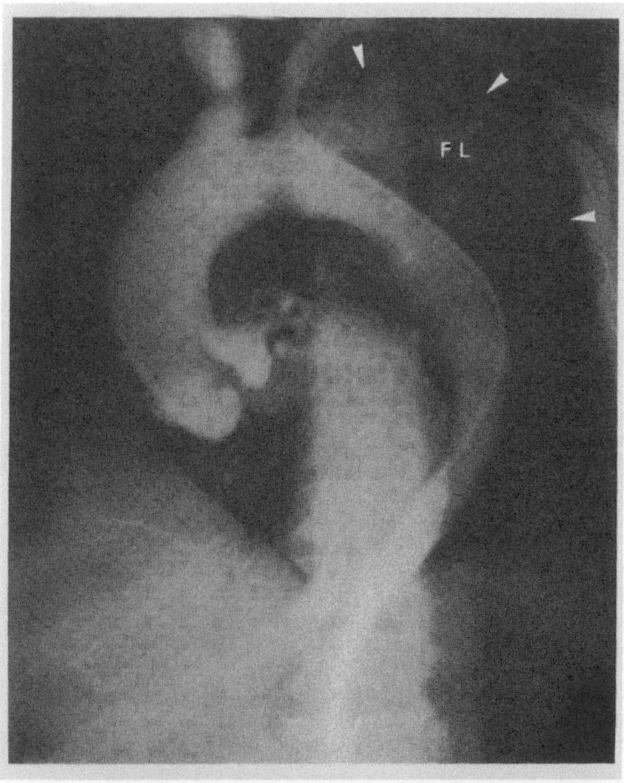

a

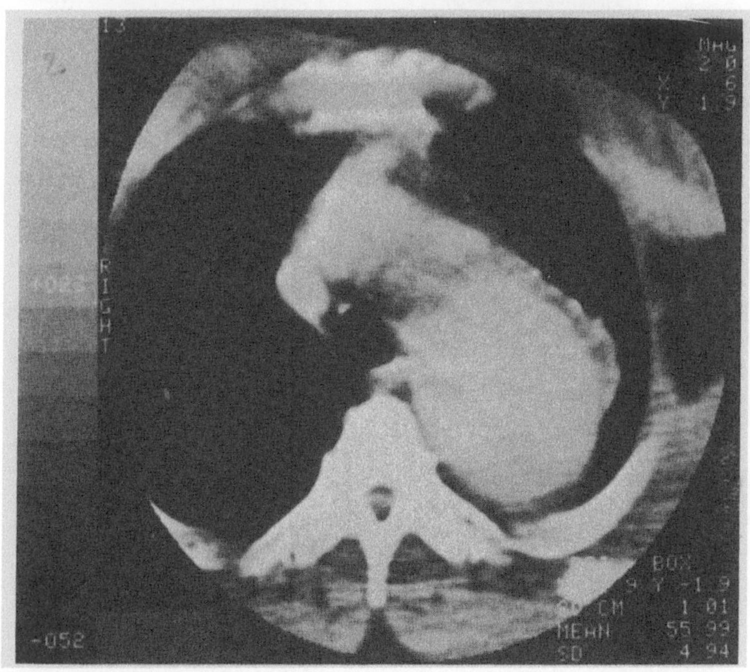

Fig. 2. a Chronic type III AD with ectasic evolution. On aortography, the false lumen appears thrombosed. b The angioscan shows a patent and immediately opacified false lumen

Some pitfalls must be pointed out: A mural thrombus in a fusiform aneurysm may mimic a thrombosed false lumen; it is not always so easy to distinguish an aneurysm from an AD. A kinked arterial trunk or some ectopic intercostal vein may appear on a CT slice located close by the aortic arch; we have seen this misleading pattern once. The intimal flap may be visible only after a fast bolus of contrast material and indistinct during a too slow iv drip because of partial volume averaging (orientation and thickness of the slice with regard to the flap). Streaks may create false channel appearance; we must recognise this artefact by varying the window setting.

Follow-up

After medical or surgical treatment, frequent systematic controls are necessary to assess the evolutivity of the disease. We must remember that 20% of the patients will die as a result of the initial disease in spite of the treatment.

As regards therapeutic evolution, different points have to be made clear: Is the false lumen patent or not and is it therefore likely to become ectasic? Is there a new spread of the disease, for instance a retrograding process transforming a type III AD (according to Debakey classification) into a type I, which change the nature of the treatment? What is the endoluminal and anastomotic state of a graft (false aneurysm)?

In our experience, CT answers all these questions, it represents a reliable reproducible, noninvasive monitoring procedure, best deciding for a new aortographic investigation, and eventually a secondary surgical repair.

Conclusions

In our experience, CT seems a reliable procedure in the evaluation of AD; it contributes to a better diagnostic approach and improves therapeutic monitoring, all of which could result in a decrease of initial and secondary deaths.

Surgical Treatment of Aneurysm of the Thoracic Aorta

E. Struck, J. Laas, H. Meisner, P. Schmidt-Habelmann, and F. Sebening*

A literature review of survival rates after surgical treatment of thoracic aortic aneurysms shows rather different results. The majority of studies with a great number of cases report a mortality rate between 30% and 40% (2, 5, 7). Besides the surgical technique the course of the thoracic aneurysms is significantly influenced by special risk factors. These risks are the general condition of the patient, the range of dissection, the localization of the intima lesion, the time course of the disease, as well as aneurysm-specific complications and therapeutic strategy. Especially within the first 4 days after dissection – that is the time of highest mortality rate – a fatal complication in the spontaneous course of the dissecting aortic aneurysm can prohibit successful surgical therapy. Therefore, the classification of aortic aneurysms by Anagnostopoulos et al. (1), in which complications and risk factors of the dissection are taken into account, should be used for comparison of results. A_1 and B_1 aneurysms are anterior and/or posterior aneurysms with complications, whereas A_2 and B_2 aneurysms are those without complicating factors.

In our institution, so far, we have operated upon 100 patients with aneurysms of the thoracic aorta, 97 of whom were evaluated in this study. Age of patients was in a range of 9 to 67 years. The largest group of patients, 26 of the 97 patients, was 40-49 years of age when undergoing surgery; 25.7% of all patients were female. According to the surgical technique used (Fig. 1) the patients were divided into seven groups:

1) Plastic correction of the ascending aorta (N = 13),
2) replacement of the ascending aorta (N = 9),
3) replacement of the ascending aorta and aortic valve (N = 14),
4) aneurysm correction using a conduit with implantation of the coronary arteries (N = 29),
5) aneurysm correction with revascularization of the supraaortic branches (N = 6),
6) replacement of the descending thoracic aorta (N = 20), and
7) wrapping of the ascending or descending thoracic aorta using a vascular prosthesis (N = 6).

Mortality was especially high in patients with isolated replacement of the ascending aorta (66.8%) and in patients with aneurysm correction including revascularization of supraaortic branches (83.3%). Mortality in patients with aortic conduit with coronary implantation was 41.7%, whereas separate replacement of the ascending aorta and aortic valve had a mortality of only 7.1%. Plastic correction of an aneurysm of the ascending aorta had a mortality of 7.7%. None of the patients with wrapping of the aorta with a vascular prosthesis died.

*German Heart Center Munich, Division of Cardiovascular Surgery, Lothstr. 11, D-8000 Muenchen 2

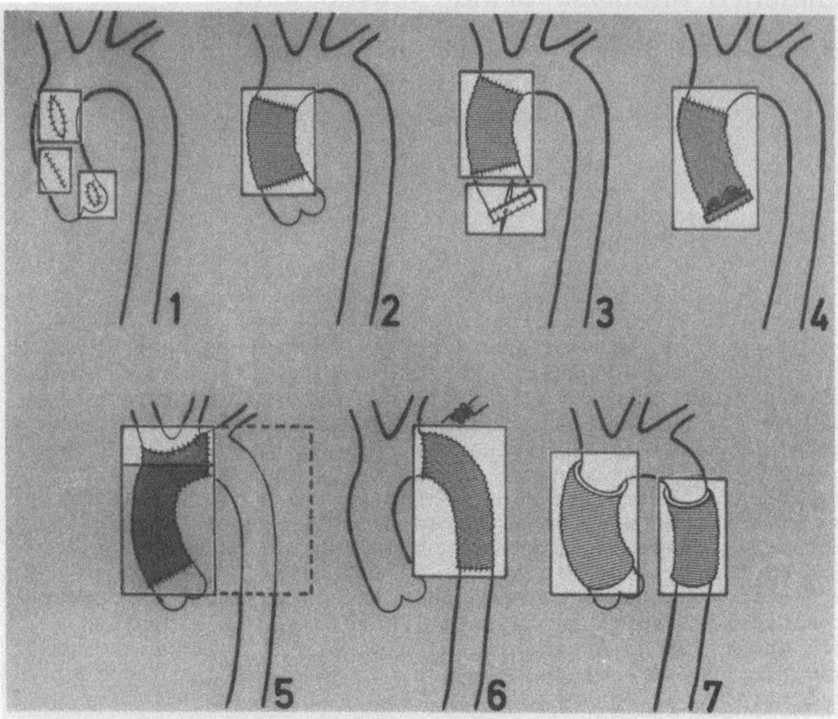

Fig. 1. Schematic drawing of surgical techniques for correction of thoracic aortic aneurysm

Using the Anagnostopoulos' classification (1) we saw the best results in A_2 and B_2 aneurysms; all patients in these two groups survived. Patients with A_1 aneurysms had a mortality of 37%; all eight patients operated upon for a B_2 aneurysm died. Four patients in our series had C aneurysms and, retrospectively, were not candidates for surgery. In correlating mortality with special complicating factors as mentioned before it can be shown that the extension of dissection into the orifice of coronary arteries, significant organ failure, pericardial tamponade, as well as special intraoperative events considerably increased the risk of the disease.

Retrospectively, 81 of our patients were evaluated according to their individual risk factors. For each patient the course of the disease was evaluated regarding the patient's preoperative clinical status, special conditions during surgical intervention, and postoperative complications. All findings were validated according to the score-system shown in Table 1, in which angiographic findings, histological examinations, course of the disease, damage of other organs, surgical technique, number of blood transfusions, and postoperative complications are taken into account. Evaluation resulted in a preoperative and in an intra/postoperative risk number. All patients having a total risk number less than 18 survived. In patients with high preoperative risk numbers, the surgical intervention should not include additional complicating factors. This evaluation cannot be based on a mathematical analysis. Evaluation was done in part according to data from the literature and in part from empiric values. For data derived from the intra- and postoperative course, no significant risk was calculated

Table 1. Score system for validation of complicating factors in aortic aneurysm disease

Parameter	0	1	2	3	4
Type of aneurysm	Dilatation	B_2	A_2	B_1	A_1
Add. diseases	Diabetes	CHD, VSD			Multitrauma
Dissection	None	Incision	At resection	To coronaries	Into coronaries
Operation	Wrapping	Suture	Prosthesis + CABG	Conduit, coron.-impl.	Conduit + CABG
Age (years)	Up to 29	30-39	40-49	50-59	Over 60
Body weight	Ideal	Normal	10% overweight	20% overweight	More than 20%
Histology	Normal	Media-necrosis	Arteriosclerosis		
Hemodynamics	Normal	Valve disease	Hypertension	Shock	
Genesis		Trauma (chron.)		Trauma (acute)	Iatrogenic
Complications preoperative	None	Pulmonary, endocrine, renal-hepatic disease	Pregnancy, CNS-sympt., renal-hepatic damage, pericard. tamp., rupture, hematothorax		renal insufficiency
Course	Chronic	Subacute (3 mo.)	Acute without diag. delay	Acute with diag. delay	Peracute with diag. delay
ECC (min)	0-179	180-239	240-299	300-359	Over 360
Hypotension (min)	Up to 29	30 - 39	40 - 59	60 - 69	Cver 70
Op.-time (hours)	Up to 7	7.5 - 12	12.5-15	15.5-20	Over 20.5
Units-blood	Up to 19	20 - 29	30 - 39	40 - 49	Over 50
Postop. course		Rethoracotomy	Shock-lung, gastro-int. bleed., pericard. tamp., anuria, hepatic insuff.	Infection	Brain edema

for ECC duration up to 3 h, hypotension of up to 29 min under 60 mm Hg, operation time of up to 7 h, and the need of less than 20 blood units. In respect to the total risk number, a significant difference between surviving and non-surviving patients can be seen.

All non-surviving patients had an increased pre- and intraoperative risk especially due to complications. This can also be shown by comparison of mean values of pre- and intraoperative risk numbers having highly significant ($p < 0.001$) differences (Fig. 2). Changes of treatment strategy have only a limited influence on preoperative risk and complications. Operative results could possibly be improved by a faster decision whether there is an indication or contraindication for surgery. Hypotension should be avoided intraoperatively, duration of operation and extracorporeal circulation should be diminished and blood loss with a need for additional transfusions should be reduced.

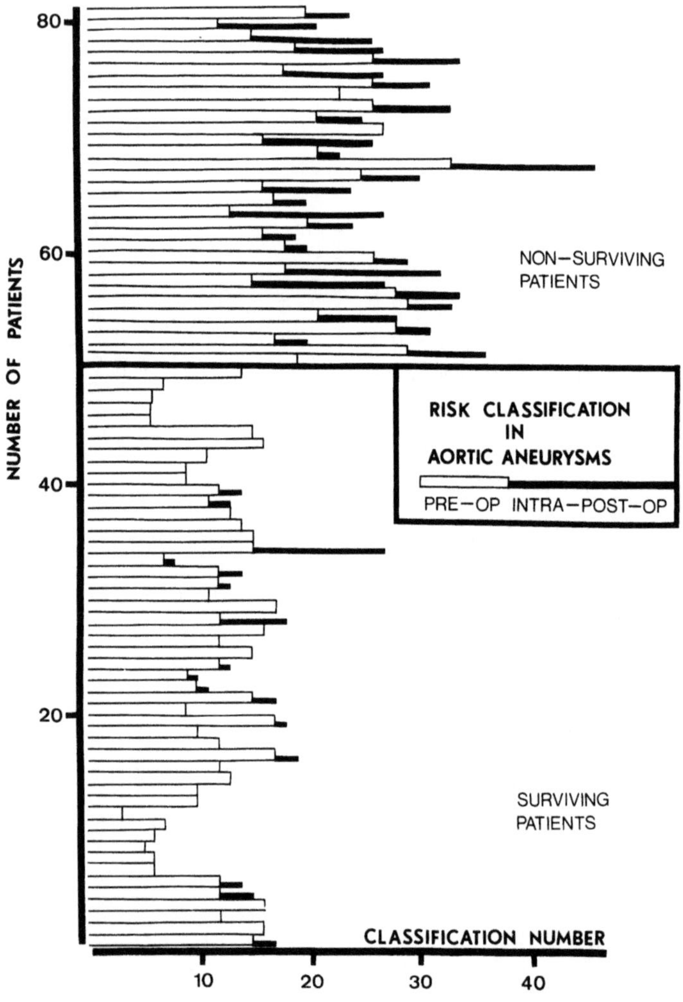

Fig. 2. Risk classification in aortic aneurysms. Comparison of surviving and non-surviving patients

To demonstrate measures to reduce the risk of surgery of thoracic aortic aneurysms, attention should be drawn to three important factors of surgical therapy. These are the local use of substances to seal sutures and vascular prostheses, the application of myocardial protection with cardioplegic solutions, and improved techniques of ECC.

By using fibrinogen glue since 1977, we were able to considerably reduce the need for blood transfusions and duration of operation. The effect of the so-called fibrinogen glue is based on the local transmission of fibrinogen into interlinked unsoluble fibrin (6). In addition the glue has a plasmin-inhibiting substance which avoids local fibrinolysis. First fibrinogen glue which contains fibrinogen and factor 13 is applied to the suture lines of vascular prostheses. This is followed by adding a second substance which contains thrombin, calcium, and aprotinin. Thrombin stimulates the activation of factor 13 and the formation of fibrinmonomers from fibrinogen-linked unsoluble fibrin. Aprotinin counteracts the solution of this sealing fibrin. By use of "fibrinogen glue" for preclotting of the vascular grafts and for sealing of the suture lines, the mount of blood units during and after surgery could be reduced drastically. In patients with replacement of the ascending aorta ($N = 51$), the use of blood transfusions was reduced from 30 ± 12 units to 18 ± 7 units per operation. This reduction was statistically significant ($p < 0.01$).

Since 1977, we also used cardioplegic solution according to Bretschneider for myocardial protection in an increasing number of patients. The action of the solution is based on an acute sodium depletion of the extracellular space. Tolerance of ischemia could be increased and the myocardium is protected during the time of surgery. The use of specific techniques of ECC makes the operation easier and safer.

For surgery of aneurysms of the descending thoracic aorta we cannulate the ascending aorta and the descending aorta and/or a femoral artery. Direct connection of these cannulas provides physiologic circulatory conditions for the lower part of the body. For reasons of safety, in some cases, these cannulas are additionally connected as inflow cannulas with a heart-lung machine. However, extracorporeal circulation is only started when the patient's own circulation cannot provide adequate perfusion during surgery. Comparing results in our institution obtained from 1974 to 1976 with the results obtained from 1977 to now, the operative risk especially for aneurysms of the ascending aorta could be reduced markedly. None of the patients with a chronic aneurysm of the ascending aorta died within the last 3 1/2 years, while mortality of these patients was 46.7% in the years 1974 to 1976. For acute aneurysms of the ascending aorta, mortality could be diminished from 77.8% to 27.8%. The number of cases with aneurysms of the aorta in other locations is still too small to be evaluated in this respect.

Summary

Since 1974, 100 patients with aneurysms of the thoracic aorta were operated on in our institution, 97 of whom were evaluated for this study. Aneurysms were classified according to the classification of Anagnostopoulos. All patients with A_2 or B_2 aneurysms survived; mortality in patients with A_1 or B_1 aneurysms was 45.2%. All patients with C aneurysms died.

Additionally, all patients were divided in groups according to the surgical technique used for correction. Regarding aneurysms of the ascending aorta, best results were obtained in patients with separate replacement of the ascending aorta and the aortic valve, with a mortality of only 7.1%. Mortality in patients with aortic conduit with coronary implantation was 41.7%. Within the last 3 years, mortality of patients with aneurysms of the ascending aorta could be reduced from 77.8% to 27.8%.

Factors of improvement are the use of fibrinogen glue for preclotting of the prosthesis and sealing of the suture lines, the application of cardioplegic solutions, and improved techniques of extracorporeal circulation.

References

1. Anagnostopoulos CE, Athanasuleas CL, Garrick RG, Paulissian R (1975) Acute aortic dissections. University Park Press, Baltimore London Tokyo
2. Bircks W (1978) Das dissezierende Aortenaneurysma. Schweiz Med Wochenschr 108: 1686-1695
3. Miller DC, Stinson EB, Oyer PE, Rossiter SJ, Reitz BA, Griepp RB, Shumway NE (1979) Operative treatment of aortic dissections. J Thorac Cardiovasc Surg 78/3: 365-382
4. Spängler HP (1976) Gewebeklebung und lokale Blutstillung mit Fibrinogen, Thrombin und Blutgerinnungsfaktor XIII. Wien Klin Wochenschr 88/4:3-18
5. Wheat MW (1980) Acute dissecting aneurysms of the aorta: diagnosis and treatment 1979. Am Heart J 99/3:373-387

Operative Treatment of Acute Aortic Dissections

P. Jaumin, V. Arena, J. Dautrebande, R. Ponlot, and Ch.-H. Chalant*

Thirty-one patients underwent operative repair of acute aortic dissections.

The patients were classified according to the de Bakey classification. Overall operative mortality rate was 40%.

The diagnostic approach, the surgical indications, the operative techniques, and the results are presented. The risk factors are discussed.

*Université Catholique de Louvain, 1200 Bruxelles, Belgium

Three-Year Clinical Experience With the Gelatine-Resorcine-Formol Biological Glue in Acute Aortic Dissection

J. Bachet, F. Gigou, C. Laurian, O. Bical, B. Goudot, and D. Guilmet*

Because of the extreme severity of spontaneous evolution of acute dissection involving the ascending aorta, there is no controversy about the necessity of urgent surgical treatment (1-6). However, hospital mortality rate remains high in most reported experiences (1, 4, 6-9).

The gravity of this accident is related to two main causes: 1) the extension of the dissecting process along the vessel, threatening the patient with severe ischemia or sudden rupture; 2) the weakness of the dissected tissues, responsible for the looseness of the sutures, the important bleeding, and, thus, the duration or repetition of cardiopulmonary bypass, the massive blood transfusion, and the frequently complicated postoperative course.

Since the first reported prosthetic replacement of the ascending aorta (10), many technical refinements have been described (1, 11, 12) to reduce the surgical difficulties. They all tend to reinforce the weak aortic layers and they generally consist in placing teflon felt inside and/or outside the dissected cylinders. Aortic valve replacement with or without a conduit has also been suggested. Despite these technical improvements, operative procedures are often difficult and mortality rate important.

Therefore the idea of using an adhesive agent in acute aortic dissection, already suggested by Anagnostopoulos (1), became logical after the reported experiments with Gelatine-Resorcine-Formol (GRF) glue (13, 14). After a 1-year experimental study in dogs (15, 16), our clinical experience started in January 1977. The operative technique and the preliminary clinical results have already been published (17, 18).

Methods and Material

Between 1970 and 1979, 40 patients suffering from acute dissection involving the ascending aorta were operated on in our institution. All underwent emgergency operation within 15 days following the onset of symptoms.

The patients can be divided in two groups: 1) Twenty-five patients were operated on between 1970 and 1976, according to "classical" techniques (CT group) (4). 2) Fifteen patients were operated on between January 1977 and December 1979, using the GRF glue to reinforce the aortic stumps before securing a Dacron prosthesis. To assess the advantages of the latter technique, this study compares the immediate and long-term results of the two groups.

*Department of Cardio-vascular Surgery, C.M.C. Foch-Universite Paris-Ouest, 40 rue Worth, 92151 Suresnes, France

The CT group consisted of 19 men and six women from 20 to 69 years old (mean age 46.5 years); the GRF group consisted of 12 men and three women from 15 to 71 years old (mean age 47.5 years). Table 1 summarizes the preoperative clinical condition of the patients of each group.

Table 1. Preoperative clinical condition of the patients of the CT and GRF groups

	CT group (25 patients)	GRF group (15 patients)
Marfan syndrome	9 (36%)	5 (33%)
Arterial hypertension	10 (40%)	6 (40%)
Iatrogenic dissection	1 (4%)	1 (6.6%)
Cardiogenic shock	18 (72%)	13 (86%)
Aortic regurgitation	20 (80%)	13 (86%)
Ischemic disorders		
Heart	9 (36%)	5 (33%)
Brain	9 (36%)	3 (20%)
Abdomen	1 (4%)	0
Limbs		
abolished pulse	10 (40%)	6 (40%)
clinical ischemia	2 (8%)	1 (6%)

Diagnosis

In the CT group the diagnosis was confirmed by veinous angiogram (pulmonary artery) in 28% of the patients, or aortogram (Seldinger technique) in 32% of the patients. Ten patients (40%) were considered too critically ill to undergo angiogram and were operated upon on clinical evidences. In the GRF group 14 patients (93%) underwent aortogram (Seldinger technique) prior to operation. In the remaining patient the aortic dissection was diagnosed at emergency reoperation, necessitated by massive bleeding 2 h after a double coronary bypass procedure.

Operative Techniques

Sixty percent of patients of the CT group and 75% of patients of the GRF group were operated on within 24 h following the onset of symptoms. Operations were carried out with the aid of cardiopulmonary bypass, one femoral artery being systematically cannulated. Since 1976, general hypothermia (25°C) is preferred to normothermia. The techniques of myocardial preservation evolved with time, as summarized in Table 2.

The aortic valve was replaced in 12 patients (48%) of the CT group (four cases of complete replacement of the aorta with a valved conduit and eight cases of simple replacement of the valve). Eight of the replaced valves were considered normal but systematically changed to avoid further aortic regurgitation. The aortic valve was replaced only once (6.6%) in the GRF group (complete replacement of the ascending aorta with a conduit for severe Marfan syndrome).

The coronary arteries were reimplanted in the Dacron prosthesis in four patients (16%) of the CT group. In the GRF group, the coronary arteries were reimplanted once, two previously implanted saphenous grafts were reimplanted in one patient, one double coronary bypass was performed in one patient, gluing of a dissected coronary ostium was performed in two patients.

Table 2. Techniques of myocardial preservation during surgery

		CT group	GRF group
Coronary perfusion	(1970-1977)	19 (76%)	4 (26%)
Local deep hypothermia (Shumway)	(1976-1977)	6 (24%)	4 (26%)
Cold cardioplegia (Bretschneider)	(1978-)	0	7 (48%)

Results

Mean duration of operative procedures was not different in the CT group (6.30 h) and in the GRF group (6 h). Nor was the mean duration of cardiopulmonary bypass different – CT group: 142 min; GRF group: 130 min. But the ranges in each group are quite different (CT group: 80 to 420 mn; GRF group: 90 to 220 mn).

Intraoperative bleeding after weaning from cardiopulmonary bypass was much more important in the CT group than in the GRF group. Blood transfusion volumes ranged from 750 to 14 000 cc in the CT group (mean volume 5900 cc) and from 800 to 5000 cc in the GRF group (mean volume 2600 cc).

Because of intractable hemorrhage and/or prolonged or repeated cardiopulmonary bypass, operative mortality affected four patients in the CT group and none in the GRF group.

Postoperative Complications

Twenty-one patients (84%) of the CT group and 15 patients (100%) of the GRF group survived operation. Bleeding was more important in the CT group than in the GRF group (mean volume 1100 cc versus 800 cc). One patient of the CT group required emergency reoperation for postoperative bleeding. Cerebral ischemia affected seven patients (33%) of the CT group: two transient focal defects, one transient coma associated with regressive hemiparesis, and four stage III coma leading progressively to death. Six patients of the GRF group showed evidence of cerebral disorders: three transient stage II coma, one paraplegia, and one sudden stroke with progressive stage IV coma due to recurrent dissection of the aortic arch 12 days after the first procedure. Acute renal failure was observed in 10 patients (40%) of the CT group. Among them, five required peritoneal dialysis or hemodialysis. Only one patient of the GRF group showed evidence of renal failure which did not require dialysis. Abdominal ischemia was the cause of one death in the CT group and was not observed in the GRF group. Ischemia of the lower limbs requiring prosthetic aortobifemoral bypass was present in one patient of the CT group.

Postoperative infection was observed in six patients of the CT group (three septicemia, three mediastinitis). It was the cause of two deaths. No infection affected patients of the GRF group. So, postoperative complications were more frequent and severe in the CT group than in the GRF group. They were the cause of eight deaths in the CT group and of one death in the GRF group. Overall hospital mortality affected, therefore, 12 patients (48%) of the CT group and one patient (6.6%) of the GRF group.

Long-Term Results

Thirteen patients of the CT group were discharged from hospital. One patient died 4 months later from stroke. Four patients had to be reoperated 6 to 42 months following the first procedure (Table 3). One died during reoperation.

Among the 11 survivors (44%), eight patients are in good condition 4 to 8 years after operation. But three of them had to be reoperated at least once. Two of the remaining patients have a moderate aortic regurgitation medically supported (one perivalvular leak, one valvular regurgitation). One patient had a stroke 9 months after discharge.

Fourteen patients (93%) of the GRF group were discharged from hospital. Follow-up ranges from 4 to 36 months (average follow-up 20 months). There was no late death. One patient has a moderate aortic regurgitation medically supported. The same patient was reoperated on 2 years after the first procedure, for vertebrobasilar insufficiency related to complete thrombosis of the left subclavian artery.

Table 3. Causes, type, and results of reoperation in patients of the CT group

First procedure	Cause of reoperation	Delay	Second procedure	Result
Replacement of AA	Aortic regurgitation	2 years	AVR	Died
Replacement of AA	Aortic regurgitation	1 year	AVR	Good
Replacement of AA, AVR	Perivalvular leak	6 months	Reinsertion	Poor
	Perivalvular leak	18 months	AVR A. annulus reconstructed	Poor
Bentall	Recurrent dissection (type III)	4 years	Replacement of Thoraco-Abd. A	Good

AA = ascending aorta; AVR = aortic valve replacement; Thoraco-Abd. A = thoraco-abdominal aorta

He underwent carotidosubclavian bypass. Two patients have neurological sequellae (one case of paraplegia, one case of psychological disorders after prolonged coma). One patient suffers from important residual arterial hypertension despite maximal medical therapy. The remaining 10 patients (66%) are in excellent clinical condition and have resumed their previous occupations. Ten patients of the GRF group underwent 11 postoperative angiograms 2 to 24 months following surgery (Figs. 1 and 2). The results are summarized in Table 4.

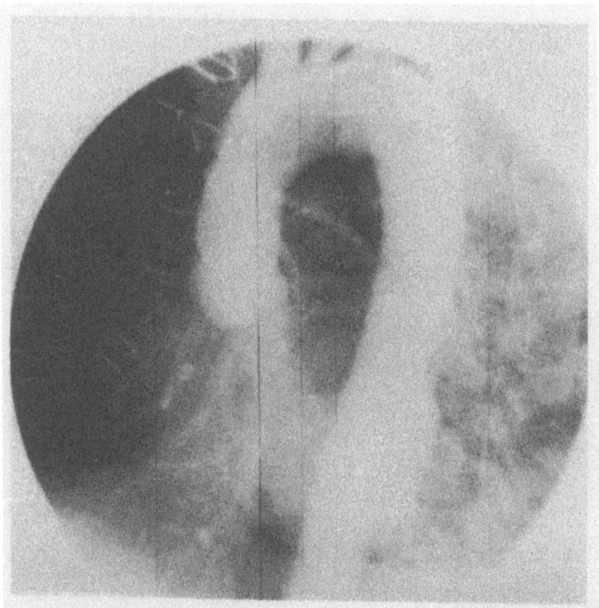

Fig. 1. Acute aortic dissection (type II): excellent surgical result. Three months after surgery the aortic morphololy appears to be normal. Two saphenous grafts can be seen on the side of the ascending aorta

Discussion

The results of the two groups must be criticized from three points of view: the homogeneity and comparability of the groups, the validity of the statistical analysis, and the interpretation of the differences. It seems obvious that criteria of homogeneity of the groups have been met. There are no differences between the patients of each group concerning the age, the sex, the clinical and anatomical data. The patients have been operated on by the same surgical team and the same medical team was in charge of the postoperative cares.

Conversely, the main objection relies on the fact that it is a retrospective study, and that results of the GRF group have certainly benefited from the general progress in pre- and postoperative medical management, better radiologic exploration, better myocardial protection during surgery. In fact, for the 12 last patients of the CT group operated between 1973 and 1976, operative mortality rate was 16% and hospital mortality 35%. Intra- and postoperative bleeding was also reduced, reaching an average volume of 4000 cc instead of 5900 cc in the whole group. This tends to prove that regardless of the surgical technique, the results improve with time. However, the gluing technique appears to bring a sudden undeniable progress in the surgical management of aortic dissection.

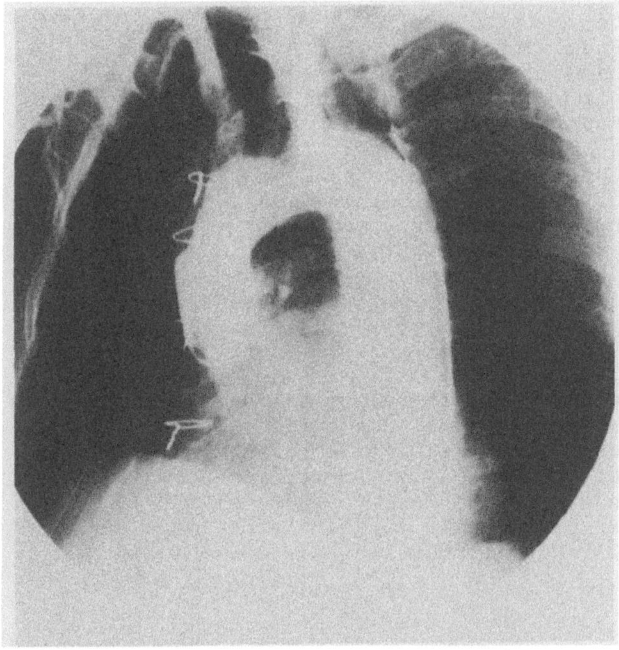

Fig. 2. Acute aortic dissection (type I) in Marfan syndrome: good surgical result. Twelve months after surgery, there is neither persisting dissection nor aortic regurgitation

Table 4. Results of postoperative angiograms in patients of the GRF group

No.	Delay (months)	Repair of AA	Persisting diss.	Aortic regurg.	Coronary abn.
1	24	Excellent	No	No	Reimplanted veinous grafts
2	6	Excellent	No	No	No
3	5	Excellent	No	No	No
4	3	Dilated valsalva S	Yes	No	Thrombosis of RCA
5	3	Dilated valsalva S	Yes	Yes	No
	24	Dilated valsalva S	Yes Left subclavian thrombosis	Yes	No
6	6	Excellent	No	No	Double bypass
7	8	Excellent	No	No	No
8	12	Dilated valsalva S	Yes	No	No
9	9	Excellent	No	No	No
10	8	Excellent (Bentall)	No	No	No

AA = ascending aorta; Diss. = dissection; Regurg. = regurgitation; Abn. = abnormality; S = sinuses; RCA = right coronary artery

Because of the small number of patients in each group, statistical validity can be discussed. Some differences between the two groups, such as operative mortality and postoperative infection, are not significant. Conversely, there is a large statistical significance regaring hospital mortality, postoperative bleeding, and long-term results.

Anyhow, there is no doubt that the operative procedures were much more simple using the GRF glue. Prolonged or repeated CPBP was never necessary to achieve surgical hemostasis in this group. This resulted in no operative death and certainly easier postoperative course (reduced blood transfusions, absence of infection and renal failure). Accordingly, the quality of adhesion of the two layers and the tightness of the sutures reduce the risk of persisting or recurrent dissection as documented by late postoperative angiograms. This probably explains the reduced amount of persisting cerebral and peripheral ischemia in the GRF group.

It also explains the absence of aortic regurgitation in most patients, despite our conservative attitude. The patient with postoperative aortic regurgitation has a congenital bicuspid aortic valve, the conservation of which was certainly abusive. In fact, abnormal or dilated aortic valves (as found in severe Marfan syndrome) should be replaced. In such cases the use of a valved conduit is the more advisable technique (12, 19), the GRF glue being used only for the distal stump.

Conclusion

This comparative study demonstrates that the use of the GRF biological glue in the treatment of acute aortic dissection: significantly reduces the necessity of aortic valve replacement, significantly reduces the intra- and postoperative bleeding because of the immediate surgical hemostasis, accordingly reduces the blood transfusion volumes, and reduces the severity of postoperative complications. So, the hospital mortality rate has been reduced from 48% to 6.6%.

Lastly, although it is presently impossible to prove that this technique reduces the risk of persisting or recurrent aortic dissection in operated patients, it certainly reduces the severity of its consequences. Therefore, the late survival rate has been raised from 40% in the CT group to 93% in the GRF group and the rate of excellent clinical condition has been raised from 30% (CT group) to 66% (GRF group).

Summary

From January 1977 to December 1979, the GRF biological glue was used for tissue reinforcement in 15 patients operated on for acute dissection involving the ascending aorta. The results of these patients (GRF group) were compared to the results of 25 patients operated on between 1970 and 1976 with "classical" techniques (CT group). There were no significant differences between the two groups regarding the age, the preoperative clinical and anatomical data.

The ascending aorta was replaced in all patients; the aortic valve was replaced once (6.6%) in the GRF group and in 12 cases (48%) in the CT group; the coronary arteries were bypassed or reimplanted in 25% of patients of each group. Average peroperative blood transfusion rate was 5800 ml in the CT group and 2500 ml in the GRF group. Four (16%) peroperative deaths were registered in the CT group and none in the GRF group.

Postoperative renal failure, cerebral ischemia, persisting peripheral ischemia, and infection were more frequent in the CT group. They were responsible for eight hospital deaths in this group and for one in the GRF group. Hospital mortality was therefore reduced from 48% (CT group) to 6.6% (GRF group). Two late deaths were registered in the CT group and none in the GRF group, all survivors being in good clinical condition.

Ten patients of the GRF group underwent eleven control angiograms, 2 to 24 months following surgery, which documented one moderate aortic incompetence (7%), three persisting dissections of the descending aorta, but good and stable repair in the other patients.

In conclusion, the use of the GRF glue significantly reduces: the number of aortic valve replacements, the per- and postoperative bleeding, and the frequency and severity of postoperative complications. Therefore, long-term (3 years) survival rate has been raised from 40% to 93%.

References

1. Anagnostopoulos CE (1976) Acute aortic dissections. University Park Press, Baltimore
2. Appelbaum A, Karp RB, Kirklin JW (1976) Ascending vs descending aortic dissections. Ann Surg 183/3:296-300
3. Dalen JE, Alpert JS, Cohn LM, Black H, Collins JJ (1974) Dissection of the thoracic aorta. Medical or surgical therapy. Am J Cardiol 34/7:803-808
4. Guilmet D, Liebeaux M, Dhainaut JF, Goudot B, Gandjbackch I, Francoual M, Bachet J (1977) Traitement chirurgical des dissections aigües de l'aorte ascendante. Arch Mal Coeur 70/6:639-644
5. Hirst AE, Johns VJ, Kimes SW (1958) Dissecting aneurysms of the aorta: a review of 505 cases. Medicine (Baltimore) 37:217-279
6. Wolfe WG, Moran JF (1977) The evolution of medical and surgical management of acute aortic dissection (Editorial). Circulation 56/4:503-505
7. Wheat MW, Palmer RF, Bartley TD, et al. (1973) Treatment of dissecting aneurysms of the aorta: current status. Prog Cardiovasc Dis 16:87-101
8. Liotta D, Grady LH, Milam JP, Cooley DA (1971) Surgical treatment of acute dissecting aneurysm of the ascending aorta. Ann Thorac Surg 12:582-592
9. Thomas CS, Alford WC, Borrus GR, Frist RA, Stoney WS (1965) The effectiveness of surgical treatment of acute aortic dissection. Ann Thorac Cardiovasc Surg 50:364-373
10. De Bakey ME, Henley WS, Cooley DA, et al. (1965) Surgical management of dissecting aneurysms of the aorta. J Thorac Cardiovasc Surg 49:130-148
11. Cachera JP, Loisance D, Carlier M, Maillet FX, Slama R, Bouvrain Y (1974) Progrès techniques dans le traitement chirurgical des dissections aortiques aigües totales de type I. Arch Mal Coeur 67:125-131
12. Bachet J (1978) Traitement des dissections aigües de l'aorte. Inform Cardiol 1: 127-137
13. Cooper CN, Falb RD (1968) Surgical adhesives. Ann NY Acad Sci 146:214-224
14. Braunwald NS, Gay W, Tatooles CJ (1966) Evaluation of cross linked gelatin as a tissue adhesive and hemostatic agent: an experimental study. Surgery 59: 1024-1030
15. Laurian C, Gigou F, Guilmet D (1977) La colle gélatine-résorcine, formaldéhyde en chirurgie vasculaire. Nouv Presse Med 6:3221-3223
16. Laurian C, Gigou F, Bical O, Barbagelata M, Bachet J, Goudot B, Guilmet D (1979) Traitement chirurgical des dissections aortiques aigües par l'utilisation d'une colle biologique. Etude expérimentale. J Chir (Paris)
17. Bachet J, Goudot B, Laurian C, Gigou F, et al. (1979) Dissection aigüe de l'aorte: nouvelle technique chirurgicale utilisant une colle biologique. Nouv Presse Med 8:1421-1425

18. Guilmet D, Bachet J, Goudot B, Laurian C, Gigou F, Bical O (1979) The use of a biological glue in acute aortic dissection. A new surgical technique. Preliminary clinical results. J Thorac Cardiovasc Surg 77:516-521
19. Bentall H, Bono AD (1968) Technique for complete replacement of the ascending aorta. Thorax 23:338

Surgical Experiences of Chronic Dissecting Aneurysms of the Aorta

A. Hashimoto and J. Wada*

Recently, the treatment of dissecting aneurysms of the aorta has made great strides, but there are still many problems to be solved. At the Heart Institute of Japan, Tokyo Women's Medical College, there were 40 cases of dissecting aneurysms of the aorta which have been operated on, while about 80 cases of this entity have been treated medically. The purpose of this presentation is to describe the surgical experiences of dissecting aneurysms, especially of the chronic type dissections, and its long-term results in comparison to those of medically treated cases, and to emphasize the superiority of surgical treatment to medical treatment of this entity.

Clinical Materials

From 1967 through March 1980, 40 cases underwent surgical treatment, of whom 24 were male and 16 female, ages ranging from 20 to 67 years, with average age of 42.3 years. Among these 40 cases, only three had acute type dissections; these were operated on during 1968 and 1969 and died from bleeding during or after operation. Out of 37 cases of chronic type dissection, 11 died after surgery, meaning a 29.7% mortality rate, while only five fatalities were encountered among 28 surgical cases since 1972, realizing a mortality rate of 17.9%. This progress in surgical proficiency is mainly due to improvement of surgical techniques which will be described later on, and those 28 chronic dissections will be also presented in detail.

In the 28 cases, 13 were found to have type I dissection with two postoperative deaths, while five had type II dissection with one postoperative death; the remaining ten with type III dissection resulted in two deaths after surgery. Each case in types I and II, as well as two cases in type III had to be reoperated in their subsequent follow-up periods (Table 1).

Surgical Techniques

In the type I and II dissections, cardiopulmonary bypass with moderate hypothermia (rectal temperature of 25°C) and arterial return, usually through a femoral artery, would be the case; however, in some cases the distal ascending aorta or aortic arch would be utilized. Coronary perfusion was used until 4 years ago; since then cold and chemical

*Department of Surgery, The Heart Institute of Japan, Tokyo Women's Medical College, 10 Kawada-cho, Shinjuku-ku, Tokyo, 162, Japan

cardioplegia has been used, and more recently this cardioplegic technique has been reinforced by continuous low flow (2-3 ml/min) coronary perfusion with cold blood or cold glucose-insulin-potassium solution to maintain an intended myocardial temperature. By this cardioplegic technique with continuous low flow coronary perfusion, aortic cross-clamping of more than 4 h is well tolerated for myocardium.

If aortic cross-clamping between the brachiocephalic artery and the left carotid artery is necessary for any case with type I dissection, a temporary bypass graft between these two neck vessels is created just before the pump bypass starts or even on the day before surgery. By this technique, extracorporeal circulation is simplified without perfusion to neck vessels.

For the type III dissection, a left heart bypass, a partial heart bypass with the femoral vein and artery cannulation, or a temporary long external bypass grafting was utilized.

In the surgical techniques, all cases had aneurysmal replacement with artificial prosthetic grafts. In the type I and II dissections with aortic regurgitation, only one case had an aortic annuloplasty, with remaining cases aortic valve replacement in combination with the replacement of the dissected aorta.

Since 1972, the graft inclusion technique (2) has been used in which an aneurysm is opened longitudinally, and the dissected pseudolumen is closed by interrupted mattress sutures reinforced by a strip of Dacron felt placed inside the intima, and an artificial graft is implanted intraluminally. If annuloaortic ectasia was combined with type I and II dissections, Bentall's technique (1) would be utilized to perform a composite replacement of the aortic valve and the ascending aorta. In the type III dissection, most cases received replacement of the thoracic descending aorta except one case where a thoracoabdominal aortic replacement had taken place. Since 1973, the graft inclusion technique as described earlier was used.

Table 1. Surgical results of aortic dissections

	1967 - March 1980		1972 - March 1980
Type	Acute cases	Chronic cases	Chronic cases
I	1 (1)	14 (3) [AAE, 7 (1)]	13[a] (2) [AAE, 7 (1)]
II	1 (1)	6 (2) [AAE, 5 (1)]	5[a] (1) [AAE, 5 (1)]
III	1 (1)	17[a] (6)	10[a] (2)
Total	3 (3)	37 (11) 29.7%	28 (5) 17.9%

( ) = hospital death; AAE = annuloaortic ectasia

[a]One case had a reoperation

Surgical Results and Causes of Surgical Deaths

As explained so far, overall operative mortality rate of the 37 cases with chronic dissections was 29.7% which by 1972 was reduced to 17.9%. The reasons for this improvement were analyzed by reviewing the causes of death.

Before 1971, principal causes were intra- or postoperative bleeding, but since 1972, postoperative deaths could be attributed to acute myocardial damage, further aortic dissection, postoperative hepatitis, and pulmonary hemorrhage. These findings and improvements were due to least preparation to expose the aneurysm, and to the technique of replacing the graft intraluminally. Postoperative long-term results of the 26 survivors with chronic aortic dissections revealed that they have recovered and returned to their jobs for a minimum of 2 months to a maximum of 11 years 3 months after operations. Four of them had to be reoperated during their follow-up period. In one case with type I dissection, pseudoaneurysm formation at the ascending aorta due to suture insufficiency necessitated an operation again 6 years and 5 months after the initial surgery, but this case died of low cardiac output syndrome postoperatively. One case of type II dissection with annuloaortic ectasis turned to type I dissection postoperatively and showed a huge abdominal aneurysm which was replaced with a graft. One case of type III dissection revealed annuloaortic ectasia 10 years after surgery, and the patient had a Bentall's operation. Another case of type III dissection showed aneurysmal dilations at the proximal and distal anastomotic portions due to further dissection and suture insufficiency. This case received reoperation 6 years after the initial surgery and died after the reoperation.

In the 37 cases of surgically treated chronic dissection, 29.7% resulted in hospital deaths after surgery, two cases died after reoperations about 6 years after the initial operations, and the remaining 24 cases have been well for 2 months to 11 years and 3 months after surgery. Their actual survival rate was 69% at 3 years and 5 years after surgery, and 57% at 7 years after surgery. While in the 43 cases of medically treated chronic dissections in our Institution, the 1-year survival rate was 60%, 3-year survival was 39%, and 5-year survival was only 32% (3) (Fig. 1). These results clearly reveal the superiority of surgical treatment to medical treatment in the chronic dissections.

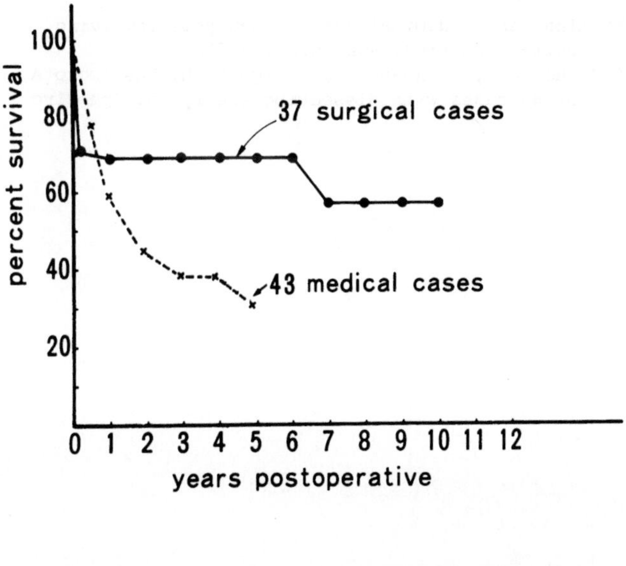

Fig. 1. Actuarial survival in surgically and medically treated cases with chronic aortic dissections

Comment

In our Institution, 43 cases of medically treated chronic dissections were followed up for 5 years after the diagnosis of each case was established (3), enabling the long-term survival rate to be presented now. The survival rates of types I and II without annuloaortic ectasia were compared with type III which revealed the latter to have seemingly done little better than the former, but both showed almost the same outcome (3). In the group of types I and II, if annuloaortic ectasia was combined, they resulted in a very poor outcome (3). From these data, it is evident that whether type I, II, or III chronic dissections, they should be operated upon at the proper time for each case, and if combined with annuloaortic ectasia, they should be operated on as promptly as possible after the diagnosis has been established. In 30 cases of acute type dissections treated medically in our Institution, the survival rate revealed 50% at 2 weeks after onset, 42% at 1 year, 32% at 3 years, and 15% at 5 years (3). The mortality rate at the acute stages is very high and we are now beginning surgical treatment of these cases with acute type dissections more aggressively.

Conclusion

Surgically treated 40 cases of aortic dissections were reviewed. Among them 37 cases had chronic type dissections. The immediate surgical results of the chronic type dissections were improved by the graft inclusion technique. The surgical treatment of the chronic aortic dissections gave much better survival rate than did the medical treatment. Also by reviewing the reoperated cases in the follow-up period, better long-term results are considered to be obtained through careful surgical techniques at the initial operations of each case.

References

1. Bentall HH, De Bono A (1968) A technique for complete replacement of the ascending aorta. Tnorax 23:338-349
2. Crawford ES (1974) Thoraco-abdominal and abdominal aortic aneurysms involving renal, superior mesenteric, and celiac arteries. Ann Surg 179:763-772
3. Yamaguchi I, Komatsu Y, Niimi S, Horie T, Takahashi S, Sekiguchi M, Hashimoto A, Hirosawa K (1978) The prognosis of 80 cases with dissecting aneurysms. Jpn Circ J 42:913-918

Variants and Surgical Treatment of Chronic Dissecting Aortic Aneurysms

A. V. Pokrovsky and V. I. Ermolaev*

In this presentation we wish to share our experience with treatment of patients with chronic dissecting aortic aneurysms, which has been gained at the Vascular Department of the Bakulev Institute of Cardiovascular Surgery of the USSR AMS, as well as to discuss several considerations of the surgical classification of this pathology.

At the present time the most widely accepted classification is that of De Bakey proposed in 1965 (1). However, in our opinion, it must be supplemented, since it does not reflect several essential conditions, defining tactics of the present-day surgical intervention. To such conditions one may refer such complications as aortic insufficiency and detachment from the true lumen of the main aortic branches. Of special interest is inclusion of the dissecting abdominal aorta which is rarely seen.

In connection with this we find it possible to introduce a classification based on De Bakey's classification which distinguishes such complications as aortic insufficiency and detachment of the main aortic branches (Tables 1 and 2). We have examined 42 patients with the dissecting aortic aneurysms. All but two patients had an acute stage of disease before hospitalization.

Table 1. Classification of dissecting aortic aneurysms

Type	Subtype	Variant
I	A	I
Dissection begins in the ascending aorta at various distances	Dissection is confined to the thoracic aorta	Dissection of the aorta is complicated with aortic insufficiency
II	B	II
Dissection is confined to the ascending aorta	Dissection extends to the abdominal aorta	Dissection is confined to the detachment of major aortic branches
III		
Dissection begins distal to the left subclavian artery and extends distally		

*The Bakulev Institute of Cardiovascular Surgery, Leninsky pr. 8, Moscow M49, USSR

Table 2. Distribution of patients with dissecting aortic aneurysms

Type I	10		
	Subtype A	2 (20%)	
		Variant I	2 (100%)
	Subtype B	8 (80%)	
		Variant I	2 (25%)
		Variant II	6 (75%)
Type II	9		
		Variant I	6 (66.66%)
Type III	23		
	Subtype A	2 (8.70%)	
	Subtype B	21 (91.30%)	
		Variant II	14 (66.66%)

Aortography is a decisive diagnostic method. At present, isotope angiography is acquiring definite value in the diagnosis of the dissecting aneurysms; in several cases it reveals a false aortic lumen (Fig. 1). In case of the dissecting aortic root, echocardiography is of value. Figure 2 shows an echogram of a patient with the dissecting ascending aortic aneurysm. Two echoes reflected from the posterior wall of the ascending aorta.

The ascending aortic aneurysms of types I and II were complicated with aortic insufficiency in 52.6% of the patients. It is worth noting that both patients with subtype A of type I aneurysms have aortic insufficiency and only two of eight patients with subtype B of type I aneurysms have aortic insufficiency. That is, distal extension of the dissection may prevent development of aortic insufficiency.

Type I dissecting aneurysm was associated with the dissecting aortic arch branches in two patients with subtype A and in two with subtype B.

In type I and III dissecting aneurysms the dissection involves the abdominal aorta in most patients. This is subtype B [eight of ten patients (80%) of type I and 20 of 23 patients (91%) of type III]. In 14 patients (48%) the dissection involves iliac arteries, six (43%) having bilateral lesions, and eight (57%) unilateral.

In subtype B (with the dissection extending to the abdominal aorta), 19 of 29 (66%) patients have ostia of the main aortic branches detached from the true lumen, eight (44%) having multiple lesions. It is worth noting that renal arteries were detached from the lumen (55%) approximately equally often on both sides (ten from the right and nine from the left). Then come detachment of coeliac trunk (seven) and superior mesenteric artery (four).

It is interesting to analyse hemodynamic changes in the case of renal artery detachment. Renal arteries originated from the false lumen in 16 patients. During pain attacks significantly elevated arterial pressure was noted in two patients. In two normotensive patients vasorenal hypertension developed following dissection, in four of 11 patients with a history of hypertension it was of a malignant nature. It is worth noting that in spite of the fact that renal arteries detached from the true lumen, three patients were normotensive. Thus,

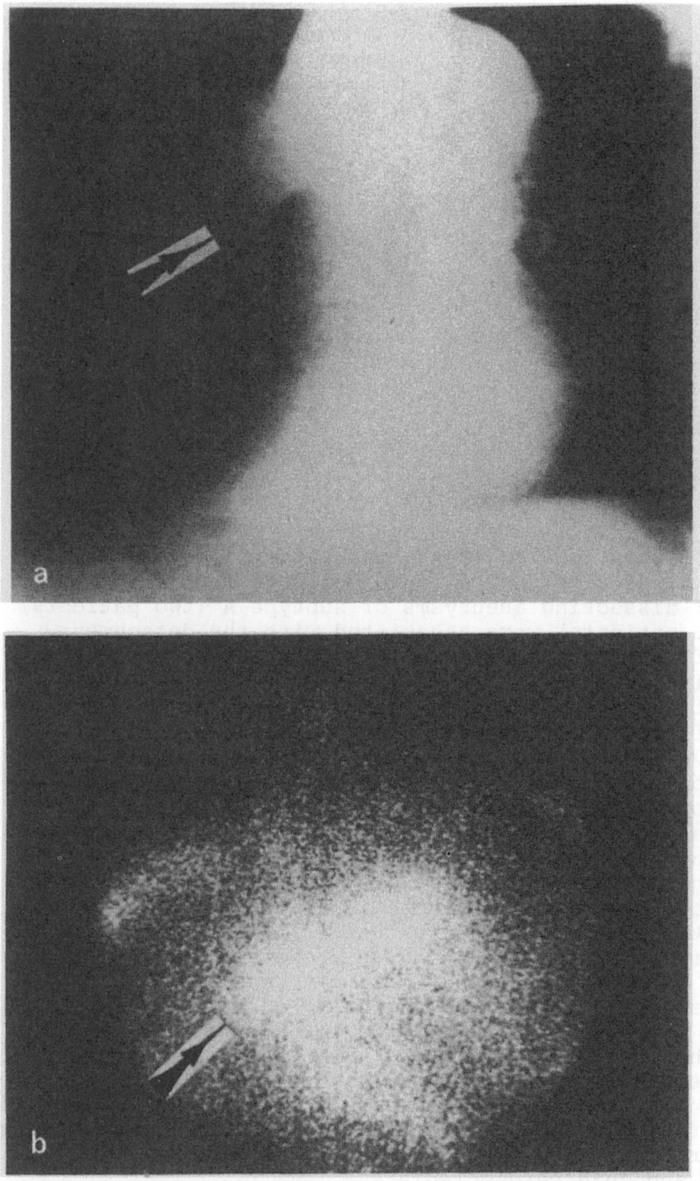

Fig. 1. a Angiogram of patient with type I B dissecting aneurysm. b Isotope angiogram of the same patient. Arrows show the opacified blood shunting into the false aortic lumen

detachment of the renal arteries resulted in hypertension or in the aggravating clinical course of hypertension in six (38%) of 16 patients.

At the chronic stage these patients had complaints of elevated arterial pressure (13 of 16 patients), more rarely of more or less marked lumbar pain (four of 16 patients). In eight patients, there was a significantly depressed renal function as defined by the isotope renography.

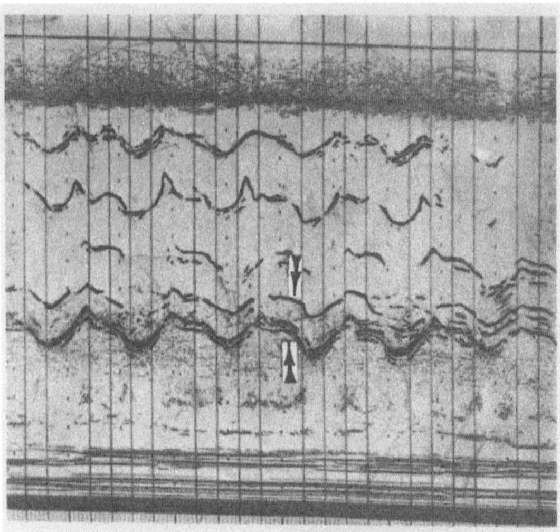

Fig. 2. Echogram of patient with the ascending aortic dissecting aneurysm. Arrows show double echo from the dissected aortic wall

In case of the affected coeliac trunk, one patient had abdominal syndrome, reminding clinical signs of acute cholecysto-pancreatitis.

In type I and III dissecting aneurysms of subtype A (two patients) and subtype B (eight patients) were associated with the detachment of the true lumen of intercostal arteries. In none were there ischemic signs in the spinal cord.

Without treatment chronic dissecting aneurysms are, as a rule, fatal. This was confirmed with our data. Four patients died in the hospital preoperatively. Anamnestic duration in these patients was from 3 weeks to 5 months. Two died from congestive heart failure, the third from pulmonary hemorrhage due to aneurysmal rupture into the left pleural space and tracheobronchial tree, the fourth, in whom there was the detached left renal artery, had hypertonic crisis with subsequent hemorrhagic stroke. Of five patients discharged for different reasons without operation, only one is alive.

On the basis of the above, we believe that all patients with dissecting aortic aneurysms must be operated upon. We have gained surgical experience with 32 operations done in 28 patients.

Seven patients had operation on the ascending aorta. Of four in whom the dissecting aneurysm was complicated with aortic valvular insufficiency, three had one-stage aortic valvular and ascending aortic replacement. At present, we hold to the opinion that it is expedient to use a previously prepared single prosthesis, as proposed by Bentall in 1968. Replacement of the ascending aorta only was performed in four patients. These operations were done under extracorporeal circulation, coronary perfusion, and cold cardioplegia.

Twenty-one patients were operated on the descending aorta; three of them had the left subclavian artery reconstructed. All patients were operated under total moderate hypothermia or left atrial-femoral shunting. One patient was operated on under normothermia without bypass.

In the follow-up period, four patients required repeated correction of the lesion in the dissecting distal segments.

1. Patient M, 46-year-old women. Eight months after dissection she underwent resection and replacement of the descending aorta for type III B aneurysm. Following operation stable hypertension has been sustained due to detachment from the true lumen of the right renal artery. In May 1980, resection of the inter- and infrarenal aortic segments

and replacement with implantation of both renal arteries into the graft was performed (Fig. 3). Postoperative patient is normotensive.

2. Patient P, 46-year-old man. In April 1977, 8 months after dissection resection and replacement of the descending aorta with implantation of the left subclavian artery into the graft was performed. Following operation malignant hypertension has been sustained due to detachment of the left renal artery. In December 1977, the remaining part of the descending aorta was replaced, abdominal aorta was replaced as well and plastic procedure was done on all visceral branches (Fig. 4). (The intervertebral and left subclavian arteries were implanted into the graft.)

3. Patient L, 43-year-old man. In March 1974, 6 months after dissection resection of the dissecting ascending aortic aneurysm was done and it was replaced. In September 1974, resection of the infrarenal aortic segment was done for secondary abdominal aortic aneurysm (Fig. 5).

4. Patient B, 39-year-old man. In September 1976, 7 months after dissection resection and replacement of the dissecting descending aortic aneurysm was done. In December 1979, resection of the distal anastomosis and replacement of the distal descending aortic segment was done for the developed fenestration in the distal anastomosis.

Table 3. Operations for dissecting aneurysm of the ascending aorta

Resection and replacement of the ascending aorta	4
Resection of the ascending aorta and aortic valvular replacement	3
Total	7

Table 4. Operations for the dissecting aneurysm of the descending aorta

Resection and replacement of the descending aorta	18
Resection and replacement of the descending aorta and replacement of the left subclavian artery	3
Additional reconstruction of the descending and abdominal aorta	4
Total	25

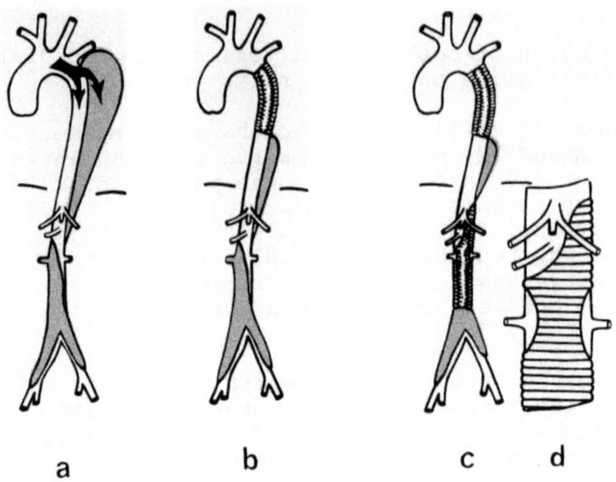

Fig. 3. a Scheme of pathology; b first stage of operative intervention; c second stage of operative intervention; d multiplied scheme of the second stage of operative intervention

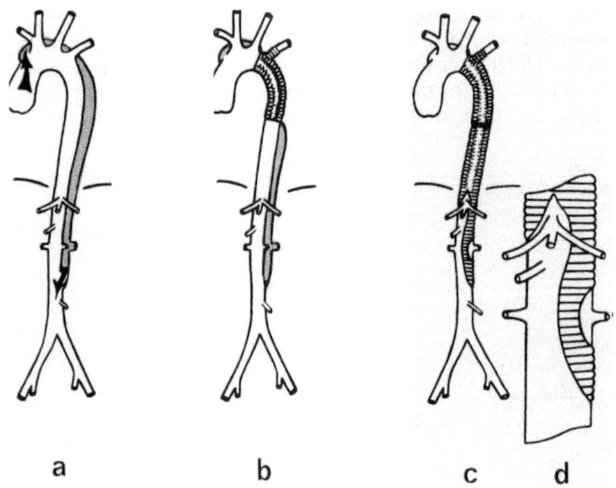

Fig. 4. a Scheme of pathology; b first stage of operative intervention; c second stage of operative intervention; d multiplied scheme of second stage of operative intervention

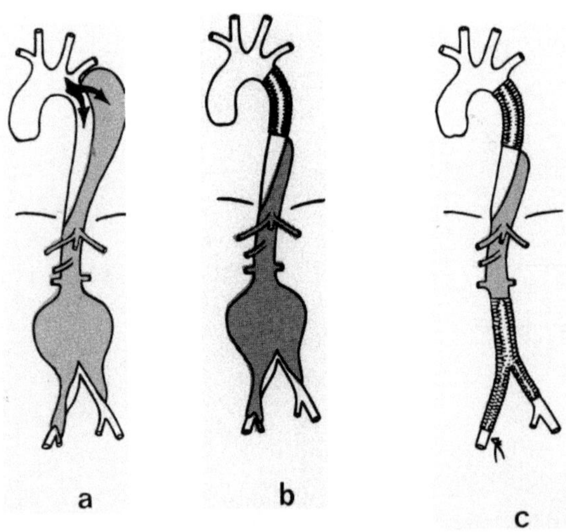

Fig. 5. a Scheme of pathology; b first stage of operative intervention; c second stage of operative intervention

During replacement of the long descending aortic segments, we implant the most large intervertebral arteries into the graft as a preventive measure against spinal cord ischemic lesions.

Thus, proposing this classification we emphasize such complications which require surgical correction (aortic insufficiency, detachment of the main aortic branches). The experience gained with surgical correction of subtype B lesions and reconstruction of the abdominal aorta and visceral arteries evidences the necessity and efficacy of these operations.

References

1. De Bakey ME, et al. (1965) Surgical management of dissecting aneurysms of the aorta. J Thorac Cardiovasc Surg 49/1:130-150

Dissecting Aortic Aneurysm: Ten Years Experience and Long-Term Results of Surgical Treatment

V. Gallucci, V. Valfré, G. Caruso, G. Panizzon, G. Aru, A. Mazzucco, and P. G. Cévese*

Acute dissection of the thoracic aorta is a lethal condition (6) demanding urgent and well-planned treatment, once the diagnosis is made with certainty. During the past 20 years, the better knowledge of its clinical manifestation and the easier access to sophisticated diagnostic facilities brought up to almost 100% the number of cases where a correct diagnosis was made in the hospitalized patient (2). Therefore, the main problem remains the choice of the most appropriate therapy, be it medical or surgical, and its quick employment in each case (3,5,7,12).

In a 10-year period (1970-1979), at the Department of Cardiovascular Surgery, University of Padua, Medical School, 84 cases of dissecting aneurysm of the thoracic aorta were observed and treated. Twenty-seven of them were treated by medical means only, through the diagnostic phase and beyond, following Wheat's method (9-11) of reducing both mean systemic arterial pressure and dP/dT, with trimethaphan, reserpine, and guanethidine, aiming to the conversion of the acute dissection into a subacute or chronic process. In this way better tissues would be available for the surgical intervention which was meant in each case, by reducing the edema and fragility of the aortic wall, developing fibrotic processes and stabilizing the lesion. Other pharmacologic agents were also employed during that phase, such as sodium nitroprusside (8), β-blockers, diuretics, etc.

The medical (hypotensive) treatment was used in each patient under close medical and nursing surveillance, continuous monitoring of all vital parameters, and readiness of operating room facilities. Unfortunately 26 out of 27 such treated patients died, mostly from rupture of the aneurysm or from complete heart block, or the consequences of cerebral and visceral aortic branch occlusion. Fifty-seven other patients instead underwent surgical treatment, once the diagnosis was established, mostly on an emergency basis.

The operations performed, different according to the type of dissection, to the site of intima laceration, and to the peripheral extension of the hematoma, were the "classical" ones proposed by De Bakey (4). In every instance a portion of dissected aorta was resected including the "entrance" to the false lumen and replaced with a Dacron prosthesis, obliterating the false lumen as carefully and completely as possible. Extracorporeal circulation, moderate hypothermia, cardioplegia were used with techniques and degrees varying with time and better knowledge of cardiac metabolism and physiology.

The two ways of treatment gave quite different results, statistically highly significant (Table 1), with a hospital mortality for the medical treatment alone, as said, close to 100%. The mortality after surgery, very high during the first years, has steadily declined, being about 20% in 1978-1979 (Table 2). Medical (hypotensive) therapy

*Clinica Chirurgica dell'Università di Padova, Centro di Chirurgia Cardiovascolare, Policlinico, via Giustinian, Padova, Italy

as the only treatment of the acute dissecting aneurysm has therefore been abandoned at our Center.

Furthermore, the constant improvement of our results with the surgical therapy, due certainly to a better surgical technique but also to the widespread experiences with a more complete myocardial protection (hypothermia and cardioplegia) and safer arterial prostheses (low porosity Dacron), made us adopt the following current policy:

a) Each patient suspected of having an acute dissecting aneurysm undergoes early intensive medical treatment (either hypotensive and/or supportive) during the diagnostic phase.

b) Once the diagnosis is established, with special reference to the site of initial dissection (ascending or descending thoracic aorta) (1), the status of the coronaries (13), the visceral aortic branches, and the limbs, the patient is taken to surgery without delay.

A good number of associated procedures were performed in the 54 operated patients, mostly in type I and II dissection (Tables 3, 4), the aortic valve being replaced numerous times. In fact, all kinds of conservative procedures on the acutely insufficient valve gave unsatisfactory results. Most recently, several patients underwent aortic valve replacement and reimplantation of the coronary arteries on the prostheses, with good outcome: these are not included in the present series. All of the operated patients who were discharged from the hospital have been followed regularly and many had repeated catheterization and angiography.

Table 1. Dissecting aneurysm of the thoracic aorta, 1970 - 1979 (N = 84)

Medical treatment only	=	27 († 96.3%	70% C.L. = 88.0%-99.5%)
Surgical treatment	=	57 († 43.8%	70% C.L. = 36.4%-51.6%)
p = 0.000001			

Table 2. Dissecting aneurysm of the thoracic aorta

Surgical mortality changes with time (1970-1979)

Year	No.	Hospital mortality (%)
1970	1	-
1971	3	66
1972	4	75
1973	6	50
1974	5	60
1975	4	50
1976	5	60
1977	10	30
1978	9	22
1979	10	20

Table 3. Type of operation and associated procedures in dissecting aneurysms of the ascending aorta

Type I: 21 pat. (20 acute stage)

Replacement of the ascending aorta (RAA)	12	† 10	(all deaths before 1978)
RAA + commissural resuspension	2	-	(1 AVR after 1 year)
RAA + aortic valve replacement (AVR)	6	† 5	(all deaths before 1978)
RAA + AVR + R. coron. bypass	1	-	(patent bypass after 2 years)
	21	† 15	

Type II: 19 pat. (9 ac., 3 subac., 7 chr. stages)

Patch closure intima laceration	1 (subac.)	† 1	
RAA	5 (2 ac.)	† 2	(2 ac.)
RAA + AVR	7 (4 ac.)	† 1	(chr.)
Asc. aortaplasty + AVR	1 (ac.)	-	
RAA + coartectomy	1 (chr.)	† 1	
RAA + AVR + MVR	1 (ac.)	-	
RAA + AVR + MVR + R. coron. reimpl.	1 (chr.)	† 1	
RAA + R. + L. coron. reimpl. (AVR 1 year earlier)	1 (ac.)	-	
RAA + AVR + R. coron. bypass + R. Valsalva sinus sut.	1 (subac.)	-	
	19	I 6	(3 ac.)

Table 4. Type of operation and associated procedures in dissecting aneurysms of the descending aorta

Type III: 17 pat. (11 ac., 1 subac., 5 chr. stages)		
Descending aorta replacement (DAR)	9	⊕ 3 (3 ac.)
DAR + L. subclavian artery reimplant (L. SAR)	2	⊕ 1 (ac.)
DAR + L. subcl. art.-R. femoral art. bypass	1	- (ac.)
DAR + no heparin.; Gott shunt	4	- (2 ac.)
DAR + Gott shunt + L. SAR	1	- (ac.)
	17	⊕ 4 (4 ac.)

From the clinical point of view, some interesting observations have been made:

1) The actuarial survival at 10 years is about 91% (Fig. 1) which seems to be quite satisfactory, indeed, for a disease usually lethal if untreated.

2) The clinical conditions of the survivors are presently excellent and most of them are asymptomatic 1 to 10 years postoperatively.

3) As far as the arterial hypertension is concerned, all of the hypertensive patients remained such, despite adequate treatment.

4) Three patients died during the 10-year follow-up period, one of them after reoperation for aortic insufficiency and two others of unknown causes.

However, these encouraging clinical findings are only partially in agreement with those of cardiac catheterization and angiography which show that only about 50% of the patients show "normal" appearing thoracoabdominal aorta and branches. The remaining 50% presented some very interesting features such as aneurysmal dilatation of the sinuses of Valsalva, aortic insufficiency, further dilatation of the distal false lumen, new dissection, compression of the true lumen, and occlusion of previously open aortic branches.

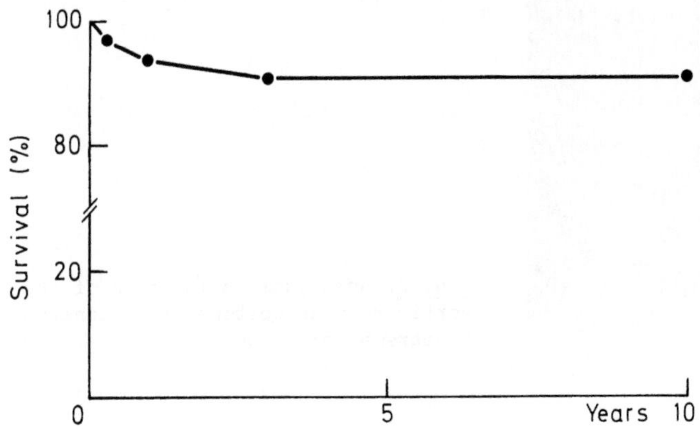

Fig. 1. Actuarial survival curve of operated dissecting aneurysms of the thoracic aorta

There must be no doubt therefore that the acute episode of dissection represents only one phase of the natural history of a profoundly altered aortic wall and this is proved by the facts that:
a) the aortic root, left behind at the time of resection of the ascending aorta in type I and II, has the tendency to dilate and become aneurysmatic, thus involving also the coronary ostia and the aortic valve (Fig. 2);
b) the valve itself, even when initially intact and well functioning, can become insufficient not only because of annular dilatation but also with degeneration of the cusp tissues;
c) despite any attempt to obliterate it, the false lumen, beyond the distal anastomosis of the aortic prosthesis, can stay open or become further dilated, giving origin to a fusiform aneurysm;
d) a true new dissection can originate at the site of distal anastomosis with new intimal laceration (Fig. 3);
e) the true aortic lumen can be compressed from outside by thrombi or hematoma present in the false lumen, so as to be stenosed (Fig. 4);
f) both the thoracic and abdominal aortic branches can become occluded by thrombosis, intimal flaps, etc. (Fig. 5).
Little correlation can therefore exist sometime between the clinical status of the operated patient which can be very satisfactory, and his anatomic situation, potentially most dangerous.

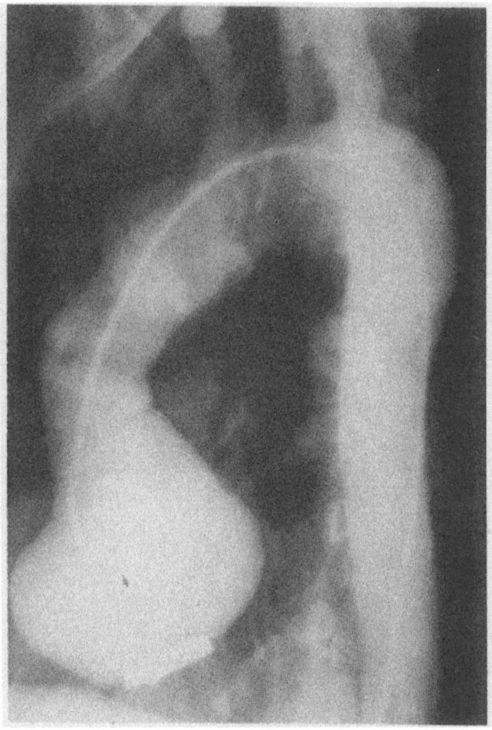

Fig. 2. Aneurysmal dilatation of the aortic root at postoperative control 6 years after surgery

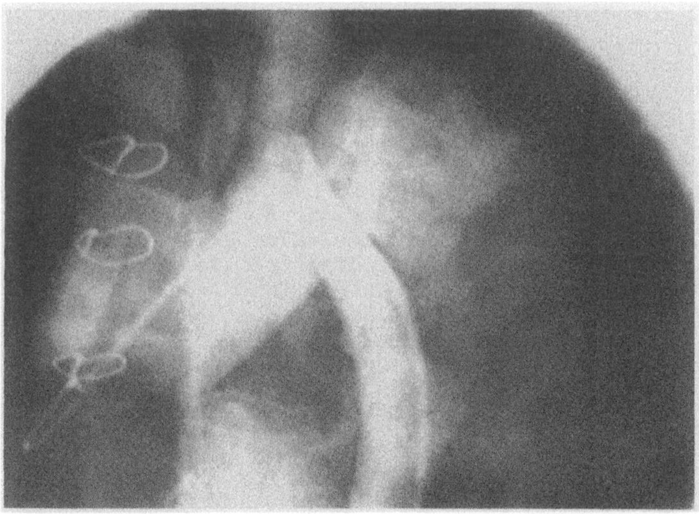

Fig. 3. New dissection originating distal to the prosthetic anastomosis; control 1 year after surgery

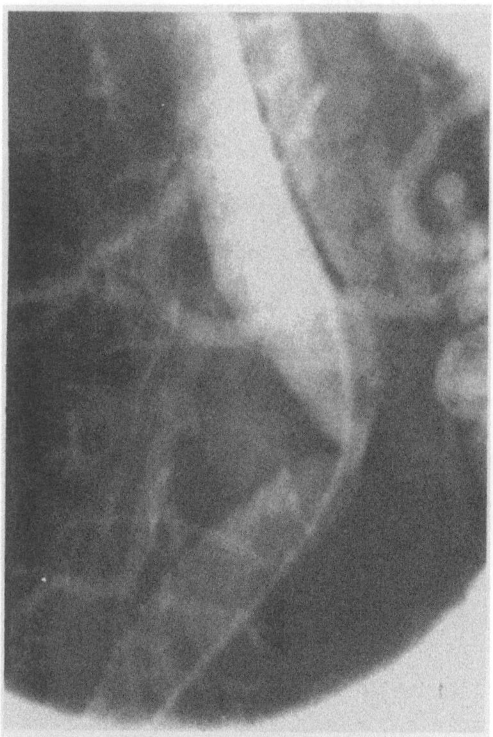

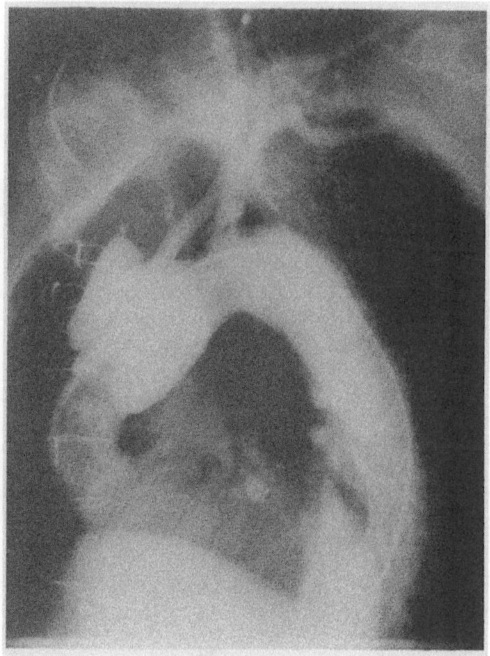

Fig. 4

Fig. 4. Stenosis of the true lumen by extrinsic compression due to the false lumen thrombosis

Fig. 5. Late obstruction of the innominate artery by intimal flap in aneurysmal dilatation just distal to the prosthetic suture line

As a consequence of the above observations, a few changes in our surgical technique have been made and routinely applied, hoping they might contribute to change the spontaneous evolution of these patients. As far as the distal suture line is concerned, where new dissection, intimal laceration, or aneurysmal dilatation has been shown to occur, we now reinforce it from the outside with a tight band made of a flattened Dacron arterial prosthesis. This besides the usual sandwich of teflon felt, pledgeting, etc.

In a good many cases of type I and II dissections, consideration is given to a routine replacement of the aortic valve and reimplantation of the coronary arteries ostia, by utilizing premade ascending aorta prostheses mounted with a mechanical valve. This is aimed to prevent both the dilatation of the residual aortic root as well as aortic regurgitation, causing reoperation in a few years. In our recent series, this last procedure did not increase surgical mortality.

References

1. Appelbaum A (1976) Ascending vs descending aortic dissection. Ann Surg 21:298
2. Cèvese PG (1977) Aneurismi dissecanti dell'aorta. Piccin, Padova
3. Daily PO (1970) Management of acute aortic dissection. Ann Thorac Surg 10:237
4. De Bakey ME (1965) Surgical management of dissecting aneurysm of the aorta. J Thorac Cardiovasc Surg 49:130
5. Gallucci V (1978) Aneurismi dissecanti dell'aorta. Indicazioni chirurgiche e terapia. VII Congr Naz Soc Ital Chir Urg e Pronto Socc
6. Hirst AE (1958) Dissecting aneurysm of the aorta. A review of 505 cases. Medicine (Baltimore) 37:217
7. Kidd JN (1976) Surgical treatment of aneurysm of the ascending aorta. Circulation 54:6
8. Siegel P (1971) Sodium nitroprusside in the surgical treatment of cerebral aneurysm and arteriovenous malformation. Br J Anaesth 43:790
9. Wheat MW (1965) Treatment of dissecting aneurysm of the aorta without surgery. J Thorac Cardiovasc Surg 50:364
10. Wheat MW (1971) Surgical treatment of aneurysm of the aortic root. Ann Thorac Surg 12:593
11. Wheat MW (1977) Dissecting aneurysm of the aorta. Gibbon surgery of the chest. Saunders, Philadelphia
12. Wolfe WG (1977) The evolution of medical and surgical management of acute aortic dissection. Circulation 56:4
13. Zubiate P (1976) Surgical treatment of aneurysm of the ascending aorta with aortic insufficiency and marked displacement of the coronary ostia. J Thorac Cardiovasc Surg 71/3:415

Late Surgical Results of Ascending Aortic Dissections

R. Nottin, Ch. d'Allaines, Ph. Blondeau, A Piwnica, A. Carpentier, A. Brunet, C. Farge, A. Deloche, P. Donzeau-Gouge, and Ch. Dobust*

As various types of surgical treatment have been applied to ascending aorta dissections during the last 20 years, interest of their long-term evaluation is obvious. This is the purpose of the subsequent study.

Material

Between 1960 and 1979, we have operated on 98 patients for ascending aorta dissection; 64 were type I and 34 type II (De Bakey's classification). Hospital mortality (first postoperative month) was 32 of 60 patients operated for acute dissection and seven of 38 patients operated for chronic dissection. Thirteen of the 59 discharged patients died in the late follow-up. These late deaths occurred between 6 months and 7.5 years after operation (mean 3.5 years). Six of them were sudden and unexplained because no postmortem examination could be performed. Three late deaths were secondary to subacute bacterial endocarditis, two secondary to myocardial failure, and one to myocardial infarction. The last case of late death followed a reoperation for a recurrent aneurysm after resection anastomosis. Only one discharged patient was last to follow-up.

The 45 remaining patients are alive at the present time and have been restudied between 1 and 14 years postoperatively (mean 6 years). Seven of them were successfully reoperated for aortic regurgitation (two patients), coronary ostial stenosis (one patient), recurrent ascending aorta dissection (one patient), and dissecting aneurysm of the descending aorta (three patients).

The 10-year actuarial survival rate is 24% for acute dissections and 54% for chronic dissections. This difference is only related to early hospital mortality as evident on actuarial survival curves (Fig. 1).

Aortographic study has been performed in 24 patients (53% of survivors) an average of 5 years (range 6 months to 12 years) after operation: 14 of 22 acute dissections long-term survivors and 10 of 23 chronic dissections survivors. Seven patients have a residual or recurrent aneurysm of the aortic root. Persistent dissection of the transverse aortic arch is present in all type I dissections (16 patients), but dissecting aneurysms of the arch observed only in one of them. In this group, four patients have a huge dilatation of the descending aorta. In type II dissections (eight patients) no secondary dissection of transverse arch or descending aorta is observed. One patient has an aneurysmal dilatation of the entire transverse arch.

---

*Clinique de Chirurgie Cardiovasculaire, Hôpital Broussais, 96, rue Didot 75014 Paris, France

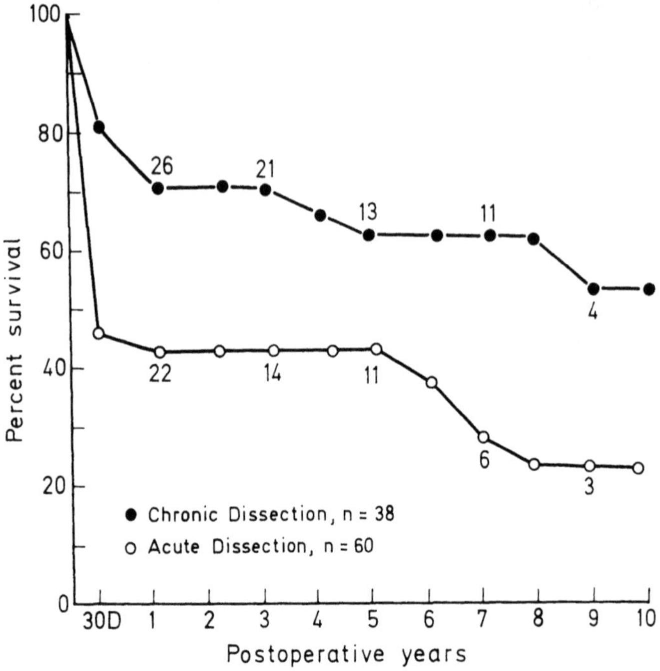

Fig. 1. Ascending aortic dissections, actuarial survival

Comments

Long-term results are closely related to initial surgical management of aortic insufficiency and ascending aorta lesions. In cases in which aortic regurgitation is absent at the time of operation, valve replacement appears unjustified. No aortic insufficiency developed in the follow-up of the nine patients that we operated in these conditions. Conservative treatment of aortic insufficiency, as done in seven patients, seems hazardous as four have persistent moderate to huge aortic regurgitation and one required valve replacement.

On the other hand, patients with valve prosthesis (42 cases) are at risk of prosthesis endocarditis (two cases) or paravalvular leak (one case). But no significant emboli episode occurred in this series and incidence of sudden deaths is not increased (4/42 valve replacement versus 2/16 conservative management).

In relation to treatment of ascending aortic lesions, comparison of long-term angiographic results is available for two techniques: resection followed by direct anastomosis (seven patients) and supracoronary tubular graft replacement (17 patients). Incidence of recurrent aneurysm of the ascending aorta appears very high in the first group (5/7) and relatively low in the second group (2/17). Moreover, in this last group dilatation of the aortic root remains stable on repeated distent controls (10 at 12 years for the first patient, 5 at 14 years for the second patient) and no patient had to be reoperated for such a reason.

It is concluded that:
1) resection anastomosis is obsolete and must be abandoned;
2) supracoronary tubular graft replacement gives long-term satisfactory results;
3) clinical superiority of more radical procedures like Bentall's needs further assessment.

In relation to long-term prognosis, more disturbing than residual aortic root dilatation are the persistency and evolution of associated transverse and descending aortic dissection. None of the 16 type I dissections studied by angiography shows healing of the dissecting process in these segments of the aorta. Progressive and symptomatic dilatation of the descending aorta have led to successful reoperation in three cases.

An original technique proposed by Carpentier (1, 2) has been used in two cases: aortic bypass from ascending to abdominal aorta with postsubclavian aortic exclusion (Fig. 2). In case of asymptomatic dilatations (four cases), a conservative attitude has been observed but remains questionable.

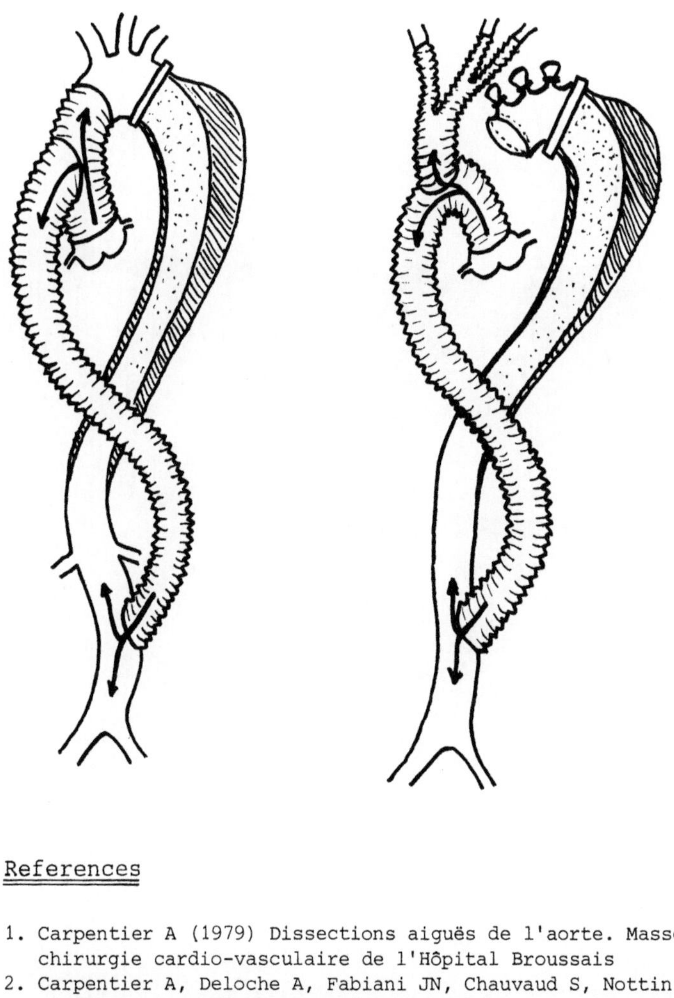

Fig. 2. Two cases of dissecting aneurysm of the descending aorta treated successfully by thromboexclusion

References

1. Carpentier A (1979) Dissections aiguës de l'aorte. Masson, Paris, Actualités de chirurgie cardio-vasculaire de l'Hôpital Broussais
2. Carpentier A, Deloche A, Fabiani JN, Chauvaud S, Nottin R, Relland J, Dubost C (1980) A new approach to the treatment of aortic dissection. 60th Annual Meeting of the American Association for Thoracic Surgery, San Francisco, April 29th 1980

Session VIII Vascular Surgery

Vascular Forum I

Chairman: A. Thevenet, Montpellier; Co-Chaiman: U. Ruberti, Milan

Surgical Treatment of Chronic Intestinal Ischemia

V. Paredero-del Bosque, A. del Río, J. López-Parra, V. Martin-Paredero, G. Pastor, and A. Vidal*

Chronic intestinal ischemia or "abdominal angina" is characterized by postprandial abdominal pain. The patient reduces the food intake and in a few weeks or months the weight loss is very profound. Weight loss is the most common finding. In fact, the diagnosis of intestinal ischemia is in doubt if the patient has had no significant decrease in weight. The malabsorption syndrome is another finding. However, it has been disappointing to most authors to discover that this syndrome was not a common feature of visceral ischemia.

The most important symptom is the patient's abdominal pain pattern. The pain is tpyically located near the epigastrium or the midabdomen. It usually occurs after a meal and is characterized by a continuous ache changing sometimes to recurrent colicky pain. The duration and the intensity of the pain correlate with the amount and the quality of food ingested. It rarely takes more than 1 h. Sometimes a systolic bruit may be heard in the abdomen but such a finding is very common in arteriosclerotic patients.

In general laboratory studies are unrewarding although the physiologic function of the small bowel can be studied by stool examination and all the variety of the absorption studies. The stool analyses for fat, nitrogen, and the urinary excretion of orally administered D-xylose, as well as vitamin B12 absorption, vitamin A tolerance, and the serun carotene level have been found to be of very limited value. Barium contrast studies of the small and large bowel are usually normal in these patients.

The arteriogram is essential and the only way to make a definitive diagnosis. The origins of the intestinal arteries should be well visualized by lateral films. Most of the patients have two-vessel obstruction. However, a few patients with a single-vessel occlusion have been shown to have attacks of abdominal angina.

The diagnosis is most difficult because the presence of intestinal visceral ischemia is rare, but the alert physician will make the diagnosis before a bowel infarction occurs, requesting a visceral artery arteriogram, after other more common abdominal diseases have been excluded.

The vascular surgical service of the Jiménez Díaz Foundation of Madrid has treated 12 patients having a chronic intestinal ischemia because of occlusive arteriosclerotic disease of the visceral intestinal arteries (Table 1).

Of these 12 patients, nine had some important obliterative arteriosclerotic disease of the aortoiliac segment. Occlusion of the superior mesenteric artery was found together with obstruction of the celiac axis. The other three cases showed a thoracoabdominal aneurysm involving the visceral abdominal arteries. In three of these patients a bilateral renal Dacron bypass graft had also to be inserted because of important bilateral ostial renal stenosis.

---

*Department of Vascular Surgery, Universidad Autónoma de Madrid, Spain

Table 1. Surgical treatment of chronic intestinal ischemia

Superior mesenteric artery revascularization		6 patients
Bilateral renal and sup. mesenteric artery revascularization:		
Thoracoabdominal aneurysms	3	
Extensive aortoiliac mesenteric and renal obstructive disease	3	6 patients

In all 12 patients the aortoiliac arterial segment was replaced by a Dacron double velour bifurcated aortoiliac or femoral graft. The thoracoabdominal aneurysms were partially resected and a bypass Dacron graft placed with side arm branches to the visceral abdominal arteries. The revascularization of the superior mesenteric artery was accomplished by the insertion of a 8 mm knitted Dacron graft from the side of the aortic graft.

Eight of our patients had a profound weight loss (15 kg) associated with abdominal angina. One patient also presented hypertension and renal insufficiency. Three thoracoabdominal aneurysms have no intestinal symptoms (Table 2). Three of the most significant cases are presented in this paper.

The first case is a patient, 65 years old, with a history of abdominal angina during the last 5 months. He had a profound weight loss of 24 kg. In the last month the only food he had was milk. The arteriogram showed a complete occlusion of the celiac axis and the superior mesenteric artery. The inferior mesenteric artery of the increase side was the only intestinal artery presented (Fig. 1).

He was operated upon and an aortobifemoral graft was done with an 8 mm knitted Dacron side arm branch graft to the superior mesenteric artery. The inferior mesenteric artery was reimplanted into the graft.

A postoperative arteriogram was carried out. The aorto mesenteric graft was patent with a good visualization of the superior mesenteric artery. The inferior mesenteric artery was also patent, the size of this artery was reduced, and there was an inversion of the flow through the marginal artery.

The second case was a 43-year-old male with an 8-month history of abdominal angina, profound weight loss, and arterial hypertension not well controlled by medical therapy. The arteriogram showed a complete obstruction of the celiac, superior, and inferior mesenteric arteries and a bilateral renal artery stenosis (Fig. 2).

Table 2. Symptoms in intestinal angina

Weight loss (15 kg) abdominal angina	8 patients
No abdominal angina	3 patients (thoracoabdominal aneurysms)
Weight loss, hypertension, renal insufficiency	1 patient (obst. of sup. mesenteric artery bilateral renal stenosis)

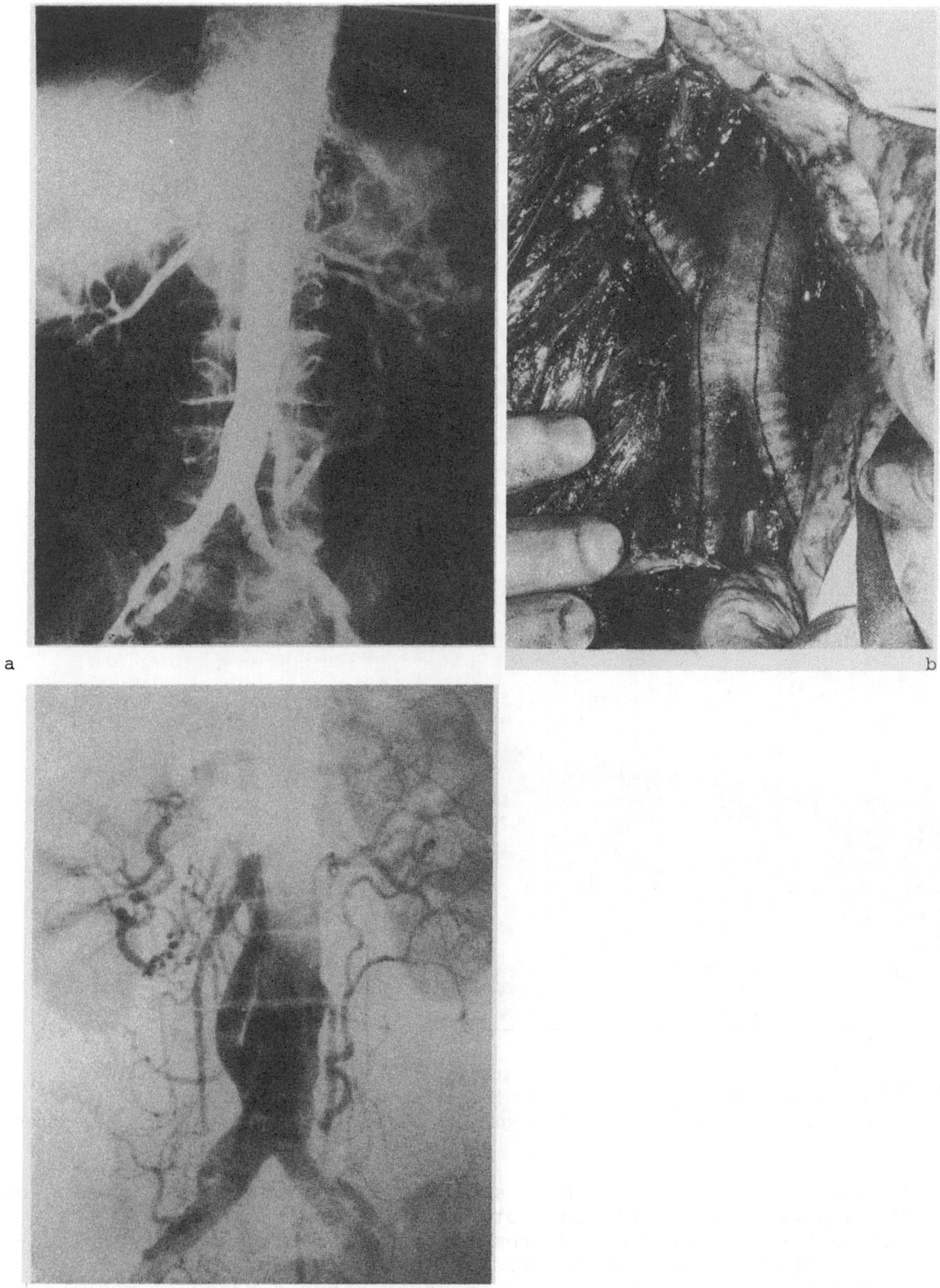

Fig. 1. a Occlusion celiac and superior mesenteric arteries. Inferior mesenteric artery of increase side with a large marginal artery. b Aortobifemoral bypass graft. Side arm branch graft to the superior mesenteric artery. c Aortomesenteric graft patent. The superior mesenteric artery is well visualized. Reduced side of the inferior mesenteric and marginal artery

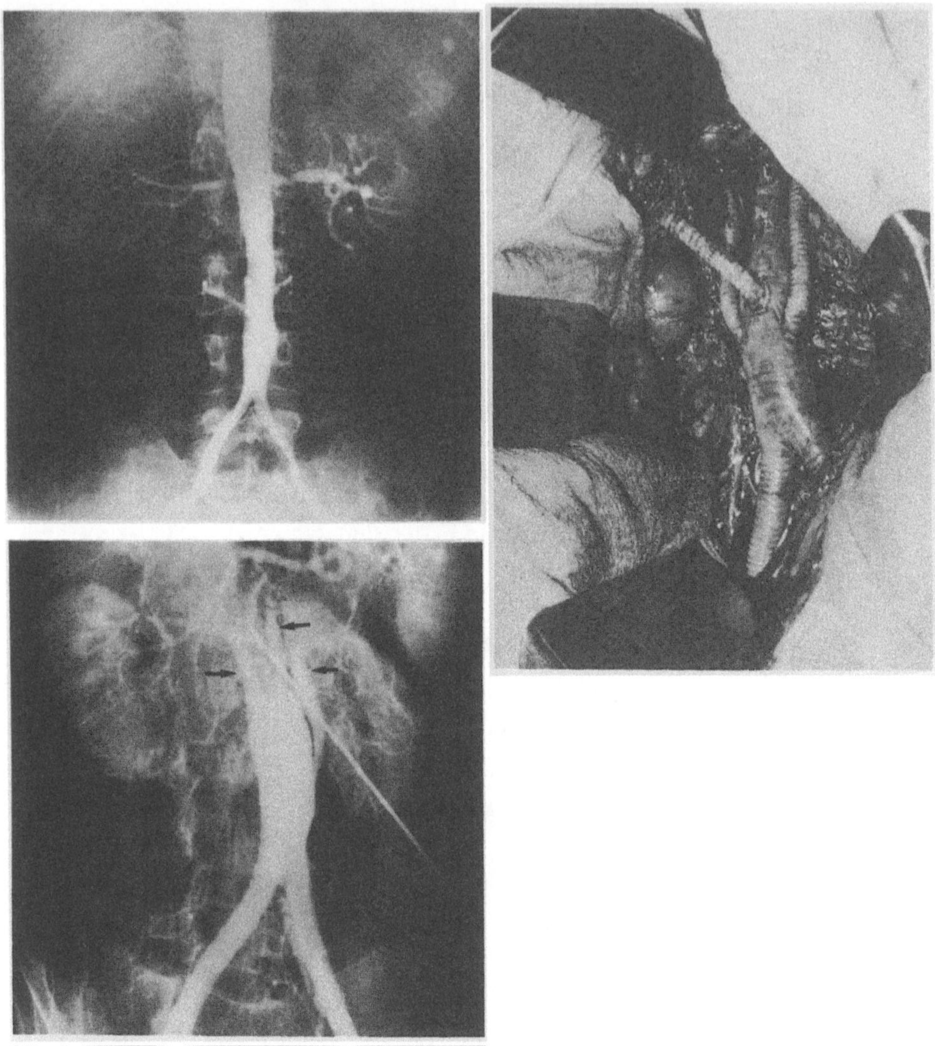

a b c

Fig. 2. a Bilateral renal stenosis. Occlusion of all the intestinal arteries. b Aortobifemoral bypass graft. Side arm branches to both renal and superior mesenteric arteries. c Postoperative arteriogram showing all the visceral branches patent

An aortobifemoral Dacron bypass graft with Dacron side arm branches to the superior mesenteric and both renal arteries was carried out.

The patient was discharged from the hospital without abdominal angina and normal blood pressure treated only with a restricted salt diet. The renal function was also improved after surgery. A postoperative arteriogram showed a patent graft.

The third case was a 47-year-old male with a history of an abdominal pulsating mass, associated with abdominal angina during the last 5 months. Angiogram studies showed a thoracoabdominal aneurysm involving the visceral arteries (Fig. 3).

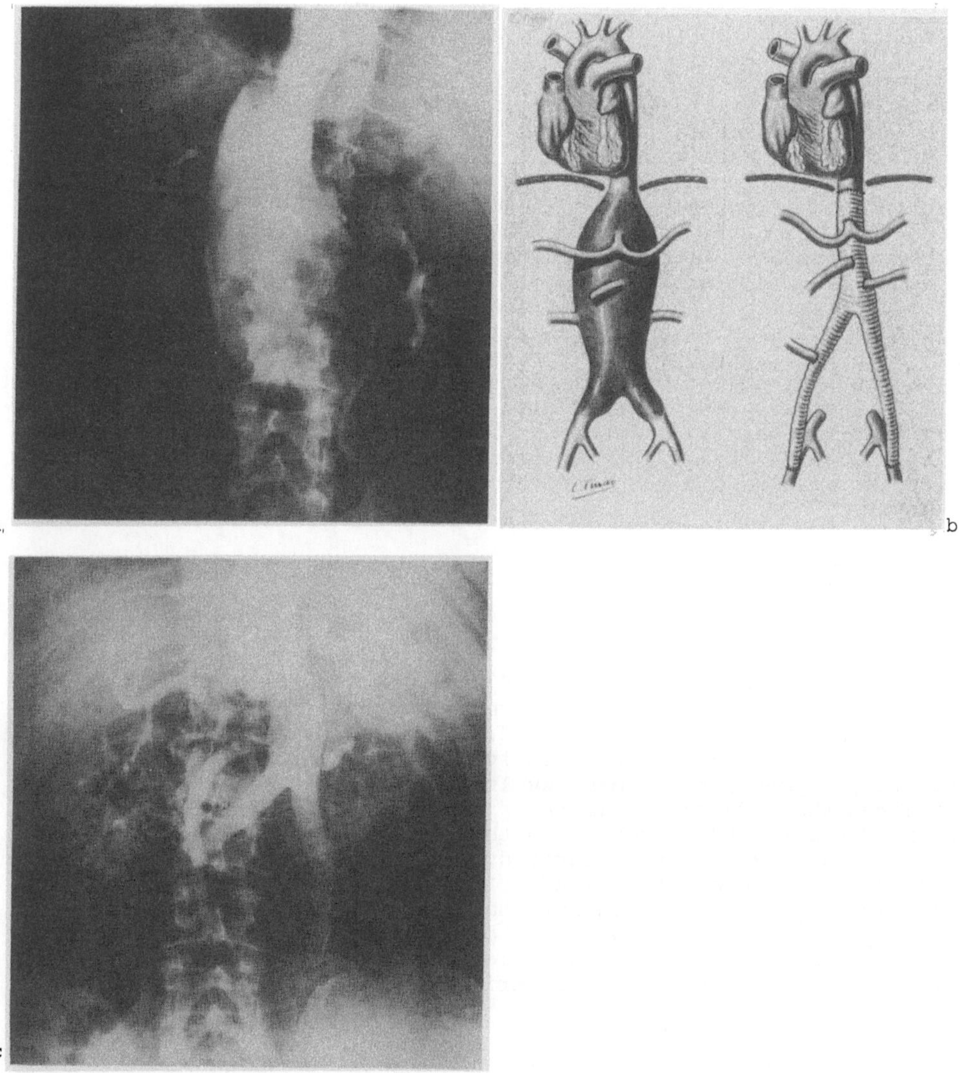

Fig. 3. a Thoracoabdominal aneurysm. b Partial resection of the aneurysm. Thoracic aorta bifemoral bypass graft. All the visceral arteries reimplanted into the graft. c Postoperative arteriogram showing the patency of the visceral arteries

The aneurysm was partially resected and a thoracic aorta bifemoral graft placed. The celiac, superior mesenteric and both renal arteries were reimplanted into the graft.

An intravenous pielogram showed normal elimination of the contrast by the two kidneys. A 6-month postoperative arteriogram was done showing the celiac superior mesenteric and renal arteries well functioning.

Results

Good results with complete relief of the abdominal angina and gaining of weight were obtained in 11 patients (91.6%). One patient died in the immediate postoperative period of an acute myocardial infarction. So the mortality rate was 8.3%.

The 11 patients had a 6-month to 5-year follow-up with these late results: One patient had an occlusion of the right limb of the aorto-femoral bypass graft. The patient was reoperated and a thrombectomy plus profundoplasty were carried out with complete relief of the ischemic symptoms of the extremity.

One patient was readmitted to the hospital because of recent post-prandial abdominal discomfort. An arteriogram was done showing an occlusion of the aortomesenteric graft. The patient was reoperated and a new graft was placed maintaining the aorto and the superior mesenteric anastomosis. One patient died 2 years after operation because of an acute myocardial infarction. One patient was readmitted to the hospital because of a right hemiparesia. Arteriograms of the supraortic trunks disclosed a complete thrombosis of the left internal carotid artery.

Discussion

All our patients having symptoms of abdominal angina had at least two intestinal visceral arteries involved. Symptoms rarely appear with only one intestinal vessel affected. For this reason and also because most of our patients had an extensive arteriosclerotic disease of the aortoiliac segment, sometimes involving both renal arteries, we only considered the revascularization of the superior mesenteric artery. Only in the patients presenting with a thoracoabdominal aneurysm was the celiac axis also revascularized. This was sufficient in our patients to obtain complete relief of the intestinal symptoms.

However, recently some authors have recommended, due to recurrence of the symptoms after a few months or years, the complete revascularization of all the intestinal arteries. Actually we think that if feasible at least two intestinal arteries should be revascularized.

References

1. Boley SJ, et al. (eds) (1971) Vascular disorders of the intestine. Appleton Century Crofts, New York
2. Connolly JE, Kwaan JM (1979) Prophylactic revascularization of the gut. Ann Surg 190:514
3. Crawford ES, Morris GC, Myhre HO, Roehm JOF (1977) Celiac axis, superior mesenteric artery, and inferior mesenteric artery occlusion. Surgical considerations. Surgery 82:856
4. Crawford ES, Saydr DM, Cho GC, Roehm JOF (1978) Progress in treatment of thoraco-abdominal and aortic aneurysms involving celiac, superior mesenteric and renal arteries. Ann Surg 188:404
5. Eidemiller LR, Nelson JC, Porter JM (1979) Surgical treatment of chronic visceral ischemia. Am J Surg 138:264
6. Marston A, Kieny R, Szilagyi DE, Taylor GW (1976) Intestinal ischemia. Arch Surg 11:107

7. McCollum CH, Graham JM, De Bakey ME (1976) Chronic mesenteric arterial insufficiency: Results of revascularization in 33 cases. South Med J 69:1299
8. Morris GC, De Bakey ME (1961) Abdominal angina diagnosis and surgical treatment. JAMA 176:88
9. Morris GC, Crawford ES, Cooley DA (1962) Revascularization of the celiac and superior mesenteric arteries. Arch Surg 84:95
10. Reul GJ, Wukasch DC, Sandiford FM, Chiarillo L, Hallman GL, Cooley DA (1974) Surgical treatment of abdominal angina, review of 25 patients. Surgery 75:682
11. Stoney RJ, Ehrenfeld WK, Wyile EJ (1977) Revascularization method in chronic visceral ischemia caused by atheroesclerosis. Ann Surg 186:468

Management of Acute Mesenteric Vascular Disease (60 Cases)

R. Kieny, J. Cinqualbre, C. Peter, and H. El Badawy*

Most of the recent papers dealing with intestinal infarction agree on the extreme severity of this condition and that there has been little recent therapeutic progress. Some authors feel that revascularization is contraindicated and consider intestinal resection the only useful procedure. However, it appears that systematic diagnostic (and sometimes interventional) angiography, in conjunction with reconstructive vascular procedures on the arteries of the digestive tract, may modify the disease.

Evaluation of this more aggressive approach requires separation of two different pathological stages in intestinal ischemia: 1) Intestinal infarction (II), where irreversible lesions require intestinal resection and in which case a vascular procedure is only able to limit the length of the resection; 2) acute ischemic mesenteric syndrome (AIMS), where the intestine presents macroscopic changes but is still viable and can benefit from a revascularization procedure.

Material

Included are 60 patients treated in our unit from 1964 to 1979. This group comprises ten cases of atherosclerotic occlusive disease (ASOD), 20 cases of superior mesenteric embolism (SME), and 30 cases of non-occlusive ischemia (NOI). Classification according to etiology and anatomical stage is represented in Tables 1 and 2.

Table 1. Etiology of 60 cases of acute intestinal ischemia

	1964-1968	1969-1973	1974-1979	
ASOD	3	5	2	10
SME	1	4	15	20
NOI	2	6	22	30
Total	6	15	39	60

*Service de chirurgie cardiovasculaire, C.H.U., Strasbourg, France

Table 2. Pathologic stage at time of diagnosis in 60 patients with acute intestinal ischemia

	1964-1968	1969-1973	1974-1979	
II 23 (infarction)	5	5	10	ASOD: 3 SME: 8 NOI: 12
AIMS 37	1	10	26	ASOD: 7 SME: 12 NOI: 18
Percent seen before infarction	1/6 = 16%	10/15 = 66%	26/39 = 66%	

Remarks

Systematic angiography has been available since 1970. Patients with atherosclerotic disease and infarction have not been treated by arterial revascularization since 1969. Since 1976, patients with NOI have not been operated upon immediately. Pathological stage was assessed on the basis of the clinical course (a patient was supposed not to have an infarction when the length of clinical course was more than 1 week). Our results are summarized in Table 3.

Table 3. Survival in 60 patients considering etiology and pathological

	II		AIMS	
	Cases	Survivors	Cases	Survivors
ASOD	3	(0)	7	(7)
Embolism SME	8	(0)	12	(7)
NOI	12	(0)	18	(5)
Total	23	(0) 0%	37	(19) 51%

Discussion

AIMS precedes intestinal infarction, and therapeutic procedures are efficient only if performed at this early stage. Unfortunately, emergency of this condition contrasts with diagnostic difficulties at this time. Pain is variable in location, duration, and severity. Abdominal examination is also not diagnostic. The only way to find these patients is to be aware of the possibility of a such condition in the presence of any abdominal symptom occurring in "high risk" patients. Patients with a history of atherosclerosis, systemic embolism, or cardiac disease should have mesenteric angiography at the slightest suspicion of bowel ischemia, because proper therapy requires the recognition of the exact cause of ischemia (ASOD, SME, and NOI).

ASOD

Atherosclerosis is diffuse, segmental, and progressive. On the basis of chronic circulatory insufficiency, the AIMS is related either to decreased perfusion in the collateral circulation or to the progression of the proximal stenotic lesions.

Abdominal pain in the presence of peripheral arterial disease is highly suggestive of intestinal ischemia when pain occurs after an episode of hypotension as caused by a surgical procedure or aortography (three cases in our series) or when a previously noted epigastric murmur disappears. Prior demonstration of a dilated inferior mesenteric artery (Riolan's arcade) strongly increases the index of suspicion.

Since the diagnosis is tremendously difficult when the chronic disease becomes acute, we indicate early operation for abdominal angina, but also strongly advocate "preventive" intestinal revascularization in selected cases: Operation may be advised in patients presenting double or triple lesions of the arteries of the digestive tract. But where the diagnosis of multiple intestinal arterial obstruction is made, mesenteric revascularization is mandatory in the presence of an aortoiliac or renal disease requiring correction. Application of this concept in 22 mesenteric revascularization since 1969 was gratifying. We observed no mesenteric ischemic complication in more than 1000 aortoiliac reconstructive procedures performed during the same period of time. Treatment of choice is bypass graft or reimplantation of the SMA into the aorta below the level of the left renal vein. Only if the hepatic pulse is still weak or not felt after this procedure do we also do an aortohepatic artery bypass.

SME and NOI

Both must be considered together because they are similar in many respects. Both occur acutely in a previously normal vascular system, without any possibility for development of collateral circulation. Both, embolism and nonocclusive ischemia, occur in patients with cardiac diseases. Clinical symptoms are even less impressive than in intestinal ischemia due to ASOD. Increased risk is associated with a recent history of cardioversion, digitalis treatment, or discontinuation of long-term anticoagulant therapy in cardiac valve patients. A previous recent history of peripheral arterial embolism, of myocardial infarction, or an episode of cardiac failure may precede these conditions.

Angiography in these cases is necessary. Radiological features of SME and NOI are specific and provide the diagnosis at an early stage when clinical and laboratory date are of little or no benefit. Angiography differentiates embolism and NOI without the necessity of laparotomy and provides the basis for a rational therapeutic approach. Furthermore, the same patient may present either an embolism or an NOI at different occasions in his life. Two personal cases, unique to our knowledge, demonstrate this fact.

In case of embolism, treatment is embolectomy of the SMA, using a Fogarty catheter after exposure of the artery in the infracolic mesentery. If an intestinal resection is required, it should be done during the same operation.

Treatment of NOI is not yet clearly defined. Results from "diagnostic laparotomies" at an early stage are well known: almost 100% mortality (10 deaths in 11 patients in our series). This operation on an unstable patient does not improve the splanchnic circulation and moreover aggravates the shock.

General supportive therapy of the cardio-circulator function is useful and sometimes is sufficient for recovery. However, the treatment of choice is the direct intraarterial injection of vasodilator drugs into the SMA. This can be done according to two procedures: bolus injection or prolonged infusion. If after infusion therapy there is no evidence of improvement as demonstrated by a repeated angiography, a laparotomy must be performed in spite of its poor prognosis. Usually, it reveals a massive infarction and is followed by death. On the opposite, when infusion therapy is effective, the place of "security laparotomy" after complete normalization of the hemodynamic parameters can be considered.

Treatment of Infections After Arterial Reconstructive Procedures: Possibilities and Results

J. Koning, and R.J.A.M. van Dongen*

Introduction

Infection is the most serious complication following arterial reconstructive surgery. It occurs in approximately 1% to 6% of all procedures and it often leads to the loss of a limb or even the life of a patient (1, 2). For this reason, prevention of infection is of the greatest importance.

Prevention of Infections

Preoperative

In the preoperative period, the patient should stay in the hospital as briefly as possible. If necessary his general condition should be improved. Diabetes mellitus, distal necrotic lesions, or infections elsewhere in the body have to be taken care of. Especially important are the measures related to the groin, the most common site of infections in vascular surgery. It has to be stressed that Seldinger arteriography should not be carried out prior to exploration of the femoral artery because of the risk of haematoma.

Peroperative

During the operation, it is important to use atraumatic surgical techniques. Care has to be taken to avoid lesions of the lymph nodes. In our opinion, electrocoagulation should not be used in the groin. Especially important is to prevent the use of allograft material in the groin, since the majority of infections occur in patients where allograft material has been used. For this reason in our hospital an iliac graft is always anastomosed with the distal external iliac artery instead of with the common femoral artery. Adequate drainage of the wound is important for the prevention of haematoma, whereas meticulous closure of the different layers prevents the formation of dead space.

---

*Department of Vascular Surgery, University Hospital "Wilhelmina Gasthuis", University of Amsterdam, 1e Helmersstraat 104, 1054 EG, Amsterdam, The Netherlands

Postoperative

In the postoperative period, the wounds should be covered adequately. In the first 5 to 7 days, the patient is immobilized. Antibiotic therapy is started when indicated. We do not use prophylactic antibiotic therapy systematically. Patients with distal gangrene or infections elsewhere in the body are treated with antibiotics after cultures and sensitivity testing.

Diagnosis

Infection of the repaired artery is often difficult to diagnose. Sometimes an abscess occurs around the graft. When a draining fistula develops in the scar at the side of an anastomosis (mostly in the groin), infection is certain. But sometimes, especially in infections in the retroperitoneal area, the diagnosis is very difficult. Unexplained fever, leucocytosis, and elevated ESR can be the only symptoms. When suspicion exists urography, sonography, computed tomography, and angiography can be of help.

Recently, we started to use the indium-111 labelled-leucocyte scanning method to diagnose or rule out infections. We attained good results as will be explained elsewhere in this volume (Rövekamp et al., see this volume p. 573). Sometimes surgical exploration is necessary to confirm the diagnosis of infection. During this procedure, cultures and Gram stains can be of help.

Therapy of Infections

In the extremities, most superficial infections involving the dermis and the subcutaneous tissue (grades I and II according to Szilagy) heal without causing infections of the reconstructed arteries (4). Szilagy's grade III infections, however, that is infections in which the repaired vessels are involved, form a real problem.

The patient is in danger of complications like sepsis, haemorrhage, or thrombosis. In relation to the therapeutic possibilities, we made a classification as shown in Figure 1, mainly based on the degree in which these complications occurred.

Classification of Infections

Stage I Infections

These are infections of the graft in which no bleeding or thrombosis occurred. The patient is treated with antibiotics and irrigation-drainage is started. In this way, the infection often can be diminished, but cure was seldom achieved when a prosthesis was implanted. The treatment was more often successful when only autologous material was used.

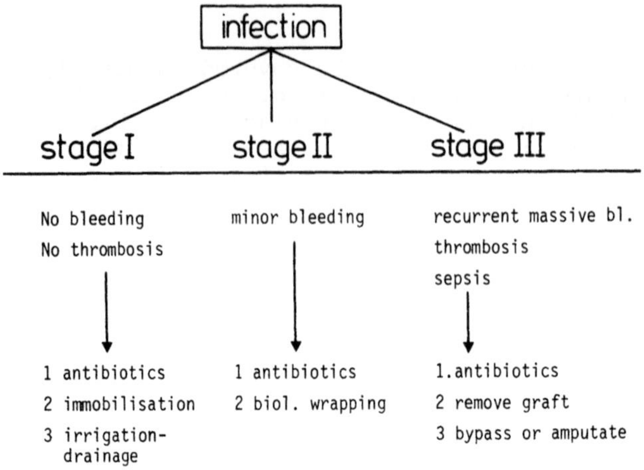

Fig. 1. Classification of infections

Stage II Infections

These are infections complicated by minor bleeding episodes. In this situation, definite healing can be achieved with the help of well-vascularized tissue, preferably the omentum. We call this biological wrapping. Originally we used biological wrapping in infections in the groin but the technique can also be used in the aortoiliac area.

Technique of biological wrapping: After removal of the infected haematoma, the leak in the suture line is closed with the help of a supporting saphenous vein strip instead of by primary suture. Then a well-vascularized pedicle is made of the great omentum via a supra-inguinal incision. This pedicle is led subcutaneously via a wide tunnel to the groin. Here it is fixed around the graft and the anastomosis. Finally the skin can be closed by primary suture, if necessary with the help of relaxing incisions, or the defect can be closed with a split skin graft.

Stage III Infections

These are infections complicated by recurrent bleeding, sepsis, or thrombosis of the graft. In this case, the graft has to be removed to cure the patient. This is also the case in stage I and II infections when the above outlined therapy fails. In general, especially in early postoperative infections, the allograft has to be removed. Partial removal of the graft is sometimes possible if an infection occurs at the site of an anastomosis in the late postoperative period when the graft is already rigidly fixed in the surrounding tissue. In this case, the graft is explored and cut in an area far away from the infected side. Later, in a second operation, the infected part of the graft is removed, mostly via the groin.

Progressive Ligature

A non-functioning, thrombosed graft can be removed safely, but when a functioning graft has to be removed, the circulation of the extremity is often endangered. In order to avoid an amputation, an extra-anatomic bypass has to be made, preferably of autologous material like the saphenous vein. However, a good saphenous vein is not always available. Sometimes severe ischaemia of an extremity is likely to occur after removal of the graft. This can be assessed by direct clamping of the graft or by intraluminal occlusion prior to surgery.

If ischaemia occurs, we first try to stimulate the development of collaterals by using a slowly progressive ligature. A slowly progressive ligature consists of slowly swelling material, Ameroid, which is contained in a metal ring. The Ameroid swells with the uptake of water, causing narrowing of the lumen. The graft is compressed in about 2 weeks and in the meantime collaterals can develop, so that the graft can be removed safely. The angiogram in Figure 2 shows the compression of the artery by the ligature after 14 days.

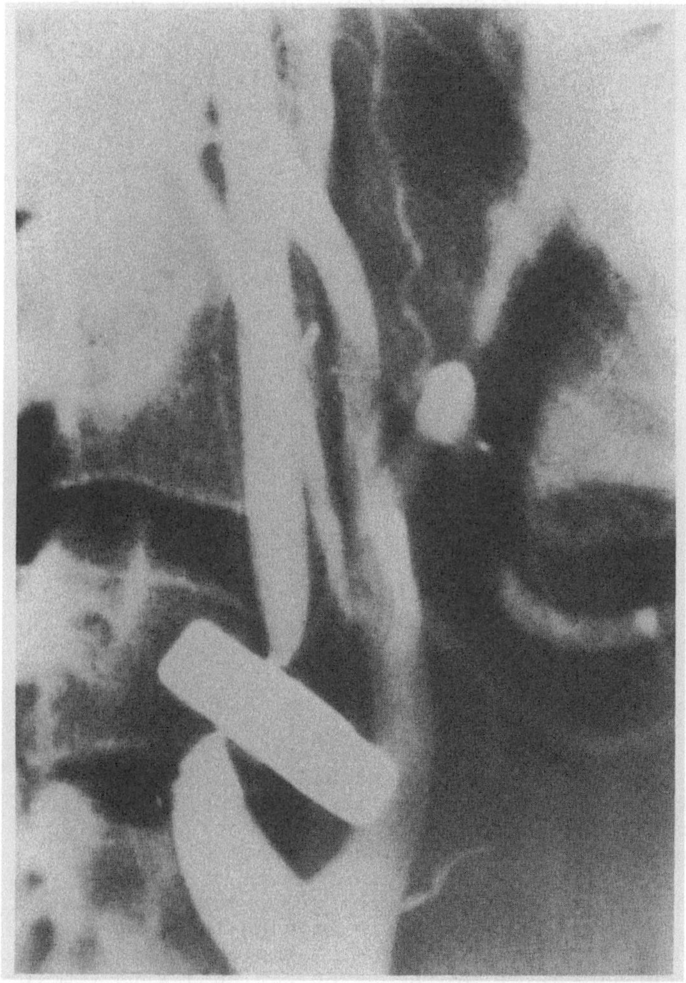

Fig. 2. The artery is severely compressed by the progressive ligature 14 days after application

When the infected graft is localized in an inaccessible area, it is impossible to use the progressive ligature. Than it is possible to obstruct the graft with an intraluminally placed balloon catheter. When the collateral circulation is sufficiently well developed, the graft can be removed safely. Otherwise choice has to be made between extraanatomic reconstruction or direct amputation.

Results

In the last 6 years, 21 patients with infections of the repaired arterial system were treated in our hospital. Seven patients were referred to us from other hospitals. In our own patient material of 1800 reconstructions during this period, we therefore had 14 infections which is 0.8%.

According to our own subdivision, the patients could be classified as shown in Table 1. Eight patients were without complications, three had minor bleedings, and ten patients had severe bleeding or sepsis.

Table 1. Stages of infection

Operation type	No. pat.	Stage		
		I	II	III
Bifurcation graft	7	2	-	5
Aortoiliofemoral	3	2	1	-
Iliac reconstr.	2	1	-	1
Femoropopliteal				
saphenous vein	4	2	1	1
prosthesis	2	-	1	1
TEA	1	-	-	1
Supraaortic	2	1	-	1

In half of the aortoiliac reconstructions the whole graft was involved. In five of the 12 patients in this group, the infection was initially localized in the groin. These were all patients with femoral anastomoses of the prosthesis. One patient had an infection of the proximal part of the graft. In the femoropopliteal region, three of seven infections occurred in the groin. In three patients, the infection occurred in the upper leg, whereas one haemorrhage occurred in the lower leg.

The incidence of reoperation was high in the group were infections occurred. Seventy-five percent of the patients with an infected aortic bifurcation graft had had several reoperations of the aortoiliac system before infection occurred. Three of the seven patients with femoropopliteal infections also had redo surgery.

The results of our therapy in relation to mortality and amputation rate are shown in Table 2. The highest mortality of 71% was recorded in patients with infected aortic bifurcation grafts. In the femoropopliteal reconstructions there was no loss of lives, but the amputation frequency was 30%. The overall mortality in our series is 28%, whereas the overall amputation frequency is 15%.

Table 2. Mortality and amputation rate

Operation	No. pat.	Mortality	Amputation
Bifurcation graft aortoiliac	7	5 = 71%	1 = 14%
Iliofemoral iliac	5	1 = 20%	0 = 0%
Femoropopliteal	7	0 = 0%	2 = 30%
Supraaortic	2	0	0
Total	21	6 = 28%	3 = 15%

Summary and Conclusion

Infection after arterial reconstructive surgery is a surgical catastrophe. The overall mortality of 28% and the amputation rate of 15% in our series are in accordance with the findings of other authors and point to the severity of the complication (3, 5). Therefore, prevention of infections is of the utmost importance. However, when infection does occur, the treatment depends on the degree to which complications developed. In this regard, a classification in three different stages is proposed. The use of biological wrapping and the possibility of stimulating the development of collaterals with the help of a progressive ligature is discussed.

References

1. Bernhard VM (1975) Management of infected vascular prostheses. Surg Clin North Am 55:1411
2. Jamieson GG, De Weese JA, Rob CG (1975) Infected arterial grafts. Ann Surg 181: 850
3. Liekweg WG, Greenfield LJ (1977) Vascular prosthetic infections: collected experience and results of treatment. Surgery 81:335
4. Szilagy EM, Amith RF, Elliott JP, Vrandecic MP (1972) Infection in arterial reconstruction with synthetic grafts. Ann Surg 176:321
5. Trede M, Rückert K, Lanbach K (1977) Septische Gefäßkomplikationen. Med Welt 28:838

Septic False Aneurysms After Vascular Operations

W. Hohenberger and D. Raithel*

Introduction

Reconstructive measurements in vascular surgery are burdened with a certain risk of infection, especially if alloplastic material is implanted. In the literature the incidence is reported to be between 0.4% and 6% (3-6).

Infection appears clinically in different forms such as wound abscess with or without bleeding, bypass thrombosis, upper gastro-intestinal bleeding, or septic embolization. Clinical symptoms are pain, subfebrile or even septic temperatures. Only occasionally infection presents as a false aneurysm.

Material and Method

Until April 1980, we saw 13 septic false aneurysms. Thus, the incidence in our patients was 0.2%. Two patients were operated on previously in other hospitals.

When regarding different courses, we could discern four different types of septic false aneurysms in our series: (1) in primary wound infection, (2) in primary healing, (3) as localized *Salmonella* infection, and (4) as aortoduodenal fistula.

Septic False Aneurysms in Primary Wound Infection

In two patients, within 3 weeks after a femoropopliteal saphenous bypass and 8 weeks after femoral thrombendarterectomy, a septic false aneurysm developed with rapid growth and profuse bleeding. In both cases, there was primary wound infection. No antibiotics were used in either of these two cases.

Septic False Aneurysms in Primary Healing

In another eight patients, septic false aneurysms occurred after implantation of allografts with primary healing in all cases. Antibiotics were always used. The operation had resulted in an aortobifemoral bypass in four cases, a unilateral aortofemoral bypass in two, which was combined with a femoropopliteal bypass in further operations, and finally, two grafts in femoropopliteal position alone. Seven aneurysms were localized in the groin, one at the aortal anastomosis.

*Chirurgische Universitätsklinik, Maximiliansplatz, D-8520 Erlangen

The interval until the development of a septic false aneurysm was between 1 and 84 months, and 21.5 months on an average. Three patients had up to three secondary operations at the localization of the later aneurysm.

The clinical symptoms were acute ischemia of the extremity and retroperitoneal encapsulated perforation in each case. Subcutaneous rupture of the aneurysm, as well as rapidly growing and pulsating tumor were seen in three.

Salmonella Infection and Aortoduodenal Fistula

One patient presented a subcutaneously ruptured aneurysm 80 months after a femoropopliteal saphenous bypass. The diagnosis of *Salmonella* infection was confirmed by culture. Two patients were hospitalized with upper gastro-intestinal bleeding from an aortoduodenal fistula 3 and 11 years, respectively, after aortobifemoral bypass.

Therapy

In four patients, infection was ignored. One tried to control the situation with local treatment. Within a few weeks, abscesses and profuse bleeding occurred at the site of the femoral anastomosis. In another patient, the femoral bifurcation was ligated because of bleeding from a septic aneurysm of a saphenous bypass. Two patients were reconstructed by extraanatomic bypass. In three cases, explantation of a limb of a bifurcation graft was the only measure taken.

In one patient, the aneurysm was resected and the aortal anastomosis resutured. Two patients with an aortoduodenal fistula were treated by resecting the aneurysm, interposition of an aortoaortal graft, and closing the duodenal fistula.

Results

Both patients with an aortoduodenal fistula died, one postoperatively of sepsis and the other from recurrent bleeding 8 months afterwards. All other patients in whom a bifurcation graft had been implanted have also died. One of these survived 18 months with recurrent abscesses in the groin. In the end he died after explantation of the graft. The patients with extraanatomic bypass did well for some months. But bypass thrombosis and recurrent infection finally led to amputation or rest pain. The latter patient died from intracerebral bleeding a short time later.

Actually only three patients achieved acceptable conditions. Nevertheless, one of them died after 14 months of lung cancer, one suffers from claudication, and the last one, with previous aneurysm of the aortal anastomosis, has no complaints till now but that is 3 months after the operation (Fig. 1). All the others have died or have undergone amputation.

Aortoduodenal fistula	2	†
In other bifurcation grafts	3	†
Extraanatomic bypass	2	†
		amputation
Local therapy in the groin	1	no complaints † (lung cancer)
	1	claudication
	2	amputation
	1	?
Resuture of aortal anastomosis	1	no complaints

Fig. 1. Results after septic false aneurysms

Discussion

The mean interval between primary operation and development of an aneurysm was 21.5 months in our patients. In contrast to the interval of non-septic false aneurysms where we found a mean of about 60 months in the groin it is much shorter.

The diagnosis of a *septic* false aneurysm is not always a simple one. Besides aortoduodenal fistulas, only in seven patients was the infection evident. Clinically, a septic false aneurysm should be suspected if there is an interval of less than 2 years since the primary operation. Furthermore, edemous tissues, thrombotic bypass occlusion, and an easily dissectible graft during operation make infection apparent.

The proof of bacterial contamination was a similar problem. Though infection sometimes presented as manifest abscesses, bacterial cultures taken intraoperatively were positive in only seven cases.

Whereas 50% of cryptogenic mycotic spontaneous aneurysms are induced by *Salmonella* (1), we found this agent as a rare cause in only one patient. Furthermore, the interval of development differred considerably from the others. It was 80 months, so that in this case secondary infection is evident.

As early as 1967, Spratt et al. (2) reported the poor prognosis of septic false aneurysms. Six of seven cases ended in amputation. Nevertheless, conservative treatment is not justified. Intraoperative diagnosis of septic false aneurysm demands removal of all alloplastic grafts. In isolated cases, extraanatomic reconstruction can be omitted. If, however, an extremity becomes ischemic, alternative bypass measures become mandatory.

Patients in poor general condition and who present a high risk because of multimorbidity may be in danger of succumbing these operations. In these cases, early decision to amputate an ischemic extremity might be life-saving.

Septic false aneurysms without allografts may be operated on only locally. However, if perfusion of the extremity is not sufficient, extraanatomic bypass must follow, taking into account the actual vascular status.

References

1. Davies OG Jr, Thorburn JD, Powell P (1978) Cryptic mycotic abdominal aneurysms. Am J Surg 136:96
2. Spratt EM, Doran ML, Baird RJ (1967) False aneurysms in the lower extremity. Surg Gynecol Obstet 124:562
3. Haimovici H (1976) Vascular surgery. Principles and techniques. McGraw-Hill, New York
4. Seybold-Epting W (1974) Rekonstruktion eines infizierten Nahtaneurysmas in der Kniekehle durch subcutanes fibulares Venentransplantat. Thoraxchirurgie 22:178
5. Szilagyi DE, Smith RF, Elliott JP, Vrandecic MP (1972) Infection in arterial reconstruction with synthetic grafts. Ann Surg 176:321
6. Hoffert PW, Gensler S, Haimovici H (1965) Infection complicating arterial grafts. Arch Surg 90:427

Secondary and Late Repair in Arterial Injury

H. Nüllen, W. Sandmann, G. Florack, D. A. Loose, and K. Kremer*

Introduction

Emergency reconstruction after arterial injury has shown sufficiently good results because many of these patients are young without degenerative lesions in their arteries. The prognosis is less favorable if the reconstruction is delayed. This possibly may occur if there is no experience in vascular surgery at the place of primary treatment or if the diagnosis of vascular injury was overlooked. Another group of patients with arterial trauma requires late repair as well because the reconstruction performed primarily has failed. In both groups of patients either secondary or late arterial reconstruction is often possible because according to the arterial segment in some patients, collaterals develop sufficiently to prevent necrosis of organs or extremities. Those patients suffer from intermittent claudication, traumatic arteriovenous (AV) fistula, or aneurysms and require reconstructive vascular surgery.

Material and Methods

From January 1959 to December 1979, 170 cases of major arterial injury underwent reconstruction in our clinic. Nearly 50% of these cases have been followed-up. Included in this series are 36 patients who underwent late or secondary repair of arterial trauma. All these patients were admitted to our hospital because primary repair performed elsewhere had failed or diagnosis of vascular injury had been made 2 weeks to 35 years later, when secondary complications like myocardial insufficiency, traumatic AV fistula with aneurysm or intermittent claudication occurred. War injuries and their late results are still present among these cases even 35 years after the end of World War II in Germany (Table 1). The majority of patients, however, had iatrogenic lesions and it is very interesting to notice the high number of successful late repair in this particular group. The average age of the patients was 39 years; excluding the war injuries the average age was only 34 years.

Twenty-one patients (Table 2) underwent 27 reconstructive operations for late repair of arterial injury. Eighteen patients with 19 reconstructions had an uneventful recovery. The hemodynamic results were excellent. In two patients an early thrombosis occurred. After thrombectomy and repair of technical failure, further recovery was without other complications. In one patient mycotic bleeding appeared after reconstruction of a cubital artery in primary infected tissue. Ligation

*Chirurgische Universitätsklinik A, Moorenstr. 5, D-4000 Duesseldorf

Table 1. Cause of injury (N = 36)

Shell splinter injury	9
Knife stab injury	6
Gunshot injury	2
Car accident	2
Metal splinter injury	1
Blunt trauma	1
Horse-inflicted injury	1
Sport accident	1
Cardiac catheterisation	7
ECC cannulation	1
Bassini's operation	1
Babcock's operation	1
Appendectomy	2
Intervertebral disk operation	1

of the artery was performed without fatal complication. Some typical examples are given by case reports.

Case 1: A 39-year-old woman sustained injury of the femoral artery during Babcock's operation. The lesion had been noticed immediately after the end of the operation, but except conservative treatment with anticoagulants, no other therapy was applied. She was admitted to our hospital 3 months later because of intermittent claudication. The occluded segment of the ligated femoral artery was excised and replaced by a segment of the great saphenous vein from the other leg. Complete repair of the femoral bifurcation was achieved by anastomosing a branch of the saphenous vein with the profundal femoral artery. After the vein valves were destroyed, the venous bifurcation was inserted in the orthopic direction. The hemodynamic result was excellent and normal anatomy was seen in the postoperative angiography.

Case 2: A 24-year-old man showed a false aneurysm of the axillary artery 14 days after gunshot injury. This injury was reconstructed by saphenous vein replacement. The course was uneventful and the hemodynamic result was very good.

Case 3: A 31-year-old Turkish man was the victim of attempted murder by his rival. The knife stab injury in the right groin was managed primarily by local wound care. The femoral AV fistula had been overlooked. Six weeks later, he was admitted to our vascular unit with a pulsating tumor in the right groin. Angiography showed two fistulas, one between the superficial femoral artery and the vein, the other into the profunda system. The aneurysms were excised and a direct end-to-end anastomosis of the two arteries and the two veins was performed. The recovery was uneventful with a normal arteriogram and phlebogram.

Case 4: A 23-year-old student developed a spurious aneurysm of the right popliteal artery and occlusion of the other caused by car accident with knee joint luxation. The arterial trauma was not recognised until 2 years later, when he complained of claudidation during dancing.

Table 2. Late repair after arterial injury (N = 21)

No.	Cause	Findings	Localisation
2	Shell splinter injury	AV fistula	Popliteal, axillary artery
4	Knife stab injury	Spurious aneurysm, occlusion	Axillary, femoral artery
1	Gunshot injury	Spurious aneurysm	Axillary artery
1	Car accident	Spurious aneurysm	Popliteal artery
1	Metal splinter injury	Spurious aneurysm	Cubital artery
1	Blunt trauma	Occlusion	Brachial artery
1	Intervertebral disk operation	AV fistula	Common iliac artery
1	Bassini's operation	Stenosis	Common femoral artery
1	Babcock's operation	Occlusion	Femoral artery
1	Appendectomy	Stenosis	Iliac artery
7	Cardiac catheterisation	Spurious aneurysm, occlusion	Cubital, femoral artery

Table 3. Secondary repair after arterial injury (N = 15)

No.	Cause	Findings	Localisation
7	Shell splinter injury	Occlusion, aneurysm of fistula artery	Femoral, popliteal artery
2	Knife stab injury	Occlusion	Femoral artery
1	Gunshot injury	Graft infection	Iliac artery
1	Car accident	Stenosis of anastomosis	Carotid artery
1	Sport accident	Graft occlusion	Femoral artery
1	Horse-inflicted injury	Graft occlusion	Femoral artery
1	Appendectomy	Graft occlusion (15 years)	Femoral artery
1	ECC cannulation	Graft occlusion	Femoral artery

The aneurysm was replaced by a saphenous vein graft; on the left side a vein bypass was performed. The recovery was uneventful and the hemodynamic result was excellent.

The second group consists of 15 patients in which 26 reoperations for secondary repair after arterial trauma had been necessary (Table 3). In these cases primary reconstruction had failed or was followed by late complications. In each of eight patients, one reoperation was performed and two patients underwent two reoperations with good hemodynamic results finally. In one case an early thrombosis occurred; after thrombectomy the further recovery was uneventful. Three other patients showed an unsatisfactory result and one patient died.

In one patient with acute thrombosis of the dilated fistula artery, the reconstruction failed and subsequent amputation was necessary. In a second patient the iliac-popliteal segment was dilated because of long persisting AV fistula after gunshot injury. When the diseased artery occluded it was replaced by a Dacron graft which became infected and had to be excised. Finally, the dilated iliac artery had to be ligated, fortunately without amputation. The third patient developed infection of the left limb after aortofemoral bypass. The prosthesis had been implanted after excision of an aneurysmatic iliac artery due to AV fistula. The leg was saved by femoral-femoral crossover bypass. In the last case of this series a gunshot injury of common iliac artery with some injuries of small bowel was found; a Dacron graft reconstruction was performed in another hospital. Graft infection occurred and despite successful extraanatomic bypass procedure, the patient died from septic complications. Two typical cases will be presented.

Case 5: A typical butcher knife stab injury of the right femoral vessels in an 18-year-old man had been reconstructed primarily with Dacron prosthesis in another hospital in 1960. Early occlusion of the prosthesis occurred. Nineteen years later, he developed intermittent claudication. The angiogram showed that the femoral artery was occluded just distal of the profundal bifurcation. The occluded prosthesis was resected and reconstruction using autogenous vein graft was performed. The postoperative angiography showed a normal anatomy.

Case 6: In a second case, reconstruction of a similar injury with defects in femoral artery as well as in femoral vein was started in another hospital. The disastrous result showed that there was no experience in vascular surgery. Twenty-one hours after the accident, the patient reached our hospital in circulatory arrest. Arterial and venous reconstruction was performed with autogenous vein. The hemodynamic result was excellent.

AV Fistula

It is well known that dilation of the artery commonly takes place proximal to an AV fistula. The size of this increase can be of extraordinary magnitude and often brings up many problems and complications.

Case 7: A 60-year-old man came to our out-patient-clinic in August 1979. His right leg was swollen and showed extraordinary venous congestion and chronic ulcerations at the distal calf. Dyspnea during working occurred the last few months before admission. The former diagnosis for many years was postthrombotic syndrome with chronic venous ulcerations. The clinical signs of AV fistula of popliteal artery could be demonstrated. Anamnesis gave the information that he had sustained a shell splinter injury of his right knee in 1944. It is astonishing that this

AV fistula was identified for the first time 35 years after arterial trauma in World War II. We used Dacron bifurcation graft for replacement and resected the fistula and the dilated artery. The hemodynamic result was good.

The late results after anastomosis with a dilated artery are not satisfactory because aneurysms at the side of anastomosis may develop. In order to avoid the recurrence of aneurysm, we used a Dacron cuff which was placed around the proximal anastomosis in five cases. Anyhow, dilation may be progressive and a very close follow-up is necessary. Angiography was suggested to be the best method for reexamination but today ultrasound sonography and CT are recommended.

Conclusions

Retrospectively, we noticed only four cases with unsatisfactory results among these 36 cases. We believe that the results after secondary or late repair due to arterial injury are almost comparable to those obtained after elective reconstructive procedures.

An Improved Autogenous Vein for Bypass Grafting? An Experimental Study

H. Rostad*

In more than 20% of patients requiring vascular grafts the saphenous vein is not suitable for use. In most of these cases the vein is too small. In recent years, an extensive search for a material to be used as a small artery substitute has been carried out. However, the ideal prosthetic graft with an acceptable patency is still not available.

The aim of this study was to try to make inadequate veins suitable for bypass grafting. As the main problem is the small diameter of the vein, the purpose was to dilate the vein by use of thin-walled silastic tubes left in the vein for some time. The external diameter of the tube should be larger than that of the vein. This report deals mainly with the morphological changes that have been found in the vein wall after dilatation with the silastic tube.

The results are based on data gained from 19 mongrel dogs weighing between 14 and 20 kg. (The animals were anesthetized with an intravenous injection of pentobarbital sodium.) In both hind legs the saphenous vein was exposed at the knee and in the inguinal region. The silastic tube was mounted on the tip of a sound allowing it to be pulled through the vein by force because the diameter of the tube was reduced by stretching. The tube was mounted on the instrument which reduced the diameter of the tube by stretching. Through an incision in the lower portion of the vein the sound was guided through the vein to the inguinal region where a new incision in the vein was made. The tube was then pulled through and left in the vein rendering a constant expansion pressure on the vein wall. A ligature was then placed proximal and distal to the incisions in the vein. Prophylactic antibiotic therapy was given postoperatively.

The veins with the silastic tubes were removed 1 to 9 weeks later and studied by light, transmission, and scanning electron microscopy.

Four control veins from dogs were studied; in two of them a silastic tube was inserted before the vein was taken out. By light miscroscopy the vein wall was thin and showed a typical appearance with the endothelium as a border against the lumen. In the cannulated veins, however, the endothelium was partly lacking and some cells showed ultrastructural signs of damage. This finding is clearly related to the cannulation procedure. Occasionally small mural platelet thrombi were also observed. The media contained circularly arranged smooth muscle cells located underneath the endothelium in one to three layers. As seen by transmission, electron microscopy elastic fibres were scattered in the vessel wall. The collagen fibrils were found between the muscle cells and arranged in bundles oriented circularly or longitudinally in the adventitia.

In the veins from dogs where the silastic tube had been left for 1 to 9 weeks the changes had occurred already after the first week but were more conspicuous after 3 weeks. The differences between 3

*Rikshospitalet, Surg. Dept. A, Oslo, Norway

and 9 weeks were inconsistent and insignificant and will not be further described here.

As shown by light microscopy the vessel wall had increased markedly in thickness. The innermost layer consisted of cells forming from one to several layers. They appeared cuboid with an irregular outline. By transmission electron microscopy these cells were found to exhibit numerous cytoplasmic projections, partly with interdigitation. They were cytoplasm-rich and contained often many cisternae with granular endoplasmic reticulum. Phagocytic vacuoles were also noted. Very few filaments were present, Weibel-Palade (WP) bodies were not identified. The nuclei were often irregular in outline and many of them contained a prominent nucleolus. On the luminal side an amorphous material was present but fibrin strands were not seen. Using scanning electron microscopic technique discontinuity between cells on the luminal surface could be seen.

The media showed increased thickness and the layers of smooth muscle cells were split by bundles of collagen fibrils. There was an increased number of fibroblasts and the amount of collagen was greater than normal.

Also in the adventitia there appeared to be an increased amount of collagen. The vasa vasorum were well preserved.

Conclusion

The present findings indicate that implantation of a silastic tube in the saphenous vein in dogs for 1 to 9 weeks leads to changes in the wall with cells lining the luminal surface, proliferation of smooth muscle cells and fibroblasts, and increase of collagen. Whether the inner surface is more thrombogenic than in the intact vein is still an open question. The greater thickness of the vessel wall with increased amounts of collagen may contribute to a more solid wall and thus make the vein more suitable for bypass grafting.

Study of the Aorta by C T Scanning

C.Sanpons*

Anatomy

The thoracic and abdominal aortas are well visualized in the majority of the patients. The visceral trunks of the abdominal aorta can be well seen on the computed tomography (CT) scan: the celiac trunk, the hepatic and splenic arteries, the superior mesenteric, the renal arteries, as well as the bifurcation trunks of the aorta.

Method of Examination

The patients are placed in supino decubitus with no angulation of the gantry. The injection of contrast material is frequently used (angio-CT).

Indications

a) Study of the abdominal and thoracic aorta aneurysms.
b) Suspicion of an infected vascular graft.
c) Leaking suspicion of an aneurysm.
d) In the presence of a retroperitoneal mass the CT allows us to study the relationship between this mass and the aorta.

Pathology

In our experience the CT is a very useful method in the study and differential diagnosis of the abdominal pulsating masses. Likewise this method is useful in the study of the thoracic aorta aneurysms. In all cases it allows us to know the diameters of the descending aorta and to observe the calcifications in its wall. In Figure 1 we observe the superior vena cava, the ascending aorta, and the pulmonary artery. Behind and to its left is a large aneurysm of the thoracic aorta. In the case of an aneurysm of the abdominal aorta the CT allows us to determine its situation:

*Centro Radiológico Computarizado, c/Tavern, 82, Barcelona, Spain

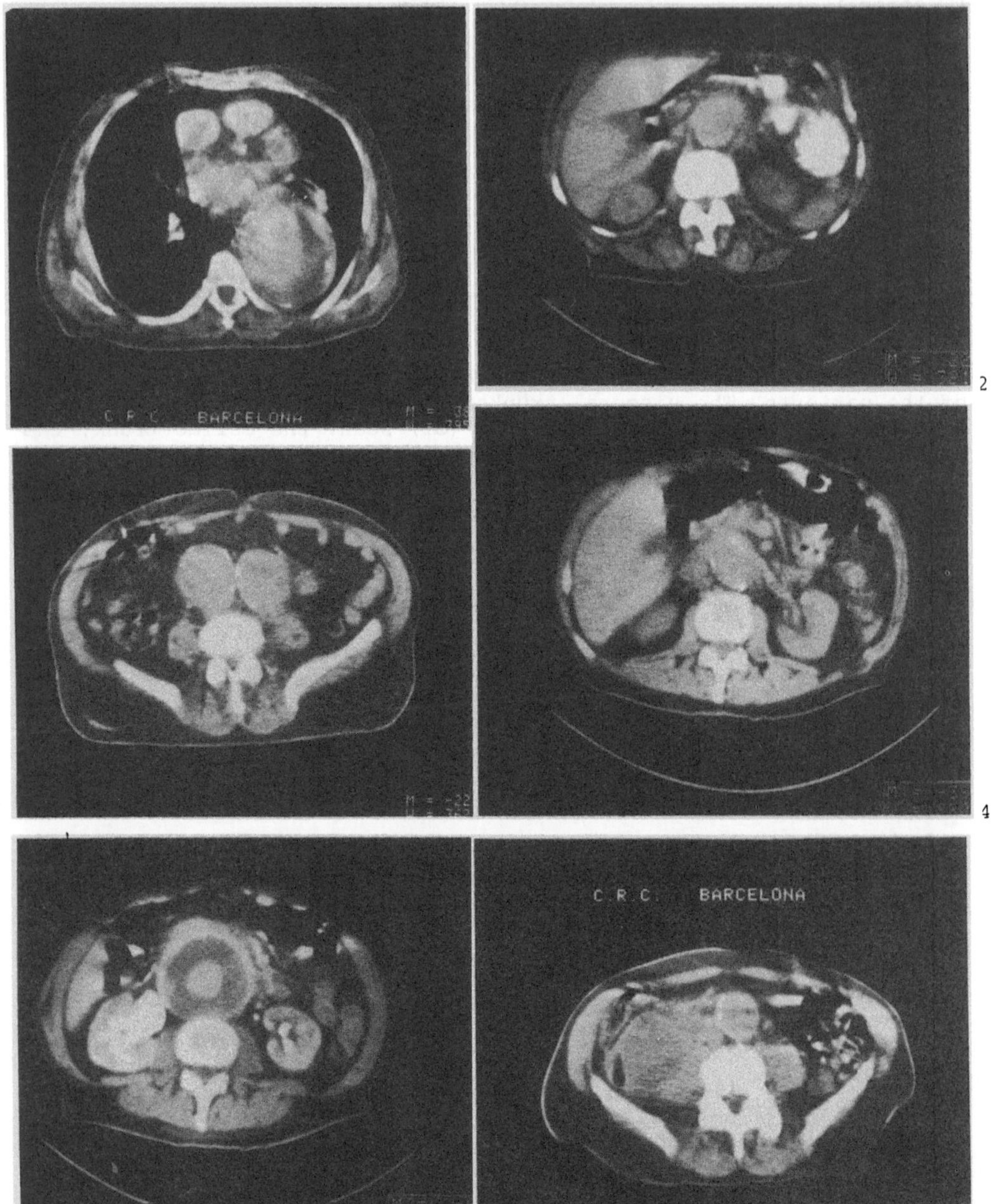

Figs. 1-6

a) Above the renal arteries and the visceral branches of the abdominal aorta. In Figure 2 at the level of the gall bladder and of the renal pole, we observe an aneurysm of the abdominal aorta.
b) What is most frequent: underneath the mentioned arterial trunks and if it extends to the iliac arteries or if it does not affect them. In Figure 3 we observe, in one transversal image practiced at the level of the iliac crest, each aneurysm of the primitive iliac arteries.
c) If it affects the origin of the visceral branches of the abdominal aorta. As we can see in Figure 4, the aneurysm of the aorta affects the origin of the left renal artery.

In every case in which it was not possible to observe an aneurysm by aortography, we obtained it by CT scanning.

The injection of a bolus of contrast material allows us to determine very clearly the light of the aorta and the intraaneurysmal thrombus. The transversal image which we appreciate in Figure 5 has been practiced after an intravenous injection of contrast which opacifies the light of the aneurysm. In case of leaking the CT allows us to demonstrate the existence of a retroperitoneal hematoma. Figure 6 corresponds to a transversal image practiced at the level of the iliac crest in which we can observe on its right and behind the aneurysm, an image which corresponds to a retroperitoneal hematoma.

In the presence of a retroperitoneal mass the CT scanning allows us to study the relationship between this mass and the aorta and the inferior vena cava. If the outlines of these vessels are blurred, the injection of a bolus of contrast medium permits us to identify them. Just as in the case when the tumor invades the inferior vena cava, an injection of contrast medium allows us to reveal it.

Conclusion

In the particular case of the aorta aneurysm, we consider that the ultrasonography is for the moment the method of selection for its study, since it offers some advantages like the lack irradiation, other of economic disposition, etc. which the CT does not have. However, the introduction of the contrast enhancement in the CT offers us some diagnostic possibilities in vascular pathology that we think should be evaluated.

Proteic Deposit and Experimental Arterial Prosthesis in the Dog

J.L. Fontaine, P. Desnoyers, J. Labaume, J.C. Plot, and G. Dupuis*

Morphological organization of experimental arterial prosthesis, especially in the dog, is actually well known. However, a few aspects of this histogenesis remain in discussion and particularly the origin, nature, and completeness of inner endothelialization of the tube. Anyhow, in this respect, there is an evident discrepancy between different animal species and mankind and it is probable that in the latter case histological maturation is never achieved: even in dogs this point may be partially true. In fact, in a previous experimental work, we showed that even after a long time of implantation fibrinolytic substances were able to produce a more or less complete lysis of the inner surfaces of the tubes. This constatation was the starting point of the present work.

Material and Methods

We exclusively used female mongrel dogs weighing about 15 kg. General anesthesia was given by intravenous injection of 0.5 ml/kg/weight of a 6% solution of pentobarbital with tracheal intubation and artificial ventilation. All these animals were submitted to the same operating procedure; through a median laparotomy infrarenal abdominal aorta was resected and replaced by a composite graft: half autologous vein proceeding from the external jugular vein and half Weavenit Dacron tube.

Twenty-four hours before sacrifice, the thyroid gland being blocked by an iv injection of a solution of IK, the dogs received an intravenous injection of 45 μCi of I 125 labeled fibrinogen. Immediately after death, the graft was taken off as well as different samples of arteries and thyroid gland. The radioactivity of the different samples was measured and related to the fresh weight of the organ.

Different fragments of the elements of the graft were submitted to an electron scanning microscopic study. During the follow-up of the dogs, the following parameters were regularly measured: coagulation time, Howell time, Quick time, fibrinogen, fibrin monomers, englobulin lysis time, platelet adhesivity, hematocrit, red cell count.

The dogs were separated in a few series according to time of sacrifice after the operation: four animals were killed 24 h after operation; four animals were killed 4 days later; four animals were killed 8 days later, five animals were killed 21 days later; three animals were killed after 2 months; and one animal was killed after 4 1/2 months.

*Hôpital Communal de Neuilly, Neuilly/Seine, France

Results

Radioactivity Measurements

For each dog the radioactivity of the following samples was measured by scintillation counter: normal aorta above and under the graft, iliac artery; the different suture lines; two samples of each component of the graft; and the thyroid gland.

The results are summarized in Figure 1 and show a maximal peak activity either in the prosthesis or in the venous graft on the fourth postoperative day. It slowly decreases afterwards and is quite absent in the vein 21 days after implantation. Anyhow, the radioactivity uptake is much higher in the prosthesis than in the vein and it persists at a significantly higher level for longer time. Four months later it is still above normal limits though really very reduced.

Biological Parameters

No significant variation of the biological parameters except a slight elevation of the fibrinogen level and a feeble decrease of the hematocrit in the immediate postoperative course was noticed. These phenomena are by no means specific and just represent the normal reaction against any important operation.

Histological Data

The scanning electron microscopic study of the venous graft showed a practically immediate desquamation of the endothelial cells probably due partly to the operating manipulations and partly to the abnormal

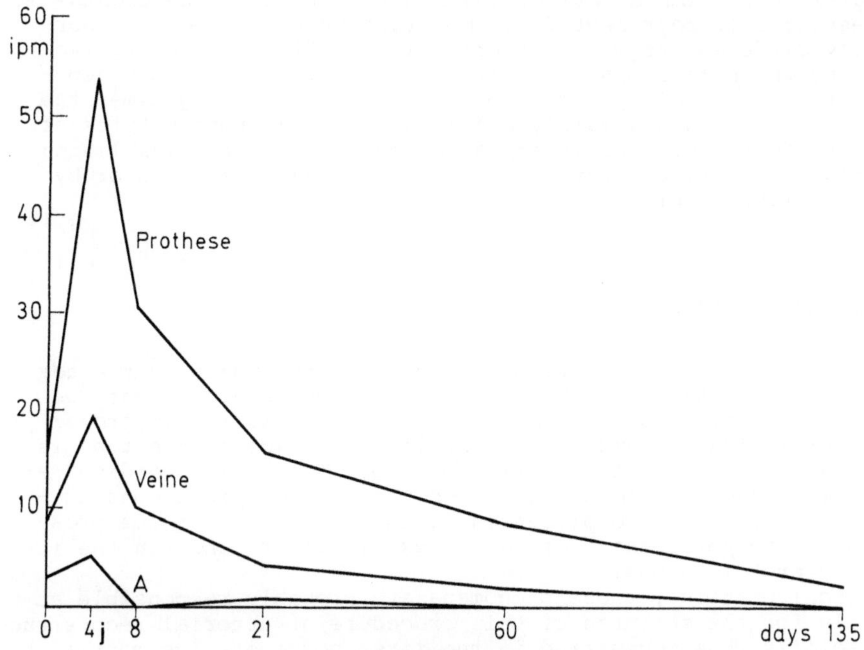

Fig. 1. Fibrinogen uptake of prostheses, vein, and normal artery

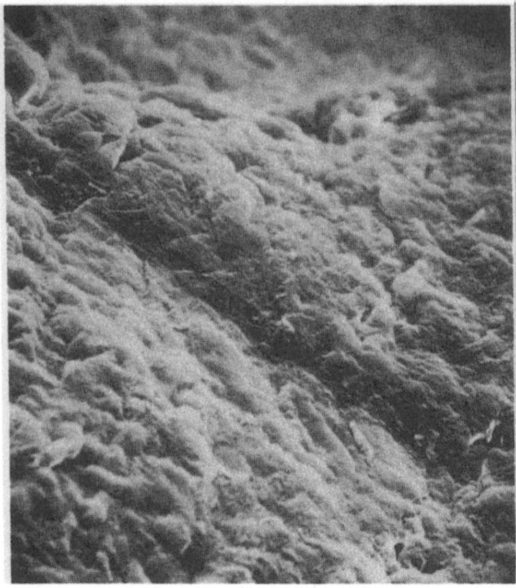

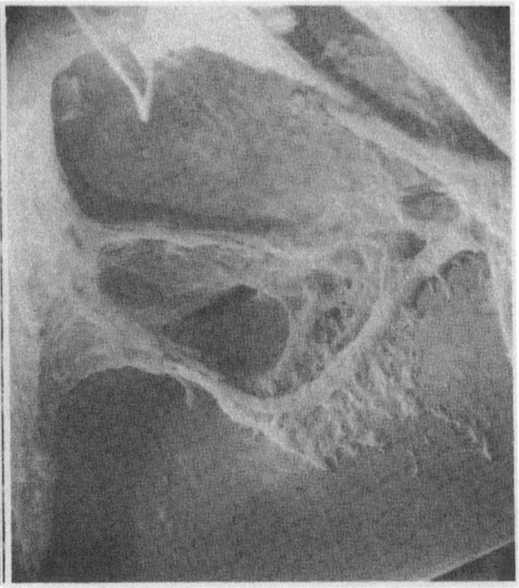

Fig. 2. Endothelial lining of a venous graft 21 days after implantation

Fig. 3. Inner aspect of Dacron arterial prosthesis 4 1/2 months after operation

high pressure to which the graft is submitted. During the first postoperative days, the endothelial lining has completely disappeared (Fig. 2). It progressively heals later but the procedure seems to be accomplished only 2 months or more after the implantation of the graft

Immediately after implantation, the inner surface of the prosthetic tubes is essentially represented by important proteic deposits, morphologically different from pure fibrin. In the first postoperative days, red and white cells and platelets are entrapped in these deposits but they rapidly disappear completely. So, for a long time, the interface blood/prosthesis mainly consists in big amorphous tufts of protein. Even four months after implantation, the endothelial lining is not continuous but, by spot, replaced by the same deposits or by naked textile fibers (Fig. 3).

Discussion and Conclusion

The general schema of organization of arterial prosthesis in the dog seemed to be well established by numerous previous publications. On the contrary, the fixation of labeled circulating fibrinogen proved that the histological maturation of the inner surface of the tube is not achieved even after a long period of time. There is a good correlation between these biological data and the microscopical constatations which showed the incompleteness of intimal lining of the prosthetic tubes, the persistance of naked textile fibers and, in the interval, huge proteic deposits.

In clinical practice, these phenomena are probably responsible at least partly for the failures of this procedure of arterial reconstruction, especially those occurring in the first postoperative months, a period during which the interface prosthesis/blood is certainly heterologous and in permanent turnover.

Vascular Forum II

Chairman: J. Sautot, Lyon; Co-Chairman: R. May, Innsbruck

Surgical Management in Patients With Embolizing Deep Vein Thrombosis

H. Nüllen, W. Sandmann, J. Lerut, and K. Kremer

Introduction

Although great progress in knowledge about pathophysiology, clinic, and prevention of deep vein thrombosis and pulmonary embolism has been made in recent years, these diseases represent a great clinical problem as far as diagnosis and treatment are concerned. In addition to this the number of these cases seems to increase.

Coon and Coller (2) in 1959 described 606 cases of pulmonary embolism among 4391 autopsies, i.e. a total of 13.8%. In Havig's study from 1977 (3) at gross examination pulmonary emboli were found in 280 cases of 508 randomized autopsies. Additional emboli were found by microscopical examination in 72 cases. Thus the total incidence of pulmonary embolism was 69.3%. It may be that this great variation of data is caused by methodical differences. The diagnosis at routine autopsy for instance may be unreliable because only large emboli in major vessels will be detected unless special methods are adopted and pulmonary emboli under such circumstances are described in only 4% to 20% of cases (3).

Similar problems arise in patients with a thrombosis of the deep veins. On a clinical basis the diagnosis of deep vein thrombosis is wrong in about half of the examined patients and this rate will increase in patients with nonoccluding thrombosis (5). Concerning the large number of patients with postthrombotic syndrome, it should be mentioned that there is an increasing need for a more aggressive management which can prevent the postthrombotic syndrome and eliminate the source of emboli.

There are different surgical concepts to protect the patients against recurrent embolism. First the classical anticoagulant therapy, second several procedures to interrupt or narrow the pathway of emboli (caval ligation, plication, clip and filters), third the venous thrombectomy to remove the source of embolism, and finally, various combined methods.

Anticoagulant therapy alone has been considered inadequate today because recurrence of pulmonary embolism is not uncommon. There are several procedures described for interruption or narrowing the inferior vena cava (see above). Many typical complications and disadvantages have been noticed. After interruption of the inferior vena cava, large collateral channels occur which allow the passage of emboli. Piccone et al. (4) published, as far as we know, the very best documented follow-up study about caval ligation. These authors found 50% recurrent embolism among 72 cases. In 16 cases, recurrent pulmonary embolism was lethal. Furthermore, we think it is important to notice that all these mentioned methods disturb normal venous hemodynamics

*Chirurgische Universitätsklinik A, Moorenstr. 5, D-4000 Duesseldorf

in the lower limbs. Instead of blocking the venous return, it seems to be better to exclude the source of embolization by removal of the fresh thrombus.

Material and Methods

In patients with occluding thrombosis of iliac and femoral veins, the ultrasound Doppler sonography in addition to case history and clinical findings offers possibilities of a safe diagnosis (5). In cases with nonoccluding thrombosis and thrombosis of the calf veins, venography should be used. After diagnosis has been established, thrombectomy is recommended.

From February 1977 to June 1980, 46 patients with acute occluding or stenosing thrombosis of iliac, femoral, or popliteal vein underwent thrombectomy in our department (Tables 1 and 2). At the time of admission, 13 patients had had one or frequent events of pulmonary embolization. In each patient with nonoccluding deep vein thrombosis, the source of emboli was found by venography. Management consisted of thrombectomy, temporary AV fistula for 3 months, and anticoagulation in the first 6-month postoperative period. Three typical case reports are presented.

Case 1: A 34-year-old woman was admitted for venous thrombectomy in May 1979. Four months before, she had to undergo emergency ileostomy because of ulcerative colitis. Two days before admission to our hospital, she felt pain in her right chest. In her home town hospital, pulmonary embolism was suspected and a phlebography had been performed. Stenosing thrombosis of left common iliac vein was seen (Fig. 1). Transfemoral catheter thrombectomy was performed with a temporary AV fistula of a branch of the saphenous vein to the femoral artery. The fistula was closed 3 months later. No further event of pulmonary embolization occurred. In the phlebogram 8 months after operation no residual thrombus was found (Fig. 2). Normal valve function was proven by ultrasound Doppler examination.

Table 1. Deep vein thrombosis, February 1977 - June 1980

Patients	46
Age	46 years (15-73 years)
Sex	Male 21; female 25
Duration of complete vein occlusion	3 days (1-7 days) (Retrospectively: five patients 14 days to 3 months)

Table 2. Embolizing deep vein thrombosis

Patients	13
Age	42 years (17-70 years)
Sex	Male 6; female 7
Anamnesis	2 days to 3 months

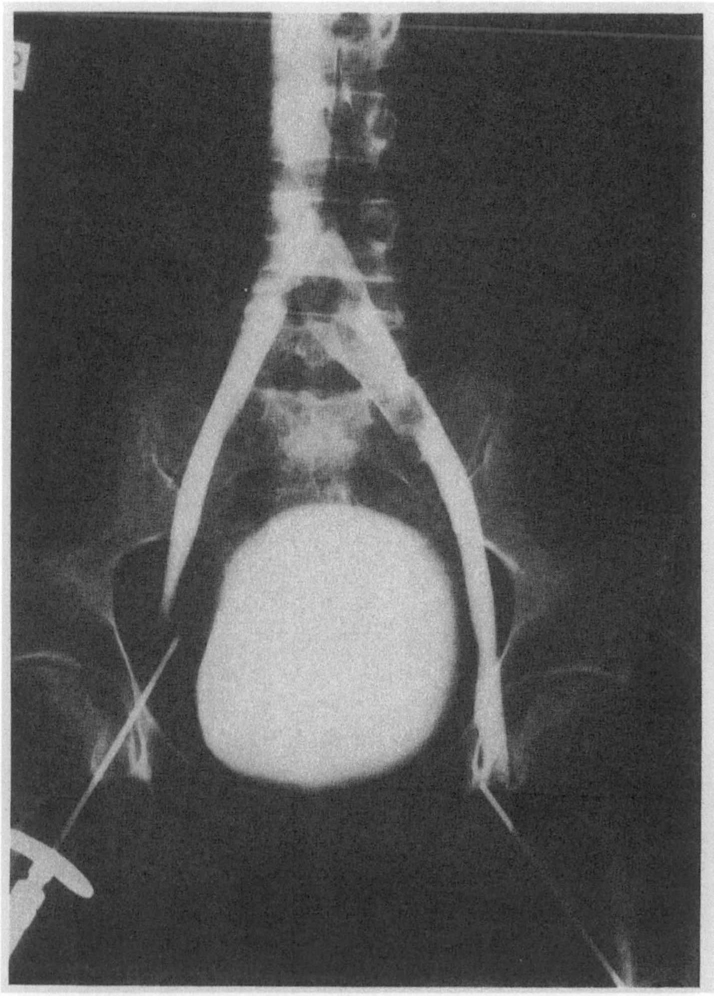

Fig. 1. Stenosing thrombosis of left common iliac vein

Case 2: A 51-year-old man underwent conservative treatment because of ulcerative colitis since January 1980. In April, he came to the hospital again with a painful and swollen leg. Diagnosis of deep vein thrombosis was established and conservative treatment started. Later clinical signs of pulmonary embolism occurred and phlebography was performed. Stenosing thrombosis of the left iliac vein was seen. Transfemoral venous thrombectomy then was done in our department in May 1980 and no further embolism occurred. The last ultrasound doppler examination 2 months after operation showed a good hemodynamic result.

Case 3: A 70-year-old man underwent Bassini's operation on the left side in May 1979. In August 1979, venous thrombosis occurred in the left leg. Although conservative treatment with anticoagulants was started with meticulous control in the laboratory, several events of pulmonary embolism were observed with impairment of lung function. In October 1979, a Kimray-Greenfield filter was inserted but despite this the frequency of pulmonary embolisms remained unchanged. Repeated

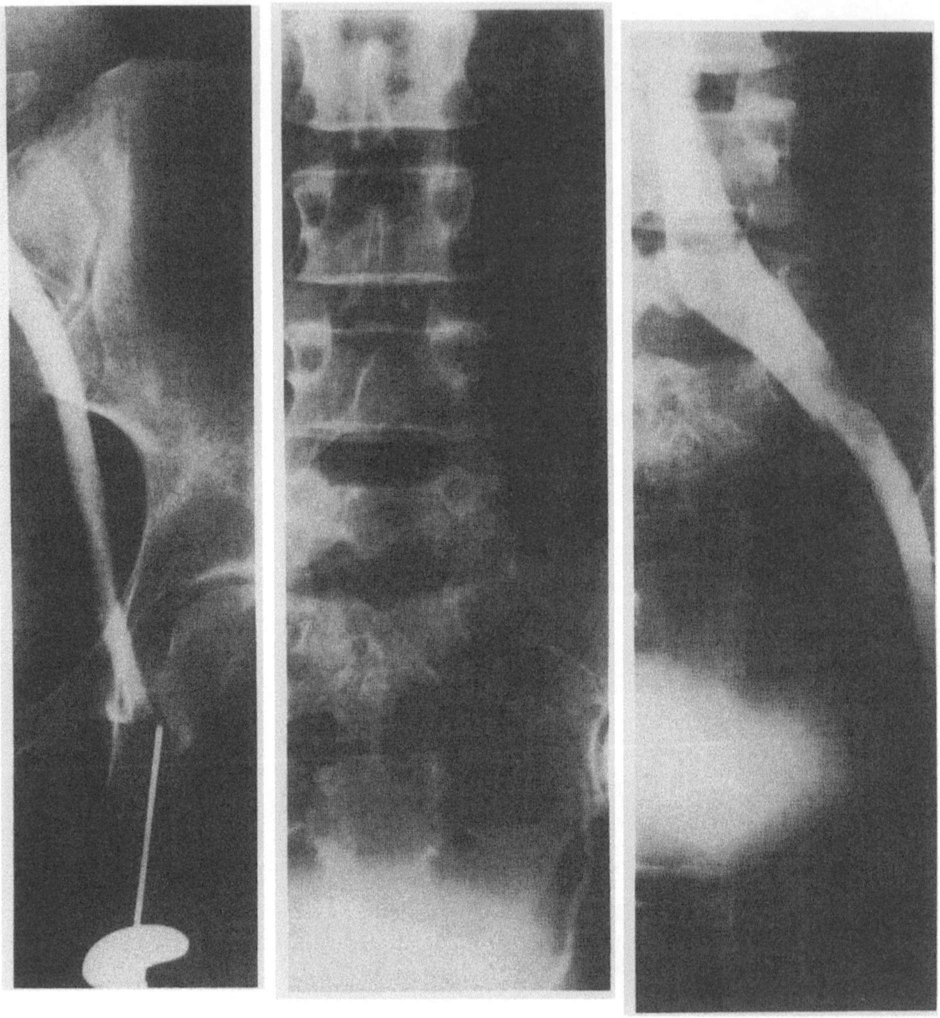

Fig. 2. Phlebogram 8 months after operation

lung scans showed increase in lung perfusion. Finally a phlebogram was performed and revealed a stenosing thrombosis of femoral and iliac vein. The patient was admitted for thrombectomy which was performed the next day together with AV fistula. Since thrombectomy, the patient remained completely free of pulmonary embolization. The femoral and popliteal vein valves were completely insufficient due to previous postthrombotic syndrome. Repeated Doppler sonography examinations after ligation of AV fistula in February 1980 demonstrated restoration of the venous iliofemoral confluence with normal venous flow signals depending on respiration.

Conclusions

In 13 patients with embolizing deep vein thrombosis who were treated in our department, surgical management consisted of venous thrombectomy, AV fistula, and high doses of anticoagulants in the postoperative period. Neither recurrent thrombosis nor recurrence of pulmonary embolism occurred. Vein valve function was preserved in all cases without previous postthrombotic syndrome. Therefore we intend to recommend this procedure as the only causal treatment in embolizing deep vein thrombosis. We think that combination of this method with caval ligation or clipping, as described by van den Berg (1), should not be recommended because disturbance of normal venous hemodynamics in the lower limb is a very important factor of Virchow's triad. In regard to the hemodynamical and clinical results, it is our opinion that thrombectomy and AV fistula are a safe method to remove the source of emboli without damaging the venous valves.

References

1. Van den Berg L (1978) Venous thrombectomies and partial interruption of the vena cava in 125 cases of thrombophlebitis. J Cardiovasc Surg 19:143
2. Coon WW, Coller FA (1959) Clinicopathologic correlation in thromboembolism. Surg Gynecol Obstet 109:259
3. Havig O (1977) Deep vein thrombosis and pulmonary embolism. Acta Chir Scand [Suppl] 478
4. Piccone VA, Vidal E, Yarnoz M, Glass P, Le Veen HH (1970) The late results of caval ligation. Surgery 68:980
5. Strandness DE, Sumner DS (1972) Ultrasonic velocity detector in the diagnosis of thrombophlebitis. Arch Surg 104:180

Surgical Treatment of Post-thrombophlebitic Syndrome of the Lower Extremities and Pelvis in the Stage of Occlusion

A.A. Shalimov and I.I. Sukharev*

The aim of this work was the development of efficient methods of surgical treatment of postthrombophlebitic syndrome of the lower extremities and pelvis in the stage of occlusion of the deep veins and indications for their use.

Materials and Methods

Analysis of the results of surgical treatment of 561 patients with postthrombophlebitic syndrome of the lower extremities and pelvis, of these 143 in the stage of occlusion of the deep veins, forms the basis of this work. The indications for reconstructive operations were the severity of clinical manifestations, the extent of impairment of regional hemodynamics, the segmentation of occlusion of the deep magistral veins, and the degree of disability.

With the aim of objective assessment of the state of the deep magistral veins and nature of collateral circulation, a functional-dynamic phlebography of the lower extremities, serial pelvic phlebography, and lymphography were carried out. This allowed separation of seven types of occlusion (1).

The access to the deep veins was defined by the state of occlusion and type of surgical intervention; specifically in occlusion of the distal superficial femoral and popliteal veins we have developed a posteromedial approach where only one muscle is dissected instead of five, in distinction from the Imperato approach (2).

In occlusion of the iliac and common femoral veins, a modified Palma operation was performed in ten patients. It consists of a preliminary thrombectomy of the common and opening of the deep femoral veins and creation of side-to-side anastomosis of the greater saphenous vein of the normal extremity to the common femoral vein of the affected extremity. Simultaneously at pressure gradient below 80 mm H_2O, a temporal end-to-side arteriovenous anastomosis is placed between the remaining stump of the greater saphenous vein of the normal leg and superficial femoral artery of the diseased one.

In the presence of occlusion of the iliac, femoral, and popliteal veins, we have developed and performed a combined operation in 30 patients which can be summarized as follows. Using a special thromboextractor, a partial semiopen thrombectomy of the common and opening of the deep femoral veins and bifurcation of the popliteal vein was carried out. Then Palma and Husne anastomoses were placed synchronously. With the aim of rethrombosis prevention in the absence of proper pres-

*Institute of Clinical and Experimental Surgery, Geroev Sevastopolja 30, Kiev 252165, USSR sure gradient, a temporal anastomosis was performed between the posterior tibial vein and artery at the level of medial malleolus.

With the occlusion of superficial femoral and popliteal veins, or one of the tibial veins, a combined operation is warranted. It involves a partial thrombectomy of bifurcation of the popliteal vein with a simultaneous placement of saphenopopliteal anastomosis in an end-to-end fashion. Nineteen patients have been operated upon by our method.

In occlusion of the superficial femoral vein, the Husne-May operation was used in 74 patients. In seven cases, this operation was associated with a lymphovenous anastomosis from the end of the deep lymphatic vessel to the side of the muscle vein.

In case of a partial recanalization of the superficial femoral vein and an inadequacy of the greater saphenous vein, an end-to-end anastomosis between the lateral and superficial femoral veins was constructed in ten patients. The suggested method has a number of important advantages thanks to the lateral vein having a significant diameter (5-9 mm) and length (average of 4.5 cm), and availability in 77% of cases of one and in 23% of cases of two functioning valves.

When segmental occlusion of the deep veins is associated with insufficiency of the communicating veins of the tibia, it is advisable to combine reconstructive procedures with a Linton or Felder operation. During the first 5-7 postoperative days, we advocate the use of an adequate regional heparinization with low molecular weight dextran, the agents improving tissue trophicity and antiinflammatory therapy.

Results

The immediate results of reconstructive operations were studied in 143 patients. Analysis of the results showed that in 104 patients (72.7%) the regional hemodynamics was compensated and the autogenous vein shunt was phlebographically functional. Satisfactory results of operation were obtained in 25 patients (16.8%), unsatisfactory in 13 (10.5%). Long-term results were studied in 122 patients 1 to 7 years after reconstructive operations. Good results were achieved in 77 patients (63.1%), satisfactory in 29 (23.8%), unsatisfactory in 16 (13.1%). Analysis of unsatisfactory results after reconstructive operations showed that the main cause of failures was shunt thrombosis. It is important to note a high effectiveness of reconstructive procedures when they are associated with a Linton or Felder operation, or with a temporal arteriovenous anastomosis. Of the 143 patients, 63.1% were able to resume their work.

Summary

Of the 561 patients with postthrombephlebitic syndrome operated upon at our clinic, 143 have been in the stage of occlusion of the deep veins. In the occlusion of the iliac and common femoral veins, our modification of the Palma operation has been used in ten patients. It consists of a preliminary thrombectomy of the common and opening of the deep femoral veins and placement of the Palma anastomosis with a temporary arteriovenous fistula.

In occlusion of the iliac, femoral, and popliteal veins, we have developed and performed a combined operation in 30 patients: a partial thrombectomy of the common and opening of the deep femoral veins and bifurcation of the popliteal vein, a simultaneous creation of the

Palma and Husne anastomoses with a temporary fistula between postero-tibial artery and vein at the level of medial malleolus.

In occlusion of the superficial femoral and popliteal veins, or one of the tibial veins, a combined operation was used in 19 patients: a partial thrombectomy of the bifurcation of the popliteal vein with a simultaneous saphenopopliteal anastomosis in an end-to-end fashion.

In occlusion of the superficial femoral vein, the Husne-May operation was used in 74 patients. In seven patients, the operation was combined with a lymphovenous anastomosis from the end of the deep lymphatic vessel to the side of the muscle vein.

In the partial recanalization of the superficial femoral vein and inadequacy of the greater saphenous vein, an anastomosis between the lateral and superficial femoral veins was placed in ten patients. Good results in the early period were obtained in 72.7% of cases and in the late period in 63.1% of cases.

References

1. Shalimov AA, Sukharev II (1975) Surgical treatment of occlusive diseases of the deep veins of the lower extremities and pelvis. Klin Khir 3:34-37
2. Imperato AM, Kim GE, Dong SC (1973) Surgical exposure for reconstruction of the proximal part of the tibial artery. Surg Gynecol Obstet 136:453-455

Randomised Trial of Bandaging After Sclerotherapy for Varicose Veins

A. J. G. Batch, S. S. Wickremesinghe, M. E. Gannon, and J. A. Dormandy*

Introduction

The injection treatment of varicose veins has been practised for at least a century. The technique fell into disrepute in the early half of this century with the realisation that significant complications and recurrence could result from spreading thrombophlebitis and damage to adjacent previously unaffected segments of varicose vein (1, 7) and for many years surgery was the treatment of choice. However, in 1963 Fegan (7) described the principles of successful compression sclerotherapy and his technique has been widely adopted since then. The basis of this technique involves the maintenance of firm uninterrupted compression for a minimum of 6 weeks, thereby preventing the formation and spread of thrombosis. As many patients find this period uncomfortable, some surgeons have modified Fegan's original principle and shorten the period of bandages, but there have been no controlled studies to evaluate the importance of the period of compression. We therefore conducted a randomised prospective trial to compare the results of compression bandaging for 3 weeks and 6 weeks after sclerotherapy.

Patients and Methods

The 148 patients (169 legs) entered into the trial presented to our varicose vein clinic between January 1976 and January 1979, with minor or intermediate varicosities of the main saphenous systems, residual or recurrent veins after previous treatment, or patients refusing surgery. (Over the period of the trial, we used compression sclerotherapy alone as the primary treatment for 37% of all new patients.)

All patients had idiopathic varicose veins. Those who had received treatment within 6 months and those with venous ulceration or signs of chronic venous insufficiency were excluded. Those with gross saphenous incompetence were considered more suitable for surgery.

At the time of injection, patients were randomly allocated to remain in bandages for 3 or 6 weeks. The two groups were well matched for clinical characteristics, type of varicosities, and number and site of injections (Table 1). Injections were all performed by one of us (S.S.W.) according to the method described by Fegan (7). Photographs of legs were taken from two positions using normal and infra-red sensitive film prior to injection, to help in the subsequent assessment of results.

*Department of Surgery, St. James' Hospital, Sarsfeld Road, London SW12 8HW, Great Britain

Table 1. Clinical characteristics

	3 Weeks group	6 Weeks group
Total numbers – patients	76	76
legs	85	84
males	19	10
females	66	57
Age – average in years	41	44
(range)	(19-66)	(15-76)
Weight – average in kg	64	66
(range)	(42-99)	(44-101)
Number with previous treatment	44	37
Average past history in years	5.8	5.8
Number with recurrent or residual veins	32	39
Average past history in years	8.2	8.4
Injections – below knee (Number of legs)	54	63
above knee (Number of legs)	1	2
both (Number of legs)	30	19
Average injections per leg	3.6	3.7

Patients were reviewed at 3 weeks after injection. Those alloted to the 3-week group received no further support, whereas those in the 6-week group were rebandaged for a further 3 weeks. Patients were subsequently assessed at 3 months and thereafter at yearly intervals by a doctor who was unaware of the original period of bandaging. A standard questionnaire was employed at each assessment and scores were allotted for the patients' comments regarding pain, mobility, and cosmetic appearance. The observing doctor scored his findings regarding phlebitis, pigmentation, induration, and the disappearance of the varicosities.

Results

Figure 1 shows the mean scores for the two groups at each assessment up to 2 years. The scores for patients' symptoms and the doctor's findings on examination are similar. Although in every case the 3-week group appeared to produce more favourable results than the 6-week group, the differences were not statistically significant. During the period of the study, 11 patients in the 6-week group (14%) and five (7%) in the 3-week group needed further treatment for recurrence after sclerotherapy (Table 2).

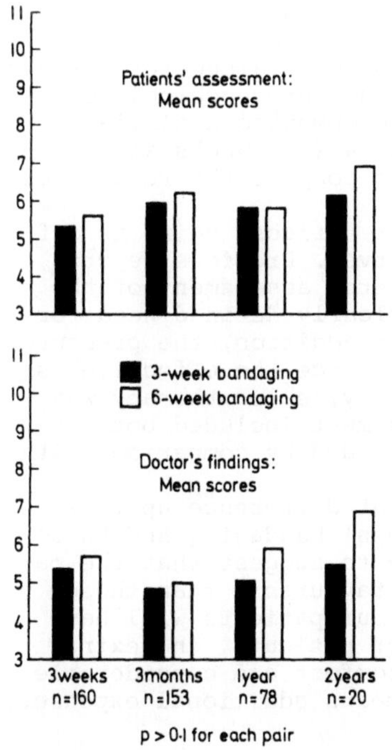

Fig. 1. Mean scores for the two groups. The vertical axes represent the actual possible score. The lowest score (3) represents the best possible result on assessment; the highest score (11) the worst. The better scores in the 3-week group are not statistically significant (P >0.1)

Table 2. Treatment failures at 2 years following injection

	3 Weeks group	6 Weeks group
Recurrent veins	5 (7%)	11 (14%)
surgery	3	2
further injections	2	5
no further treatment	-	4
Persistent pigmentation	1	2
Displeased with results	3	2

Discussion

The recent literature (2, 6, 7, 10-12, 15) suggests that sclerotherapy has become a widely accepted technique in the treatment of varicose veins, though there is still much debate about the exact indications. Fegan (7) commented on the potential dangers of sclerotherapy without compression; florid phlebitis with spread to adjacent unaffected segments of vein, consequent valvular damage, pulmonary embolism (1, 5) may all occur. In addition, fluctuations in venous pressure above the sclerosed segment may cause separation of the clot from the vein wall with consequent recanalisation and eventual recurrence of varicosities. This view is supported by the work of De Jode (3) who found the late results of sclerotherapy to be better in those patients where no intravascular thrombus was present at the site of injection.

Fegan's suggestion that compression should be maintained for 6 weeks was based on histological studies of injected and thrombophlebitic veins (7, 8). While some reports (6, 10, 15) recommended a similar period, others suggested bandaging for 3 (4) or 4 (14) weeks after injection. However, there have been no studies to compare the results of compression bandaging for different periods.

The assessment of the results of therapy for varicose veins is difficult to quantify, as McAdam et al. (13) observed. Previous reports have used patient satisfaction (4, 16), observers' assessment of the disappearance of veins (3, 11), and the more clearly defined need for retreatment (2, 6) as methods of assessment. In addition, the pressure of bandages applied by different surgeons (and hence the effectiveness of compression) can vary widely (9). In our study, sclerotherapy was all performed by one doctor, and "blind" assessment included both patient satisfaction and objective improvement, aided by comparison with pretreatment photographs.

This study has failed to show any significant difference up to 2 years between the results achieved after 6 weeks' bandaging and those after 3 weeks, and so far there is no evidence to suggest that the patients in the 3-week group will progress less favourably than those in the 6-week group. However, reassessment of our patients will have to be continued for up to 5 years at least. For patients, the extra 3 weeks in bandages represent unnecessary discomfort and considerable inconvenience, and for the Health Service it means additional expense.

References

1. Agrifoglio G, Edwards EA (1961) Results of surgical treatment of varicose veins. JAMA 178:906-911
2. Beresford SAA, Chant ADB, Jones HO, Piachaud D, Weddell JM (1978) Varicose veins: a comparison of surgery and injection/compression sclerotherapy. Five year follow-up. Lancet 1:921-924
3. De Jode LR (1970) Injection compression treatment of varicose veins. Br J Surg 57:285-286
4. Dee R, Finkelstein JE (1977) Treatment of varicose veins; sclerotherapy with compression or stripping and multiple ligations. Angiology 28:223-227
5. Dodd H, Cockett FB (1979) The pathology and surgery of the veins of the lower limb, 2nd edn. Churchill Livingstone, London
6. Doran FSA, White M (1975) A clinical trial designed to discover if the primary treatment of varicose veins should be by Fegan's method or by an operation. Br J Surg 62:72-76
7. Fegan WG (1963) Continuous compression technique of injecting varicose veins. Lancet 2:109-112
8. Fegan WG (1960) Continuous uninterrupted compression technique of injecting varicose veins. Proc R Soc Med 53:837-840
9. Fentem PH, Goddard M, Gooden BA, Yeung CK (1976) Control of distension of varicose veins achieved by leg bandages, as used after injection sclerotherapy. Br Med J 2:725-727
10. Hobbs JT (1974) Surgery and sclerotherapy in the treatment of varicose veins. Arch Surg 109:793-796
11. Hobbs JT (1968) A random trial of injection compression sclerotherapy. Br J Surg 55:889-895
12. Jakobsen BH (1979) The value of different forms of treatment for varicose veins. Br J Surg 66:182-184
13. McAdam WAF, Horrocks JC, De Dombal FT (1976) Assessment of the results of surgery for varicose veins. Br J Surg 63:137-140

14. Miller SS (1955) Investigation and management of varicose veins. Ann R Coll Surg Engl 55:245-252
15. Reid RG, Rothnie NG (1968) Treatment of varicose veins by compression sclerotherapy. Br J Surg 55:777-780
16. Stother IG, Bryson A, Alexander S (1974) The treatment of varicose veins by compression sclerotherapy. Br J Surg 61:387-390

Stereoflebografic Study of the Insufficient Perforating Veins, Dependent on Deep and Superficial Femoral Veins

J. S. Marques, A. Coito, and M. Korn*

The authors have chosen the above subject because this type of perforating vein has not been properly studied, contrary to the perforating veins of the leg. Their role in the pathogenesis of the essential varices is not disputed.

The stereophlebography carried out according to Cid dos Santos' techniques and principles was and still is the only method which permits the following statements to be made:

a) Some types of varices in the I.S. system are a consequence of the incompetence of perforating veins of the superficial femoral vein. Not so frequently, avalvulation of the venous duct of the postero-external side of the thigh, is also due to incompetence of perforating veins of the superficial femoral vein.

b) The importance of the incompetence of the deep femoral perforating veins is stressed as the cause of varices in the venous duct postero-external side of the thigh but not so often in certain varices of the internal, saphenous system.

The authors, after stating the importance of the above-mentioned principles in the planning of chirurgical treatment concluded by presenting final conclusions.

*Centro Angiologia R. Dos Santos, Faculd. Medicina, Lisboa, Portugal

Impedance Plethysmography and Its Limitations (Remarks Based on 79 Cases)

S. Milingos, J. Tassopoulos, C. Alexiou, and M. Gerazounis*

It is well known that the clinical diagnosis of deep vein thrombosis (DVT) is not simple, while pulmonary embolism as a consequence of DVT is a potential hazard for any patient. Various methods have been developed for the detection of DVT, the best of which is venography.

Nevertheless, it is an invasive, expensive, and time-consuming method, needing special equipment, highly trained personnel and is unsuitable for bedside screening. The need for a reliable, non-invasive, and simple method as well as early encouraging reports concerning impedance plethysmography have cast interest on the method.

With the above in mind the authors attempted an evaluation of this method by comparing its findings with those of venography, to discover its value and limitations in the detection of deep vein thrombosis.

Materials and Method

Seventy-nine patients hospitalized for general surgical problems underwent occlusive impedance plethysmographic (IPG) studies during the past 2 years; 49 were males and 30 females. The mean age was 49 years. All patients underwent minor or major surgical procedures and were referred for venography after completion of the IPG studies.

For the plethysmographic studies, a Model 200 impedance plethysmograph (cintor) was used. A mid thigh pneumatic cuff was applied and inflated to 45 cm H_2O, to occlude venous return for 45 s, and was then rapidly deflated. This maneuver produces changes in blood volume of the calf and consequently changes in impedance which are detected by a pair of electrodes applied to the calf and recorded as a tracing rise during calf inflation, and a tracing fall after deflation. The rise of the tracing and fall in the presence of venous obstruction will be reduced depending on the severity of the obstruction. Patients were tested in the supine position. The lower limb was elevated to 25° with the knee flexed to 15-20°. The ankle was 10 cm higher than the knee and, before starting every single test, it was assured that the patient was comfortable and totally relaxed (Fig. 1).

Alternatively and in the same patients, we performed tests with the knees overflexed, with the limb horizontal, with the knee straight, and the limb elevated. The results were plotted on a graph and the one showing the highest rise and greatest fall of the tracing was chosen as the representative IPG.

*Aghios Panteleimon Hospital of Nikea-Piraeus, Stournara 32, Athens, 103, Greece

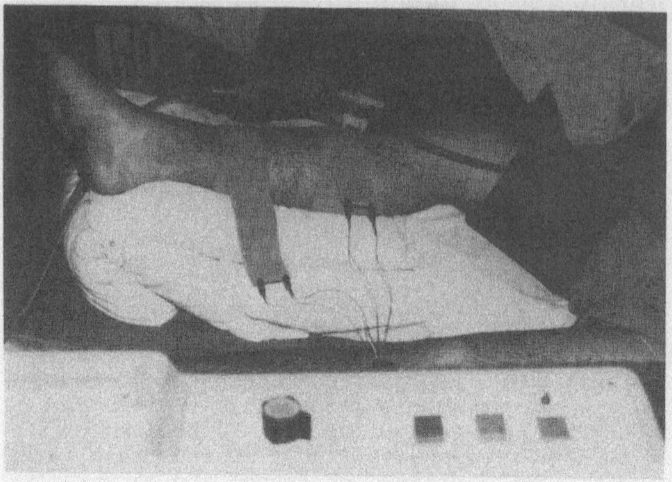

Fig. 1. Patient's position for plethysmographic studies

Results

A total of 79 patients underwent both venography and impedance plethysmographic studies; 59 patients showed normal or abnormal in both IPG and venographic studies, while in 20 patients IPG results disagreed with the venographic findings. In five of the latter, despite normal IPG, venography showed small thrombi in the calf veins and in one in a soleus vein. In 14 patients the absence of thrombi, as shown by venography, could not justify the abnormal IPG test; however, four suffered from cardiac insufficiency, three patients suffered from arterial insufficiency secondary to diabetes mellitus, two were debilitated, and in five patients the absence of DVT led to a repetition of the IPG studies after exercise and results were normal (Table 1).

The optimal IPG studies were achieved with the patient in the supine position, relaxed, with the knee flexed from 15-20°, the limb elevated to 25° and externally rotated, and with the ankle 10 cm higher than the knee.

Table 1. Number of patients studied by venography and IPG, and results

Patients	Abnormal		Normal	
	Venograms	IPG studies	Venograms	IPG studies
23			O	O
36	O	O		
14		O	O	In five after exercise
6	O			O
79	42	50/45	37	29/34

Comment

The questions a surgeon is quite often called to answer are whether or not a patient has DVT and whether or not chest X-ray findings, postoperatively, are due to some sort of pulmonary embolism secondary to DVT. Venography has been shown to be able to answer these questions once performed but, on the other hand, it has the disadvantages that it cannot be performed at bedside and is not suitable for the follow-up of patients with DVT. A non-invasive, simple, reliable, and rapid method is required to assess the risk of pulmonary embolism. For this purpose, occlusive impedance plethysmography has been developed and its reliability evaluated in previous reports by Wheeler et al. (6) and Dmochowski et al. (4).

The present study aimed at evaluating the reliability of this method in the detection of DVT by comparing its findings with those of venography. In the 79 patients in our series studied by both IPG and venography, we observed that this non-invasive method is not capable of detecting early DVT or small thrombi in the calf veins or old venous thrombosis without any fresh clot if it does not produce any significant haemodynamic changes in the limb. We encountered such false negative impedances results in six of our patients (7.6%). False positive results are often encountered in chronically ill and debilitated patients in whom bedding is likely to produce thrombosis. In those cases where DVT is excluded by venography, many of the false positive results change to negative after exercise. Abnormal impedance studies are also observed when external pressure is exerted on a major vein either by a tumor or bad limb posititioning.

Changes of limb position after each single test especially in those cases where abnormal studies are encountered is thought to be the only way to obtain the best out of the method. False positive results were encountered in 14 of our patients (17.72%) but re-examination after exercise gave normal impedance studies in five.

Our results show that occlusive impedance plethysmography is a non-invasive and reliable method for detecting DVT in most of the cases were it is present. However, it always has to be borne in mind that personal factors and small thrombi in the calf veins, as well as lack of exercise in patients bedded for a period of time, cardiac and arterial insufficiency, severe cold, old venous thrombosis with well-developed venous collateral circulation, tumors, or edema, in addition to such factors as chronic lung disease, limb positioning, improper clothing, and pain may lead to faulty results.

Despite its disadvantages and limitations, occlusive impedance plethysmography is a useful method for the follow-up of patients with DVT.

Summary

During the past years, impedance plethysmography has been widely used for the detection of deep vein thrombosis of the lower extremities. Compared to venography it seems that the method is capable of giving accurate results in most of the cases.

Nevertheless, our experience with the method during the past 2 years, based on 79 cases, showed that a number of limitations in its use should be taken into account to lessen the encountered false positive and false negative results. Faulty results are encountered in 10%-15% of the cases.

Factors leading to faulty results as well as the limiting factors, external pressure on the major vein, bedding, soft tissue pressure, small thrombi in a soleus vein, and a different technique during the examination constitute the method unsuitable for detection of deep vein thrombosis.

In conclusion, the authors believe that much care should be given to the interpretation of impedance plethysmography results because of the above limitations.

References

1. Browse NL (1974) Current thoughts on venous thromboembolism. Surg Cardiac Dis 54:229-238
2. Connolly JE, Gazzaniga AB (1974) Newer techniques to detect venous thrombosis with special reference to electrical impedance plethysmography. Surg Clin North Am 54:69-75
3. Deuvaert FE, Dmochowski JR, Couch NP (1973) Positional factors in venous impedance plethysmography. Arch Surg 106:53-55
4. Dmochowski JR, Adams DF, Couch NP (1972) Impedance measurements in the diagnosis of deep venous thrombosis. Arch Surg 104:170-173
5. Mullick SC, Wheeler HB, Songster GF (1970) Diagnosis of deep venous thrombosis by measurement of electrical impedance. Am J Surg 119:417-422
6. Wheeler HB, O'Donell JA, Anderson FA Jr, Benedict K Jr (1974) Occlusive impedance phlebography: a diagnostic procedure for venous thrombosis and pulmonary embolism. Progr Cardiovasc Dis 27:199-205

High Aortoiliac Occlusion: Treated by Bypass Grafting from the Thoracic Aorta to Femoral Arteries

G. Lakner and L. Lukács*

In the presence of arteriosclerotic occlusive disease of the aortic bifurcation, the infrarenal aorta is sometimes unsuitable for proximal grafting. In these cases, axillofemoral bypass grafting is recommended for use in poor-risk patients; however, this method has some drawbacks beside its advantages. If the patient's general condition is good, we prefer a revascularization procedure of greater value. We suggest the use of a Dacron bifurcation bypass graft extending from the descending thoracic aorta to the common femoral arteries in the treatment of high aortoiliac occlusive disease if the suprarenal aorta is unusable for grafting. Review of the literature showed few reports concerning the use of thoracic aorta-to-femoral arteries bypass grafting.

Blaisdell et al. (1) reported a bypass graft from the descending thoracic aorta to the left common femoral artery which included an extension to the right femoral artery. This procedure was performed to replace an infected and bleeding aortobifemoral prosthesis. The aorta was exposed through thoracotomy and the prosthesis was brought extraperitoneally to the femoral artery. The patient died due to sepsis.

Nunn and Kamal (4) described the first aortobifemoral bypass grafting from the thoracic aorta to femoral arteries for high occlusion of aortic bifurcation. The infrarenal portion of the aorta was unsuitable for grafting in all of the three cases reported. One patient had a saphenous vein graft inserted additionally between the aortic portion of the Dacron graft and the celiac artery because of significant narrowing of the celiac artery.

Frantz et al. (3) reported an ascending aorta-bilateral femoral artery bypass through a midline abdominal incision and median sternotomy. The prosthesis was brought subxiphoid through the gastrohepatic ligament into the retroperitoneum and sutured to the femoral arteries.

Cleveland (2) described a simultaneous mitral valve replacement and ascending aorta to left common femoral artery bypass with extension to the right common femoral artery for occlusion of the distal aorta. The 10 mm Dacron graft was brought through a subcutaneous tunnel to the femoral arteries.

Operative Technique

The patient is placed in a supine position and the femoral arteries are exposed in order to evaluate their status. A midline abdominal incision is made simultaneously. If the infrarenal abdominal aorta is found to be unusable, the incision is extended to the left eight intercostal space for exposure of the thoracic aorta. A partial occlusion

*Postgraduate Medical School, 1st Department of Surgery, 1135 Budapest, Szabolcs u. 35, Hungary

clamp is applied to the distal descending thoracic aorta and a vertical aortotomy is made. The aortic end of a Cooley double velour graft measuring 16 x 8 x 8 mm is sutured end-to-side to the aorta with continuous No. 4-0 Prolene sutures. The prosthesis was brought through the aortic hiatus, placed in a retroperitoneal position along the course of the arteries, and sutured to the common femoral arteries bilaterally with No. 5-0 Prolene sutures. The left pleural cavity is drained (Fig. 1).

During the operation and the postoperative period, ECG, blood pressure, CVP, urine excretion monitoring, electrolyte, and blood gas analysis are advisable. This procedure is rather an atypical bypass than an extraanatomic one because the prosthesis is brought along the course of the arteries.

Case Reports

The technique mentioned above was performed in two patients.

Case 1. A 45-year-old woman, a heavy smoker, had a left lumbar sympathectomy because of claudication 4 years prior to admission. At the time of admission, the patient was able to walk only 10-15 m before the onset of pain. There was no history of rest pain. Physical examination revealed an absence of pulses in the lower extremities. Blood pressure was recorded as 150/90 mm Hg in both arms. A translumbar aortogram showed complete occlusion of the infrarenal aorta.

Surgery was performed on September 19, 1978. The infrarenal aorta was exposed through a median laparotomy and found to be a thin fibrous cord with no lumen and was unsuitable for proximal grafting. The in-

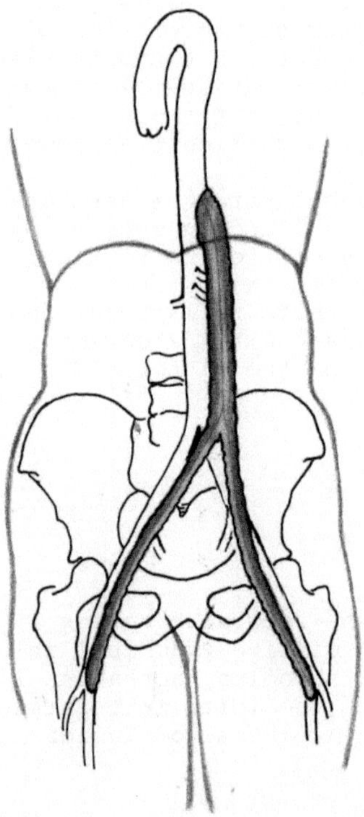

Fig. 1. Diagram of the surgical procedure

cision was extended and the prosthesis anastomosed to the descending thoracic aorta and distally to the common femoral arteries.

The postoperative period was uneventful and good peripheral pulses were palpable bilaterally. The follow-up aortogram showed a patent graft (Fig. 2). At 1 1/2 years, the patient continues to be asymptomatic.

Case 2. The patient was a 52-year-old obese woman who complained of claudication in the lower extremities. Physical examination revealed a normally developed female with no pulses in either leg. The blood pressure was 145/85 mm Hg. The abdominal aortogram showed complete occlusion of the abdominal aorta just below the renal arteries. The patient was put on a low calorie diet and following weight loss was readmitted. On March 15, 1979, the patient underwent operation. The infrarenal aorta was found to be unsuitable for grafting. The midline abdominal incision was extended to the chest with a left-sided thoracotomy and a descending thoracic aorta to common femoral arteries bypass graft was inserted. Good pedal pulses were noted bilaterally following the operation. The postoperative course was uncomplicated.

The postoperative aortogram showed a well-functioning graft (Fig. 3). One year postoperatively the patient is asymptomatic.

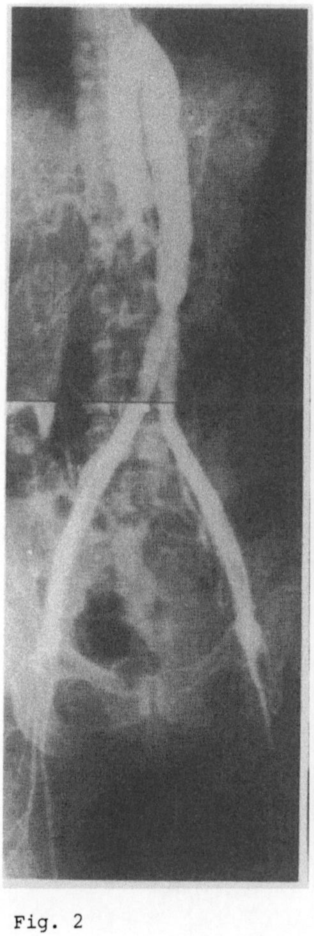

Fig. 2

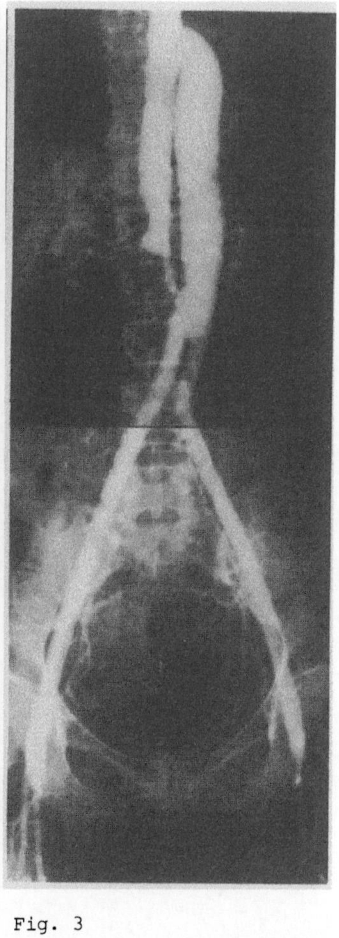

Fig. 3

Fig. 2. Postoperative aortogram showing well-functioning bypass graft

Fig. 3. Postoperative aortogram revealing a patent graft

Discussion

The complete occlusion of the proximal infrarenal aorta can present a great problem to the vascular surgeon who is attempting to perform an aortobifemoral bypass. In some patients the abdominal aorta is an unsuitable proximal take-off point for revascularization of the lower extremities. The descending thoracic aorta to femoral arteries bypass grafting is a suitable procedure for treating relatively good-risk patients with disabling claudication. The opening of the abdominal and pleural cavities does not cause any complications in the postoperative period.

"Steal effect" caused by the bypass graft was not observed in the splanchnic circulation and the review of the literature failed to disclose any report concerning this problem. It is our feeling that this technique offers several advantages and good results for the treatment of high aortoiliac occlusive disease.

References

1. Blaisdell FW, De Mattei GA, Gauder PJ (1961) Extraperitoneal thoracic aorta to femoral bypass graft as replacement for infected aortic bifurcation prosthesis. Am J. Surg 102:583-587
2. Cleveland JC (1980) Ascending aorta to common femoral artery bypass: An unusual but successful method for revascularization of the lower extremity: Report of a case. Cardiovasc Dis 7:74-77
3. Frantz SL, Kaplitt MJ, Beil AR, Stein HL (1974) Ascending aorta-bilateral femoral artery bypass for the totally occluded infrarenal abdominal aorta. Surgery 75: 471-475
4. Nunn DB, Kamal MA (1972) Bypass grafting from the thoracic aorta to femoral arteries for high aortoiliac occlusive disease. Surgery 72:749-755

Management of Subclavian and Common Carotid Lesions by Transposition

J. Lerut, W. Sandmann, M. Hennerici, A. Aulich, and K. Kremer

Introduction

In the period from 1976 to June 1980, 279 operations were performed upon the supraaortic vessels in 226 patients. Twenty-two patients underwent transposition of the subclavian into the carotid artery (21 patients) and of the common carotid into the subclavian artery (one patient). The results of this technique are presented and discussed in this paper.

Patients and Method

Twenty-one patients from 38 to 67 years old had cerebral and/or peripheral vascular insufficiency in the presence of the subclavian steal syndrome. There were 11 women and ten men; in all but one the lesion was left-sided (Table 1). A total of 57% (12/21 patients) suffered from cerebrovascular insufficiency, 76% had peripheral arm and/or hand symptoms (16/21 patients).

Three patients underwent correction of an asymptomatic lesion in order to prevent neurological complications after repair of the associated aortoiliac occlusion disease. Each patient had a multivessel supraaortic disease. Ten patients had a typical subclavian steal syndrome with vertebrobasilar TIA and peripheral ischemic symptoms; one of them had a gangrene of the fifth left finger. Two patients had a permanent neurological deficit, caused by an associated high-grade internal carotid stenosis. Six patients were operated on because of ischemic hand or arm complaints.

Table 1. Transposition surgery

21 Subclavian artery occlusions/stenoses			
Sex	11	10	
Age	38-67 years		mean age 50.5 years
Location	20 left	1 right	
1 Common carotid artery occlusion			
	1	left	mean age 66 years

*Chirurgische Klinik A der Universität Düsseldorf, Moorenstr. 5, D-4000 Düsseldorf

One patient presenting an occlusion of the left common carotid artery in association with a severe bilateral internal carotid stenosis and a moderate bracheocephalic trunk stenosis suffered from poststroke symptoms. All patients underwent an extensive continuous-wave ultrasound Doppler examination of the extracranial arteries (bidirectional Doppler flowmeter/system Delalande) (UDS).

Sixteen patients presented an occlusion of the subclavian artery; five had a severe stenosis. All these lesions caused a reversal of the ipsilateral vertebral flow with steal phenomenon. It should be remarked that seven patients (33%) did not have a cervical bruit. Blood pressure gradients between both brachial arteries varied from 25 to 100 mm Hg. In case of a clear non-invasive diagnosis, in 12/22 patients as proven later by surgery, invasive diagnostic procedures, especially angiography, could be omitted. Nine out of 22 patients underwent further retrograde brachial and/or percutaneous carotid or aortic arch angiography, seven patients because of a UDS multivessel disease and two patients because of a redo subclavian artery surgery after carotid-subclavian bypass which was performed in other institutions.

As can be seen in Table 2, nine patients (41%) had an additional, simultaneous or staged intervention for a significant lesion in other extracranial vessels; the majority of them were thromboendarterectomies of the internal carotid arteries (7/12 operations). In case of an ipsilateral haemodynamically significant internal carotid arterial stenosis (four patients in the series), carotid *thromboendarteriotomy* was done first, using an intraluminal shunt followed by transposition of the subclavian artery. During the transposition operation, the shunt was left in place.

Two cases underwent additional desobliteration of the ipsilateral stenosed vertebral artery using the eversion method. Additional aortic surgery was performed in seven patients, coronary artery surgery in one. Simultaneous corrections (three patients) did not influence the morbidity or mortality.

Table 2. Associated extracranial vascular interventions in 22 patients submitted to transposition surgery

Thromboendarterectomy (TEA)	N	Simultaneous	Staged
Ipsilateral int. carotid art.	4	4	-
Contralateral int. carotid art.	3	-	3
Brachioceph. trunk	1	1	-
Ipsilateral common carotid art.	1	1	-
Ipsilateral vertebral art.	2	2	-
Contralateral vertebral art.	1	-	1
	12 operations in nine patients (41%)		

Operative Technique

After supraclavicular skin incision, the subclavian artery and the carotid artery are dissected down to the origin of the aortic arch or to the brachiocephalic trunk, respectively. The subclavian artery is ligated near the aortic arch and transected. If the stenotic lesion involves the origin of the vertebral artery, the subclavian artery can be everted and endarterectomy is possible under direct vision. The distal subclavian segment is shortened obliquely, leaving a longer caudal part, in order to construct a natural bifurcation. After clamping of the common carotid artery, an elliptic excision of the wall at the dorsolateral side is performed. The subclavian artery is anastomosed with two running sutures of 6-0 Prolene. This anastomosis mostly takes about 5-20 minutes. The clamping time is without danger if the blood pressure is kept constant and if the other supraaortic vessels are free of haemodynamic significant lesions. In case significant lesions are present, correction should be done previously, either simultaneously or in a staged procedure. In case of ipsilateral internal carotid artery stenosis, we used a Javid shunt.

Results

The transposition surgery caused a very low morbidity and no mortality. One patient developed a haematoma without clinical significance. There was one chylothorax requiring transthoracic drainage and the leakage of the lymphatic duct was repaired by a vascular suture. Nine patients presented a temporary phrenic nerv paresia. One patient presented a TIA, probably caused by microembolization into the brain stem region. UDS was normal but the patient had a severe arrythmia which may be responsible for this embolization. One superficial secondary wound healing (*Staphylococcus albus*) occurred and required no special therapy. All patients underwent repetitive UDS examination of the supraaortic vessels during the postoperative period (Table 3). In the first part of this series, postoperative angiography was performed in each patient (Fig. 1) but later control angiography was performed only in case of abnormal Doppler findings or if a remaining brachial pressure gradient was measured. Only one patient out of the series again presented a subclavian steal phenomenon due to a stenosis at the anastomosis. This happened at the beginning of the series; no further intervention was required because the patient was free of symptoms. Two patients presented an alternating vertebral flow. This phenomenon was seen during the early postoperative period and changed some weeks later into normal flow direction. Two patients presented an important postreconstruction blood pressure gradient between both brachial arteries. The first had previously overlooked atherosclerotic plaque in the peripheral segment of the subclavian artery, the second presented a stenosis at the origin of the common carotid artery. Repair by endarterectomy was successful in both patients. The one patient with transposition of the common carotid into the subclavian artery postoperatively had a normal Doppler flow pattern and a normal angiography (Fig. 2). Simultaneous intraoperative pressure and quantitative flow measurement in the proximal carotid artery, in the common carotid artery distal to the anastomosis, and in the subclavian artery showed a total flow reduction of about 20% through the peripheral segment of the common carotid artery after restoration of the circulation. This blood flow reduction correlated well with the simultaneous flow reversal and augmentation in the ipsilateral vertebral artery; thus it can be stated that transposition surgery does not cause carotid steal. Measurement of blood flow perturbation by spectral Doppler analysis assured us that the flow at the anastomosis was undisturbed or slightly disturbed, indicating a haemodynamically favourable anastomosis (6).

Table 3. Postoperative ultrasound Doppler findings

Patients	Type of reconstruction	Extracranial circulation		
		Normal	Abnormal	Brachial
21	Subclavian-carotid transposition	20	1	2
1	Carotid-subclavian transposition	1	0	0

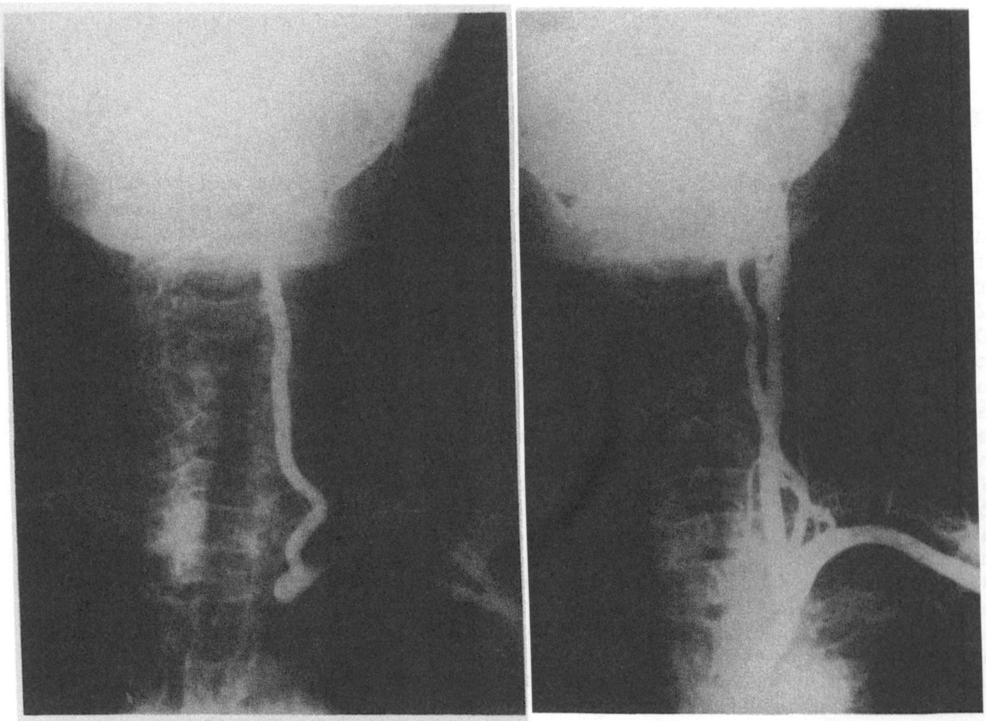

Fig. 1. Original figure of subclavian transposition from Parrot (1964 [4])

Discussion

The operative technique used for transposition was described in 1964 by Parrot (4) (Fig. 3) who had already transposed the subclavian into the common carotid artery with simultaneous ipsilateral thromboendarterectomy of the internal carotid artery. Recently, there were the works of Mehigan et al. (3), Edwards and Mulherin (2), Cormier et al.

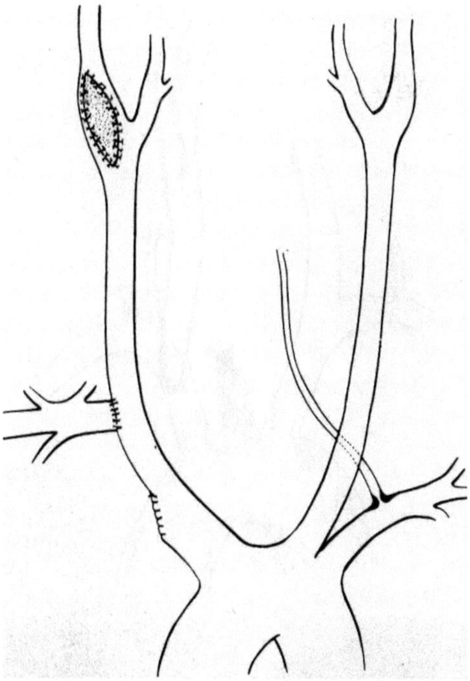

Fig. 2. Pre- and postoperative retrograde transbrachial angiography in a patient with left subclavian artery occlusion managed by transposition of the subclavian artery to the common carotid artery

(1), and our own group (5) who described their experience with this technique and the results. The whole procedure can be performed through a supraclavicular incision and is especially recommended for patients at high risk. Lesions of the proximal subclavian artery can be treated by transthoracic subclavian endarterectomy, by transthoracic or transmediastinal prosthetic reconstruction, and by a variety of extraanatomic bypass techniques. The first two methods have the advantage of an in situ repair: the original flow direction is restored and reoccorrence of the disease is rare.

The variety of extraanatomic bypass techniques, for instance carotid-subclavian, subclavian-subclavian, and axillo-axillo bypasses can also be performed in high-risk patients. The methods have, nevertheless, some disadvantages: prosthetic material, frequently a large Dacron tube, is used causing abnormal flow patterns at the level of the peripheral anastomosis to the subclavian artery (6), and the arterial segment between the distal anastomosis and the origin of the vertebral artery may even become thrombosed. The method of Parrot (4) has several advantages making it the procedure of choice for the operative management of proximal subclavian lesions: no graft material is used, just one vascular anastomosis is necessary, receptor and donor arteries are approached by the same extrathoracical incision, an eventual source of embolization is excluded, the flow pattern is restored to normal, there is a low morbidity and no mortality in the series reported so far, and the hospitalization time is reduced in comparison to other methods. The donor arterial system must be free of any stenotic disease; this is one of the major conditions to avoid unnecessary brain ischaemia. Care should also be given to peripheral subclavian lesions. Haemodynamic significant lesions of the ipsi- or contralateral supraaortic vessels can easily be detected by extensive continuous-wave Doppler sonography and should be repaired before subclavian transposition is performed.

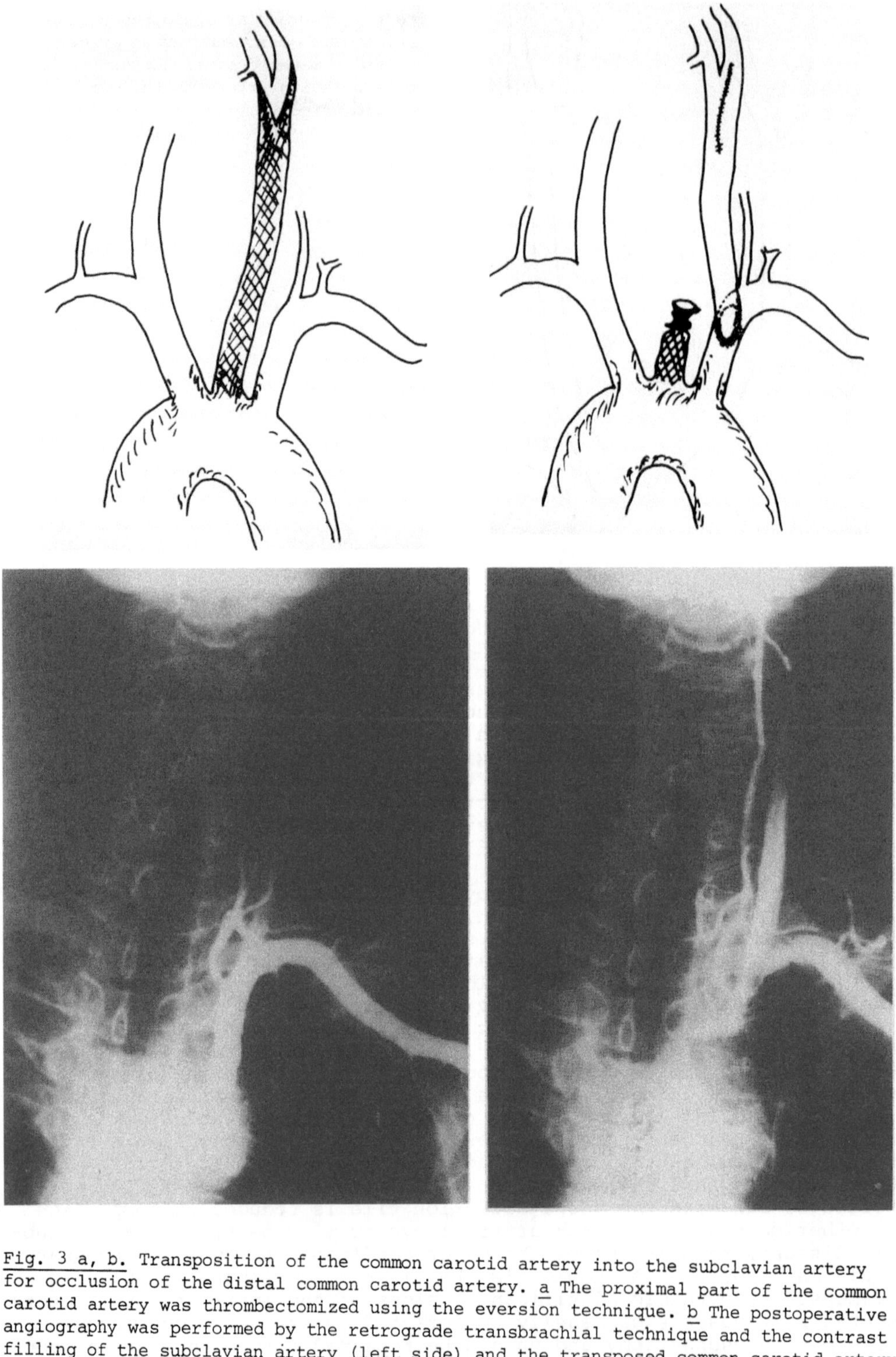

a

b

Fig. 3 a, b. Transposition of the common carotid artery into the subclavian artery for occlusion of the distal common carotid artery. a The proximal part of the common carotid artery was thrombectomized using the eversion technique. b The postoperative angiography was performed by the retrograde transbrachial technique and the contrast filling of the subclavian artery (left side) and the transposed common carotid artery (right side) as well as the maintained vertebral artery can be seen

Our intraoperative flow measurements did not reveal any carotid steal phenomenon after transposition. The flow reduction of about 20% in the common carotid artery correlates well with a simultaneous flow reversal in the ipsilateral vertebral artery, so the net flow to the brain is augmented. Turbulence measurements by analysis of the Doppler spectrum revealed a haemodynamically favourable anastomosis which has almost a normal bifurcation.

In case of associated major vascular surgery, the asymptomatic subclavian steal syndrome is only corrected in case of multivessel disease in the supraaortic arteries. Pre- and postoperative angiography is only mandatory in case of unclear Doppler findings or in case of multivessel diseases. The good results of this technique influenced us to perform this operation in two patients who had already undergone carotidosubclavian prosthetic bypasses previously in other institutions. In a third case, we performed the technique in the reversed way, transposing the common carotid artery which was distally occluded, into the subclavian artery. The results in these particular three patients were also excellent.

The subclavian-carotid transposition became the method of choice for us in the surgical treatment of proximal subclavian lesions. Some patients have now follow-up results longer than 2 years and their haemodynamic results continue to confirm this concept. The use of the transposition surgery for occlusion of the common carotid artery certainly in the high-risk patients should be kept in mind.

Summary

Lesions of the proximal subclavian artery can easily be treated by transposition of this artery into the common carotid artery. The main advantages of this method are a short operation time with only one vascular anastomosis, avoidance of graft material, and the construction of a haemodynamic favourable anastomosis. Careful selection of patients is necessary using the ultrasound Doppler sonography for examination of the extracranial cerebral vessels. Angiography is required if the Doppler examination shows a multivessel disease or leaves some uncertainty about the extent of the disease. Twenty out of 21 patients had a normalization of vertebral blood flow after this procedure (success rate 95%); one additional patient had a successful transposition of the common carotid into the subclavian artery. Because of these results and in respect to the low morbidity, the transposition operation became the method of choice in patients with subclavian steal syndrome and in those suffering from distal common carotid artery occlusion.

References

1. Cormier JM, Ricco JB, Franceschi C (1979) 82 cas de réimplantation de la sons-clavieu on de la vertêbrale dans la carotide primiture. Chirurgie 105/7:592-596
2. Edwards WH, Mulherin JL (1980) The surgical approach to significant stenosis of the vertebral and subclavian arteries. Surgery 87/1:20-28
3. Mehigan JT, Buch WS, Pipkin RD, Fogarty TJ (1978) Subclavian-carotid transposition for the subclavian steal syndrome. Am J Surg 136/1:15-20
4. Parrott JD (1964) The subclavian steal syndrome. Arch Surg 88:661-666
5. Sandmann W, Kremer K, Lerut J, Hennerici M, Aulich A (1980) Subclavia-Carotis Transposition zur Behandlung der Subclavia-Verschlußerkrankung mit Anzapfsyndrom. Chirurg 51/4:228-234
6. Sandmann W, Peronneau P, Schweins G, Bournat J, Hinglais J (1978) Turbulenzmessung mit dem Doppler-Ultraschallverfahren: eine neue Methode der Qualitätskontrolle in der Arterienchirurgie. In: Kriessmann A, Bollinger A (eds) Ultraschall Doppler-Diagnostik in der Angiologie. Thieme, Stuttgart, p 77

The Surgical Treatment of Atherosclerotic Occlusion of the Innominate and Subclavian Arteries. Long-Term Results

G. P. Deriu and E. Ballotta*

Introduction

The ischemic syndromes due to different kinds of stenotic or occlusive lesions of the supra-aortic trunks have by now assumed precise physiopathologic, diagnostic, and therapeutic aspects in the field of cerebrovascular insufficiency (1-26).

Materials and Methods

Among 78 patients operated on for occlusive disease of subclavian, innominate, and common carotid artery, we studied 34 patients affected by the disease operated on by the senior author at the Vascular Surgery Department of the Institute of Surgical Pathology I of the University of Padua during the period October 1970 to October 1975. Of these, 27 (79.4%) were male and seven (20.5%) were female; the average age was 60 years (Table 1). The innominate artery was affected in six cases (17.6%); one case (2.9%) was a common left carotid-subclavian trunk which is included in this report among the innominate trunk lesions as "left innominate artery".

Table 1. Sex distribution

	34 Patients		Subclavian artery		Innominate artery	
Sex	No.	%	No.	%	No.	%
Male	27	79.4	21	77.7	6	85.7
Female	7	20.5	6	22.3	1	14.2

Of these seven cases, X-rays showed six (85.7%) as stenosis of the lumen, only one case (14.2%) as complete obstruction (Table 2). The subclavian artery was affected in 27 cases (79.4%), 23 (85.1%) on the left and four (14.8%) on the right. Of these 27, X-rays showed 15 (55.5%) as occlusion, 13 on the left and two on the right; the remaining 12 (44.4%) were stenoses, ten on the left and two on the right (Table 2). Therefore, the lumen occlusion of the involved artery occurred in 16 cases (47.1%), stenosis in 18 (52.9%) (Table 3).

*Istituto di Patologica Chirurgica Ia, Padova, Italy
Cattedra di Chirurgia Vascolare, Padova, Italy

Table 2. Pattern of obstruction

	34 Patients		Stenosis		Occlusion	
	No.	%	No.	%	No.	%
Right subclavian artery	4	11.7	2	11.1	2	12.5
Left subclavian artery	23	67.6	10	55.5	13	81.2
Innominate artery	6	17.6	5	27.7	1	6.2
Left innominate artery	1	2.9	1	5.5	-	-

Table 3. Location and extent of lesions

	34 patients		Subclavian artery		Innominate artery	
	No.	%	No.	%	No.	%
Occlusion	16	47.1	15	55.5	1	14..2
Stenosis	18	52.9	12	44.4	6	85.7

The symptoms noted (usually very light and discontinuous), in order of frequency, were vertigo in 19 (55.8%) cases, visual disturbances in 13 (38.2%), paresthesias in 11 (32.3%), headache in eight (23.5%), tinnitus in seven (20.5%), pallor and hypothermia of the fingers of the limb corresponding to the side of the arterial lesion in four (11.7%), and trophic lesions of the fingers in three (8.8%) cases. On three occasions, the patient was completely asymptomatic (Table 4).

Table 4. Symptoms of obstruction

	34 patients		Subclavian artery		Innominate artery	
	No.	%	No.	%	No.	%
No symptoms	3	8.8	2	7.4	1	14.2
Vertigo and dizzines	19	55.8	15	55.5	4	57.1
Blackout	3	8.8	2	7.4	1	14.2
Visual disturbances	13	38.2	11	40.7	2	28.5
Tinnitus	7	20.5	5	18.5	2	28.5
Finger tip necrosis	3	8.8	3	11.1	-	-
Upper extremity chronic ischemia	4	11.7	3	11.1	1	14.2
Paresthesia	11	32.3	11	40.7	-	-
Headache	8	23.5	6	22.2	2	28.5
Pressure gradient						
<30 mm Hg	18	52.9	15	55.5	3	42.8
>30 mm Hg	16	47.0	12	44.4	4	57.1

A pressure difference was noted between the two upper limbs in all the patients (100%). All the patients were studied with angiography in all cases but one. Subclavian or innominate artery steal was documented in 16 cases.

Noteworthy is the association of the lesions of the supra-aortic trunks with other pathology: 18 patients (52.9%) complained, among other things, of a peripheric obliterating arteriopathy; 14 (41.1%) a cardiopathy; four (11.7%) hypertension; in three (8.8%) a nephropathy (Table 5).

Table 5. Other symptoms

	No.	%
Hypertension	4	11.7
Diabetes	3	8.8
Aortoiliac a/o femoropopliteal disease	18	52.9
Heart disease	14	41.1
Kidney disease	3	8.8

In 22 patients (64.7%), the operation consisted in a carotid-subclavian bypass for lesions all located at level with the subclavian; in six (17.6%) in an aorto-carotid bypass, always involving lesions of the innominate artery; two (5.8%) were endarterectomies of the subclavian, while only once (2.9%) an endarterectomy of the innominate artery was performed (Table 6).

Table 6. Type of operation

	34 patients		Subclavian artery		Innominate artery	
	No.	%	No.	%	No.	%
Carotid subclavian bypass	22[a]	64.7	22	81.4	-	-
Aortocarotid bypass	6	17.6	-	-	6	85.7
Subclavian endarterectomy	2	5.8	2	7.4	-	-
Innominate endarterectomy	1	2.9	-	-	1	3.7
Exploration	1	2.9	1	3.7	-	-
Others	2	5.8	2	7.4	-	-

[a]Five patients had a combined homolateral carotid endarterectomy

Other operations were a subclavian-axillary bypass with a vein graft brought subcutaneously above the clavicle to the axilla (once) and an extra-anatomical axillobifemoral-axillary Dacron bypass graft in a very high risk patient with contemporary lower limb severe ischemic disease.

Results

All the treated patients have been followed-up in the postoperative period. The operative results, divided into immediate (within the first postoperative month) and long-term (from 3 years to 8 years, since the check was done at the end of 1978) were considered good if the patient experienced complete remission of the symptoms, poor if the symptoms were aggravated by operation or if the subject encountered significant complications connected to the operation. After 1 month, 16 (50%) patients experienced complete remission of symptoms; 11 (34.3%) recovered very well, while in three (9.3%) patients the symptoms were unchanged after the operation (Table 7). In all the cases, the blood pressure was normalized and no variation was found by postoperative examinations.

Table 7.

	Immediate results No.	1 month follow-up on 32-34 patients 1 hospital death %
Asymptomatic	16	50
Improved	11	34.3
Unimproved	3	9.3
Neurological complications	2[a]	6.2

[a]All in patients with combined homolateral carotid endarterectomy

Two cases (5.4%) developed neurologic complications in the immediate postoperative period. Aphasia and paresis of the upper limb contralateral to the operated side developed in patients treated with the subclavian revascularization by carotid endarterectomy due to the concomitant stenosis of the internal extracranial carotid (Table 7). Of the 32 patients considered in Table 7, 31 have been postoperatively examined.

Of the operative complications, the aphasia completely regressed; however, the motor deficiency of the upper limb, even if very slight, remained (Table 8). Of the 31 patients considered in Table 8, 27 were postoperatively examined after more than 3 years. One patient died from a cancer of the esophagus, three patients of myocardial infarction. One patient was operated on with excellent results for contralateral carotid endarterectomy (Tables 9 and 10).

Conclusions

The bypass operation, such as the carotid-subclavian or the aortocarotid bypass, represents the surgical conclusion of choice we have proposed in most cases of subclavian or innominate lesions. Unlike stenotic lesions precisely located at the carotid bifurcation which

Table 8.

	6 months follow-up No.	31 patients 1 patient dead for unknown reason %
Asymptomatic	12	38.7
Improved	14	45.1
Unimproved	4	12.9
Worsened	-	-
Neurological complications	1	3.2

Table 9.

Total deaths	6
Hospital death	1
Unknown reason	1
Cardiac	3
Cancer	1

Table 10.

	Late results (28 patients) (3-10 years) No.	%
Asymptomatic	12	44.4
Improved	13	48.2
Unimproved	2	7.4

require a precise endarterectomy and patch with relatively long clamping time, in the bypass carotid clamping time (restricted moreover only to the common carotid and therefore with preservation of the external carotid-internal carotid communication) necessary only for performing an end-to-side anastomosis between prosthesis and artery is only about 10 minutes. On this subject our case report is significant with reference to the operating risk which is practically nil and reappears when the presence of a concomitant lesion of the carotid bifurcation requires a double carotid-subclavian bypass and carotid endarterectomy operation.

Following this consideration, we began in 1975 in such circumstances to use an internal shunt, either for all the clamping duration or, as we prefer, only for the time following the carotid endarterectomy. On the basis of the follow-up results (from more than 3 to 8 years), we felt impelled to affirm that the carotid-subclavian bypass should be performed even on subjects scarcely symptomatic in order to prevent the development of cerebrovascular insufficiency which, even in these cases, though to a lesser degree, could follow that of cerebrovascular insufficiency due to stenosis of the internal carotid artery in its extracranial tract.

Summary

Among 78 patients operated on for occlusive disease of supra-aortic trunks in the period 1970-1978, 34 patients who underwent carotid-subclavian bypass (64.7%), aortocarotid bypass (17.6%), endarterectomy of subclavian artery (5.8%), or endarterectomy of innominate artery had follow-up studies for 3-10 years since surgery. All patients demonstrated originally a differential in systolic blood pressure in the upper extremities. The surgical indications were posed on the basis of neurologic symptoms of vertebrobasilar insufficiency and the angiographic evidence of "subclavian" (79.4%) or "innominate" (20.6%) steal.

The carotid-subclavian bypass has been the preferred surgical treatment technique in patients with "subclavian steal". This operation is indicated also in nearly asymptomatic patients in order to prevent the natural history of vertebrobasilar insufficiency. In our experience, operative risk in carotid-subclavian bypass is not present, unless an associated lesion of carotid bifurcation exists which needs an endarterectomy with patch-graft angioplasty. Long-term results are considered satisfactory in surgically treated patients.

Session IX Joint Session

Infections in Cardiovascular Surgery

Chairman: C. Hahn, Geneva; Co-Chairman: G. Poulias, Athens

Leriche Lecture

On the Management of the Ichaemic Limb

P. Martin*

When presented with a patient suffering from the effects of an obstructed artery, in the great majority of instances the cause is arteriosclerosis. We are presented therefore with a symptom of a generalised disease, and there is little we can do as regards the latter, but with modern techniques we can in most relieve the symptom, though often for only a relatively short time. It is interesting that in the more elderly, the results are very much better than in the younger patient (Tables 1 and 2). This suggests that in the younger group the disease process is more active. Royle of Melbourne (personal communication) showed that in dietary induced atheroma in rabbits, simple suture of the femoral artery led to atheromatous obstruction, as did simply passing a needle through the vessel wall. McManus (2) in his textbook of pathology noticed that in the 80-year-old patient a previous atheromatous plaque was often represented by fibrous tissue. This seems to show that the disease becomes less active or tends to regress in the elderly.

Table 1. Longest patency of femoropopliteal reconstruction in different age groups of patients

Age	Longest patency time (mo.)
33-40	47
41-50	96
56-60	120[a]
61-70	120[a]
71-83	72[a]

[a]Still patent when last seen.

Table 2. Femoropopliteal vein grafts patent for 5 years or more

Age (yr.)	Total femoropopliteal vein grafts	No. of grafts patent after 5 yr.	Percent
33-40	9	0	0
41-50	41	3	7.3
51-60	117	18	15.4
61-70	106	29	27.4
71-84	27	Follow-up unreliable	
All	300 (273 + 27)	50	18.3

It seems too that vessels of supply such as the renal or mesenteric arteries are relatively free from disease except at their origins where they arise from a vessel of conduction. The profunda femoris artery, largely an artery of supply to the thigh muscles, is similarly free from disease except at its origin from the common femoral artery or in

*Royal Postgraduate Medical School, London, and Chelmsford Hospital, Great Britain

its most proximal course to the level of the first perforating artery. Beales et al. (1) described a method of lateral angiography of this vessel which reveals the orifice and proximal profunda (Fig. 1).

We thought it reasonable therefore to use the profunda femoris artery as more suitable to replace the obstructed femoral and even the popliteal artery. I have never seen distal arteriosclerotic obstruction of the profunda femoris artery, except in association with diabetes. Its anatomy (Fig. 2) shows anastomoses above with the internal iliac system, and below with the tibial vessels, and as it is not affected by atheroma, its dilatation, given a good proximal flow of blood, is such that it readily replaces the femoropopliteal trunk. A number of operations have been described (Fig. 3) to achieve this, but we prefer the "boomerang" patch method using a segment of saphenous vein, with the ends cut square stitched over a grooved metal dilator to avoid any stenosis (Figs. 4 and 5).

We rarely do a femoropopliteal graft, except sometimes in patients over the age of 65. If there is a profunda orificial stenosis, this is dealt with, and in most this completes the operation; but if the popliteal is relatively healthy a femoropopliteal graft can be added. We have not done a femorotibial graft for the last 7 years, but in those where it might be considered, we find a profundoplasty more successful as time passes, though symptoms may not be greatly relieved initially. The operation is indicated after failure of a previous femoropopliteal graft. In fact, if there is a stenosis, even a minor one, of the orifice of the profunda artery, it seems to us that as the years after operation pass, a profundoplasty is more satisfactory. It is a relatively minor operation which can be done under local anaesthesia. Sometimes there is disease of the iliac vessels, and in such we extend the incision proximally, dividing the inguinal ligament and the abdominal wall along the outer border of the rectus abdominis muscle and approaching the iliac system retroperitoneally. By passing a malleable stripper upwards, the diseased intima is separated and divided proximally by a retrograde knife and then removed by special forceps (Fig. 6). Should the aortic bifurcation be affected, then a major operation is required.

The results of the operation are not so immediately impressive as after a femoropopliteal graft, though after a few weeks symptoms improve as the profunda dilates because of the improved inflow of blood. Results vary with the severity of the condition when the patient presents and are as follows Tables 3 and 4. Many such patients would have been suitable only for a distal tibial anastomosis on bypass grafting. The long-term results (5-9 years) show an improvement in the profundoplasty group particularly as regards later amputation and are as follows Table 5. Surely some claudication in the elderly is a small price to pay for retaining a lower limb till death.

This talk is dedicated to the memory of René Leriche, a great Frenchman with a wide interest in disease, and one who was particularly concerned with the physiology of the surgical patient. His work on the sympathetic nervous system led to sympathectomy being a valuable and indeed the only surgical measure for patients with limb ischaemia. Many thousands of such operations were done throughout the world with benefit. It is sad that his death occurred before the age of direct arterial surgery, a conception in which he was always interested. He was a man of remarkable intellect and ability with a great devotion to the service of others and was properly honoured by his surgical colleagues throughout the world. He was a great and gentle man.

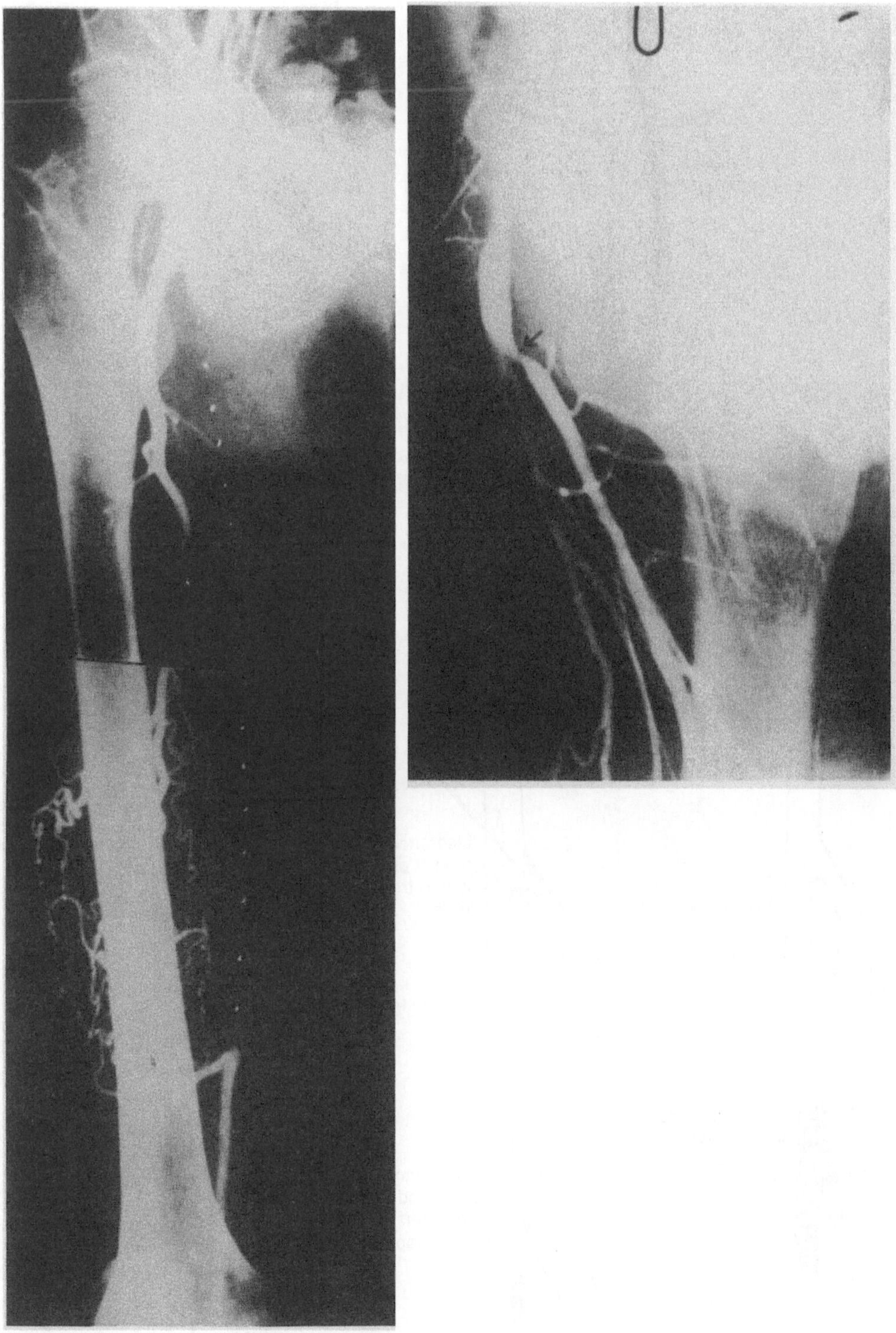

Fig. 1. Lateral angiography

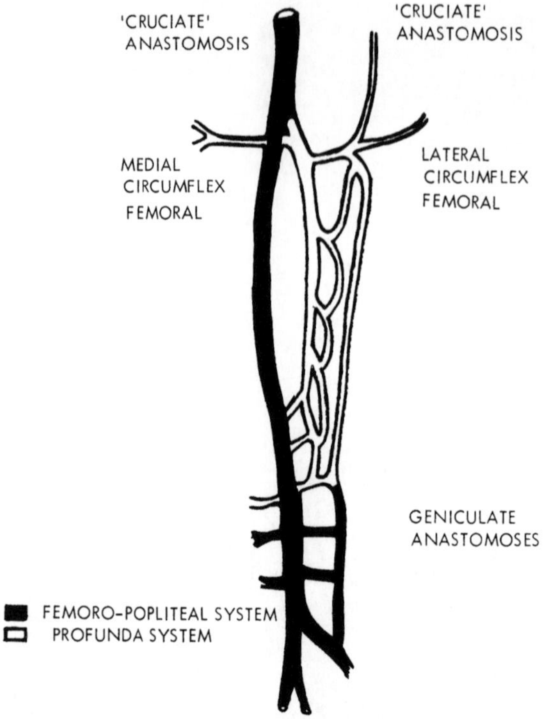

Fig. 2. Anatomy of profunda femoris artery

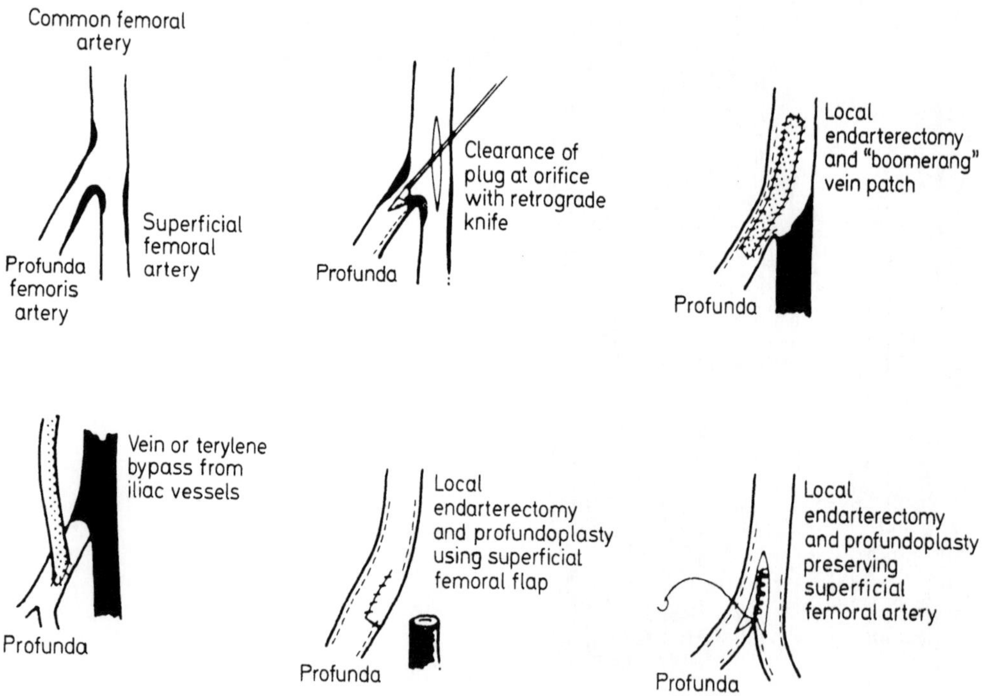

Fig. 3. Operation methods

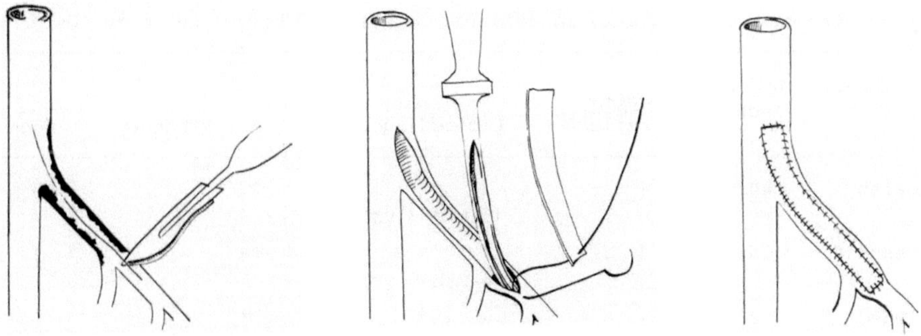

Fig. 4. "Boomerang" patch method

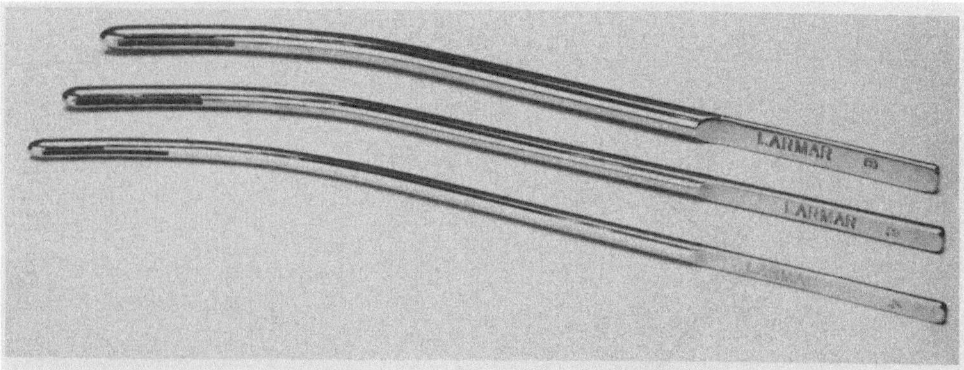

Fig. 5. Metal dilators (these and all special instruments in this paper can be obtained from Chas. F. Thackray & C., Leeds, Great Britain

Table 3. Amputations related to presenting symptoms

Symptom	No. of legs	No. of amputations
Intermittent claudication at 200 m	8	0
Intermittent claudication at 100 m	10	0
Intermittent claudication at 20-50 m	34	5 (0-2 yr postop.)
Rest pain	37	6 (0-5 yr postop.)
Gangrene of toes	18	5 (0-6 yr postop.)
Total	107[a]	16

[a]Five legs not included (patients died within 1 month of operation)

Table 4. Results of profundoplasty in relation to state of below-knee arteries

State of three main vessels	No. of legs	Result			
		Failure	Limited success	Satisfactory	Good
Three healthy	44	-	2 (6 mth-3 yr)	24	18
Three stenosed	35	3	4 (4 mth-5 yr)	25	3
One occluded	2	-	-	1	1
Two occluded	16	2	-	14	-
Three occluded	7	-	5 (1-5 yr)	2	-
Unknown	3	-	-	2	1
Total	107[a]	5	11	68	23

[a]Five legs not included (patients died within 1 month of operation)

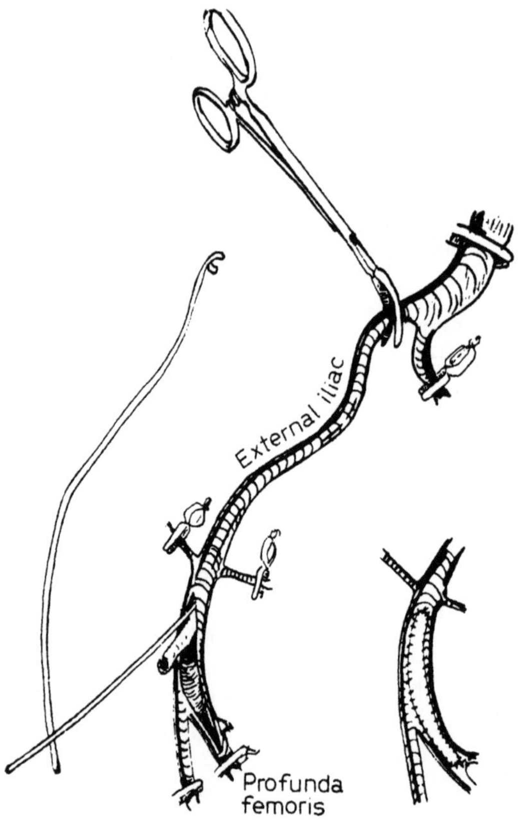

Fig. 6. See text

Table 5. Amputation rates

After femoropopliteal graft at 5 years	34.6%
After profunda surgery at 5-9 years	12 %
Death rates	
In either group from cardiovascular or other causes at 5 year follow-up	25 %

References

1. Beales JSM, Adcock FA, Frawley JS, Nathan BE, McLachlan MSF, Martin P, Steiner RE (1971) Br J Radiol 44:854
2. McManus JFA (1966) General pathology. Chicago, p 407

General Hospital Hygiene and Wound Infections After Heart Surgery

R. Panzner and H. Neef*

We would like to impart our experience in two hospitals concerning conditions of general hygiene. This was made possible by the construction of a new university hospital. The Surgical Clinic of the university hospital of Halle was opened 100 years ago. Its founder, Richard Volkmann, had adopted and carried on Lister's methods since 1867, thus establishing antisepsis in Germany. All knowledge of hospital hygiene available at that time had been taken into account in constructing the building of the Clinic. Due to the advances in surgery made over the last 30 years, the building eventually housed seven special surgical departments as well as the department of anaesthesia. This resulted in overcrowded wards and high patient frequency. Unfortunately another consequence was also an increase in infections.

We have been performing open cardiac surgery since 1962. For checking the standards of hygiene, which was first done sporadically and later on sytematically, we put up sedimentation plates in the operating theatre and in the wards. Smears were taken from the patients before, during, and after operation. The instruments and drains used for the same patients as well as the suture material removed from them were examined for bacterial invasion. The bacteriological investigations, more than 3000 of which were carried out in cooperation with the Institute of Microbiology, also included water pipes, towels, and staff uniforms, as well as hand prints of staff members. Pathogenic germs were found above all on the hands and clothes of staff members when the protective clothing was worn for more than 2 days. In the operative theatre predominantly instruments which had been exposed for a longer time were invaded. Samples taken from the Priming-volume of the heart-lung machine before and after bypass always proved to be sterile. In two instances conserved blood was infected. In most cases the mode of infection could not be proved, in some only assumed. After these investigations educational steps toward better hygiene were taken. Undoubtedly there are more factors that could be considered regarding infection; a routine programme, however, is restricted to a certain extent. In order to determine the rate of infection, we evaluated the findings of 499 patients with cardiac surgery. Among these, 62 had infections with serious clinical consequences (12.5%); seven patients died of septic complications, in six of these the sepsis was due to mediastinitis after primary healing.

After the Department of Cardiac and Thoracic Surgery had moved to its new premises in autumn 1979, all disturbances in wound healing were recorded. So far, 170 patients have been operated upon, the infection rate being 3%. In three cases, we observed seroma formation, twice mediastinitis occurred due to *Staphylococcus aureus* and *Klebsiella* (these two cases occurred on the same day). There has not been any fatality caused by infection.

*Chirurgische Klinik und Poliklinik der Martin-Luther-Universität Halle-Wittenberg, Halle-Wittenberg, GDR

In the new hospital the patient wards are in special buildings separated by a tract containing the operating theatres, the intensive care unit, and most of the functional rooms.

In the old hospital building we carried out a total of 68 investigations. Of 340 blood plates set up in the operating theatre, 34 remained sterile, while 273 plates were covered with apathogenic germs with more than five colonies after 48 h aerobic cultivation. Thirty-three plates showed populations of pathogenic germs, the number of colonies ranging from 4 to 24.

In the new hospital building our microbiologists performed 111 investigations with a total of 333 blood plates. Of these, 76 blood plates did not show any growth, 245 plates had populations of one or two colonies, and nine plates had three colonies. In one case the number of colonies amounted to 41, among them two colonies of *Staphylococci*. Both patients had infections. The cause of the severe contamination was found to be a filter improperly installed in the air-conditioning system.

How to explain this drastic decrease in infection to one-quarter of that in the old hospital building?

As far as prophylaxis with antiobiotics is concerned, we may say that we have been using a constant scheme since 1976. This year, we reduced the administration of antibiotics. Since that time, patients have been receiving a combination of two antibiotics only on 2 days, or on 3 days in the case of foreign-body implantation. So far, we have not been able to prove on our patients that this has influence on the infection rate. We got the impression that there have been fewer late infections.

The conditions regarding the staff of the wards have remained unchanged, since doctors, nurses, and cleaning personnel have all moved over from the old hospital building. The anaesthetists are also the same. The patients come from the same institutions of pre-treatment as before. There have not been any changes in methods of hand disinfection, surgical techniques, machine fillings, suture material, disinfectants, and laundry.

More favourable conditions prevail in the accommodation of patients. The wards for cardiac and thoracic patients were separated. Changes were also introduced in the operating theatres with closed adjoining rooms.

Linen and instruments are now packed up according to a set system which I consider to be an essential factor. All nurses who come from different hospitals have to submit to a strict uniform regime of hygiene introduced by the senior nurse. The building conception enables us to practise a strict air-lock system. Changes have also been introduced with regard to skin disinfection, the formerly used iodine spirit having been replaced by 0.2% peracetic adic.

The greatest advantage in the new building, however, seems to be the air-conditioning system in the operating theatres and in the intensive care unit. We believe that the continuous replacement of the germ-infected air has been contributing substantially to the decrease in infection.

Summarizing we may state that the number of infections has been reduced by three-fourths since we moved into the new hospital premises. We hold that this is in the first place due to the new operating tract. The rigorous air-lock system compels all members of the staff to an antiseptic mode of behaviour. It is, however, mainly the air-conditioning system and the consequent reduction in the number of germs and dust that have brought about the improvement in our situation. This is also supported by a phenomenon observed in patients operated on for a lung disease.

These primarily not aseptic patients revealed an approximately constant rate of infection in both hospital buildings. The major task, however, remains constantly to encourage all staff members to keep to a strict regime of anti- and asepsis.

Penetrability of Four Cephalosporins Into Skeletal Muscle and Subcutaneous Fat of the Ischaemic Leg

R. C. Kester, C. H. Ramsden, and B. R. Bullen*

Introduction

The use of the cephalosporin antibiotics in the management of infection has increased greatly because of their safety and broad spectrum of bactericidal activity. The use of prophylactic antibiotic cover in peripheral vascular surgery is now commonplace either to prevent postoperative infection in an amputation stump where natural resistance is necessarily reduced or to prevent postimplantation infection of a prosthetic vascular graft – a most serious complication which threatens both life and limb. This study has investigated the tissue concentrations of four cephalosporin antibiotics achieved in the relatively ischaemic lower limbs of such patients.

Patients and Methods

Patients

One hundred and three patients aged from 40 to 88 years underwent either arterial reconstruction (44 cases) or amputation (59 cases) either above or below the knee for ischaemia of the lower limb due to occlusive arterial disease.

Dosage Regimens

Cephazolin: 1 g intramuscularly (im) with premedication (approximately 1 h preoperation)
1 g intravenously (iv) with induction of anaesthesia

Cefuroxime: 0.75 g im with premedication
1.5 g iv with induction of anaesthesia

Cefamandole
Cephradine: either (Group I)
1 g im with premedication
+ 1 g iv with induction of anaesthesia
or (Group II)
2 g iv with induction of anaesthesia.

*University Department of Surgery, St. James' University Hospital, Leeds, Great Britain

Samples Taken

Ten ml of blood were taken from a peripheral vein either at the time of division of the limb's blood supply in amputation cases or immediately prior to the application of occluding clamps in reconstruction cases. Specimens of approximately 2 g of subcutaneous fat were taken from the groin wounds of patients undergoing arterial reconstruction. Specimens of 2 g each of subcutaneous fat and skeletal muscle were taken from the amputated limbs proximally at the level of section and distally from the level of the Achilles tendon after above-knee amputation or from the sole of the foot after below-knee amputation. These samples were taken without delay to the laboratory where tissue samples and spun serum were then stored at -20°C for later batch assay of cephalosporin concentration.

Cephalosporin Assay

Assays were carried out by an agar plate diffusion technique previously described by Kester et al. (5). The tissues were homogenised in phosphate buffer pH 7.0 and the sera diluted 1 in 15 in pooled human serum prior to assay. Appropriate reference standards were prepared using cephalosporins supplied by the manufacturers and the assay organism used was *Bacillus subtilis*.

Results

Time Intervals between Dosage and Sampling

The mean time elapsed for each group of patients is shown in Table 1.

Serum Concentrations

The serum concentrations at the time of operation were well in excess of the minimum inhibitory concentrations (MIC) for the majority of commonly encountered gram-positive and gram-negative organisms (taken as 8 µg/ml) in all cases except some of those in group I of the patients receiving cephradine (Tables 2 and 3).

Tissue Concentrations

1. Muscle

a) *Proximal muscle* concentrations (Table 2) exceeded 8 µg/g in all patients who received cefuroxime and the single iv doses of cephradine and cefamandole, five out of eight patients given cephazolin and eight out of ten patients given cefamandole in divided doses.
b) *Distal muscle* concentrations (Table 2) exceeded 8 µg/g in eight of ten patients given cefuroxime, seven of 11 given cephradine in divided doses compared to eight of ten given a single large iv dose, and six of ten given cefamandole in divided doses compared to eight of ten given a single large iv dose.

2. Fat

a) *Proximal fat antibiotic concentrations* (Tables 2 and 3) in the subcutaneous fat of the groin wounds of patients undergoing reconstructive surgery exceeded 8 µg/g in nine of ten patients given cefuroxime, seven of nine patients given cephazolin, and eight of ten given a single large iv dose of cephradine compared to only four of 15 patients given cephradine in divided doses. Tissue concentrations in the subcutaneous fat at the level of amputation exceeded 8 µg/g in all ten patients given cefuroxime, six of eight given cephazolin, eight of ten given a single large iv dose of cefamandole compared to only two of nine given cefamandole in divided doses, and seven of ten patients given cephradine as a single large iv dose.

b) *Distal fat concentrations* (Table 2) exceeded 8 µg/g in eight of ten patients given cefuroxime, eight of ten given cephradine as a single dose compared to one of three given divided doses, and five of ten given cefamandole as a single dose compared to four of ten given divided doses.

Wound Sepsis

The simple clinical criterion of an inflamed wound discharging infected material was taken. On this basis, seven of 59 amputation wounds (12%) became infected but there was only one wound infection out of the 44 cases (2%) which underwent arterial reconstruction. The overall sepsis rate was thus 8%.

Table 1. Time intervals (means and ranges) between administration of antibiotic and sampling of blood and tissues

Antibiotic	im to iv dose	iv dose to sampling
Cephazolin	96 (60-138)	60 (30-180)
Cefuroxime	90 (40-160)	42 (10- 70)
Cefamandole - Gp I	66 (30-110)	21 (10- 44)
- Gp II	-	21 (13- 30)
Cephradine - Gp II	-	39 (10-175)

Discussion

There is little published information regarding the concentrations of cephalosporin antibiotics occurring in the tissues as opposed to body fluids and in our interpretation of results we have assumed that a unit concentration in µg/g of tissue is equivalent to a unit concentration in µg/ml of body fluids in terms of antibacterial activity. From the work of Selwyn (6, 7), Williams and Geddes (8), Eykin et al. (2), Barry et al. (1), Gaya et al. (3), and Goto (4) it seems reasonable to assume also that a concentration of 8 µg/ml of the cephalosporins studied will exceed MIC of the majority of common pathogens likely to be of importance to the vascular surgeon. Serum concentrations of

Table 2. Serum and tissue concentrations: amputation cases (means and ranges)

Antibiotic	Serum (µg/ml)	Skeletal muscle (µg/g)		Subcutaneous fat (µg/g)	
		Proximal	Distal	Proximal	Distal
Cephazolin	96 (72-158)	14 (4-33)		12 (7-21)	
Cefuroxime	128 (60-287)	26 (12-59)	18 (2-45)	19 (0-31)	13 (2-40)
Cefamandole - Gp I	105 (38-201)	12 (7-20)	10 (2-24)	7 (4-13)	7 (1-15)
- Gp II	164 (84-285)	19 (12-35)	13 (2-22)	13 (6-22)	9 (2-23)
Cephradine - Gp I	68 (10-165)		13 (2-22)		6 (1-8)
- Gp II	119 (49-285)	22 (12-60)	14 (0.5-26)	14 (3-30)	13 (2-21)

Table 3. Serum and tissue concentrations: reconstruction cases (means and ranges)

Antibiotic	Serum (µg/ml)	Subcutaneous fat (µg/g)
Cephazolin	89 (49-135)	13 (6-26)
Cefuroxime	87 (52-210)	15 (5-22)
Cephradine - Gp I	55 (4-205)	5 (1-18)
- Gp II	71 (12-122)	11 (4-21)

all four cephalosporins at the time of operation exceeded this value in all cases except two – both in group I of those given cephradine.

Prosthetic vascular grafts commonly traverse the subcutaneous fat of the groin. Antibiotic concentrations in this fat were adequate for antibacterial prophylaxis in most patients given cefuroxime, cephazolin, or the single large iv dose of cephradine but in only four of 15 patients given cephradine in divided doses. This is, perhaps, not surprising since cephradine is one of the least fat-soluble cephalosporins and is therefore relatively poorly absorbed when given by the intramuscular route.

Tissue concentrations at the level of section of amputated limbs were again adequate for prophylaxis in the majority of cases, the principal exception being cephradine which was only adequate in the subcutaneous fat of four cases out of the 15 who received the drug in divided doses. When given as a single 2 g iv bolus, however, cephradine was adequate in 80% of cases.

Tissue concentrations in the distal parts of amputated limbs are probably not relevant to antibacterial prophylaxis but are of interest when one is considering treating soft tissue infections in critically ischaemic areas. Despite this critical reduction in perfusion it was somewhat surprising to find that concentrations of the cephalosporins in this distal muscle exceeded 8 µg/g in 37 of 51 amputated limbs. Similarly subcutaneous fat levels were greater than 8 µg/g in 26 of 43 samples from these distal ischeamic areas.

Conclusions

These findings confirm that the cephalosporins we have studied may have a place in the prophylaxis against infection of patients undergoing vascular surgery. Furthermore, the concentrations achieved in the critically ischaemic distal areas of amputated limbs suggest that these antibiotics may also be of use in the treatment of soft tissue infections in these sites.

Summary

Concentrations of cephradine, cephazolin, cefamandole, and cefuroxime were measured in peripheral blood and in skeletal muscle and subcutaneous fat samples taken from 103 patients undergoing either reconstructive arterial surgery or amputation of the leg for severe ischaemia. Tissue concentrations of cephalosporins in both groups of patients were adequate for antibacterial prophylaxis in the majority of cases even in critically ischaemic tissues. Based on these findings we suggest that any of these cephalosporins may be of value for antibacterial prophylaxis in patients undergoing vascular surgery.

References

1. Barry AL, Thornsberry C, Jones RN, Fuchs PC, Gaven TL, Gerlach EH (1977) Cefuroxime, an in vitro comparison with six other cephalosporins. Proc R Soc Med [Suppl 9] 70:63-71
2. Eykin S, Jenkins C, King A, Phillips I (1976) Antibacterial activity of cefuroxime, a new cephalosporin antibiotic, compared to that of cephaloridine, cephalothin, and cefamandole. Antimicrob Agents Chemother 9:690-695
3. Gaya H, Brown EM, Friedman P, Cox SE (1977) Comparative in vitro activity of cefuroxime and its interactions with aminoglycoside antibiotics. Proc R Soc Med [Suppl 9] 70:51-55
4. Goto S (1977) The in vitro and in vivo antibacterial activity of cefuroxime. Proc R Soc Med [Suppl 9] 70:56-62
5. Kester RC, Ramsden CH, Matharu SS (1979) The penetrability of cephazolin into the subcutaneous fat and skeletal muscle of ischaemic lower limbs with atherosclerotic disease. Curr Med Res Opinion 6:44-49
6. Selwyn S (1973) Advertising of antibiotics. Br Med J 2:239-240
7. Selwyn S (1976) Rational choice of penicillins and cephalosporins based on parallel in vitro and in vivo tests. Lancet 2:616-618
8. Williams JD, Geddes AM (1973) Advertising antibiotics. Br Med J 2:613

Risk of Postoperative Infections in Cardiovascular Surgery

P. Kalmar, R. Akrami, H.-J. Krebber, and G. Rodewald*

Postoperative infections are dangerous and in minor cases at least troublesome complications of surgical procedures. While infections are accepted as a biological phenomenon when people who up to that point were healthy fall ill, one tends to look for a culprit when postoperative infections occur. This psychological problem is the reason why unbiased discussions or comparative studies are so difficult when dealing with surgical infections. The high probability of infections among patients undergoing open heart surgery was the reason for this critical analysis of infectious complications started many years ago (1, 3, 9).

In order to allow comparisons we needed a clear definition. This is as described earlier: infections are present when wounds heal per secundam or in seromas and hematomas, further in cases with fever above 38.5°C and leucocytosis above 13000, when at least once a bacteriological culture was positive. Using this rather broad definition, an infection during hospital stay may be without any influence to the patient's general state or to the duration of hospitalisation (11).

Table 1 depicts incidence and mortality of postoperative infections during several periods since 1963. Until 1969, all data were gained by retrospective investigation of patient's records. Since then all relevant data are prospectively processed as there are the clinical picture, wound healing, and the following bacteriological cultures: a preoperative throat swab, a wound swab (if healing per secundam), a selective aspiration of tracheal secretion during extubation, all tips of intravascular catheters and drainage tubes, blood cultures, and specimens of urine, puncture fluid etc. (5). Between 1963 and 1965, the incidence of infections was 27.34% with a mortality of approx. 2.4%. From 1969 to 1972, the incidence was 11%; nine patients died of these complications; this corresponds to a mortality of 0.74%. Between 1973 and 1975, due to several changes and measures against hospital infections, a reduction of the incidence of infections down to 4.6% with a mortality of 0.25% was achieved. As it is to be seen, there is an unchanged incidence with 4.6% and a similar mortality during the last period from 1976 to 1979.

Table 2 shows the reduction in frequency of hospital infections due to the different measures taken such as surface disinfection, construction of sluices for personnel, patients, and supply, and intensification of all kinds of minor disinfecting procedures like hands etc. (6, 7, 10, 12). In this presentation we confine ourselves to the analysis of results since 1973, as since that time the regimen of surgical treatment and postoperative care has changed only insignificantly.

*Universitätskliniken, Abt. für Herz- und Gefäßchirurgie und experimentelle Kardiologie, D-2000 Hamburg-Eppendorf

Table 1. Incidence of infection and mortality during various periods since 1963

Years	Operated N (100%)	N infections (%)	N death due to infection (%)
1963-1965	377	103 (27.3)	9 (2.4)
1969-1972	1213	134 (11)	9 (0.74)
1973-1975	1210	56 (4.6)	3 (0.25)
1976-1979	2115	98 (4.6)	7 (0.33)

Table 2. Effect of measures against hospitalism in frequency and mortality of postoperative infectious complication in cardiovascular surgery

Measure	Year	Infections	
		Frequency %	Mortality %
None	1963	37.1	2.7
Room surface disinfection	1964/5	17.8	2.1
Sluice system for operating theatre Weekly general disinfection of OP theatre, anesthesia rooms, and recovery rooms Electrical door opener connected with hand disinfection container Peri- and postoperative prophylaxis with antibiotics	1969/70	13.7	1.3
Improving of surface disinfection with great reduction of airborne organism Hand disinfection container at each bed in recovery room, ICU and regular ward Prophylaxis with antimycotics	1971/72	8.9	0.3
Sluice system for ICU	1973/75	4.6	0.25
No further changes	1976/79	4.6	0.33

Table 3 gives a synopsis over the group of patients operated upon and analysed between 1973 and 1979. It is evident that out of 735 patients undergoing valve replacement procedures, 63, that is 8.6%, became infected. The incidence of postoperative infections was 5.5% among the group of patients with coronary artery disease. It is remarkable that among the mainly younger patients with congenital heart disease operated upon with extracorporeal circulation the incidence of infections was only 1.6%. Among the remaining groups operated upon without heart-lung machine, the incidence was between 2.3% and 4% except in patients with pacemakers where the incidence of this complication was 0.5%. Nine patients with valve disease and one patient out of 730 following vascular surgery died of infectious complications. This all totals to ten patients out of 3325 corresponding to an incidence of 0.33%.

Table 3. Distribution of patients operated upon between 1973 and 1979 according to operative diagnosis and infectious complications

Diagnosis	N	Infection N (%)	Death due to infection N (%)
Acquired valve disease	735	63 (8.6)	9 (1.2)
Coronary heart disease	614	34 (5.5)	0
Congenital lesions (with ECC)	381	6 (1.6)	0
Congenital lesions (without ECC)	227	10 (4.4)	0
Others, mainly lung, heart, or great vessel disease (without ECC)	443	10 (2.3)	0
Vascular disease	730	30 (4.1)	1 (0.1)
Pacemaker	195	1 (0.5)	0
Total	3325	154 (4.6)	10 (0.3)

Table 4 shows the kinds and origins of postoperative infections in 154 patients between 1973 and 1979. In 53 cases wound infections, in 45 cases infections of the urinary tract, in 21 cases broncho-pulmonary infections were noted. Bacteraemia or septicemia were present in 23 patients, while in 12 patients other infectious complications were noted. Detection of the origin and source of the infection was performed either by bacteriological surrounding analyses and examination of the patient himself or concluded from the clinical course. We found that in 26% of the patients the infection was probably due to contamination during surgery, and in 41% to contamination or cross infection during intensive care. Finally we could prove the presence of autoinfection in 33% of the cases.

It became evident that primarily wound infections go mainly back to the time of surgery while secondary infections are acquired during intensive care. It further became evident that urinary tract infections and broncho-pulmonary infections are either originated in the intensive care unit or are so-called autoinfections, while on the other hand more than half of the cases with bacteraemia or sepsis go back to the operating theatre. Comparative studies of the rate of wound infections revealed that there is no correlation with the duration of surgery or the surgeons who performed the procedures (4, 8). In all these years, the bacteriological specimens of the perfusate of the pump taken after surgery have been sterile. From that one could draw the conclusion that the higher suction rate during valve procedures compared to coronary artery procedures is of no importance concerning the higher infection rate among the first group.

An analysis of the distribution of infections according to the duration of the aortic cross-clamping time of the patients operated between 1975 and 1980 for valve replacement or coronary bypass procedures revealed the following results.

Table 4. Source and kind of infectious complications between 1973 and 1979

Kind of infection	N[a]	Source of germs			Detection of the origin of the infection by	
		OR	ICU	Patient	Bact. culture	Clinically
Primary wound infection	35[b]	21	6	8	22	13
Secondary wound infection	18[b]	2	11	5	6	12
Urinary tract infection	45	3	31	11	15	30
Broncho-pulmonary infection	21	1	7	13	13	8
Bacteraemia, sepsis	23	10	6	7	13	10
Others	12	3	2	7	7	5
Total	154	40	63	51	76	78

[a] 154 patients with infectious complications out of 3325 patients operated upon (4.6%)

[b] The sternum was involved in 11 patients out of 53 with wound infection

Table 5 shows that out of the 1297 patients operated on during this period, in 167 – that is 12.9% of the group – the aorta was cross-clamped for more than 120 minutes. In 1130 patients (87.1%), the aortic cross-clamping time was less than 120 minutes (2).

Table 5. Duration of aortic cross-clamping time in 1297 patients with acquired heart disease

	N (%)
Cross-clamping time >120 mins.	167 (12.9)
Cross-clamping time <120 mins.	1130 (87.1)
Total	1297 (100)

Table 6 shows that in the whole group of 1297 patients, 42, that is 3.2%, died during the first 30 days postoperatively. In eight of them, the cause of death was an infectious complication. In each of the groups, the one with the aorta cross-clamped for more and the one with cross-clamping of less than 120 minutes, four patients died. That means that the postoperative infection as leading cause of death is ten times as often in the group with the aorta cross-clamped for more than 2 h than in the group with less. Statistical calculations proved the result to be significant. In each of the two groups, two patients died of hospital infections *and* autogenous infections.

Table 6. Incidence of lethal complications in relation to duration of the aortic cross-clamping time in patients with valve replacement and/or coronary surgery

Duration of aortic cross-clamping		Early mortality	
		Total N (%)	Due to infection N (%)
≥120 minutes	(N = 167)	12 (7.2)	4 (3.33)
<120 minutes	(N = 1130)	30 (2.7)	4 (0.35)
Total	(N = 1297)	42 (3.2)	8 (0.5)

Conclusions

1. The prospective collection and continuous analysis of all data on infectious complications since 1969 revealed that with introduction of suitable antiseptic measures and their strict control the incidence of infectious complications following cardiovascular procedures decreased significantly.
2. Postoperative infections occurred most often in patients following valve replacement. The specific features of this group are: long history of the disease, repeated hospital admissions, and secondary organ damage. Patients with coronary artery disease, in whom the duration of surgery was much longer, had a significantly lower incidence of postoperative infections and no mortality due to infectious complications. While operative technique and duration of the surgical procedure did not influence the incidence of postoperative infections, there was a correlation between aortic cross-clamping time and the incidence of infections noted.
3. The decrease of resistance against infections in this group, due either to the main disease or to the kind of treatment, results in a lower resistance threshold against germs, increasing the risk of infections. The origin of the infection may be either within the patient himself or in his surroundings. That means that measures against hospitalism must aim at the decrease of the number of germs in the unit where patients are treated by a great number of equally important repeated antiseptic procedures in order to avoid the infectious complications even in the face of reduced resistance against germs.

Summary

In order to assess the risk of infections following cardiovascular procedures, 4552 patients were studied for bacteriological contamination or clinical signs of infection. Classified as infections were: positive bacteriological findings of cultures of blood, urine, or wound secretion, as well as positive findings from other material when clinical signs of infections were present (leucocytosis, temperature above 38.5°C for more than 3 days, or wound inflammation). In addition, regular regional examinations of the operating room and the intensive care unit were performed. Frequent controls of air contamination revealed optimal antiseptic conditions in the OR.

In 26% of the patients, the infection originated in the OR probably due to contamination during surgery, in 41% the source was located in the ICU, while so-called autoinfections were present in 33% of the cases. When listing the infections in regard to diagnosis, one finds that the group operated upon because of valvular dysfunctions has the highest rate of infections with 8.6%, followed by the group of coronary patients with 5.5%, while the rate of infection is only 1.6% in patients with congenital heart disease operated upon with extracorporeal circulation.

Various measures taken in construction and organization such as lock chambers for personnel entering the OR or ICU, special hand and surface (room) disinfection, and prophylactic antibiotics, to mention only a few, led to a decrease of infection rate from 11% in 1969/1972 to 4.6% continuously since 1973. Lethal infections were encountered in 0.25% to 0.33% in comparison to 0.74% in 1969.

References

1. Benzer H, Rotter M (1979) Klinisch hygienische Probleme beim kardiochirurgischen Patienten. In: Klinische Hygiene und Intensivtherapie-Patient. Thieme, Stuttgart (INA, vol 18, p 40)
2. Bleese N, Darup J, Pokar H, Rödiger W, Rodewald G (1980) Causes of death in "complicated" open heart procedures. Thorac Cardiovasc Surg 28/1:35
3. Gradock PR, Yawata Y, von Santen L, Gilberstadt S, Yacob HS (1974) Acquired phagocyte dysfunction. N Engl J Med 20:1403
4. Jaballah N (1972) Wundheilungsstörungen nach Herzoperationen. Medical dissertation, University of Hamburg
5. Kalmar P (1973) Fremdkörperinfektion in der Herz- und Gefäßchirurgie. Med Mitt 47:325
6. Kalmar P, Meyer-Rohn J (1968) Erfahrungen mit einem neuen Händedesinfektionsmittel. Chirurg 39:231
7. Kalmar P, Rodewald G, Klosterhalfen H (1970) Raumplanung einer Intensivstation unter den Gesichtspunkten einer Organtransplantation. Med Mitt 44:141
8. Kalmar P, Horatz K, Rodewald G, Schassan HH, Schassek S (1976) Hospitalismus in der chirurgischen Intensivpflege. Langenbecks Arch Klin Chir [Suppl] 342:383
9. Lackner F (1975) Untersuchungen von Parametern der zellulären und humoralen Abwehr gegen bakterielle Infektion während Herzoperationen mit der Herz-Lungen-Maschine. Acta Chir Austr [Suppl] 16
10. Rodewald G (1970) Intensivüberwachung nach Herzoperationen einschließlich Aufbau und Einrichtung einer Wachstation — Probleme in der cardio-chirurgischen Intensivpflege. Herzchirurgisches Symposium, Tegernsee, May 1970
11. Rodewald G, Sagebaum H, Matz K, Kalmar P, Pokar H (1970) Infektionen nach Eingriffen am Herzen und den großen Gefäßen. Thoraxchir Vask Chir 18:4
12. Rodewald G, Kalmar P, Polonius MJ, Schassan HH (1977) Infektionen in der Herz- und Gefäßchirurgie. In: Hygiene und Asepsis in der Chirurgie. Thieme, Stuttgart (INA, vol 7, p 34)

Indium[111] – Leukocyte Scintigraphy. A New Method in Diagnosis of Infected Vascular Prosthetic Grafts. Preliminary Results

M.H. Rövekamp, E.A. van Royen, J. Koning, and M.R. Hardeman*

Introduction

In vascular surgery, infection at the site of the reconstructed arteries is a serious complication with a high morbidity and mortality, particularly in cases in which synthetic arterial substitutes are used (8, 9, 13). Diagnosis is difficult, since symptoms are variable and no specific diagnostic test is available. The onset of symptoms is often gradual. Fever, leukocytosis, and elevated ESR can be the only signs (1).

In the early postoperative period disturbed wound healing can lead to the diagnosis, especially when an abscess is drained. In some patients, bleeding from a leaking anastomosis in case of a false aneurysm or a GI bleeding in case of a fistula, leads to the diagnosis of infection (1, 2). Other patients are septic. Occasionally thrombosis is the first complication of the infected graft (3). In the early postoperative period, the whole graft is always involved. Sometimes, in infections that occur in the late postoperative period, only a localized area can be affected. Investigations to prove infection prior to surgical exploration often fail.

Angiography can reveal a false aneurysm. Urograms can be of help in retroperitoneal infections, when ureteral compression occurs. Ultrasonography and computed tomography are able to visualize localized fluid collections and aneurysms (4, 7, 10, 18). Recently some reports were published of computed tomography showing air in the aortic wall in case of an infected aortic-bifurcation graft (4, 5). Endoscopic examinations may reveal bowel wall defects and visible prosthetic grafts, in case of an aorto-enteric fistula, especially in patients with aortic-bifurcation grafts. In many cases, however, the diagnosis can only be confirmed at operation.

We recently started to use the indium-111 labeled leukocyte scintigraphy to diagnose infections after arterial reconstruction. The use of indium-111 labeled autologous leukocytes in diagnosis of infections was first described by Thakur et al. (12, 14-17). We obtained good results with a modification of this technique in patients with intra-abdominal infections (6, 11). The underlying study was performed to evaluate the indium-111 leukocyte scintigraphy in the diagnosis of infected vascular prosthetic grafts.

*Department of Surgery, Academic Hospital, Binnengasthuis, Grimburgwal 10, 1012 GA Amsterdam, The Netherlands

Patients

Thirty scintigrams were performed after arterial reconstruction in 25 patients of the department of vascular surgery, Academic Hospital University of Amsterdam. The population consisted of 18 males and seven females, of ages ranging from 41 to 76 years, with a mean of 58.

The following operations were performed: an aortic-bifurcation graft in 19, an aortic-Y patch in four, and a bypass procedure in two patients. Twenty-six scintigrams were performed within 3 months after operation. Four scintigrams were performed in patients who underwent arterial reconstruction more than 1 year earlier. In these patients, infection of the graft was suspected on clinical grounds.

Method

The leukocytes were labeled as described elsewhere (11). Fifty ml of venous blood was taken from the patients, leukocytes were isolated and incubated with indium-111 oxine. The procedure lasted about 1 1/2 h. The final preparation consisted of a 2 to 3 ml cell suspension with 300 to 500 μCi radioactivity. Scintigrams (Fig. 1a) were performed on a gamma camera, 24 h after intravenous administration of the labeled cells. Anterior and lateral views were taken from each patient during a 10-minute period. Data were stored on an on-line computer. Leukocyte accumulation at the proximal aorta and the graft was quantified by choosing regions around the various structures, with aid of a joystick (Fig. 1b). The activity was normalized for dosage, time of scanning, and surface of the involved area, and expressed in counts/100 μCi/10 min/pixel.

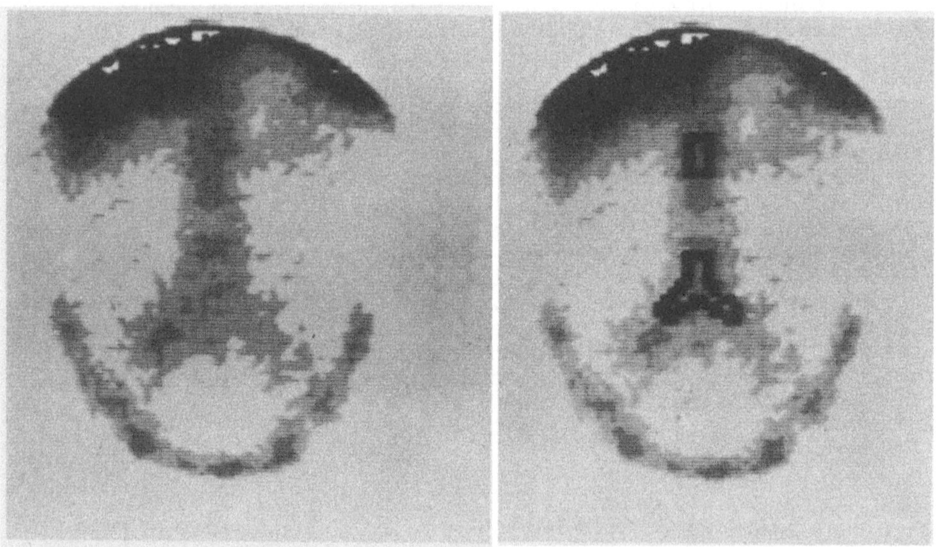

a b

Fig. 1. a Normal scan. b Regions around the proximal aorta and the graft

Results

All 30 scintigrams invariably showed high accumulations of activity in liver, spleen, vertebral bodies, and pelvic bones (Fig. 1a). Nineteen showed this normal distribution of activity, while 11 showed an abnormal activity as well. This abnormal distribution showed on seven of the 26 scintigrams performed within 3 months after operation.

A slight abnormal activity was seen on two of these scintigrams at the distal anastomosis in one and at the proximal anastomosis in the other patient. Marked abnormal activity was clearly demonstrated in the midline on the AP scintigram in another patient. On the lateral view, however, the accumulation was localized at the site of the median laparotomy and thus abnormal activity at the site of the graft excluded. This patient later developed a wound abscess. Two other scintigrams, performed in one patient, showed a marked abnormal activity at the site of the proximal anastomosis (case 1). The last two scintigrams showed an abnormal activity not related to the site of operation. An abnormal distribution was also observed on all four scintigrams performed in patients who had had their arterial reconstruction more than 1 year earlier.

The abnormal activity was observed at the proximal anastomosis in one (case 2) and at the distal anastomosis in three patients (case 3). In patients with an abnormal activity at the proximal anastomosis, this activity was quantified and compared with the quantified activity of the proximal aorta and the graft in scans with a normal distribution of activity.

Figure 2 shows that the activity over the graft is remarkably higher in these patients. In two patients the activity found over the proximal aorta was higher as well.

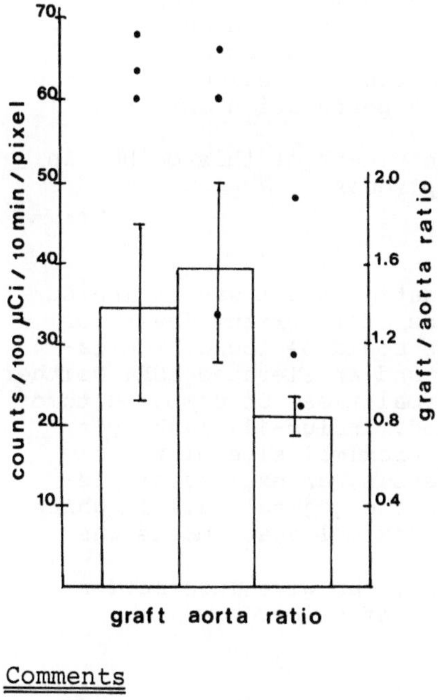

Fig. 2. Quantified activity in patients with a normal distribution and patients with abnormal activity at the proximal anastomosis of a bifurcation graft. . = values obtained in patients with the abnormal activity; ⊢·⊣ = represents the standard deviation

Comments

In all patients with a *normal distribution of activity*, clinical follow-up revealed that they were free of infection. The majority of these scintigrams were performed within 4 weeks after operation. Therefore it may be concluded that implantation of the graft itself and normal wound healing do not give rise to substantial accumulation of indium-111 labeled leukocytes, so that the correct diagnosis in case of infection is not hampered by these normal processes.

In the two patients with only a *slight abnormal activity*, repeated scintigrams after 2 weeks were normal. There were no clinical signs of infection in these patients. One patient with abnormal activity at the distal anastomotic site had a haematoma in the groin. The other patient, with the activity at the proximal anastomosis, probably had a haematoma as well. A mild leukocyte infiltration at the site of the haematoma without infection is likely in these patients. In this last patient, the graft/aorta ratio (Fig. 2) was within the normal range. In the future, when more computer analysis data become available, it may be possible to discriminate more precisely between normal activity, activity due to haematoma, and activity due to infection. In all patients with a *marked abnormal activity* on the scintigrams, infection was proved at operation or autopsy.

The possibility of diagnosing an infection with indium-111 leukocyte scintigraphy in the early postoperative period is illustrated by the following case history:

Case 1

A 66-year-old male patient in whom an aortic-bifurcation graft was implanted. In the first week after operation, he developed an abscess at the site of a suction drain. The scintigram, peformed 3 weeks after operation, showed a marked abnormal activity at the proximal anastomosis. At that time, the patient was without any clinical sign of infection. He was discharged on the 30th postoperative day. Six weeks after operation, he was readmitted with symptoms of a G-I bleeding. Angiograms and a barium enema did not reveal any abnormality. A repeated scintigram (Fig. 3b) showed the same marked activity with an extension into the left abdomen. Before further diagnostic measures could be taken, the patient died of exsanguination. Autopsy revealed a complete disruption of the proximal anastomosis with a perforation into the sigmoid colon.

The next case history illustrates the usefulness of this method in localizing the source of recurrent septic episodes.

Case 2

A 64-year-old male patient. An aortic-bifurcation graft was implanted 2 1/2 years earlier. He suffered from periods of recurrent fever for more than 1 year for which no definite cause could be found. The laboratory tests revealed a mild leukocytosis and an elevated ESR. Neither angiography nor ultrasonography showed abnormalities. On computed tomograms a retroperitoneal abscess was suggested. Indium-111 leukocyte scintigrams showed a marked activity at the proximal site of the bifurcation graft. After a period of severe sepsis, an exploratory laparotomy was performed. The graft had eroded the jejunal wall in which a defect of 2 1/2 cm diameter existed. The proximal anastomosis was unaffected. The graft was removed.

Sometimes indium-111 leukocyte scintigraphy can give information concerning the extension of an already known infection.

Case 3

A 58-year-old male patient with an aortic-bifurcation graft implanted 1 year earlier, was admitted with an abscess in the right groin. Scintigrams (Fig. 3a) showed a marked accumulation of activity at the site of the abscess, but an extension of activity into the right iliac region was visualized as well. At a consecutive exploratory laparotomy a large retroperitoneal abscess was found.

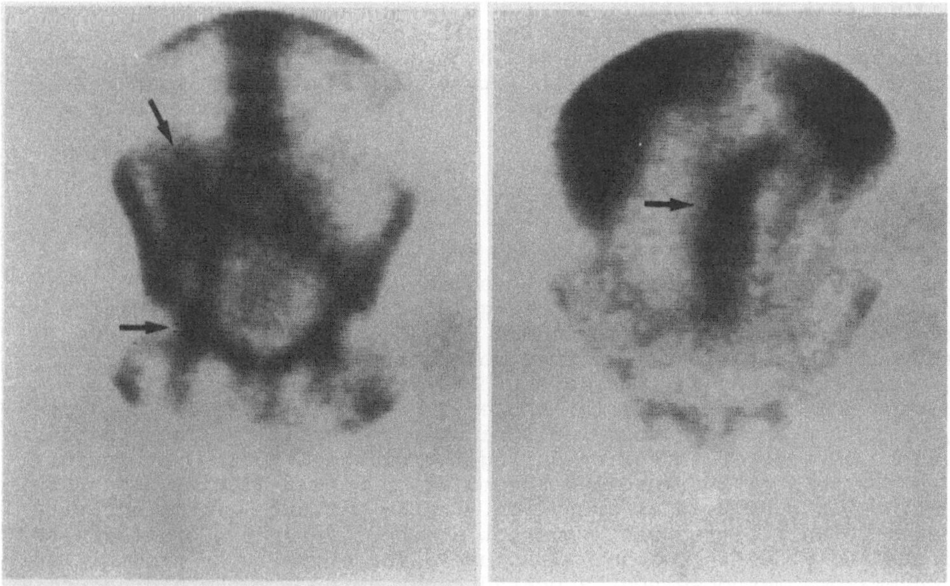

a b

Fig. 3. a Scintigram of a 58-year-old male patient 1 1/2 years after implantation of an aortic-bifurcation graft. Presenting with a groin abscess and a large retroperitoneal abscess (case 3). b Scintigram of a 66-year-old male patient with an infected aortic-bifurcation graft, 6 weeks after operation, due to a perforation into the sigmoid colon (case 1)

Discussion

In the diagnosis of infected arterial grafts, very little help can be expected of the usual techniques. Angiography, urography, and sonography only give indirect information concerning complications (false aneurysm, ureteral compression etc.). Computed tomography can show air in the aortic wall suggesting infection. Labeled leukocytes concentrate at the site of infection. Therefore, the indium-111 leukocyte scintigraphy may offer a specific diagnostic test. It can be performed in the very early postoperative period, because of its relative noninvasive nature, with only minor discomfort for the patient. It can prove infection before complications like sepsis and haemorrhage occur, so that treatment is possible in an earlier stage when the patient is still in a good clinical condition. This may improve the results of the treatment of these critically ill patients who still have a high morbidity and mortality.

Conclusion

These results obtained with indium-111 leukocyte scintigraphy show that this test is a reliable procedure in diagnosing infections after reconstructive arterial surgery. Especially its noninvasive nature, the ease of administration, and the high accuracy make it a clinical useful test. Moreover, the possibility of earlier diagnosis in these high-risk patients is encouraging.

Summary

Scintigraphy of autologous leukocytes labeled with indium-111 oxine was used as a new test for diagnosing infections of vascular grafts. Thirty scintigrams were performed in 25 patients after arterial reconstruction. Operations performed were aortic-bifurcation grafts in 19, aortic-Y patches in four, and bypass procedures in two patients.

Eleven scans (nine patients) showed abnormal accumulation of activity. Nineteen showed a normal distribution of activity. These patients proved to be free of infection during the clinical follow-up. In four patients with a marked abnormal accumulation at the site of the graft, infection was confirmed at operation. In one patient, a high activity was seen in an infected wound but not at the site of the graft. In two patients, only a slight abnormal accumulation of activity probably due to a haematoma was observed. Repeated scans after 2 weeks did not show residual abnormal activity. In two other patients, the site of abnormal activity was not related to the site of operation. In case of infection a marked accumulation of activity was observed.

In uncomplicated cases implantation of a graft and wound healing did not give rise to substantial accumulation of activity. Some activity can be seen due to haematomas; repeated scans are then necessary. The test is less invasive than angiography and causes only minor discomfort for the patient.

References

1. Becker RM, Blundell PE (1976) Infected aortic bifurcation grafts; experience with fourteen patients. Surgery 80:544-549
2. Boyd DP (1976) Infected aortic grafts and aortic fistulas. Surg Clin North Am 56:743-747
3. Goldstone J, Moore WS (1974) Infection in vascular prostheses; clinical manifestations and surgical management. Am J Surg 128:225-233
4. Haaga JR, Alfidi RJ, Havrilla TR, Cooperman AM, Seidelmann FE, Reich NE, Weinstein AJ, Meaney TF (1977) CT detection and aspiration of abdominal abscesses. AJR 128:465-474
5. Haaga JR, Baldwin GN, Reich NE, Beven E, Kramer A, Weinstein A, Havrilla TR, Seidelmann FE, Namba AH, Parrish CM (1978) CT detection of infected synthetic grafts; preliminary report of a new sign. AJR 131:317-320
6. Hardeman MR, Roos D (to be published) In vitro granulocyte chemotactic assay; a valuable predictor for granulocyte in vivo function.
7. Hill BA, Yamaguchi K, Flynn JJ, Miller DR (1975) Diagnostic sonography in general surgery. Arch Surg 110:1089-1094
8. Jamieson GG, DeWeese JA, Rob CG (1975) Infected arterial grafts. Ann Surg 182: 850-852

9. Liekweg WG Jr, Greenfield LJ (1977) Vascular prosthetic infections; collected experience and results of treatment. Surgery 81:335-342
10. Pripstein S, Cavoto FV, Gerritsen RW (1979) Spontaneous mycotic aneurysm of the abdominal aorta; case report. J Comput Assist Tomogr 3:681-683
11. Rövekamp MH, Hardeman MR, van der Schoot JB, Belfer AJ (1981) Indium 111 labeled leukocyte scintigraphy in the diagnosis of inflammatory disease; first results. Br J Surg 68:150-153
12. Segal AW, Arnot RN, Thakur ML, Lavender JP (1976) Indium-111 labeled leucocytes for localization of abscesses. Lancet 2:1056-1058
13. Szilagyi DE, Smith RF, Elliott JP, Vrandecic MP (1972) Infection in arterial reconstruction with synthetic grafts. Ann Surg 176:321-333
14. Thakur ML, Coleman FE, Mayhall CG, Welch MJ Jr (1976) Preparation and evaluation of indium-111 labeled leukocytes as an abscess imaging agents in dogs. Radiology 119:731-732
15. Thakur ML, Coleman RE, Welch MJ (1977) Indium-111 labeled leukocytes for the localization of abscesses; preparation, analysis, tissue distribution, and comparison with Gallium-67 citrate in dogs. J Lab Clin Med 89:217-228
16. Thakur ML, Lavender JP, Arnot RN, Silvester DJ, Segal AW (1977) Indium-111 labeled autologous leukocytes in man. J Nucl Med 18:1014-1021
17. Thakur ML, Segal AW, Louis L, Welch MJ, Hopkins J, Peters TJ (1977) Indium-111 labeled cellular blood components; mechanism of labeling and intracellular location in human neutrophils. J Nucl Med 18:1022-1026
18. Wheeler WE, Beachley MC, Ranniger K (1976) Angiography and ultrasonography; a comparative study of abdominal aortic aneurysms. AJR 126:95-100

Serratia Marcescens Septicemia from Pressure Monitoring Chambers in Cardiovascular Operations

J. Fraile, T. Moreno, N. G. de Vega, and G. Rábago*

During March 1977, 24 consecutive patients operated on with extracorporeal circulation were exposed to a contamination via the arterial pressure monitoring chamber.

In 22 patients operated upon for valvular disease, we performed one or two prosthetic valve replacements on the left side; in the other two patients, total correction of congenital defects was done.

The bacteriological agent was Serratia Marcescens, XXVI nonpigmented with typical antibiotic sensitivity.

Blood cultures were positive in ten patients.

Hospital mortality (less than 30 days) was 37%. The nine patients died between the 5th and the 26th day of the postoperative course because of acute sepsis and severe hemodynamic impairment.

When the infection was detected, treatment with carbenicillin associated with amikacin was started.

In those patients who died, no prosthetic detachment was either suspected or confirmed.

In this paper, we review 1) the uneffectiveness of benzalkonium chloride in the sterilization of pressure chambers; 2) methods of bacteriological identification; 3) clinical response to the antibiotic treatment; 4) cause of death; 5) long-term follow-up of the surviving patients.

*Fundación Jiménez Díaz, Madrid, Spain

Factors Influencing Infection Rate of Indewelling Intravascular and Thoracic Catheters Following Cardiac Surgery

A. Barankay, I. Bartek, and A. Arvay*

In spite of aseptic surgical techniques and use of antibiotics, infection may develop in the postoperative period of cardiac operations (1-3, 6-8). To decrease the number of infections, all prophylactic hygienic measures should be taken and all factors known to initiate an infection should be excluded (4, 5, 8).

In our 1979 series of 662 cardiac operations (Table 1), the rate of fatal infections was 0.54%. In this series of patients Keflin (Lilly) was used as a prophylactic antibiotic agent for 48 h during and after operations.

Table 1. Cardiac operations and fatal infections

Type of surgery	No. operations	No. of fatal infections
Open heart	388	3
Closed heart	122	0
Pacemaker impl.	152	0
Total	662 (100%)	3 (0.45%)

The fatal infection rate of 0.45%, however, is somewhat higher than reported by Rodewald et al. who has found a fatal infection rate of 0.25% in a large series of cardiac and vascular surgical operations (8).

Searching for the possible sources of infection, we took samples regularly for bacteriological investigations from indwelling catheters postoperatively. Of the 339 samples, 12 were found infected (Table 2). Arterial catheters were less frequently infected than the venous ones, in spite of the fact that antibiotics were given through venous catheters. It should be mentioned, however, that following Freeman's advice all catheters were removed as early as possible.

The types of microorganisms isolated from removed catheter tips were: *Streptococci* (1), *Pseudomonas aeruginosa* (2), *Klebsiella* (1), *Proteus* (3), and the so-called opportunistic microorganisms such as *Propioni*, *Micrococcus*, and *Citrobacter* (5). These are generally assumed apathogenic and can be isolated from the air (7). In addition, the particle number in the air sampled in the operating theatres were found higher than allowed. After new filters had been mounted to the ceilings of operating theatres, the bacteriological investigations were repeated.

*Hungarian Institute of Cardiology, Budapest, Hungary

Table 2. Infection rate of indwelling catheters

Type of catheter	No. sampled	Infection rate
Venous	130	4/130
Arterial	112	2/112
Left atrial	48	4/ 48
Thoracic	49	2/ 49
Total	339	12/339

Table 3 shows the effect of proper air filtration on infection rate of indwelling catheters. With proper air filtration the infection rate of indwelling catheters decreased from 3.5% to 1.8%. There was no fatal infection in this period. We think that the infection rate of removed intravascular and thoracic catheters – among others – may represent the efficiacy of all hygienic measures connected to surgery and postoperative care.

It is important to review periodically the infection rate at each hospital to discover and eliminate the possible sources of infection and to determine whether it is necessary to change the antimicrobal regimen too.

Table 3. Effect of proper air filtration on infection rate of indwelling catheters

	Without a new filter	With a new filter
Number sampled	339	109
No. of infected samples	12	2
Infection rate	12/339	2/109
Infection rate (%)	3.5	1.8

References

1. Amoury RA (1972) Infection following cardiopulmonary bypass. In: Norman JC (ed) Cardiac surgery. Appleton Century Crofts, New York, pp 55-68
2. Freeman R (1976) Microbiological aspects of open-heart surgery. In: Ionescu MI, Wooler GH (eds) Current techniques in extracorporeal circulation. Butterworth, London Boston, pp 369-380
3. Hornick RB (1977) Source of contamination in open-heart surgery. In: Duma RJ (ed) Infections of prosthetic heart valves and vascular grafts. University Park Press, Baltimore London Tokyo, pp 81-97
4. Kalmar P (1977) Organisatorische Probleme in der Hospitalismusbekämpfung. In: Eckert P, Rodewald G (eds) Hygiene und Asepsis in der Chirurgie. Thieme, Stuttgart, pp 9-17

5. Kluge RM (1974) Sources of contamination in open-heart surgery. JAMA 230: 1415-1419
6. Myerowitz PD, et al. (1977) Antibiotic prophylaxis for open-heart surgery. J Thorac Cardiovasc Surg 73:625-631
7. Norenberg RG, et al. (1976) Opportunistic endocarditis following open-heart surgery. Ann Thorac Surg 19:592-597
8. Rodewald G, et al. (1977) Infektion in der Herz- und Gefäßchirurgie. In: Eckert P, Rodewald G (eds) Hygiene und Asepsis in der Chirurgie. Thieme, Stuttgart, pp 34-41

The Blood-gas Analyzer and Disposable Pressure Monitoring Systems as Sources of Infection

J. Dankert, J. N. H. van der Heide, and A. Eijgelaar*

During a *bacteriological study* to detect the various sources of infection in open-heart surgery, we frequently sampled, amongst others, the surgical wound area during surgery and the oxygenator after surgery.

In March 1978, *Pseudomonas aeruginosa* was cultured from the *surgical wound area*. The same micro-organism was cultured from the *oxygenator*. Cultures from the nose, throat, skin, faecal material etc., taken at admission and just before surgery from these patients, had always been negative for this micro-organism. Furthermore, this bacterium was found on *sedimentation* plates which had been left open in the operating theatre during surgery. This indicated that *P. aeruginosa* was present in the air.

Pyocine typing showed that all strains isolated were of the same type. This suggested a common source of contamination. Culture results of throat and faecal samples of the personnel involved in cardiac surgery revealed that *P. aeruginosa* was present in the gastro-intestinal tract of one of the 22 subjects studied. The pyocine type of this strain differed, however, from that isolated from the patients and the environmental samples. Further investigation showed that the patient-type strain could only be cultured from the floor of the operating theatre on one side of the operating table and in the vicinity of the oxygenator.

A new type of blood-gas analyzer [Analysator D. Eschweiler en Co., Kiel (DBR)] had been installed just before samples showed the presence of *P. aeruginosa*. This analyzer was connected to the disposable oxygenator. Cultures taken from the blood-gas analyzer and the tube connecting this apparatus to the oxygenator showed that the same pyocine type as that isolated from the patients and the oxygenator was present. The organism was found on the *electrodes*, the *thermostat*, and the *inside of the waterbath*. The analyzer therefore seemed to be the source of contamination and was treated with 2% glutaraldehyde. Cultures taken *afterwards* showed that the apparatus was sterile. However, in the next surgical procedure *P. aeruginosa* of the same pyocine type was again cultured from the oxygenator and also from the blood-gas analyzer.

We concluded that the source of infection lay elsewhere. The fluids used to standardise the electrodes of the apparatus were cultured and, to our surprise, *P. aeruginosa* was isolated from these commercially bought fluids in a concentration of 10^5 to 10^6 organisms per ml. Pyocine typing showed that this type was identical to that found in patients, air, and floor samples. The use of contaminated standardising fluids explained why after disinfection the apparatus was once more contaminated.

The conclusion of this study is that all materials and apparatus used in connection with the oxygenator should be sterile since *retro-*

---

*University Hospital, Department of Surgery, Groningen, The Netherlands *grade* contamination from such in-line apparatus to the patient can easily occur, as demonstrated by our findings. The patients involved received gentamycine and did not develop septicaemia or any other infection.

A second and more or less identical finding was the detection of *Serratia marcescens* bacteriaemia in three of our patients during treatment in the intensive care unit. These three episodes occurred postoperatively over a period of 3 months. Biotyping revealed that the same strain caused all three bacteriaemias. The identical strain was sometimes present in the environmental samples taken sporadically in the intensive care unit from sinks, floor, etc. The strain was not isolated in material cultured at admission or during surgery. This meant that the contamination was exogenous and that the source of infection had to be present in the intensive care unit. The results of culturing various sites pinpointed the pressure monitoring device (Statham) as the most probable source. We use disposable domes in the pressure monitoring system and a 5% sterile glucose as flush solution. It was therefore difficult to find an explanation for the contamination. However, from a non-selected number of patients, we found that *S. marcescens* could be cultured from nearly 50% of the complete pressure monitoring devices (Table 1). The organism was isolated from the outside of the tap, the outside of the continuous flow device, and from the *inside* of the dome itself. This finding suggested that contamination of the domes occurred due to handling of the monitoring device in the intensive care unit since domes were sterile before use. This assumption was strengthened by the presence of *S. marcescens* on the fingers of some of the staff.

Table 1. Culture results of disposable domes in use

	Positive sample sites			
Dome connected to	Tap	Flow device	Inside dome	Total
Arterial line (N = 20)	2	3	3	8
Venous line (N = 19)	4	2	4	10
Left atrium line (N = 12)	0	1	2	3
Total 51	6	6	9	21

Further culturing revealed that clamps in which the domes were fixed were contaminated by *S. marcescens*. These armatures are frequently handled, so that organisms were transferred to the taps and the flow devices of the domes of the pressure monitoring system. The clamps are made of non-disposable material and are disinfected by cleaning with chlorhexidine in ethanol, whilst still attached to their metal stand. In the small space between the clamps and this metal stand, the disinfectants could, however, not penetrate, so organisms survived and the holders remained contaminated. In addition, during use, 5% glucose solution dripped into the holder, providing favourable conditions for a rapid growth of micro-organisms and especially *S. marcescens*.

In conclusion, contamination of the blood circulation of patients again occurred from in-line systems. The source of this serious infection was the holder for fixation of the domes of the monitoring device which was inadequately cleaned or sterilized. This finding underlines the fact that in conjunction with the use of disposable sterile domes other sub-parts of the pressure monitoring system should be cleaned or sterilized adequately. Contamination of such devices cannot be prevented as they are a regular part of the normal intensive treatment room furniture, but the risk of contamination would be decreased if they were changed regularly. The three patients showed symptom of septic shock and received intensive supportive therapy in combination with antibiotics. They were discharged in good health.

The lesson of our experience is: *retrograde* infection through in-line monitoring devices, even with a centrifugal uni-directional flow, is a real danger for the patient and all materials used for standardising or even the simple furniture in close connection with the monitoring device should be clean or sterile because contamination can take place by handling!

Are the Inguinal Lymph Nodes Responsible for Infections of Angioplastic Procedures in the Groin?

P. Balas, E. Giamarellou, and N. Pagratis*

Infection of an angioplastic procedure might result not only in severe complications but might also threaten the patient's life (1, 4, 6, 7). The more common site of development of infection is the groin (5).

The early recognition of an infection as well as the vigorous treatment with massive administration of antibiotics, systematically and locally, could stop the infective process. However, it is more important, by knowing the etiology and the pathogenetic mechanism of the development of this complication in the groin, to prevent it. This study was planned to explore the possible etiologic involvement of the inguinal lymph nodes in the development of an infective process of the angioplastic procedures in the groin.

Material and Method

Eighty-four patients who were submitted to various angioplastic procedures with 135 angioplasties of the femoral arteries were included in the present investigation (Table 1). In all these procedures plastic arterial substitutes from Dacron or expanded polytetrafluoroethylene were used as tubes or patches except for eight saphenous femoropopliteal bypasses. In 12 patients who were submitted to bilateral femoral angioplasty lymph node was taken from both inguinal areas. Also, 20 patients who were submitted to crossectomy in the groin for varicose veins extirpation were included and were used as controls.

Table 1. Surgical procedures performed in the mentioned group of patients

Angioplastic procedures	No. patients	No. femoral angioplasty
Aortobilateral femoral bypass	41	82
Axillofemoral bypass	6	6
Femoral-femoral bypass	10	20
Femoropopliteal venous bypass	8	8
Angioplastic of the femoral bifurcation	19	19
Total	84	135

*First Department of Surgery and the Infectious Diseases Laboratory of the First Department of Propedeutic Medicine, Athens University Medical School, 4 Hiraclitou st., Athens 136, Greece

Preparation before surgery. Twelve hours prior to surgery after shaving of the groin and vigorous cleaning with soap and warm water, the whole area was cleaned with Betadine (Ethenyl-2-pyrrolidinone homopolymer compound with iodine) ointment for 3-5 minutes. After drying with a sterile towel, Betadine ointment was applied and was left overnight and the area was covered with a sterile towel. After induction of anaesthesia, the inguinal area was cleaned vigorously with Betadine scrub for 3-5 minutes and was dried; finally it was covered with a fine coat of Betadine solution.

Of the 84 patients who were submitted to angioplastic procedures, 34 had received antibiotic intramuscular 6-8 g cephalosporin during the 24 h prior to surgery (group a), while the remaining 50 patients did not receive any prophylactic (group b) administration of antibiotics.

During operation. After performing the inguinal incision, one lymph node was excised. From the group of 34 patients, 36 lymph nodes were taken, while from the group of 50 patients 60 lymph nodes were examined. The lymph nodes were cut into small pieces; they were subsequently placed in a bottle of 50 ml of trypcade diphasique solution which was sent to the bacteriology department. The bacteriologic study was performed as follows: Lymph nodes cut into three or four pieces were put into Castaneda bottles containing CO_2 under vacuum (BBL). Cultures were performed immediately by withdrawing 1 ml sample of the inoculated broth and culturing 0.5 ml into solid media. After 24 h of incubation at 37°C, solid media were recultured as previously. If cultures proved positive, bottles were discarded; otherwise they were left for another 5 days in the incubator and a final reculture was done. Microorganism identification was performed according to the American Society of Microbiology (Leynette et al., 1974). Sensitivities of the isolated microorganisms were determined by the agar diffusion Kirby-Bauer technique.

Also, immediately before making the inguinal incision, skin cultures were taken from the groin area in 20 cases in which femoral arterioplasty was subsequently made.

Results

In 84 femoral angioplastic procedures in which 96 lymph nodes were examined, 53 positive cultures were found (55.20%), while in the remaining 43 lymph nodes the cultures were negative (44.79%). In 50 femoral angioplastic procedures in which the patients had not received antibiotics and in which 60 lymph nodes were excised, sterile cultures were found in the lymph nodes of 23 procedures (38%), while in 34 procedures with the administration of antibiotics to the patients and in which 36 lymph nodes were excised, cultures were found sterile in 20 (55%) (Table 2). These results are not statistically significant. The bacteria isolated in the lymph node cultures included *Staphylococcus epidermidis*, *S. aureus*, *Streptococci* Spp. (non group A), and *Acinectobacter* Spp. *S. epidermidis* and *S. aureus* were isolated in skin cultures. The skin cultures were found sterile in 90.9% of the cases.

In 20 normal individuals submitted to crossectomy, the cultures of the lymph nodes were sterile in 14 cases (Table 3). In this series no Betadine ointment was applied before surgery. In the case where the *S. aureus* was found, a venous ulcer was present. These findings are not statistically significant.

Table 2. Results of bacteriologic study of lymph nodes taken from the inguinal area of the arterioplastic procedures

Prophylactic administration of antibiotics	No. femoral angioplastic procedures	No. examined lymph nodes	Sterile culture ($X^2 = 2.69$)
Yes	34	36	20 (55%)
No	50	60	23 (38%)
Total	84	96	43 (44.79%)

Table 3. Results of bacteriologic study of lymph nodes taken from the inguinal area at crossectomy

Cultures	No. cases
Positive	6 (30%)
Sterile	14 (70%)
Total	20

Bacteria isolated in the cultures:	*Staphylococcus*	*Albus*	3
		epidermidis	2
	Staphylococcus	*aureus*	1

In two femoral angioplastic procedures out of 135 submitted to the study, infections of various types, according to the classification of Szilagyi et al. (6),developed. In one case which received antibiotics prophylactically, the injection was type II (Szilagyi's classification) and the same microorganism, *S. epidermidis*, was found in the lymph node and in two consecutive wound cultures. In another case of injection of type III, the culture of two lymph nodes taken from both inguinal areas (aortobilateral femoral bypass) was sterile. Prophylactic antibiotics were not administered and the case was considered sterile. In this case, the number of infected groins was small in a series of 135 cases of femoral angioplastic procedures (1.48%). In one case, in spite of the prophylactic administration of antibiotics, a wound infection had developed. However, the difference in the incidence of groin infection in cases with or without prophylactic administration of antibiotics was not statistically significant.

In the cases with infection of the groin, only in one out of two cases did the bacteria found in the cultured lymph nodes taken during surgery correspond to the bacteria found in the cultures from the infected wound. Therefore, in most of the cases with infected groins causes other than the infected lymph nodes were responsible for the infection. Only in one case could the lymph nodes be considered responsible for the infection of the inguinal area and this incidence is not statistically significant.

Discussion

Many causes and pathogenetic mechanisms are responsible for infections of the various angioplastic procedures. The incidence varies between 1.3% and 6% (3, 6). The pathogenetic mechanisms include two broad categories: first the *intrinsic infection* which usually develops on an existing hemorrhage or hematoma around the area of angioplasty and, second, the *extrinsic infection*. An *early* (first days and weeks) or a *late* (month and years) infection following the angioplastic procedure can develop.

The angioplastic procedure in the femoral artery bifurcation is the most common site of infections. Whether or not inguinal incision per se are responsible for this higher incidence has not been clearly shown. Szilagyi et al. (6) in 40 patients with groin infection, considered that the inguinal skin appeared to be the source of infection in 23. In our study the cultures taken from the skin of the inguinal area were negative for bacteria in an incidence of 90.9%. Among the bacteria found one was pathogenic. Also, the more common development of false aneurysms in this area seem to be a predisposing factor or the main cause (5).

The investigation of the possible etiologic role of the inguinal lymph nodes for the development of infection of the angioplastic procedures in that area was based on the following. Some of the patients undergoing angioplastic procedures of the femoral artery had broken the continuity of the skin or open ulcer in the ipsilateral foot. These lesions could be a potential source of contamination of the ipsilateral inguinal lymph node chain and through their cut surfaces of the area of femoral angioplasty.

In our study a higher incidence of positive cultures in the lymph nodes taken at the angioplasty of the femoral arteries (55.20%) in comparison to the incidence of the cultures taken from the lymph nodes excised at the crossectomy (30%) was found, in spite of the more strict skin preparation of the inguinal area in the angioplastic procedures (Table 4). This difference has statistical significance. The skin breaks or the ulcerations of the ipsilateral ischemic foot might be responsible for the higher incidence of lymph node contamination in the cases of angioplasty. Another operative finding supporting this hypothesis is the existence of large inguinal lymph nodes showing histologically reactive lymphadenitis in the groin of the patients undergoing femoral angioplastic procedure, while small nodes were found at crossectomy.

However, although positive cultures were found in 53 (55.20%) of the examined lymph nodes excised at the femoral angioplastic procedures, only in one case did groin wound infection develop. In this case, *S. aureus* was found in the culture of the lymph node and consequently in the cultures of the infected wound secretions. This correlation is statistically significant.

In conclusion, the present investigation, still in evolution, has shown that the inguinal lymph nodes might be the source for the development of an infection of the angioplastic procedures of the femoral arteries.

Table 4.

Lymph node culture	Femoral angioplasty No. cases	%	Crossectomy No. cases	%
Positive	53	55.20	6	30
Negative	43	44.80	14	70
Total	96		20	

Summary

An investigation of the possible etiologic role of the inguinal lymph nodes for the development of infection of the angioplastic procedures of the femoral arteries was carried out. This study was based on the culture of lymph nodes taken from the inguinal wound. Positive cultures were obtained in 53 (55.20%) of the examined lymph nodes. In one of the groin wounds from which excised and cultured lymph nodes had positive culture, infection developed. In this case, *Staphylococcus aureus* was found in the lymph node culture and in the culture of the wound secretions. The present investigation has shown that the inguinal lymph nodes might be the source for the development of an infection of the angioplastic procedures of the femoral arteries.

References

1. Carter SC, Cohen A, Whelan TJ (1963) Clinical experience with management of infected Dacron graft. Ann Surg 158:249
2. Fry WJ, Lindenauer SM (1967) Infection complicating the use of plastic arterial implants. Arch Surg 94:600
3. Hoffert PW, Gensler S, Haimovici H (1965) Infection complicating arterial grafts. Arch Surg 90:427
4. Javid H, et al. (1962) Complications of abdominal aortic grafts. Arch Surg 85:650
5. Sawyers JL, Jacobs JK, Sutton JP (1967) Peripheral anastomotic aneurysms. Arch Surg 95:802
6. Szilagyi DE, Smith RF, Elliot JP, Vrandecic MP (1972) Infection in arterial reconstruction with synthetic grafts. Ann Surg 176:321
7. Willwerth BM, Waldhausen A (1974) Infection of arterial prostheses. Surg Gynecol Obstet 139:446

The Hepatitis Risk After Operations Using Extracorporeal Circulation (ECC) – A Prospective Study

R. Stute, W. Franzen, H. D. Schulte, and H. Brüster*

Introduction

Although diagnostic tools have been improved very much during recent years, hepatitis is a serious postoperative problem after open-heart procedures using extracorporeal circulation (1-4). To reduce the risk of hepatitis after cardiac surgery, we have chosen a specific program of blood donor selection, of repeated donor control, and a differentiated investigation set-up before transfusion of any donated blood.

In a former retrospective study between January 1974 and December 1976, we looked into the incidence of this complication in all adults who had undergone open-heart procedures and found a hepatitis rate of less than 2% (7). For control of our fairly low incidence of hepatitis, we continued our efforts in a prospective study using another test system associated with hepatitis B infection, the anti-core determination (5).

Material and Methods

Our donors feel closely associated to the bloodbank and some of them have been donating for 30 years in our center. They usually live in intact families, work regularly, and boast an above-average standard of life. Nearly 50% of them have telephones. Even before sensitive tests for the detection of HB_S Ag were available, all donors who were involved in a case of hepatitis were marked with an "H". If a donor was involved in a second case of hepatitis, he was excluded from blood donation. Our entire laboratory program is organized in such a manner that we are able to finish all determinations for donors' examinations within 3 h. The donors arrive between 6 and 8:30 a.m. Already at 9 o'clock, we can release the first donated fresh blood, for instance for cardiopulmonary bypass in open-heart surgery. Due to this, no hemorrhage complications arise which otherwise could force us to administer pool preparations. We only could obtain this assigned method by shortening those methods which were most time-consuming and performing all essential tests at the same time early in the morning. To save time for the coagulation, we chose methods which could proceed from heparin plasma.

The major unit of the complete diagnostics was a highly sensitive method for the detection of HB_S Ag. For this purpose, we equally deem applicable both our modified radioimmunoassay (RIA) AUSRIA II as well

*Institute for Blood Coagulation and Transfusion Medicine, Department Surgery B, University of Duesseldorf, Moorenstr. 5, D-4000 Duesseldorf 1, FRG

as the HEPANOSTIKA (5). Anti-HB_s and anti-HB_c were determined by radioimmunoassay (RIA) (AUSAB, CORAB).

With the aid of a Coulter counter, we can do the routine blood examinations, with an automatic photometer the GPT UV test, and furthermore the TPHA test. The representation is closed up by a yearly X-ray screening of the thorax, examination of urine, and control of the blood sedimentation rate (BSR). In our unit no blood will be transfused which points out any pathological affection.

Results

To determine the incidence of hepatitis infections, 302 adult patients wo had undergone open-heart surgical procedures between July 1977 and June 1978 were investigated. All patients were informed about the hepatitis symptoms and their family doctors were asked to send a blood sample each month for 6 months postoperatively. We examined the following parameters pre- and postoperatively from all samples: GPT, HB_s Ag, anti-HB_s, and anti-HB_c.

Out of the 302 chosen patients, wo got at least four samples from 203 patients for examination and three or less from another 30 patients. Two persons out of this group proved to be carriers of HB_s Ag. In 36 patients (15%), anti-HB_s could be detected preoperatively; in 49 patients (21%), we found anti-HB_s after the operation, caused by transfusion of anti-HB_s positive blood.

Two hundred and one patients (86%) never had elevated transaminase, 20 patients (8.6%) had slightly elevated transaminases pre- and postoperatively (GPT less than 50 IU), 12 persons (5%) had a value of above 50 IU one or more times. Of these 12 patients, only seven (3%) had a hepatitis. The other five had either elevated GPT values before the operation or other complications, such as swelling of the liver or metabolism disturbances.

We found three cases of hepatitis B and four cases of non-A-non-B hepatitis. None of the donors involved in these cases of hepatitis B showed an isolated anti-HB_c antibody at the time of giving blood or later. None of these donors became later HB_sAg positive. So, these infections must be caused by other sources than blood transfusion. The four patients with the non-A-non-B hepatitis were negative for hepatitis B markers and developed their symptoms 8 weeks after the operation. In all cases no pathological affections could be proved in the given blood. So we found a hepatitis rate of 3% which is a fairly low result compared to those of other centers. The negative result for anti-HB_c of all donors involved in the hepatitis B cases demonstrates that it is necessary to look into other ways of infection. Only the four patients of non-A-non-B hepatitis seem to be caused by blood transfusion (1.7%).

But the main reason for these exceptionally good results in this study – in our opinion – are exact and repeated controls of continuous blood donors, modern and improved laboratory test methods, no application of blood with increased transaminase, no use of pool blood preparations at all, and a strict indication for blood transfusions.

Summary

In a prospective study the incidence of hepatitis after open-heart surgical procedures using ECC was investigated. During July 1977 and June 1978, 302 operated adult patients were chosen for this study.

Preoperatively blood samples were taken for anti-HB_s, HB_s Ag (RIA), and optimized transaminases (SGPT). After instruction, only 233 of these patients sent one blood sample every month postoperatively for further investigation. The mean transfusion rate in this group was 6.2 transfusions of whole blood and/or plasma per patient. Two hundred and one patients (86.9%) had no increase of transaminases. In 20 patients (8.6%), there was a moderate increase (SGPT <50 IU). In 12 patients (5.2%), a distinct increase of SGPT (>50 IU) was detected, but only in seven patients (3%) was the reason a hepatitis: hepatitis B – three patients (1.3%); presumably non-A-non-B hepatitis – four patients (1.7%). This fairly low incidence of hepatitis in our patients depends on exact and repeated controls of the blood donors, improved laboratory test methods, no application of blood with increased transaminases, no use of pool blood preparations, and strict indication for blood transfusion.

References

1. Glinz W, Knoblauch M, Rothlin M (1972) Häufigkeit und Verlauf der ikterischen und anikterischen Transfusionshepatitis. Helv Chir Acta 39:303-308
2. Lee AKY, Tse TF, Mock CK (1974) Australia antigen in open-heart surgical unit in Hongkong. Aust NZ J Med 4:8-11
3. Slater SD (1974) Allo-antibodies and Australia antigen after open-heart surgery. J Clin Pathol 27:45-49
4. Ohlmeier H, Dahmen E, Hoppe J (1979) Hepatitisrisiko von humanen Gerinnungspräparaten aus gepoolten Plasmen. Dtsch Med Wochenschr 103:1701
5. Overby LR, Ling CM (1976) Radioimmune assay for anti-core as evidence for exposure to hepatitis B virus. Rush-Presbyterian St Luke's Med Bull 15:83-92
6. Stute R, Luxem T, Brüster H (1979) Untersuchungen zur Bestimmung des Hepatitis-B-Oberflächenantigens (HB_s Ag) im Enzymimmunoassay. Lab Med 3:47-49
7. Stute R, Krian A, Staudacher B, Schulte HD, Brüster H (1979) Frequency of hepatitis B after open-heart surgery: A retrospective study over a three-year period (1974-1976). Thorac Cardiovasc Surg 27:238-240

Hepatitis After Open Heart Surgery

P. Satter and W. Blum*

Hepatitis after open-heart surgery is a well-known problem with a frequency between 0.9% and 52% (1-8) (see Table 1). Until a few years ago, blood transfusion was thought to be the main cause of postoperative hepatitis type B, and many studies considered only this possibility.

Most efforts to prevent hepatitis were aimed in the direction of reducing the use of blood and screening the donors for hepatitis B (HB) antigens. Unexpectedly, however, the incidence of hepatitis did not decrease particularly in our institution (Fig. 1). While the incidence from 1973 to 1975 was between 6% and 7%, we found a sharp increase to 24% in 1976 and to 32% in 1977. Since there was no significant change in operative techniques, we started a prospective study in 1978 to find out the cause and how to prevent it. A short pilot study revealed that the increase was mainly due to an increase in non-A-non-B type hepatitis and therefore could not be prevented with the available screening tests for type B (9, 10).

All blood used during the operations was produced by the regional blood bank of the German Red Cross in Frankfurt which operates on a base of volunteer donors. PPSB (factor IX concentrate) and Cohn I made from pooled plasma also produced by this institution were used rather frequently. The blood for transfusion as well as for the preparation of the factor IX concentrates was checked for HB_s antigen and discarded if positive.

Table 1. Incidence of hepatitis after open-heart surgery

Author	Year	Number of patients	Incidence (%)
Glinz	1972	145	32
Rastan	1973	29	20
Schlaak	1974	48	52
Slater	1974	102	0.9
Pandel	1976	41	32
Schricker	1976	293	7
Ohlmeier	1978	247	10
Stute	1979	588	2

*Klinik für Thorax-, Herz- und Gefäßchirurgie, Universitätsklinikum, Theodor-Stern-Kai 7, D-6000 Frankfurt/a.M. 70

Results

One hundred and ninety-eight consecutive patients were entered into the study. In order to find out if the prophylactic administration of intravenous gamma globulin is able to reduce the incidence of hepatitis, as Knodell and others reported (11, 12), 2.5 g gamma globulin was given intravenously immediately after operation to half of the patients according to their birthdates. Blood tests were performed in short intervals postoperatively up to 6 weeks and in monthly intervals up to 6 months. The blood was tested for SGOT, SGPT, γ-GT, bilirubin, and iron, HB_s antibody and different HB_s antigens with the radioimmunoassay test. A hepatitis was diagnosed if the transaminase, SGOT, and SGPT were preoperatively within normal range and rose at least 2 weeks after the operation to more than 2.5 of the normal value for more than 1 week. A hepatitis type B was diagnosed if postoperative HB_s antigen appeared or if the conversion from anti-HB_s negative to positive occurred postoperatively after an interval of 1 month together with an increase of transaminases. One hundred and fifty-four patients met all the necessary criteria to be evaluated. Under those above-mentioned strict criteria, a hepatitis was diagnosed in 61 of 154 patients which is an incidence of 39.6% (Table 2).

Table 2. Incidence and type of hepatitis 1978

Pat.	Hepatitis Yes	Hepatitis No	Incidence (%)	Type B		Type non-A-non-B	
154	61	93	39.6	5 (8%)		56 (92%)	
				Ict.	Nonict.	Ict.	Nonict.
				3	2	12 (22%)	44 (78%)

A hepatitis type B was found in only five of these 61 patients (8%) and 56 (92%) had to be considered as non-A-non-B. From 56 patients of the non-A-non-B type hepatitis, 44 or 78% were nonicteric and 12 (22%) icteric with an incubation time of 2 to 12 weeks and a maximum around the sixth week.

Eighty-four of these 154 patients received intravenous gamma globulin and 70 did not. Table 3 shows incidence and type of hepatitis with and without administration of gamma globulin. The incidence of hepatitis was 33 out of 84 with gamma globulin and 28 out of 70 without gamma globulin. As you can see, gamma globulin did not show any significant effect in preventing hepatitis. There was also no difference in incubation time or number of icteric and nonicteric cases, not even in hepatitis type B where three of the five patients with this type of hepatitis received gamma globulin intravenously. Two of them became icteric with rather severe symptoms and one later death. The most interesting but not unexpected results from this study came with the analysis concerning the mode of infection.

Table 4 shows the relationship between the number of blood transfusion and the incidence of hepatitis. With the number of blood units, the incidence of hepatitis increases. But if you cut out all patients which got pooled plasma preparations as well, the picture is completely different (Table 5).

Table 3. Incidence and type of hepatitis with and without administration of gamma globulin

	With gamma globulin	Without gamma globulin
Patients	84	70
Incidence of hepatitis	33 (39%)	28 (40%)
Type B	3 (9%)	2 (7%)
Icteric	2	1
Nonicteric	1	1
Type non-A-non-B	30 (91%)	26 (93%)
Icteric	6 (20%)	6 (23%)
Nonicteric	24 (80%)	20 (77%)

Table 4. Incidence of hepatitis in correlation with number of blood units

Units	Pat.	Hepatitis Yes	No	Incidence (%)
0	18	1	17	5.5
1-3	44	12	32	27.2
3	92	48	44	52
Total	154	61	93	39.6

Table 5. Incidence of hepatitis in correlation with number of blood units without administration of pooled plasma preparations

Units	Pat.	Hepatitis Yes	No	Incidence (%)
0	2	0	2	0
1-3	14	1	13	7
3	18	1	17	5.5
Total	34	2	32	6

The risk of blood transfusion shows no statistically significant difference between the use of 0 to 3 units and more. The incidence of hepatitis still lies around 5%. During this study, 120 patients out of a total of 154 received pooled plasma preparations, particular prothrombin complex (PPSB = factor IX concentrate) fibrinogen or Cohn I provided by the regional blood bank.

Of 120 patients, 59 (49%) developed a hepatitis, while of the remaining 34 patients only 2 (6%) came down with this disease (Table 6). In other words: from 61 patients with postoperative hepatitis, 59 or 96% received pooled plasma preparations. Similar results have been reported by Dahmen, Ohlmeier, and others (7, 13-17). This shocking result led to an abrupt change in our policy concerning postoperative blood transfusion and the use of pooled plasma preparations, as follows:
1. All pooled plasma preparations from the regional blood bank were stopped and a commercially available hepatitis-free prothrombin complex was used in selected cases (PPSB Biotest).
2. Two to three units of autologous blood is obtained 2 to 3 weeks preoperatively and immediately before installing bypass, another 500 cc is removed from the patient.
3. Intra- and postoperative blood loss is substituted mostly with autologous blood and packed and washed red cells.

Table 6. Incidence of hepatitis in correlation with administration of pooled plasma preparations

Pooled plasma preparations	Pat.	Hepatitis Yes	No	Incidence (%)
250 U. PPSB	3	1	2	33.3
500 U. PPSB	96	44	52	45.8
750 U. PPSB	21	14	7	66.6
Total	120	59	61	49.1

PPSB = factor IX concentrate

With this, the rate of hepatitis in a control group of 50 patients during the second half of 1979 dropped to 4%. Interesting is the fact that of those patients in the control group receiving blood and commercially available hepatitis-free prothrombin complex during 1979, we did not have a single case of hepatitis, while we had two incidences of hepatitis in patients who had received neither blood nor pooled plasma preparations. Therefore, other modes of infection may be more frequent than generally thought and the term "transfusion hepatitis" should be omitted (6, 18).

Summary

A sudden increase in hepatitis during the years 1976 to 1977 had two main causes:
1. The increasing incidence of a new type of hepatitis non-A-non-B which could not be excluded from blood donors by the available routine tests including radioimmunoassay. The incidence rose from 7% to 39%.
2. The most important cause of infection came from pooled plasma preparations, particularly the factor IX concentrate provided by the regional blood bank.

3. With the use of a commercially available hepatitis-free prothrombin complex (PPSB biotest), this mode of infection can be avoided.
4. Passive immunisation or prophylaxis with administration of intravenous gamma globulin is not possible. This money can be saved.

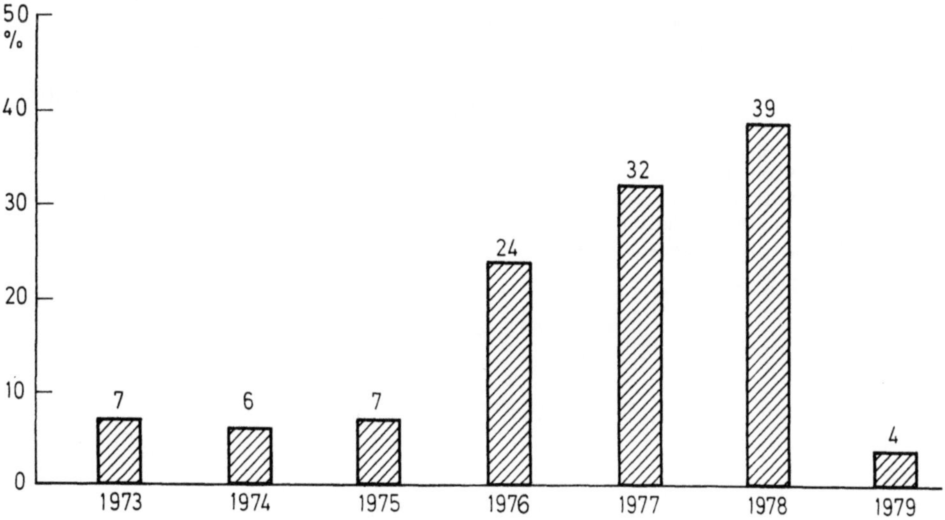

Fig. 1. Incidence of hepatitis in open-heart surgery

References

1. Glinz W, Knoblauch M, Rothlin M (1972) Häufigkeit und Verlauf der ikterischen und anikterischen Transfusionshepatitis. Helv Chir Acta 39:303-308
2. Rastan H, Schmidt G (1973) Lebererkrankungen nach Eingriffen am offenen Herzen. MMW 115:968-990
3. Schlaak M, Lehmann H, Schober A (1974) Hepatitisrisiko nach Transfusion von HB_s-Antikörper-positivem Blut. Verh Dtsch Ges Inn Med 80:469-470
4. Slater SD (1974) Allo-antibodies and Australia antigen after open-heart surgery. J Clin Pathol 27:45-49
5. Pandel E, Lehmann H, Schlaak M (1976) Die posttransfusionelle Hepatitis als Komplikation nach Operationen mit Hilfe der Herz-Lungen-Maschine im Kindesalter. Z Kardiol 65:37-41
6. Schricker KT, Jeltsch H (1976) Bedarf die Bezeichnung "Transfusionshepatitis" einer Revision? Eine prospektive Studie an 293 Herzpatienten. Forsch Ergeb Transf Med Immun Hämatol 3:115
7. Ohlmeier H, Dahmen E, Hoppe I (1978) Hepatitisrisiko von humanen Gerinnungspräparaten aus gepoolten Plasmen. Dtsch Med Wochenschr 103:1700-1703
8. Stute R, Krian A, Staudacher B, Schulte HD, Brüster H (1979) Frequency of hepatitis B after open-heart surgery: A retrospective study over a three-year period (1974-1976). Thorac Cardiovasc Surg 27:238-240
9. Feinstone SM, Kapikian AZ, Purcell RH, et al. (1975) Transfusion-associated hepatitis not due to viral hepatitis Type A or B. N Engl J Med 292:767-770
10. Kaltenbach M, Krehan L, Wolf K, Satter P (1979) Recent changes in incidence and course of hepatitis after heart surgery. In: Roskamm H, Schmutziger M (eds) Coronary heart surgery. Springer, Berlin Heidelberg New York, pp 368-370

11. Knodell RG, Conrad ME, Ginsberg AL, Bell CJ, Flannery EP (1976) Efficacy of prophylactic gamma globulin in preventing non-A-non-B post-transfusion hepatitis. Lancet 557-561
12. Katz F, Rodriguez J, Ward R (1971) Post-transfusion hepatitis-effect of modified gamma globulin added to blood in vitro. N Engl J Med 285:925-932
13. Dahmen E, Ohlmeier H, Hoppe I (1978) Eigenblutspende und Hepatitisrisiko bei kardiochirurgischen Risikopatienten. Thoraxchirurgie 26:27
14. Faria R, Fiumara N (1972) Hepatitis B associated with Konyne. N Engl J Med 287: 358-359
15. Iwarson S, Kjellmann H, Tegef-Nilsson A (1976) Incidence of viral hepatitis after administration of factor IX concentrates. Vox Sang 31:136-140
16. Nagaraja M, Joseph R (1976) Hepatitis following prophylactic administration of Konyne. Univ Mich Med Center J 42:217-218
17. O'Connor ML, Melk ES, Simmons A (1977) Detection of HB_s Ag in coagulation factor IX concentrates. Transfusion 17:44-46
18. Hoppe I, Dahmen E, Ohlmeier H (1980) Krankenhaus-Hepatitis. Dtsch Med Wochenschr 105:435-438

Prophylaxis and Therapy of Graft Infection in Vascular Surgery

W. Sandmann, J. Lerut, H. Nüllen, and K. Kremer

Introduction

Infection is the most dreadful complication in vascular surgery. The rate of primary infection in artificial grafts was reported to be in the range of 2% to 6% (3, 4). Despite strong efforts to avoid this complication, the rate of graft infection remained 1% to 3% (7, 9) for reconstructions using artificial graft material. Lately an extremely low infection rate of 0.3% was reported by Brewster and Darling (1). This excellent result was achieved in a personal series. In general, more significant progress has been made to manage graft infection itself. The mortality rate reported in the literature was 75% some years ago (3). In 1979, Ehrenfeld et al. (2) reported a mortality rate of less than 15% using autogenous tissue reconstruction in the management of infected prosthetic grafts. It is the aim of this paper to present our material of the last 10 years in regard to vascular infection and to evaluate some factors of importance contributing to this problem.

Material and Methods

During the period from January 1, 1970, to May 31, 1980, 2747 patients underwent reconstructive vascular operations for occlusive or aneurysmal disease. Since 1974, prophylactic antibiotics were not used any more except in patients with gangrene and positive culture. Plastic skin drapes were used routinely. Since 1978, open wounds during operation were covered with Betadine (Ethenyl-2-pyrrolidinone homopolymer compound with iodine) and cloths were sutured to the wound borders. Operations were performed by five experienced surgeons and by about ten surgeons to be trained in vascular surgery.

The material was analyzed concerning the primary and secondary infection rate. A primary infection was defined as a vascular infection in a patient with an uneventful postoperative course in respect to the hemodynamic result of the reconstruction, while a secondary infection was defined as infection occurring after reoperation for early failure including hematoma, leakage, and graft thrombosis. The material is summarized in Table 1. Patients with autogenous procedures were compared to those reconstructed by the use of a vascular prosthesis. The rate of both early and late infections in the former group was 0.4%, in the latter 5%; thus the risk of infection using an artificial implant is 12 times higher than in autogenous reconstruction.

*Surgical Clinic A, University of Duesseldorf, Moorenstr. 5, D-4000 Duesseldorf

Table 1. Postoperative infection rate in vascular surgery

Type of procedure	No. of cases	Primary infection %	Cases of early "redo" No.	%	Secondary infection %	Infections total %
Autogenous	1823	0.1	167	9.2	3.64	0.4
Prosthetic	924	1.5	96	10.4	34.0	5.0
Total	2747	0.5	263	9.6	9.6	1.9

The group of autogenous reconstructions contains arterial reconstructions and has included 102 operations for disease of the deep veins like iliofemoral thrombosis, traumatic AV fistula, and others. Patients with acute vascular injury, those with angioaccess for hemodialysis and patients with vascular anastomosis in organ transplantation are not included in the series, because problems of infection are not comparable to reconstructive arterial surgery.

In the group of 1823 autogenous reconstructions, the primary infection rate was very low (0.1%); nevertheless, the problem of vascular infection in autogenous reconstruction is not completely negligible, because out of 167 patients with "early redo" surgery, 3.6% became infected.

Analysis of infection rate in the various groups of autogenous procedures demonstrates that infection in the aortoiliac thromboendarterectomy group did not occur, although in about 50% of the cases Dacron patches had been used (Table 2). Reconstructions of the carotid arteries and in the supraaortic branches were free of infection, probably due to the limited use of arterial grafts and patches, for example, we did not use a Dacron patch in carotid endarterectomy. The iliac femoral TEA[a] group and the group of patients in which vein grafts had been inserted revealed a 0.5% and 0.7% infection rate, respectively.

Table 2. Infections in autogenous reconstructions

Type of reconstruction	No. of cases	Grade III infection rate (%)		
		Primary	Secondary	Total
TEA[a] aorto-iliac	146	0	0	0
TEA[a] iliac-femoral	578	0.17	3.17	0.52
Vein graft	696	0.14	4.4	0.72
Carotis	218	0	0	0
Supraaortic/ brachial	83	0	0	0
Deep veins	102	0	0	0
Total	1823	0.1	3.6	0.4

[a]TEA = Thromboendarterectomy

None of the early redo cases developed infection in the supraaortic region, while those of the iliac femoral TEA and the vein graft group had inguinal infections. The groin was the most frequent localization of infection.

Further analysis of the material was done to evaluate the influence of the type of procedure (Tables 2 and 3), the type of disease, and the experience of the institution (Table 4). The primary infection rate in the total of aortofemoral grafts – occlusive and aneurysmal – was 1%. In the group of patients with occlusive disease, it was 0.8% and decreased to 0.7% in the latest period (1978-1980). Aortoiliac reconstructions are possibly at a lower risk of infection than aortofemoral, but in our series infection in aortoiliac grafts occurred in 2.6%. In the "miscellaneous" group, the rate of early redo operations was extremely high due to graft thrombosis. It may be that there was a negative selection of candidates for amputation and only very few patients had been discarded from reconstruction because of uncorrectable disease in the outflow tract. The risk of infection in early redo cases in the miscellaneous group is high and reached 50% in our material.

Table 3. Infection of Dacron (+ Teflon) arterial grafts

Type of reconstruction	No. of cases	Grade III infection rate (%)		
		Primary	Secondary	Total
Aortofemoral	584	1.0	31.0	4.1
Aortoiliac	117	2.5	-	2.6
Miscellaneous iliac-femoral femoral extraanat. late repair of Dacron graft	222	2.3	50.0	9.0
Total	924	1.5	34.0	5.0

Table 4. Infection of aortoiliofemoral grafts (occlusive disease)

Period	No. of cases	No. of early "redo" cases	Grade III infection rate (%)		
			Primary	Secondary	Total
1970-1974	138	21 (15%)	0.9	24	4.3
1975-1977	200	16 (8%)	1.0	44	4.5
1978-1980 (15.6)	171	16 (9%)	0.7	31	3.5
Total	509	53 (10%)	0.8	32	4.1

Since 1970, we have had a total of 53 infections, the majority occurring early after reconstruction of occlusive arterial disease. Another group of 14 patients with graft infections was admitted from other hospitals during the last decade. Late graft infections appeared as an infected aneurysm or infectious drainage. A sinogram may be helpful to determine the extention of the inflammatory process, but generally the diagnosis of graft infection can be made on a clinical basis (Fig. 1). In the recent years, the double velour type of Dacron prosthesis had been used and it seems to us that the velour layer limits the expansion of infection.

Several methods had been used to manage graft infection (Table 5). Local care was completely unsuccessful; mortality rate was 100%. Ligation or excision of the graft saved the life of nine out of 15 patients, but could not prevent amputation of six out of 20 legs. Removal of the infected part of the graft and extraanatomical bypass (EAB) performed simultaneously was the most successful method of repair. The operation is performed at one time in three stages. First the infected Dacron graft is ligated and dissected in a noninfected field, second the extraanatomic graft is placed, and third the infected wound is explored and the

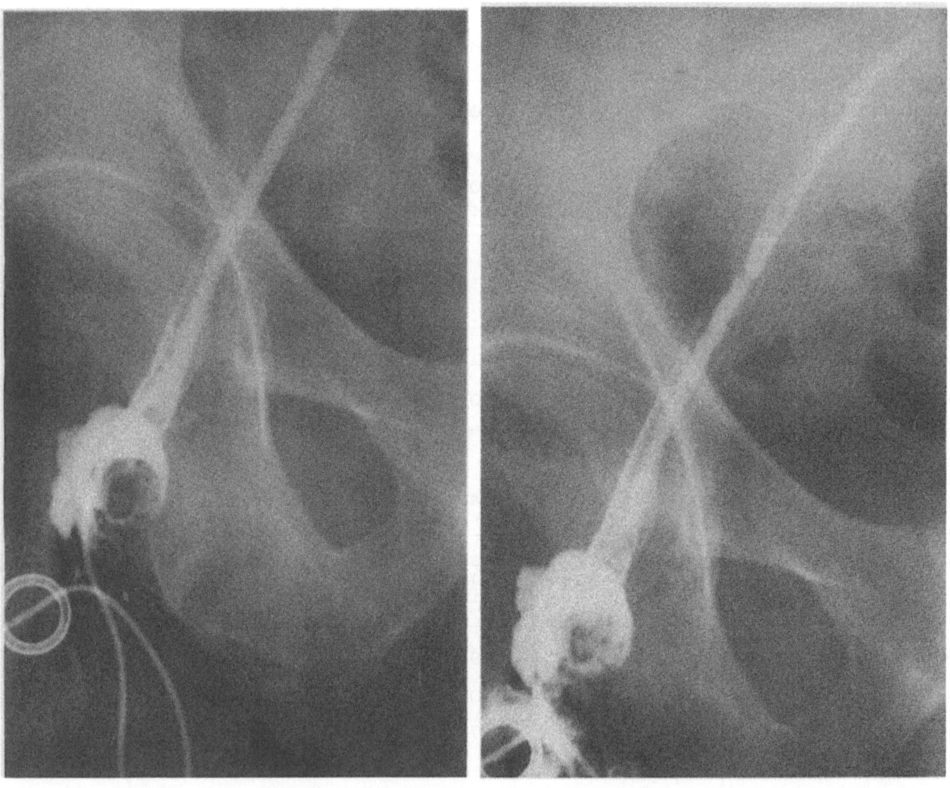

Fig. 1. Sinogram of a 65-year-old patient who maintained infectious drainage 12 weeks following implantation of an aortofemoral bifurcation graft. Infection of this Weavenit prosthesis expanded from the right femoral anastomosis to the aortal suture line; the total graft had to be removed and bilateral axillofemoral graft was performed

Table 5. Summary of results

Management	No. of patients	No. of deaths	Legs at risk	Amputation No.	Stage II No.
Local care	8	8	16	3	0
Ligation/ excision	15	6	20	6	4
EAB + removal	36	4 (11%)	62	4 (6%)	4
Omentumplasty	2	1	4	0	0
Autogenous in situ repair	6	0	7	0	0
Total	67	19 (28%)	108	13 (12%)	8 (7%)

infected part of the prosthesis is removed. Isolated Dacron limb infection in the groin caused the majority of infections. The obturator route was used most frequently but in cases with infection at or above the inguinal ligament, a femoral crossover graft was found to be equally safe (Figs. 2 and 3).

In 15 patients, autogenous tissue repair was used to manage infection. In six patients, the infected part of the arterial substitute was removed and vascular continuity was restored in situ using the great saphenous vein in three patients and a thrombectomized segment of the femoral artery or the internal iliac artery in three patients. End-to-end or end-to-side anastomoses in the infected field were performed with absorbable PGS (polyglycol acid suture) using single stitches. Each of the six patients had complete healing of infection. Nine patients with graft infection after various types of arterial reconstruction were managed by partial or total graft removal and extraanatomical bypass using the great saphenous vein. Running or single suture of Prolene were used for the anstomoses which were performed in a noninfected field. The results of autogenous tissue repair are summarized in Table 6. The mortality rate was 13%, amputation rate 12% concerning the legs at risk. The two deaths were unrelated to the infectious complication.

Table 6. Autogenous tissue reconstruction – results

Infected graft site	No. of patients	No. of deaths	Legs at risk	Amputations	Strokes
Aortofemoral	3	0	6	2	-
Aortoiliac	1	0	1	0	-
Femoral	9	2	10	0	-
Carotid	2	0	-	-	0
Total	15	2 (13%)	17	2 (12%)	0

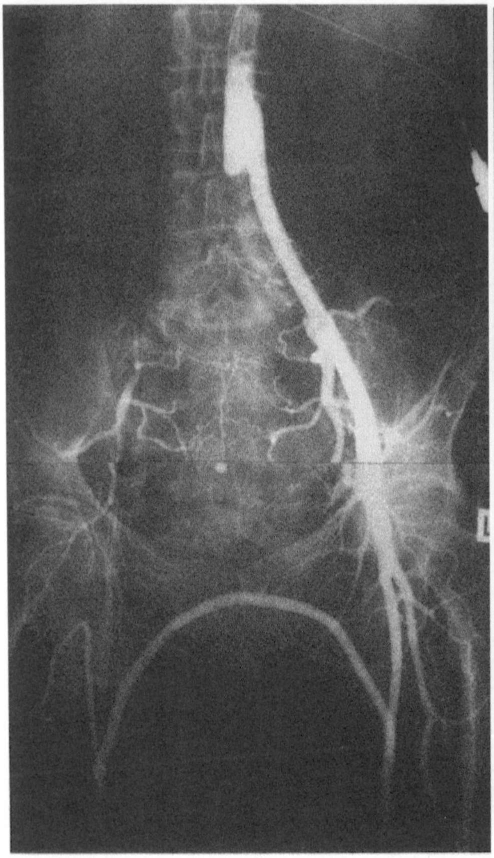

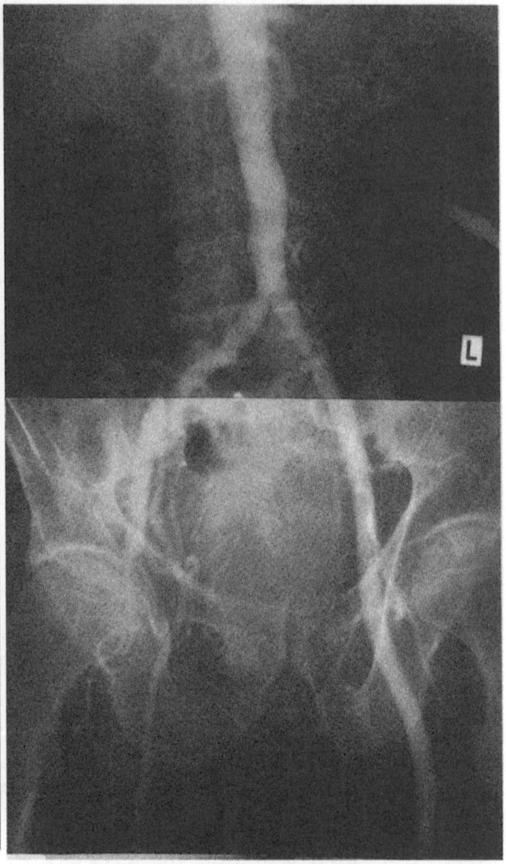

Fig. 2

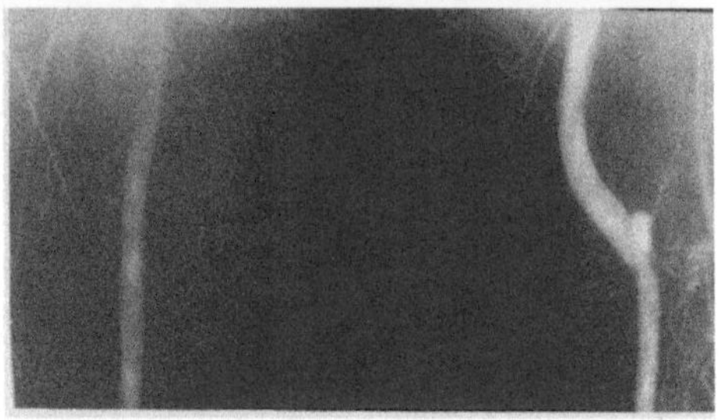

Fig. 3

Fig. 2. Angiogram of an obturator bypass graft on the right and the left side. On the left side, an 8 mm Dacron double velour graft had been used, while on the right side the obturator bypass was performed with the great saphenous vein. The extra-anatomical repair was performed after infection of a right femoral to left femoral Dacron graft. The left obturator bypass is still patent 2 years later, the right one occluded 1 year after operation

Fig. 3. Angiogram of a left femoral to right femoral Gore-Tex bypass which was inserted after infection of an aortofemoral bifurcation graft at the right femoral anastomosis. After 3 years, the cross-over graft is still patent

In our summarized material of 67 arterial infections, a total mortality rate of 28% occurred. The mortality rate in patients with the most favourable procedure of repair – as described above – was 11%, the amputation rate concerning the legs at risk 6%. In the aortoiliofemoral bypass group, local care or ligation/excision was followed by a mortality rate of 80%, while the procedure of choice, extraanatomical repair and graft removal lowered the mortality rate to 12% (Table 7).

Table 7. Aortoiliofemoral grafts – repair of infection

Management	No. of patients	No. of deaths	Legs at risk	Amputations
Local care	8	7 (80%, local care and ligation/excision together)	16	1
Ligation/ excision	7	5	14	2
EAB + removal	25	3 (12%)	50	1
Total	40	15 (37%)	80	4 (5%)

Discussion

In our presented material several factors influencing the rate of arterial and graft infection were analyzed. Two of them may have major importance. The material used for vascular replacement was significantly involved in the rate of infection. Artificial grafts are not resistant against contamination and such grafts maintain infection, because the foreign material disturbs the biological repair. Anyhow, Brewster and Darling (1) reported a very low infection rate following the use of aortoiliofemoral Dacron grafts of 0.3%. In comparison to our material, the second important factor determining the incidence of graft infection is therefore the experience of the vascular surgeon. A teaching institution like ours must have a higher incidence of vascular infection, because in the group of patients with early redo operations caused by hematoma, bleeding at the suture line, or graft thrombosis comparatively increased the infection rate. Careful selection of patients and procedures and improvement of surgical skill and technical performance should avoid the redo operations; thus the rate of graft infection will be reduced. Consequently, further specialisation in vascular surgery is absolutely mandatory in respect to the fate of the patient.

Besides the graft material it was the anatomical region which determined the risk of infection, especially in patients with early redo operations. A more lateral approach to the femoral vessels has been recommended to avoid dissection of the lymph nodes and lymph vessels.

The low rate of graft infection in the series cited above (1) is almost convincing for the use of prophylactic antibiotics, although its effectiveness has been unproven by means of a randomized study in clean vascular operations. Two years ago, we started the use of antiseptic wound covering with Betadine, mainly to protect the groin wound during operation. Additionally, cloths were sutured to the wound borders to avoid any contact of the graft to the skin. Maybe these efforts were effective in preventing aortofemoral graft infection which could be reduced from 1% to 0.7% in non-redo cases.

A total of 67 patients with arterial infection were observed, so we had to gain some experience in the management of this complication. Local care failed in every case of Dacron graft infection. This method is dangerous in the area of anastomosis and should be abandoned. Ligation of the graft, excision, and antiseptic irrigation was a method to be used in earlier years and can preserve the noninfected part of a bifurcation graft. Sometimes it may be very difficult to determine whether the collateral circulation will be sufficient or not. We have limited experience with omentumplasty recommended by Van Dongen (8) who reported good results with this procedure in bifurcation grafts at the iliac infection side. In our view, it is a major operation and leaves some uncertainty about the fate of the graft.

In general, there are two ways of management in graft infection, extraanatomical repair and removal of the infected part of the graft or in situ repair using autogenous tissue mainly advocated by Ehrenfeld et al. (2). Autogenous tissue reconstruction is the method of choice in infection of autogenous tissue reconstruction and can be applied in patients with an infected Dacron graft as well. In six patients with autogenous in situ repair, we used resorbable PGA sutures which develop fewer foreign body reactions (6) and may support a healing anastomosis of autogenous arterial substitutes in an infected field. However, not every segment of endarterectomized artery is suitable for transposition into an infected field (5), and experience in vascular surgery is obligatory to manage vascular infection. Although it remains a severe complication, there are reliable methods for repair to eliminate this "nightmare of a vasculaur surgeon".

Summary

Out of 2747 patients undergoing reconstructive vascular procedures, a total of 53 (1.9%) patients developed vascular infection. Forty-four (1.6%) occurred early within a 6-week postoperative period; nine (0.3%) were seen later from 6 weeks to 8 years after reconstruction. Until 1974, prophylactic antibiotics were used in most of the patients; since that time, only patients with gangrene and positive culture received antibiotics. Out of 1823 autogenous reconstructions, 0.1% became infected primarily, while in the group of 924 patients with a prosthetic arterial substitute the primary infection rate was 1.5%. The same difference was true in patients with early redo operations. One hundred and sixty-seven (9.2%) patients of the autogenous group had to be reoperated because of hematoma, bleeding, or thrombosis causing an arterial infection rate of 3.6%. In the prosthetic group, 96 (10.4%) patients required early redo surgery and 34% became infected. The total incidence of vascular infection was 0.4% in the autogenous and 5% in the prosthetic group.

Regarding the experience of the institution, three time periods (1970-1974, 1975-1977, 1978-1980) were compared. In patients undergoing aortoiliofemoral graft procedures, the primary infection rate decreased from 1% to 0.7%, the total infection rate from 4.3% to 3.5%.

A total of 67 patients with arterial infections has been observed, 53 out of our own material and 14 admitted for management of graft infection from other hospitals. Local care (eight patients) resulted in 100% mortality rate. Ligation and/or excision of the graft with antiseptic irrigation resulted in 40% (6/15) death rate and a 30% (6/20) amputation rate.

From our experience, two methods can be recommended for management of graft infection: extraanatomical bypass with removal of the infected part of the prosthesis performed simultaneously or autogenous tissue repair. The former was followed by a 11% (4/36) mortality rate and a 6% (4/62) amputation rate, the latter 13% (2/15) mortality rate and 12% (2/17) amputation rate. The material was analyzed in detail to evaluate factors influencing the rate of infection. More progress has been made in the management of graft infection than in prevention of that complication.

References

1. Brewster DC, Darling RC (1978) Optimal methods of aortoiliac reconstruction. Surgery 84:739
2. Ehrenfeld WK, Wilbur BG, Olcott CN, Stoney RJ (1979) Autogenous tissue reconstruction in the management of infected prosthetic grafts. Surgery 85:82
3. Fry WJ, Lindenauer SM (1967) Infection complicating the use of plastic arterial implants. Arch Surg 94:600
4. Hoffert P, Gensler S, Haimovici H (1965) Infection complicating arterial grafts. Arch Surg 90:472
5. Sandmann W, Lerut J (to be published) Autogenous grafts and absorbable suture material in management of arterial infection.
6. Sandmann W, Wildeshaus KH, Lenz P, Kremer K, Peronneau P (1979) Gefäßnähte mit resorbierbarem Nahtmaterial: röntgenologische, hämodynamische, licht- und elektronenmikroskopische Befunde. Langenbecks Arch Chir [Suppl]:1
7. Sandmann W, Kremer K, Staskiewicz V, Lerut J, Kaschner A (1979) New aspects for prophylactic and therapeutic proceedings in vascular infections. Angio 1:38
8. Van Dongen RJAM (1976) Septic complications in vascular surgery: operative treatment and results. Langenbecks Arch Chir 342:511
9. Vollmar J, Buettner-Ristow A (1976) Diagnostic and clinical aspects of septic complications in vascular surgery. Langenbecks Arch Chir 342:505

Session X Cardiac Surgery

Cardiac Forum II

Chairman: M. E. M. Macedo, Lisbon; Co-Chairman: P. Satter, Frankfurt

Comparative Hemodynamic Results of Medical and Surgical Therapy in Patients With Hypertrophic Obstructive Cardiomyopathy

B. Lösse, H. Krönert, D. Rafflenbeul, H. Kuhn, H. D. Schulte, and F. Loogen*

Considerable long-term experience in the treatment of hypertrophic obstructive cardiomyopathy (HOCM) has been sampled with two therapeutic procedures, i.e., the medical treatment with beta-blocking agents and the surgical approach consisting in ventricular septal myotomy and myectomy. Whereas the effects of both procedures on clinical status and resting hemodynamics of the left ventricle are well documented (1, 3-6, 8-10, 12-15), there is only little information available concerning the long-term effects on circulatory function during exercise (2, 3, 7, 11, 15). We have, therefore, compared the influence of medical and surgical therapy on several important circulatory parameters at rest and during maximal exercise.

Patients and Methods

The study consists of 25 patients. The diagnosis of HOCM had been confirmed by heart catheterization and left ventricular angiography in all patients. Twelve patients (six males, six females, mean age 40.3 ± 8.5 years) were treated with daily doses of 120 to 360 mg (mean 205 ± 70 mg) propranolol. The dose of the drug was adjusted to achieve a resting heart rate between 50 and 60 beats per minute. Thirteen patients (ten males, three females, mean age 38.9 ± 9.0 years) underwent transaortal subvalvular septal myectomy (10). All of them had been pretreated with propranolol without satisfactory results.

Exercise measurements were performed in supine position on a bicycle ergometer with increasing work loads being terminated by angina, dyspnea, or exhaustion. Pulmonary artery pressure, oxygen consumption, and arteriovenous oxygen difference were directly measured, enabling the calculation of cardiac output according to the Fick principle. Stroke volume was derived from cardiac output and heart rate. The exercise studies were performed in the medically treated group immediately before and after a propranolol therapy of 1 to 7 (mean 3) months duration, in the surgically treated group 1 week to 28 months (mean 7.5 months) before and 3 weeks to 35 months (mean 10 months) after surgery. Propranolol therapy had been finished in the surgically treated group at least 3 days (in most cases several weeks) before the preoperative exercise test in all patients except two who received 160 and 240 mg propranolol, respectively. At the postoperative study, six of the 13 operated patients were under sustained beta-blocking therapy with 30 to 120 mg propranolol because of rhythm disturbances or tachycardia observed in the immediate postoperative period.

*Med. Klinik B der Universität, Moorenstr. 5, D-4000 Duesseldorf

Results

Table 1 demonstrates that both the medically and the surgically treated groups were of comparable age. Likewise, there were no significant differences in heart catheterization data, though the subsequently operated patients initially expressed a tendency to higher values of left ventricular end-diastolic pressure and of left ventricular outflow tract gradient. On the other side, the surgically treated patients initially achieved lower maximal exercise loads than the medically treated patients. This was, in part, responsible for the lower maximal values of heart rate and cardiac index in the surgical group. The lower maximal cardiac index in this latter group, however, was additionally caused by a lower stroke volume during maximal exercise. Despite the lower maximal work load and the lower cardiac index, surgically treated patients initially exhibited a more pronounced pathologic increase in pulmonary artery pressure during maximal exercise than the medically treated patients.

Table 1. Initial heart catheterization and exercise hemodynamic data in 25 patients with hypertrophic obstructive cardiomyopathy subsequently treated with propranolol (n = 12) or septal myectomy (n = 13). Note that in the surgically treated group the exercise hemodynamic parameters were measured at a lower maximal work load than in the propranolol group. EDP_{LV} = left ventricular end-diastolic pressure, syst. P_{LV} = systolic left ventricular outflow tract gradient at rest and at post-extrasystolic provocation, HR = heart rate, SVI = stroke volume index, CI = cardiac index, $\bar{P}_{PA}$ = mean pulmonary artery pressure. Statistical comparisons were made by use of Student's t test for unpaired data

		Propranolol (n = 12)	Myectomy (n = 13)	p
Age	(years)	40.3 ± 8.5	38.9 ± 9.0	n.s.
EDP_{LV}	(mm Hg)	16.1 ± 7.5	18.8 ± 7.5	n.s.
Syst. P_{LV} rest	(mm Hg)	40.9 ± 34.6	65.3 ± 39.4	n.s.
post-ES	(mm Hg)	120.0 ± 41.9	130.5 ± 27.0	n.s.
Max. working capacity	(watts)	72.7 ± 28.4	59.6 ± 16.3	n.s.
HR (at max. exercise)	(min^{-1})	140.9 ± 23.6	118.2 ± 19.0	<0.025
SVI (at max. exercise)	($ml \cdot m^{-2}$)	51.3 ± 9.8	44.7 ± 11.0	n.s.
CI (at max. exercise)	($l \cdot min^{-1} \cdot m^{-2}$)	7.27 ± 2.12	5.26 ± 1.61	<0.025
$\bar{P}_{PA}$ (at max. exercise)	(mm Hg)	37.7 ± 11.3	45.8 ± 13.8	n.s.

All these findings express a somewhat stronger hemodynamic impairment of the subsequently operated patients. This is reflected in the initial functional classification, too (Fig. 1). Three of the medically treated patients initially belonged to NYHA class II, the majority of nine patients to class III. In the surgically treated group, initially only one patient was of class II, ten patients belonged to class

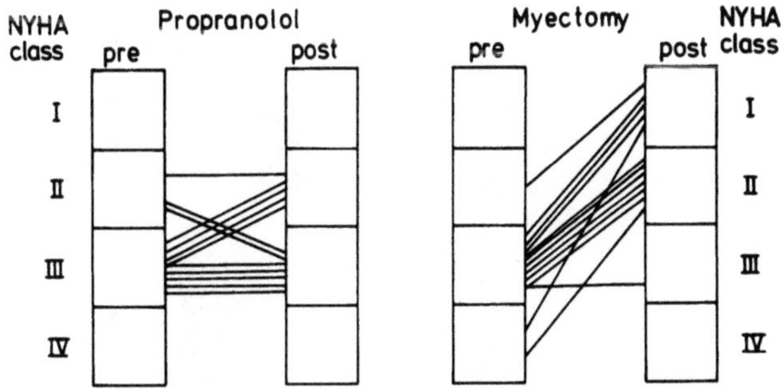

Fig. 1. Clinical classification of 25 patients with hypertrophic obstructive cardiomyopathy before and after medical therapy (propranolol, n = 12) or surgical therapy (myectomy, n = 13)

III, and two patients to class IV. After medical therapy, six of the 12 patients remained in the same functional class (Fig. 1). Only four patients improved by one class, whereas two patients deteriorated by one class. Concomitantly, the maximal exercise capacity was, on an average, not changed in this group (72.7 ± 28.4 watts before treatment, 72.9 ± 24.9 watts after treatment). In contrast, 12 of the 13 operated patients improved, seven of them by one class, four by two classes, and one by three classes. Only one patient remained unchanged and no patient deteriorated. This was accompanied by a significant increase in maximal exercise capacity from an average of 59.6 ± 16.3 watts before to 80.8 ± 20.8 watts after surgical therapy ($p < 0.005$).

The hemodynamic changes induced by the two different therapeutic procedures are illustrated for the individual patients in Figure 2 and summarized for both patient groups in Table 2. As intended, propranolol induced a significant decrease in heart rate. Since stroke volume, despite marked individual differences, on an average did not show a significant change, this was accompanied by a significant decrease in cardiac output. Despite this decrease in cardiac output, mean pulmonary artery pressure was, however, not lowered but tended in most patients, especially during exercise, to yet higher values. Myectomy induced, in contrast, no change in heart rate. Stroke volume could be increased during exercise significantly better than before operation. Consequently, cardiac index tended to higher values, too. This increase would probably have been more significant if not six patients, versus two at the preoperative test, had received propranolol at the postoperative measurement. Despite these concomitant increases in cardiac output, most patients exhibited substantial decreases in mean pulmonary artery pressure, averaging 3.8 mm Hg at rest and 12.7 mm Hg during exercise.

Discussion

Both therapeutic procedures used in this study have the same aim, i.e., the reduction or abolition of the left ventricular outflow tract obstruction. Propranolol is thought to reach this aim by its negative inotropic action. In fact, acute administration of propranolol or other beta-blocking agents has been shown to diminish left ventricular outflow tract pressure gradients (4, 15). But it has been shown, too, that this reduction in outflow tract obstruction persisted in only some patients during sustained propranolol therapy (5, 8, 15). Further-

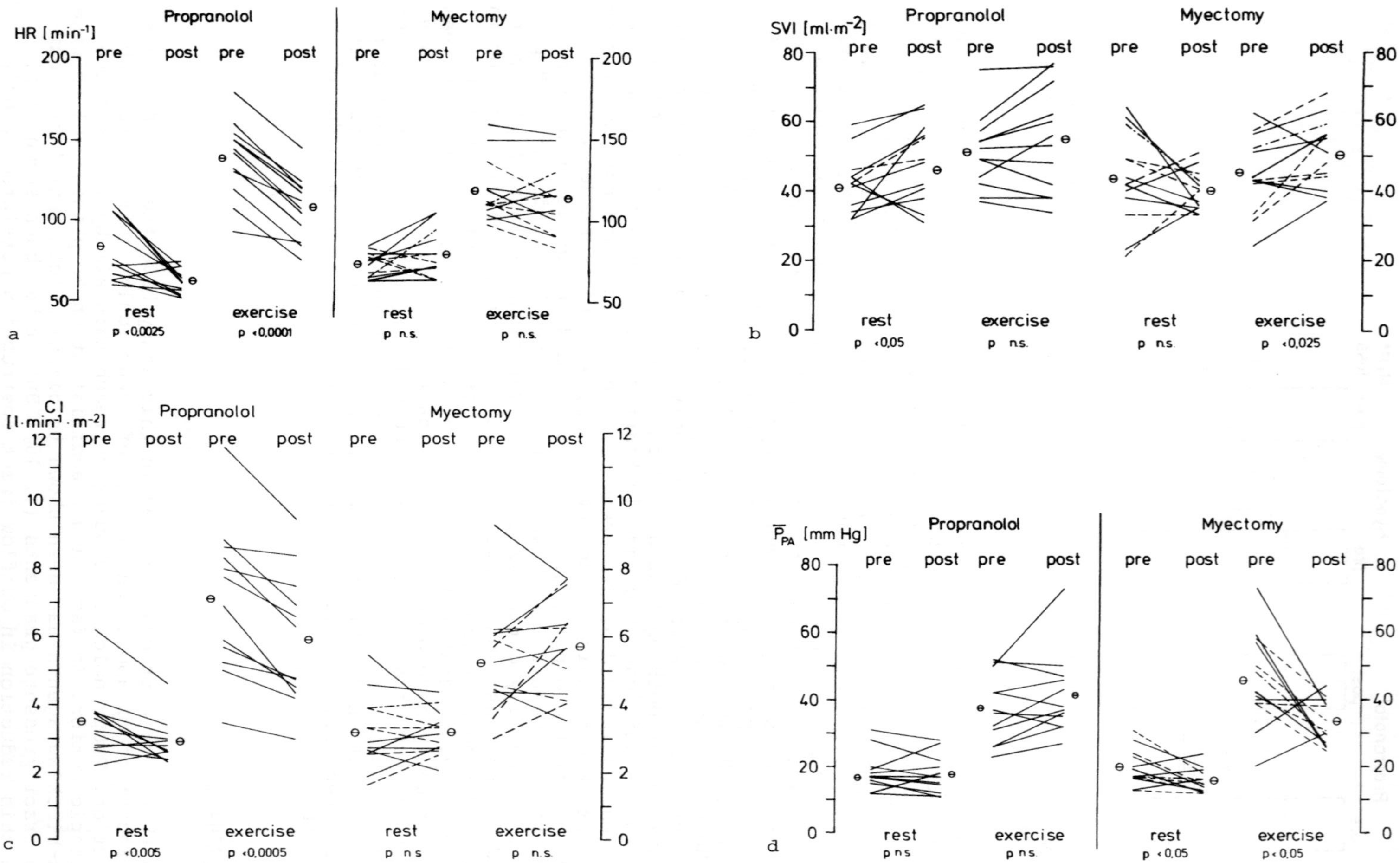

a
HR [min⁻¹]
Propranolol
Myectomy
pre
post
200
150
100
50
rest
p <0,0025
exercise
p <0,0001
rest
p n.s.
exercise
p n.s.
b
SVI [ml·m⁻²]
80
60
40
20
0
rest
p <0,05
exercise
p n.s.
rest
p n.s.
exercise
p <0,025
c
CI [l·min⁻¹·m⁻²]
12
10
8
6
4
2
0
rest
p <0,005
exercise
p <0,0005
rest
p n s
exercise
p n.s.
d
P̄PA [mm Hg]
80
60
40
20
0
rest
p n s
exercise
p n s
rest
p < 0,05
exercise
p < 0,05

Fig. 2 a-d

more, it could be demonstrated that the left ventricular end-diastolic pressure showed in most patients a further gradual rise despite sustained propranolol administration (8, 15). This was associated with the observation that the exercise tolerance of the patients usually remained unchanged or gradually further deteriorated (3).

The results of our study support the disappointing experiences with long-term beta-blocking treatment. As the only favorable result, we found a symptomatic improvement in four of 12 patients (i.e., 33%) consisting mainly in the reduction of palpitations which could be attributed to the reduction in heart rate. Circulatory parameters, however, did not improve. Due to the reduced left ventricular compliance, patients with HOCM are not able to increase stroke volume as normal persons do. The necessary increase in cardiac output during exercise is nearly exclusively reached by increasing the heart rate. But just this compensatory mechanism is disturbed by propranolol. Our results demonstrate that this rate dependent decrease in cardiac output invariably occurred in all propranolol treated patients irrespective of the initial cardiac output. If the initial cardiac output was high, this decrease had not much effect on exercise tolerance. Due to reduced subjective symptoms (palpitations, etc.), some of these patients reached even higher exercise levels than before therapy. With initially depressed cardiac output values, however, the further drug-induced decrease was of disadvantage and reduced the exercise capacity significantly. Another disadvantageous consequence of propranolol was the tendency of further rises in pulmonary artery pressure which occurred in spite of the fall in cardiac output.

The surgical approach directly reduces or abolishes the left ventricular outflow tract obstruction in nearly all patients (1, 2, 8, 9 - 15) by widening the left ventricular outflow tract through septal myotomy-myectomy. Furthermore, an improved ventricular compliance may be achieved at least in the septal area. Our results demonstrate that the operation results in significantly more favorable effects on clinical symptomatology, circulatory function, and exercise tolerance. Of special importance was the significant rise in stroke volume during exercise and the significant decrease in pulmonary artery pressure at rest and during exercise. The increase in cardiac output would have been more significant if not several patients would have been under sustained propranolol therapy at the postoperative measurement. Concomitant with these favorable effects and in contrast to medical therapy, exercise tolerance of the patients was significantly increased.

Earlier studies have demonstrated that the operation-induced reduction of the left ventricular outflow tract obstruction and the symptomatic improvement persist in the majority of patients over considerable average follow-up periods of up to more than 5 years (8-10), in individual observations up to 17 years (9). It may be assumed that the hemodynamic improvements may equally persist, but corresponding long-term observations are missing.

Operative mortality has been reduced with increasing surgical experience. In recent statistics including 30 to 124 patients, mortality rates of 0 to 8% have been reported (9, 12, 13). In our most recent series of 51 patients operated upon during 1976 and 1979, two patients (4%) have died.

<u>Fig. 2a-d.</u> Hemodynamic data at rest and during exercise at identical levels in the pre- and postoperative test (68.8 ± 26.4 watts in 12 propranolol treated patients, 57.7 ± 15.8 watts in 13 surgically treated patients). <u>a</u> Heart rate (HR), <u>b</u> stroke volume index (SVI), <u>c</u> cardiac index (CI), <u>d</u> mean pulmonary artery pressure ($\bar{P}_{PA}$). – – – – – = preoperatively no drug, postoperatively propranolol; — · — · — = preoperatively propranolol, postoperatively no drug. Statistical comparisons were made using the two-tailed Student's test for paired data

Table 2. Hemodynamic findings ($\bar{x} \pm s$) before and after therapy with propranolol (n = 12) or subvalvular septal myectomy (n = 13) in 25 patients with hypertrophic obstructive cardiomyopathy. HR = heart rate, SVI = stroke volume index, CI = cardiac index, $\bar{P}_{PA}$ = mean pulmonary artery pressure, p = error probability in Student's t test for paired data. The exercise values were measured at identical exercise levels averaging 68.8 ± 26.4 watts in the propranolol treated patients and 57.7 ± 15.8 watts in the operated patients

		Propranolol (n = 12)				Myectomy (n = 13)			
		pre	post	change	p	pre	post	change	p
HR	rest	83.7 ± 21.2	62.5 ± 6.9	-25.3%	<0.0025	73.7 ± 7.9	79.6 ± 14.7	+ 8.0%	n.s.
[min^{-1}]	exercise	138.3 ± 23.8	107.9 ± 19.4	-22.0%	<0.0001	118.2 ± 19.0	113.8 ± 21.2	- 3.7%	n.s.
SVI	rest	40.7 ± 6.9	45.7 ± 10.3	+12.3%	<0.05	43.5 ± 13.3	39.9 ± 5.8	- 8.3%	n.s.
[$ml \cdot m^{-2}$]	exercise	50.9 ± 10.5	54.7 ± 15.2	+ 7.5%	n.s.	44.7 ± 11.0	50.6 ± 10.1	+13.2%	<0.025
CI	rest	3.50 ± 1.02	2.91 ± 0.63	-16.9%	<0.005	3.18 ± 1.07	3.17 ± 0.66	- 0.3%	n.s.
[$l \cdot min^{-1} \cdot m^{-2}$]	exercise	7.12 ± 2.20	5.91 ± 1.94	-17.0%	<0.0005	5.26 ± 1.61	5.73 ± 1.45	+ 8.9%	n.s.
$\bar{P}_{PA}$	rest	17.7 ± 4.9	17.8 ± 5.7	+ 0.6%	n.s.	19.7 ± 5.4	15.9 ± 3.5	-19.3%	<0.05
[mm Hg]	exercise	37.3 ± 10.2	41.3 ± 12.1	+10.2%	n.s.	45.9 ± 13.8	33.2 ± 6.6	-27.7%	<0.05

Considering the significantly better symptomatic and functional results as well as the reduced operative risk, surgical therapy should be taken into consideration earlier and not be confined to only the most severely ill patients of functional class IV.

Summary

Of 25 patients with hypertrophic obstructive cardiomyopathy, 12 were treated with propranolol (mean dosage 205 mg, mean duration 3 months) and 13 underwent transaortal septal myectomy. Based on clinical symptoms and measurements of heart rate, stroke volume, cardiac output, and mean pulmonary artery pressure, surgical therapy turned out superior to medical therapy concerning significant improvements in clinical symptoms and circulatory function.

References

1. Bigelow W, Trimble AS, Wigle D, Adelman AG, Felderhof C (1974) The treatment of muscular subaortic stenosis. J Thorac Cardiovasc Surg 68:384
2. Borer JS, Bacharach SL, Green MV, Kent KM, Rosing DR, Seides SF, Morrow AG, Epstein SE (1979) Effect of septal myotomy and myectomy on left ventricular systolic function at rest and during exercise in patients with IHSS. Circulation [Suppl 1] 60:82
3. Edwards RHT, Kristinsson A, Warrell DA, Goodwin JF (1970) Effects of propranolol on response to exercise in hypertrophic obstructive cardiomyopathy. Br Heart J 32:219
4. Flamm MD, Harrison DC, Hancock EW (1968) Muscular subaortic stenosis. Prevention of outflow obstruction with propranolol. Circulation 38:846
5. Frank MJ, Abdulla AM, Canedo MI, Saylors RE (1978) Long-term medical management of hypertrophic obstructive cardiomyopathy. Am J Cardiol 42:993
6. Kuhn H (1979) Hypertrophische obstruktive Kardiomyopathie. In: Bolte HD (ed) Therapie mit Beta-Rezeptorenblockern. Springer, Berlin Heidelberg New York, p 71
7. Lösse B, Kuhn H, Krönert H, Rafflenbeul D, Kirschner P, Schulte HD, Loogen F (1980) Hämodynamische Auswirkungen konservativer und operativer Therapie bei hypertrophischer obstruktiver Kardiomyopathie. Z Kardiol 69:470
8. Loogen F, Kuhn H, Krelhaus W (1978) Natural history of hypertrophic obstructive cardiomyopathy and the effect of therapy. In: Kaltenbach M, Loogen F, Olsen EGJ (eds) Cardiomyopathy and myocardial biopsy. Springer, Berlin Heidelberg New York, p 286
9. Maron BJ, Merrill WH, Freier PA, Kent KM, Epstein SE, Morrow AG (1978) Long-term clinical course and symptomatic status of patients after operation for hypertrophic subaortic stenosis. Circulation 57:1205
10. Morrow AG, Reitz BA, Epstein SE, Henry WL, Conkle DM, Itscoitz SB, Redwood DR (1975) Operative treatment in hypertrophic subaortic stenosis: Techniques and the results of pre- and postoperative assessments in 83 patients. Circulation 52:88
11. Redwood DR, Goldstein RE, Hirshfeld J, Borer JS, Morganroth J, Morrow AG, Epstein SE (1979) Exercise performance after septal myotomy and myectomy in patients with obstructive hypertrophic cardiomyopathy. Am J Cardiol 44:215
12. Reis RL, Hannah H, Carley JE, Pugh DM (1977) Surgical treatment of idiopathic hypertrophic subaortic stenosis (IHSS): Postoperative results in 30 patients following ventricular septal myotomy and myectomy (Morrow procedure). Circulation [Suppl 2] 56:128
13. Rothlin M, Arbenz U, Krayenbühl HP, Turina J, Senning A (1976) Spätresultate nach Operationen bei muskulärer subvalvulärer Aortenstenose. Z Kardiol 65:501

14. Shah PM, Adelman AG, Wigle ED, Gobel FL, Burchell HP, Hardarson T, Curiel R, de la Calzada C, Oakley CM, Goodwin JF (1974) The natural (and unnatural) history of hypertrophic obstructive cardiomyopathy, Circ Res [Suppl 2] 34/35:179
15. Stenson RE, Flamm MD, Harrison DC, Hancock EW (1973) Hypertrophic subaortic stenosis: Clinical and hemodynamic effects of long-term propranolol therapy. Am J Cardiol 31:763
16. Webb-Peploe M (1971) Management of hypertrophic obstructive cardiomyopathy by beta-blockade. In: Wolstenholme GEW, O'Connor M (eds) Hypertrophic obstructive cardiomyopathy. Ciba Foundation Study Group No. 37, London, p 103

Fibrin Glue for Treatment of Bleeding in Cardiac Surgery

A. Haverich and H. G. Borst*

Introduction

Bleeding control in surgery requires an intact physiological coagulation system with any method used. In open-heart surgery, however, the extracorporeal circulation with the need of heparinization, coagulation may be disturbed, especially after prolonged cardiopulmonary bypass. The drop of both the platelet count and the concentration of proteins like thrombin and fibrinogen may result in oozing and bleeding from the heart and great vessels which can be difficult to stop. In such cases it seems logical to apply a clotting-factor-containing biological tissue glue which has been already used successfully as a tissue adhesive in vascular, bone, and plastic surgery (1, 2).

Method and Application

The mechanism of glueing is an imitation of the final pathway in the physiological coagulation system (Fig. 1). Thus, the compounds needed are fibrinogen (Fibrin-Kleber) which is transferred into fibrin by adding calcium and thrombin (Topostasin). This initial fibrin formation is then stabilized by factor XIII (Fibrogammin); fibrinolysis is inhibited by ε-amino-capronic acid (ε-Aminocapronsäure).

For local application of the glue collagen fleece (Kollagen-Vlies) is used which has a certain hemostatic effect by itself activating platelet adhesivity at the bleeding site (3). The fibrinogen which can be stored at a temperature of -20°C for up to 6 months, has to be warmed to body temperature immediately before application. A small pledget of collagen fleece is soaked with the fibrinogen and is then placed onto the bleeding site which has been dried carefully. The activator solution containing thrombin, calcium, ε-amino capronic acid, and factor XIII is sprinkled onto the pledget. A dry sponge, a forceps, or any other suitable instrument is pressed onto the pledget for about 60 s. The whole procedure takes about 5 minutes.

*Klinik für Thorax-, Herz- und Gefäßchirurgie, Medizinische Hochschule Hannover, Karl-Wiechert-Allee 9, D-3000 Hannover 61

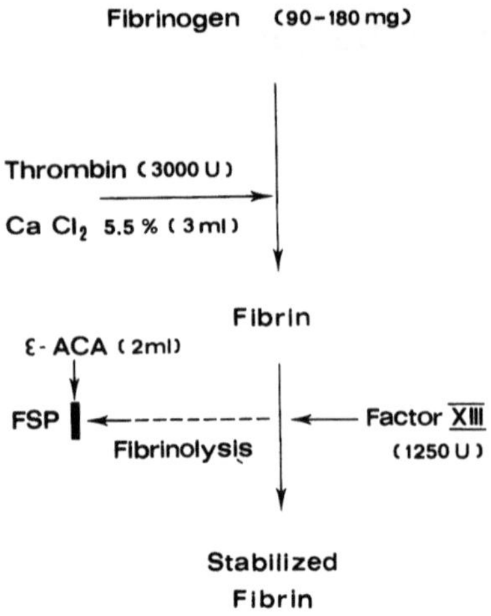

Fig. 1. Fibrin glue mechanism

Results

We have used the fibrin glue now in 68 cases of arterial bleeding sources, for example to secure bleeding from stitch holes and bleeding from coronary anastomoses (Table 1). Most cases of non-successful glueing were performed during the first 2 months after introduction of this method. The overall rate of successful glueing in this series was 86%, but now – after composition and concentration of the activator solution was adapted for use in cardiac surgery including extracorporeal circulation – we can secure bleeding from almost any arterial source of less than 1 mm^2 in size.

In a series of 26 cases of capillary and venous bleeding involving diffuse epi- and myocardial sources after reinterventions as well as epicardial venous bleeding near coronary anastomoses glueing was succesful, except for one right ventricular perforation which first was mistaken for a coronary vein hemorrhage (Table 2).

We have not seen any recurrent bleeding when fibrin glueing had secured bleeding in the first place. The fibrin glue was also found to be absolutely reliable for preclotting prostheses or stopping oozing from prosthetic fabric. It was used in eight patients undergoing combined aortic valve and ascending aorta replacement with optimal results.

Discussion

As outlined in the Introduction, conventional means of bleeding control, such as oxycellulose or microfibrillar collagen alone often are not effective in cardiac surgery of disturbed coagulation after cardiopulmonary bypass. This is caused by loss of clotting factors and platelets as well as a delayed re-establishment of physiological clotting times by adding protamine chloride after heparinization. Additional sutures, such as in coronary anastomoses, may be difficult or even dangerous, or may result in recurrent bleeding from stitch holes.

Table 1. Hemostasis by use of fibrin glue

Site (Arterial bleeding)		N	Successful Yes	Successful No
Asc. Aorta		39	32	7
Cannul.	18			
Aortotomy	14			
Prosthesis	3			
Patch	3			
Aortic root	1			
Coronary bypass anastomosis		26	23	3
Proximal	12			
Distal	14			
LV aneurysmect.		2	2	-
LV perforation		1	-	1
Total		68	57 (84%)	11

Table 2. Hemostasis by use of fibrin glue

Site (Venous bleeding)		N	Successful Yes	Successful No
Epicardial	17	21	20	1
Myocardial	4			(RV perf.)
RV patch		1	1	-
RA cannul.		1	1	-
LA cathet.		1	1	-
Liver decapsulation		2	2	-
Total		26	25 (96%)	1

In cases of diffuse epicardial bleeding in reinterventions, fibrin glueing offers the opportunity of atraumatic bleeding control covering large areas without the risk of damage to coronary vessels or the myocardium. Other methods to achieve hemostasis, such as laser, electric, or infra-red coagulation, do not exclude such risks. In our experience fibrin glueing is a superb method for stopping punctual or diffuse bleeding, particularly after prolonged extracorporeal circulation.

References

1. Stemberger A, Fritsche HM, Primbs P, Blümel G (1978) Fibrinogenkonzentrate und Kollagenschwämme zur Gewebeklebung. Med Welt 29:720-724
2. Pearl RM, Wustrack KO, Harbury C, Rubenstein E, Kaplan EN (1977) Microvascular anastomosis using a blood product sealant-adhesive. Gynecol Obstet Invest 144: 227-231
3. Abbott WM, Austen WG (1975) The effectiveness and mechanism of collagen-induced topical hemostasis. Surgery 78:723-729

Assessment of Right Ventricular Preservation During Cold Cardioplegic Arrest

M. V. Braimbridge and S. Canković-Darracott

Background

During the past 14 years at St. Thomas' Hospital, left ventricular biopsies taken routinely at surgery from 680 patients have been studied by cellular chemical methods. Cold cardioplegic arrest with the St. Thomas' solution was adopted as the method of myocardial protection 5 years ago.

Results obtained from the biopsies assisted in optimising the protective effects of cardioplegia in our hospital in two ways:
1) The cellular chemical results on the biopsies showed that patients in whom aortic clamp times exceeded 80 minutes with a single infusion of cardioplegic solution, showed a higher incidence of deterioration and postoperative low cardiac output than those with shorter aortic clamp times. Hourly infusion of the St. Thomas' cardioplegic solution resulted in good protection irrespective of the period of aortic clamping.
2) They showed that although the endocardial regions were now well preserved, the epicardium was at risk of damage due to inadequate cooling of the outer surface of the heart. The operative technique was modified to ensure efficient cooling of this region, and damage now occurs rarely.

If deterioration of the outer part of the left ventricle tended to occur with cardioplegia, it appeared to us likely that deterioration might well be occurring in the thinner right ventricle which was exposed to the warmth of the operating room lights and out of the pericardial cooling pool.

Having achieved consistently good left ventricular protection, we therefore became interested in comparing protection of the right ventricle in the same patients.

Material and Method

In 1975 in the initial series of patients undergoing surgery with St. Thomas' Hospital cardioplegia, no patient received special attention to right heart protection. An increased incidence of supraventricular dysrhythmia led to the addition to the protocol of right heart cooling. This was accomplished by laying the ventricular cooling catheter spraying 4°C Hartmann's solution over the right ventricle rather than the left, so that the cold fluid covered both. In addition an infant feeding catheter was inserted into the right atrium, isolated from the

*Heart Research (Surgical Cytochemistry), The Rayne Institute, St. Thomas' Hospital, London SE1, Great Britain

systemic circulation by establishing total bypass with caval snares, and 4°C Hartmann's solution run into that also. All biopsies discussed in this presentation were done with this protection.

Left and right ventricular biopsies have been obtained from 64 patients. The groups of patients were: mitral valve replacement (MVR) ± coronary artery bypass grafting (CABG) or tricuspid valvoplasty n = 9 (average duration of aortic occlusion 96 minutes); aortic valve replacement (AVR) n = 17 (average aortic occlusion 90 minutes); aortic and mitral valve replacement (A + MVR) n = 2 (average aortic occlusion 140 minutes); CABG n = 25 (average aortic occlusion 99 minutes); miscellaneous (atrial-septal defect, ventricular septal defect, subvalvar aortic stenosis, pulmonary valvotomy, Tetralogy of Fallot, patent ductus arteriosus + aneurysm) n = 11 (average aortic occlusion 74 minutes).

Full thickness core biopsies were obtained from the left and right ventricles by a Tru-cut biopsy needle and these were chilled by precipitate immersion in n-hexane at -70°C. The biopsies were then sectioned at 8 μm in a cryostat at -30°C and the cellular chemical assessments were completed within 3 h of the end of bypass.

Cytochemical Tests

1) Succinate dehydrogenase activity, a mitochondrial enzyme and marker of Krebs cycle activity. 2) Myosin adenosine triphosphatase activity. 3) The presence of unsaturated fatty acids of phospholipids, demonstrated by the acid haematein reaction. Semiquantitative gradings were ascribed to the activities of the three tests, 0 for the most normal appearance, 3 for the most abnormal, and 1 or 2 for intermediate responses.

Quantitative Polarization Microscopy

A freshly cut section was mounted and examined under a polarizing microscope. The birefringence of the muscle fibres was measured quantitatively by a rotating calibrated compensator. A drop of buffer containing ATP (2 mM) and calcium (0.036 M) was placed on the section causing an immediate increase in birefringence due to increased orientation of the myosin micelles. The birefringence of the same muscle of the fibres was measured again. The "incremental birefringence" of the muscle fibres, i.e. the change in birefringence in response to the addition of ATP and calcium was obtained by subtracting the values obtained in air from those obtained after the addition of ATP and calcium.

Experimental and clinical experience has shown that in healthy myocardium the response to ATP and calcium buffer is significantly higher than that of poorly functioning myocardium; these responses have been validated in bioptome biopsies obtained at cardiac catheterization which show a highly significant correlation with physiological measurements of function ($p < 0.001$). To assess the efficacy of myocardial protection during open-heart surgery, comparative biopsies were obtained from patients at the beginning and end of bypass and the cellular chemical gradings were compared in the two biopsies.

Results

Left Ventricular Protection

The results are shown in Table 1. Sixty-one patients (95.3%) had good left ventricular preservation; three showed deterioration in cellular chemical assessment during the bypass period and two of these had subsequent low cardiac output. The two patients with low cardiac output were both undergoing aortic valve replacement, and one of these had a grossly hypertrophied heart (LV 2 inches thick). One patient undergoing ASD closure showed LV deterioration after an aortic occlusion time of 29 minutes; no pericardial cooling was used in this patient, possibly accounting for the LV deterioration.

Table 1. Results

n = 64	Cellular chemical assessment				Postoperative cardiac output	
	LV Good	LV Deterioration	RV Good	RV Deterioration	Good	Low
MVR (n = 9)	9	0	9	0	9	0
AVR (n = 17)	15	2	16	1	15	2
A + MVR (n = 2)	2	0	0	2	2	0
CABG (n = 25)	25	0	23	2 1 temporary heart block	25	0
Miscellaneous (n = 11)	10	1	10	1	11	0

Right Ventricular Protection

Six patients showed right ventricular deterioration only during the bypass period. None had low cardiac output postoperatively. In one patient undergoing coronary artery bypass graft x 4, the right heart cooling catheter slipped out, accounting for the poor preservation. He had temporary heart block postoperatively. Both patients undergoing aortic and mitral valve replacement showed right ventricular deterioration; one had right coronary artery disease and therefore probably received inadequate infusions of the cardioplegic solution and thus inadequate protection during the bypass period.

Discussion

Previously protection of the left heart was the foremost concern. This has now been achieved and has resulted in a much reduced mortality, but morbidity from other problems has begun to appear. One of these is unexplained right heart failure with or without supraventricular dysrhythmias.

We have studied the incidence of right heart deterioration on cardiopulmonary bypass by selective biopsy of both ventricles and have shown that, in spite of maximal attempts at right heart cooling, both internally and externally, right ventricular deterioration still occurs even though the left ventricle has been protected. Chiu, Mulder, and Burgess in Montreal studied right ventricular haemodynamics following cardioplegic myocardial protection and showed deterioration in 25% of patients.

Therefore, right ventricular protection should not be neglected, particularly in patients with pulmonary hypertension or those with such poor myocardial function that the maintenance of sinus rhythm will make the difference between survival or death.

A Comparision Between Myocardial Protection With Nifedipine and Other Cardioplegic Techniques

O. Elert, J. Lang, P. Eigel, B. Kunkel, and S. Pomer

The currently available cardioplegic preparations may differ in their composition but they all have very similar modes of action. Practically all techniques involve infusion or perfusion methods. The ingredients of the solutions that are designed to protect the heart muscle are high potassium concentrations with or without calcium or sodium deprivation, or high concentrations of magnesium. Supplementary local anaesthetics (procaine, novocaine) block the cell membranes and thereby accelerate the paralysis of the heart and reduce the ischaemic cell oedema. They have dose-dependent toxic effects, however, and effect the lactate permeability of the cell membrane. In the future more complex constituents will be used as ingredients for cardioplegic preparations, so that such extreme unphysiological electrolyte concentrations will be avoided and the solution will be as similar in composition as possible to the extracellular fluid (1).

This report is concerned with the effect of a new cardioplegic substance that has a different mode of action. It does not rely on the alteration of the cation concentration in the cell membrane by removal or overloading of electrolytes in the way that traditional cardioplegic techniques do.

Calcium ions have been found to play a role in the excitation of the heart cell membranes and the activation of the contractile elements. As a result of this knowledge specialised slow channel calcium blockers have been experimentally tested as cardioplegic substances (2, 3). The studies described here were designed to investigate whether the electromechanical uncoupling action of calcium antagonists can effect an adequate and reversible heart paralysis under clinical conditions.

Material and Methods

Fourteen mongrel dogs weighing between 24 and 48 kg were anaesthetised with halothane-laughing gas and oxygen. The arterial pressure was measured continuously by means of a Statham element and pressure intensifier through the left femoral artery. The cardiac electrical activity was measured with the aid of an inserted electrode and displayed on an ECG monitor. Extracorporeal circulation was maintained via the right femoral artery and returned to the vena cavae by cannulating the right atrium. Steady state conditions were maintained for 10 minutes during partial bypass and then total bypass. The aorta ascendens was then clamped for 60 minutes at normal temperature and the various cardioplegic solutions were introduced into the root of the aorta using gravity as the only pressure source. The aorta clamp was removed after 60

*Chirurgische Universitätsklinik, Theodor-Stern-Kai, D-6000 Frankfurt/a.M.

minutes and in every case the extracorporeal circulation was stopped after a further 5-7 minutes.

Myocardial tissue of the left ventricle was removed from all dogs by means of a guide-puncture cannula in a modified frozen stop technique before cardiac arrest, during ischaemia and during reperfusion time. These tissues were analysed for the myocardial high energy phosphates, adenosine triphosphate and phosphocreatine, and for lactic acid. Tissue samples of all layers of the left ventricular apex were also removed at the times stated above for examination under the electron microscope.

Three cardioplegic techniques were used as follows:

Group 1. Calcium antagonist and normothermia

Perfusion of 40 ml NaCl and nifedipine* (15 µg/kg) into the coronary arteries; n = 4.

Group 2. Cardioplegic solution and normothermia

Perfusion of 400-500 ml into the coronary arteries: 5.8% hydroxyethyl starch with:

magnesium aspartate	1.47	g/1000 ml
potassium chloride	0.37	
calcium chloride	0.07	
procain HCI	1.10	
mannite	35.36	
sodium bicarbonate	20.00	mval/l

pH 7.2 - 7.4, osmolarity 310 mosmol; n = 6.

Group 3. Combination of the cardioplegia of groups 1 and 2, normothermia

Perfusion of 400-500 ml into the coronary arteries: nifedipine* (15 µ/kg) in 5.8% hydroxyethyl starch with:

magnesium aspartate	1.47	g/1000 ml
potassium chloride	0.37	
calcium chloride	0.07	
procain HCI	1.10	
mannite	35.36	
sodium bicarbonate	20.00	mval/l

pH 7.2 - 7.4; osmolarity 310 mosmol.

Results

The hearts of all experimental groups were mechanically paralysed during the initial 2 minutes. Group 1 (nifedipine alone) required the least time. In groups 2 and 3 the electrical activity disappeared at the same time as the mechanical activity. In contrast, the hearts of group 1 remained unchanged in their electrical atrial and ventricular complexes at the time of mechanical arrest and thereafter only slowly approached the base line. 15 µg/kg nifedipine was sufficient to prevent electrical and mechanical activity of the myocardium during the 60-minute period of cardiac arrest.

All hearts reactivated once the aorta was reopened by removing the aortic clamp but showed different reactions: Whereas the hearts of group 1 became electrically and mechanically active immediately after the coronary blood reperfusion, the same phenomenon was observed with the group 2 2 minutes later and with the group 3 another 2 minutes later.

*BAYER, Leverkusen, FRG

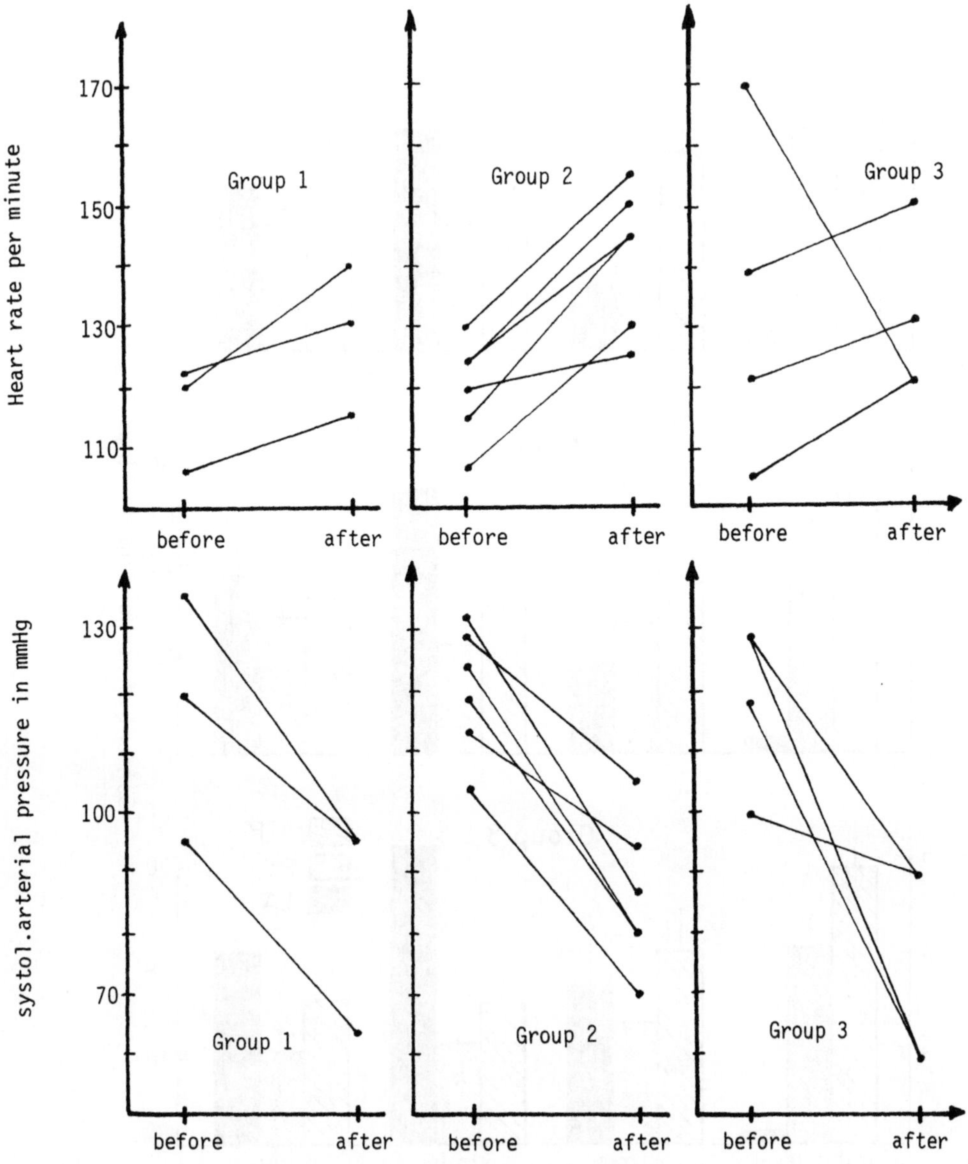

Fig. 1. Hemodynamics before and after a 60-minute cardioplegic cardiac arrest normothermia. Heart rate and systolic arterial pressure before clamping of the aorta and 10 minutes after release of the blood flow into the coronary artery. Normothermic ischaemia of 60 minutes in all three groups

Figure 1 illustrates the changes of the heart rate and arterial pressure before the ischaemia and after the termination of the extracorporeal circulation with a reperfusion of 10 minutes duration.

The phosphoadenylic acid cycle substrates (adenosine triphosphate and phosphocreatine) and the final product of anaerobic glycolysis (lactic acid) had similar acitivity curves in all cases (Fig. 2). The only obvious differences were the somewhat smaller drop in high energy phosphate levels in group 1 as compared to groups 2 and 3, and the

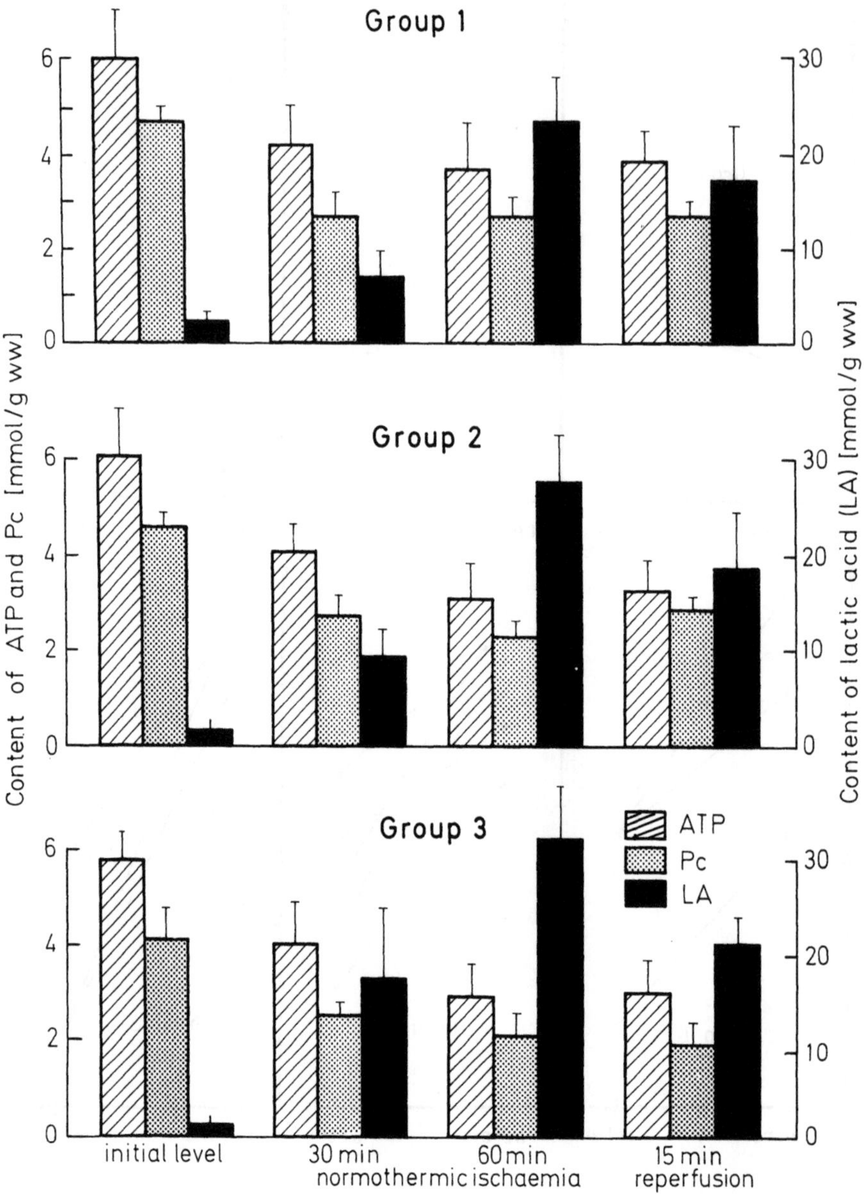

Fig. 2. Change in metabolic parameters during different cardioplegic procedures. Specimens of myocardial tissue were taken at the beginning and during a 1-hour period of normothermic arrest and during the reperfusion phase

significantly lower accumulation of lactic acid after 60 minutes of normothermic ischaemia in the presence of the nifedipine cardioplegic solution. These differences are no longer detectable in the early reperfusion phase, 10-15 minutes after release of the aortic clamp.

Electron Microscopic Alterations

Swollen cells, widened intracellular spaces, and disrupted mitochondrial cristae can be seen in all samples of the left ventricular apex (Fig. 3). After coronary occlusion of 60 minutes and whole blood reperfusion of 10 minutes duration, more marked reversible ischaemic damage to the myocardium can be demonstrated in group 2: The increase of the previously described alterations of the mitochondrial and cell separation from each other at the intercalated disc. The cell damages are even more pronounced in group 3: In one dog of this group irreversible ischaemic destruction is seen. The ischaemic alterations in group 1 disappear subsequent to 10 minutes blood reperfusion of myocardium, leaving well-preserved cell morphology, mitochondrial cristae being slightly disrupted, the cell membrane intact.

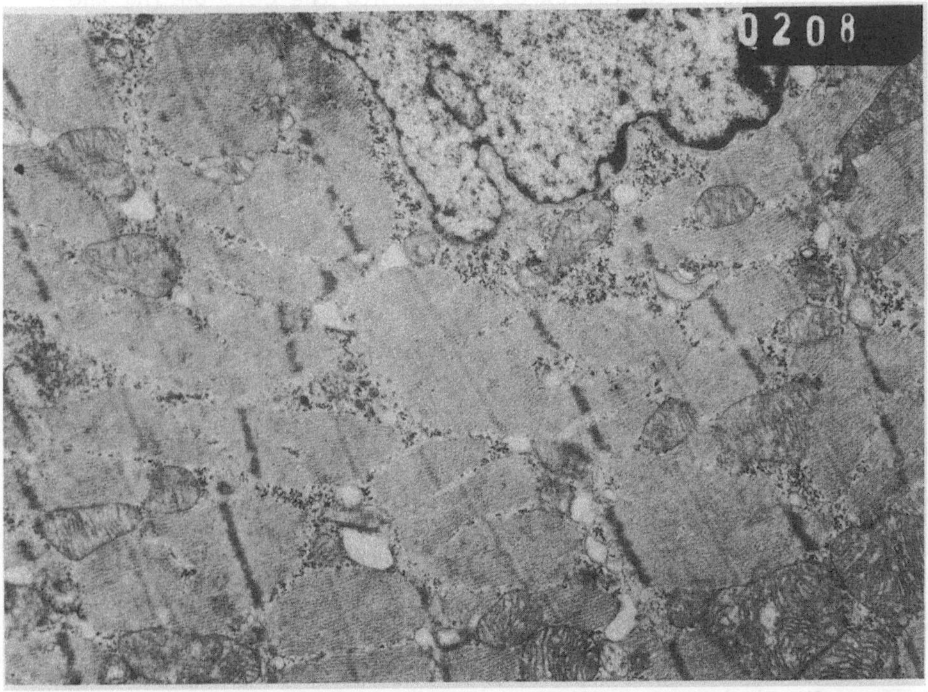

Fig. 3. Left ventricular myocardium after ischaemic arrest with normothermia and nifedipine (original magnification 15 000)

Discussion

These investigations show that nifedipine, when administered in the described dosage, effects a prompt cardiac paralysis and represents a useful drug for protection of heart muscle during normothermic ischaemia. In addition, this calcium blocking agent could effect a reduction in energy by inhibiting contractility (4) and also increase the ischaemic tolerance of the myocardium. There is, however, no advantage with respect to levels of energy phosphates during the ischaemic phase.

ATP und PC are reduced by the same amount in all three groups. This amounts to 40%-50% of the initial values determined prior to the 60-minute normothermic ischaemia. The accumulation of lactic acid as a result of long-term anoxia is increased by the supplementary use of procaine (groups 1 and 2 twelvefold, group 3 sixteenfold).

During the early reperfusion phase, 15 minutes after reopening the aorta or, in other words, at the point where the heart has completely reassumed the pumping work, the high-energy phosphates show a tendency to reaccumulate in groups 1 and 2. The highly potent calcium blocker nifedipine (5) really succeeds as a protective compound during this post-ischaemic phase. It must be remembered that the overloading of the heart muscle cell with uncontrollable, high extracellular calcium concentrations leads to metabolic and mechanical disturbances (6-8). The post-ischaemic lesions in the cell which are caused by an increased calcium influx and result from permeability changes are revealed in the form of distended mitochondria and the formation of vacuoles. An outcome of this is the inhibition of phosphorylation (9). The combination of the increased influx of water into the cell during the post-ischaemic phase and the high calcium influx leads to a more or less complete loss of function in the muscle cells. The inhibition and interruption of the calcium overloading of the cell by nifedipine is demonstrated by the results of the electron microscopic study described in this report. The nifedipine-treated hearts display clearly reduced levels of cell distension as compared to groups 2 and 3. They also have an improved retention of mitochondrial inner structure.

References

1. Iynge P, Hearse DJ, Braimbridge MV (1977) Myocardial protection during ischemic cardiac arrest. J Thorac Cardiovasc Surg 73:848
2. Clark RC, Ferguson BT, West PN, Shuchleib RC, Henry PD (1977) Pharmacological preservation of the ischemic heart. Ann Thorac Surg 24:307-314
3. Magee PG, Flaherty JT, Bixler TJ, Glower D, Gardner TJ, Burkley BH, Gott VL (1979) Comparison of myocardial protection with nifedipine and potassium. Circulation 60:151-157
4. Fleckenstein A (1977) Specific pharmacology of calcium in myocardium, cardiac pacemakers, and vascular smooth muscle. Annu Rev Pharmacol Toxicol 17:149-166
5. Fleckenstein A, Tritthart H, Döring HJ, Byon YK (1972) Bay a 1040 — ein hochaktiver Ca^{++}-antagonistischer Inhibitor der elektro-medianischen Kopplungsprozesse im Warmblüter-Myokard. Arzneim Forsch 22:22-33
6. Fleckenstein A (1964) Die Bedeutung der energiereichen Phosphate für Kontraktilität und Tonus des Myocards. Verh Dtsch Ges Inn Med 70:81-99
7. Schildberg FW, Fleckenstein A (1965) Die Bedeutung der extrazellulären Calciumkonzentration für die Spaltung von energiereichem Phosphat in ruhendem und tätigem Myokardgewebe. Pfluegers Arch 283:137-150
8. Fleckenstein A (1963) Metabolic aspects of the excitation-contraction coupling in the cellular functions of membrane transport. In: Hoffmann JF (ed) Symp. Soc. Fen., Physiol. Woods Hole/Mass. Enlewood Cliffs, pp 71-93
9. Schaff HV, Dombroff R, Flaherty JT, Burkley BH, Hutchins GM, Goldman RA, Gott VL (1978) Effect of potassium cardioplegia on myocardial ischemia and post arrest ventricular function. Circulation 58:240

Effects of Intraaortic Ballon Counter Pulsation of Collateral Blood Flow and Infarct Size*

P. Walter, F. Lübbecke, K. Müller, G. Stämmler, W. Schaper, and F. Hehrlein**

The application of the intraaortic balloon counter pulsation (IABP) has become a standard therapy in patients with cardiogenic shock or in cases of low cardiac output postoperatively. Experimental results to show a reduction of the infarct size due to the IABP are contradictory (6, 9-12). The aim of this study is to find out if an acute evolving myocardial infarction can be reduced in size by the IABP.

Methods

In order to minimize interindividual variables of coronary circulation, two infarctions were produced in the same experimental animal of which one was treated with IABP; the other one was used as control under the same hemodynamic conditions. The following suppositions for the validity of this infarct size manipulation method must be fulfilled (8): Equal amount of myocardial oxygen consumption (MVO_2) of the heart at both infarctions, equal size of the occluded vessels, and spatial separation of the perfusion areas. These presumptions were fulfilled by eight mongrel dogs. The dogs were anesthetized (4), the chest was opened in the 4th left intercostal space. Two small- to medium-sized branches of the left anterior descending coronary artery (LAD) and the left circumflex coronary artery (LC) were selected, prepared, and tied with ligatures. A balloon catheter was introduced over the femoral artery to the left subclavian artery. Balloon counter pulsation was started using a Data Scope System 80 and set with pressure-hold-exhaust-logic. The following hemodynamic parameters were registered: The electrocardiogram (EKG), the pressure in the aorta, in the left ventricle and the dp/dt max. By running the IABP, the first vessel was occluded for 90 minutes. Occlusion of branches of the LAD and the LC were performed alternatively. Five minutes before and after reopening of the vessel, radioactive tracer microspheres (TM) were injected into the left atrium for measurement of the regional and collateral blood flow (2). After the opening of the vessel, the IABP was stopped. A 15-minute recovery period was instituted for occasional reflow arrhythmias. Then the second vessel was occluded for 90 minutes, TM were injected in the same manner.

Ninety minutes after reperfusion of the second artery, the dogs were killed by AC shock, the heart was excised, and the coronary arteries were ligated at the same level. The left coronary artery was cannulated and micronized barium sulphate suspended in gelatin solution was injected by increasing pressure (from 1000 to 2000 mm H_2O) into the

*represents part of a Doctor Thesis of F. Lübbecke

**Clinic Cardiovascular Surgery, J.-Liebig-University, Klinikstr. 29, D-6300 Gießen
Max-Planck-Institut, Sprudelhof 11, D-6350 Bad Nauheim

coronary artery. The perfusion areas were excised with a wide margin of normally perfused tissue. Both perfusion areas were then sliced perpendicular to the apex base axis and incubated in the 0.1 M phosphate buffer containing p-nitro blue tetrazolium and malate (5). After demarcation of the necrotic area, the slices were photographed on a color transparency film. Slice angiograms were made with a microfocus X-ray tube to determine the borders of the perfusion areas (3). Both angiogram and color transparency were projected over each other and the outlines of the borders of the perfusion area and of the unstained necrotic area were followed with a curser of a computer-coupled graphic tablet. The integrals of both areals were compared, i.e., the quotient infarct size over perfusion area was multiplied by 100 (7). The measured tissue TM concentration could be expressed as myocardial blood flow (ml/min/100 g tissue) (2). The oxygen consumption of the heart was calculated by the Bretschneider formula (1) using the above cited hemodynamic parameters.

Results

The effect of the IABP on the myocardial oxygen consumption as well as on hemodynamic parameters was tested before the occlusion of a coronary artery. The results are demonstrated in Figure 1. The MVO_2 was reduced from 9.4 ± 2.05 under control conditions to 7.7 ± 1.3 due to the effect of the IABP. This reduction was statistically significant $p < 0.05$. The decrease of the MVO_2 is mediated by a reduction of the heart rate of about 10 beats per minute. A decrease of the left ventricular systolic pressure (LVSP) could be observed from 133 ± 18 to 127 ± 16 mm Hg due to the IABP. The IABP caused a significant increase of the diastolic aortic pressure (DAP) from 106 ± 16 to 117 ± 14 ($p < 0.05$).

The regional myocardial blood flow under control conditions and under the effect of the IABP was measured. The results are demonstrated in Figure 2. Total regional and collateral blood flow in the subendo- and subepicardial layers during the IABP and under control conditions is summarized. There is no significantly different blood flow in the nonoccluded areas during both conditions (upper part of the figure). A significant increase of collateral blood flow into the subendocardium during IABP was measured ($p < 0.05$) (lower part of the figure).

The myocardial oxygen consumption, the dp/dt_{max}, the heart rate, the left ventricular systolic pressure (LVSP), the diastolic aortic pressure (DAP), and the left ventricular end-diastolic pressure (LVEDP) were measured continuously and are summarized in Figure 3. The MVO_2

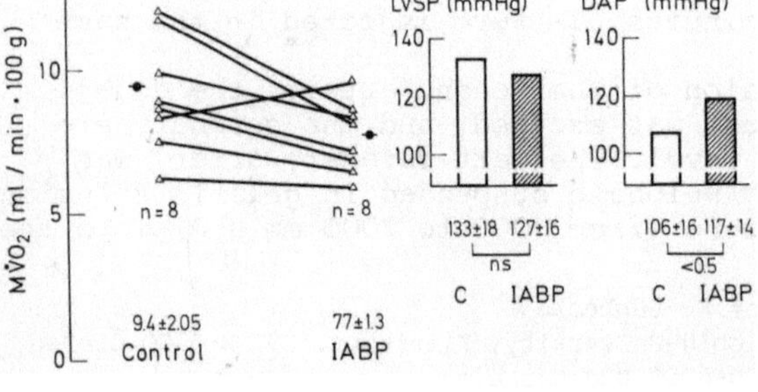

Fig. 1. Change of myocardial oxygen consumption (MVO_2), left ventricular systolic pressure (LVSP), and diastolic aortic pressure (DAP) under control and IABP condition before coronary artery occlusion

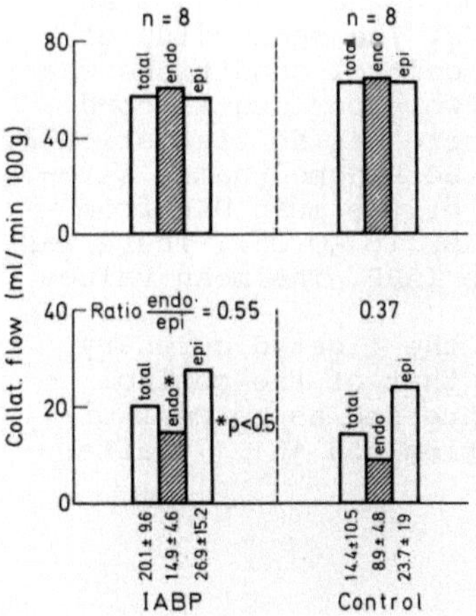

Fig. 2. Myocardial blood flow in the normal perfused myocardium (upper part) and collateral blood flow into ischemic myocardium (lower part) influenced by the IABP. Distinction between total, subendocardial, and subepicardial flow

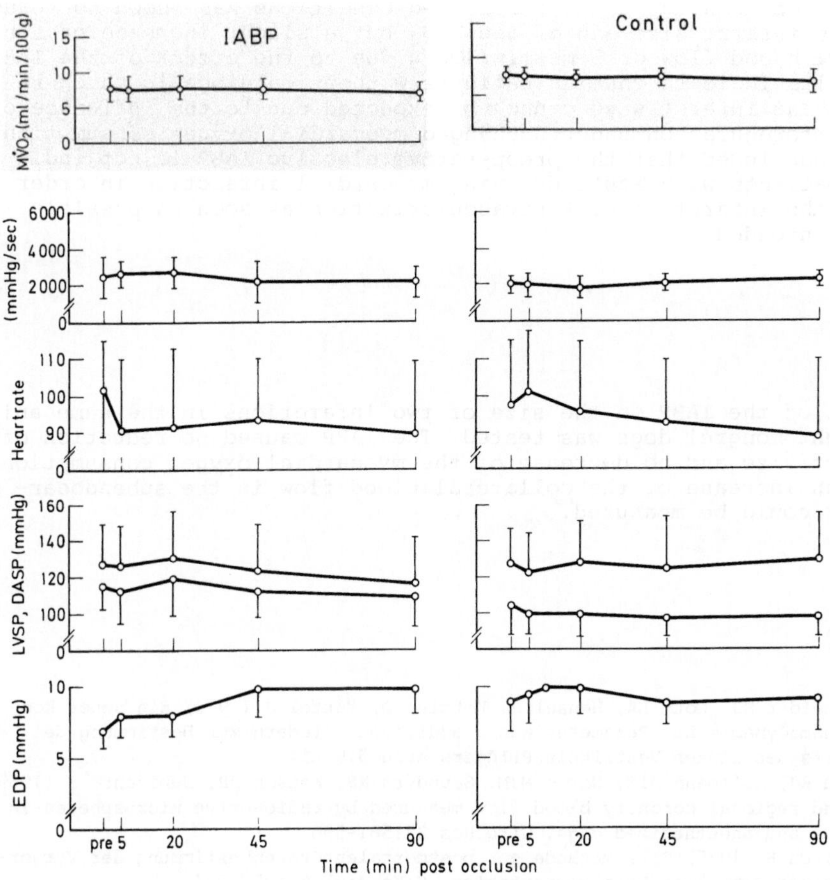

Fig. 3. Effect of IABP on myocardial oxygen consumption (MVO_2), dp/dt_{max} heart rate/ left ventricular systolic and end-diastolic pressure as well as diastolic aortic pressure during pre-occlusion and post-occlusion time

during the effect of the IABP was 7.8 ml/min/100 g whereas the mean MVO_2 during control condition was 7 ml/min/100 g. The mean value of dp/dt_{max} during IABP was 2490, the value under control conditions was 2135 mm Hg/s. The mean heart rate under these two experimental conditions was 94 and 95 beats/min, respectively. There was no statistically significant difference in the mean LVSP during both hemodynamic situations. The IABP caused a significant increase of the mean DAP from 106 mm Hg during control to 117 mm Hg during IABP ($p < 0.05$). There was no significant decrease of the LVEDP during the IABP. The mean values were 9.6 and 8.6 mm Hg, respectively.

The weight of myocardial tissue perfused by the ligated coronary artery in case of the IABP was 17.7 ± 6.3 g and that of the control condition was 15.6 ± 6.2 g. The infarct size expressed as percent of perfusion area was 18 ± 10% under control condition and 18 ± 17% after the application of the IABP.

Discussion

This experimental study under controlled conditions has shown no reduction of the infarct size and of the MVO_2 but a slight increase of subendocardial blood flow of 5 ml/min/100 g due to the effect of the IABP. These results indicate that in patients without cardiogenic shock reduction of the infarct size cannot be expected due to the influence of coronary autoregulation under unchanged myocardial oxygen consumption. It may be concluded that the preoperative elective IABP is not indicated in patients with acute evolving myocardial infarction in order to reduce the infarct size. A revascularization as soon as possible should be intended.

Summary

The effect of the IABP on the size of two infarctions in the same animal in eight mongrel dogs was tested. The IABP caused no reduction of the infarct size and no decrease of the myocardial oxygen consumption although an increase of the collateral blood flow in the subendocardial layer could be measured.

References

1. Bretschneider HJ, Gott LA, Hensel J, Kettler D, Martel J (1970) Ein neuer komplexer hämodynamischer Parameter aus 5 additiven Gliedern zur Bestimmung des O_2-Bedarfs des linken Ventrikels. Pflügers Arch 319:R14
2. Domenech RJ, Hoffmann JIE, Notle MJM, Saunders KB, Kenson JR, Subijanto S (1969) Total and regional coronary blood flow measured by radioactive microspheres in conscious and anesthetized dogs. Circ Res 25:581-596
3. Kalbfleisch H (1975) Eine Methode zur postmortalen Größenbestimmung der Versorgungsgebiete einzelner Herzkranzarterien. Z Kardiol 64:987-994
4. Kettler D, Cott I, Martel J, Bretschneider JJ (1970) Combination of Piritramide and N_2O, a new anesthetic method for studies of cardiovascular function in dogs. Pflügers Arch 319:R42

5. Nachlas MM, Schnitka DK (1963) Macroscopic identification of early myocardial infarcts by alterations in the hydrogenase activity. Am J Pathol 42:379-396
6. Powell WJ Jr, Dagget WH, Magro AE, Bianco JA, Buckley MJ, Sanders CA, Kantrowitz AR, Austen WG (1970) Effect of intra-aortic balloon counter pulsation on cardiac performance, oxygen consumption, and coronary blood flow in dogs. Circ Res 26: 753-764
7. Schaper W, Frencel M, Hort W (1979) Experimental coronary artery occlusion. I. Measurement of infarct size. Basic Res Cardiol 74:46-53
8. Schaper W, Hofmann M, Müller KD, Genth K, Carl M (1979) Experimental occlusion of two small coronary arteries in the same heart. A new validation method for infarct size manipulation. Basic Res Cardiol 74:224-229
9. Sugg WL, Webb WR, Ecker RR (1969) Reduction of extent of myocardial infarction by counter pulsation. Ann Thorac Surg 7:310-316
10. De Vivie ER (1975) Experimentelle Untersuchungen der intraaortalen Balloongegenpulsation bei verschiedenen Formen der Herzschädigung zur Frage des Wirkungsspektrums und der klinischen Indikation. Habilitationsschrift, University of Göttingen
11. Walter P, Flameng W, Seeger S, Mulch J (1975) Einfluß der intraaortalen Ballonpulsation auf die Umverteilung der Myokarddurchblutung bei Koronararterienstenose und Verschluß. Thoraxchirurgie 23:354-358
12. Wolner E (1972) Die mechanische Kreislaufunterstützung in Experiment und Klinik. Wien Klin Wochenschr [Suppl] 1:4-20

Cardiac Valve Replacement With Pericardial Xenograft

R. Deac, M. Liebhart, D. Bratu, S. Bradisteanu, and J. Benedek*

Clinical Material

From May 1977 to May 1980, 48 patients underwent cardiac valve replacement with Ionescu-Shiley pericardial xenograft (1-4). There were 20 males and 28 females with age range of 20 to 56 years; 38 patients were class III (NYHA), six class IV, and four class II. Mitral valve replacement was required in 33 patients; eight patients had isolated aortic valve replacement. Combined aortic-mitral valve replacement was required in seven patients (Table 1). The common indications of tissue valve were applied for use of pericardial xenograft: contraindications for anticoagulant treatment, women at child bearing age, difficulties in the control of chronic anticoagulant treatment (patient unreliability, occupational hazard).

Table 1. Heart valve replacement with Ionescu-Shiley pericardial xenograft

Valves replaced	No. of patients	Hospital deaths	Late death
Mitral	33	2	-
Aortic	8	-	-
Mitral and aortic	7	-	-
Total	48	2 (4.1%)	

Operative Techniques

Standard cardiopulmonary bypass at 25-30°C with disposable oxygenator was used with hemodilution, cold cardioplegia, and local cooling for myocardial protection. The valves were rinsed thoroughly in saline with special care to remove the formaldehyde solution from the suturing skirt. During the valve insertion in mitral position, a few technical precautions were taken to match the valve size to annulus and LV dimensions, to pull the valve up in LA following insertion, to avoid entrapment of the prongs by using continuous suture, and to place two prongs astride the LV outlet.

*Clinic for Cardiovascular Surgery, Institute of Medicine and Pharmacy, Mures Clinic Hospital, Tirgu-Mures, Romania

For mitral valve replacement, as shown in Table 1, the most common implantation diameters of the valve were 25 mm (14 patients) and 27 mm (21 patients). In three patients 29 mm valves were used; for aortic valve replacement, 21 mm and 23 mm (Table 2). For mitral valve replacement, continuous suture was used in 31 cases, interrupted in four, and mixed in three cases. For aortic valve replacement only interrupted sutures were employed (Table 3). Additional surgical procedures performed at the time of valve replacement are shown in Table 4. After the operation, measures to obtain the optimum cardiac output were ensured as well as measures to maintain an adequate gas-exchange/ventilation, acid-base balance, and fluid-electrolyte balance.

Table 2. Ionescu-Shiley pericardial xenograft (valve sizes)

Implantation diameter (mm)	21	23	25	27	29
Mitral	-	-	14	21	3
Aortic	7	7	-	-	1
Total	7	7	14	21	4

Table 3. Ionescu-Shiley pericardial xenograft (type of suture)

Valve replaced	Interrupted	Continuous	Mixed
Mitral	4	31	3
Aortic	15	-	-
Total	19	31	3

Table 4. Additional surgical procedures performed at the time of valve replacement

Procedure	Mitral	Aortic
Tricuspid annuloplasty	4	-
Aortic valvuloplasty	1	-
Total correction Fallot's tetralogy	-	1
Total	5	1

Results

In the group of 48 operated patients (Table 1), there was one operative death due to myocardial failure – a patient with a thrombosed Björk-Shiley valve operated upon as an emergency after cardiac arrest and resuscitation. This death could not be related to any valve abnormality. One hospital death occurred 2 months after operation with complications not related to the valve itself (the integrity of the valve was confirmed at postmortem examination). The hospital mortality was 4.1% (Table 1). All hospital survivors (46) were followed-up from 1 to 37 months after the operation (mean follow-up 12.2 months): 404 patients/months for mitral valve replacement; 95 patients/months for aortic valve replacement, and 75 patients/months for mitral and aortic valve replacement (Table 5). The majority of mitral patients were in class III before the operation and in class I after the operation (Table 6). In the aortic group before the operation, three patients were in class II, four patients in class III, and one in class IV. After the operation, all aortic patients were in class I. In the double valve group, there were six patients in class III before operation and one in class IV; after the operation, they were in classes I and II. The first 17 patients (15 mitrals, 13 in AF atrial fibrillation; one aortic, one mitral and aortic) were not anticoagulated but under chronic dipyridamole (Persantin) and aspirin treatment. There was one transient ischaemic episode of lower limb in this first group. The following 27 patients (16 mitrals, 11 in AF; seven aortics, six mitral and aortics – two in AF) were on anticoagulants (prothrombin depressant) for 6 weeks and chronic aspirin and dipyridamole treatment. Two patients with double valve replacement were on chronic anticoagulant treatment for mechanical valves (BS) in mitral position. No thromboembolic complications occurred in the second group of 29 patients. No valve thrombosis occurred in the entire group of patients (Table 7). There was no instance of valve failure or dysfunction (Table 8). No paravalvular leaks were noticed. Two patients with apical systolic murmur were fully reinvestigated but LV angiography showed competent mitral valves.

Table 5. Follow-up of 46 hospital survivors
(1 to 37 months, mean 12.2 months)

Valves replaced	Total months
Mitral	404
Aortic	95
Mitral and aortic	75
Total	574

Table 6. NYHA classification

Class	Mitral		Aortic		Mitral and aortic	
	Preop.	Postop.	Preop.	Postop.	Preop.	Postop.
I	-	25	-	8	-	3
II	1	5	3	-	-	4
III	28	1	4	-	6	-
IV	4	-	1	-	1	-
Total	33	31	8	8	7	7

Table 7. Embolism in 46 patients followed-up for 574 months

Treatment	No. of patients	Emboli
Dipyridamole and aspirin	17	1 (M) transient ischemic episode (lower limb)
Prothrombin depressant + dipyridamole + aspirin	29	-
for 6 weeks postop. 27		-
long-term 2		-
Absence of valve thrombosis		

Table 8. Complications in 48 patients with pericardial xenograft

Complication	Eearly	Late
Valve failure	-	-
Infective endocarditis	-	1
Paravalvular leak	-	-
Haemolysis	-	-

Conclusions

In our group of patients the pericardial xenograft proved to meet the expected advantages of low mortality and morbidity; very low embolic rate, limited anticoagulation; absence of valve thrombosis; and maintenance of structural and functional integrity over a period of more than 3 years. We consider the pericardial xenograft as the valve of choice for patients in whom anticoagulants are contraindicated and for patients with small aortic roots.

Addendum. Since May 1980, another ten patients were operated upon using pericardial xenograft valve (eight mitrals, one aortic, one mitral and aortic). From the first group of 48 patients, one mitral patient mentioned in Table 8 with endocarditis required reoperation. One late death occurred in the double-valve group also due to endocarditis. For the entire group of 58 patients, the hospital mortality is 3.4% and late mortality 1.7%.

Summary

Between May 1977 and May 1980, pericardial xenograft (Ionescu-Shiley valve) was used for cardiac valve replacement in 48 patients, 33 as single mitral, eight as single aortic, and seven as mitral and aortic valve replacement. The procedures were done in hypothermic cardiopulmonary bypass at 25°C with cold cardioplegia for myocardial protection. During the valve insertion, several precautions were taken: to match the valve size to LV dimensions, position the valve high up in the LA after suturing, use continuous suture to avoid entrapment of the prongs by isolated sutures and to place two prongs parallel to the outflow tract of the LV. There were one operative death due to myocardial failure and one hospital death with complications not related to the valve. The overall mortality was 4.1%. All 46 surviving patients were followed-up from 1 to 37 months after the operation. There was no late mortality. The first 17 patients were off anticoagulants with one transient ischemic attack; 29 patients were anticoagulated for 6 weeks after the operation with prothrombin depressant. No thromboembolic complications were noticed in this group. There was no instance of valve failure or valve dysfunction. One case had late endocarditis. In our group of patients the pericardial xenograft as cardiac valve replacement proved to meet the expected advantages, low valve related complications, up to 37 months of follow-up.

References

1. Ionescu IM, Tandon AP, Mary DAS, Abid A (1977) Heart valve replacement with the Ionescu-Shiley pericardial xenograft. J Thorac Cardiovasc Surg 73:31-42
2. Tandon AP, Smith DR, Mary DAS, Ionescu IM (1977) Sequential hemodynamic studies in patients having aortic valve replacement with the Ionescu-Shiley pericardial xenograft. Ann Thorac Surg 24:149-155
3. Tandon AP, Smith DR, Whitaker W, Ionescu IM (1978) Long-term haemodynamic evaluation of aortic pericardial xenograft. Br Heart J 40:602-607
4. Tandon AP, Smith DR, Ionescu IM (1978) Hemodynamic evaluation of the Ionescu-Shiley pericardial xenograft in mitral position. Am Heart J 95:595-601

Invited Lecture

Beneficial Effects of Computer-Controlled Blood Infusion in Patients Recovering from Cardiac Surgery

T. Masters, F. Robicsek, and H. Ferrari*

Postoperative management of cardiac surgical patients via computerized intensive care monitoring algorithms has been found to be a very valuable and useful application in medicine (1-18). Patients are admitted to the cardiovascular recovery unit immediately postoperatively, connected to the computer system, and monitored until all the recorded parameters have stabilized. All pertinent pressures, fluid loss and gain, respiratory parameters, temperature, and various objective (X-ray findings, ECG changes, patient appearance) inputs are entered into the computer system either by direct monitoring input or manual input. The information is stored and permanently maintained on the patient's record following high speed printouts at various timed intervals during the patient's stay.

One of the most useful algorithms in the system is that used for replacing blood. The importance of blood replacement therapy in the recovery of cardiac surgical patients is one of the most important considerations during the immediate postoperative period (19). Methods for "routine" blood replacement for an otherwise stable patient after open-heart surgery vary from maintaining left atrial pressures at an adequate level to replacing only chest drainage. The pathophysiological changes occurring during the recovery phase of cardiac surgery would tend to favor a combination of these two parameters. When the patient arrives from the operating room, the temperature is usually below normal, even though effort has been made to increase the patient's core temperature postoperatively. Most patients maintain a vasoconstriction which does not always respond to core warming. Therefore, upon completion of surgery, fluid replacement by way of the cardiopulmonary bypass is based on the left atrial pressure level which is adequate for pressure maintenance at this degree of vasoconstriction. However, it would appear that when the patient's temperature begins to increase postoperatively, there is a progressive increase in vasodilation and naturally simultaneous reduction of peripheral vascular resistance. Any decrease of the left atrial pressure resulting from blood loss will now be further potentiated by the vasodilation. This could result in a significant decrease in blood pressure and a need for blood infusion.

To investigate this particular phenomenon, we followed the recovery course of 100 cardiac surgical patients who had surgery for coronary artery occlusive disease and were monitored in a computerized intensive care recovery unit with closed-loop blood transfusion. This allowed us to follow pressure changes in response to parallel fluctuations in temperature and at the same time to evaluate the merit of closed-loop blood infusion.

*Heineman Medical Research Laboratories and Department of Thoracic and Cardiovascular Surgery, Charlotte Memorial Hospital and Medical Center, P.O. Box 32861, Charlotte, N.C. 28231, USA

Methods

For a more detailed description of our computerized intensive care system, we refer to our papers published previously (11, 21). A brief description of the system is presented below.

The computerized intensive care unit at Charlotte Memorial Hospital and Medical Center is shown in Figure 1. A diagrammatic representation of the various parts of the system is shown in Figure 2. Systolic, diastolic, and mean pressures; temperature; right and left atrial pressures; amount of blood infused; chest drainage; urine output, and respiration are measured automatically every 2 minutes or on demand. Manual input entries include arterial blood gases (Fig. 3), laboratory information, X-ray and ECG abnormalities, and medication. Fluids are automatically infused by computer-controlled pumps based on the patient's body surface area. The total input can be adjusted manually to correct for fluids not administered through the automatic infusion algorithm. It is also possible to manually correct the total amount of blood infusion when blood or blood products are administered outside the blood infusion program.

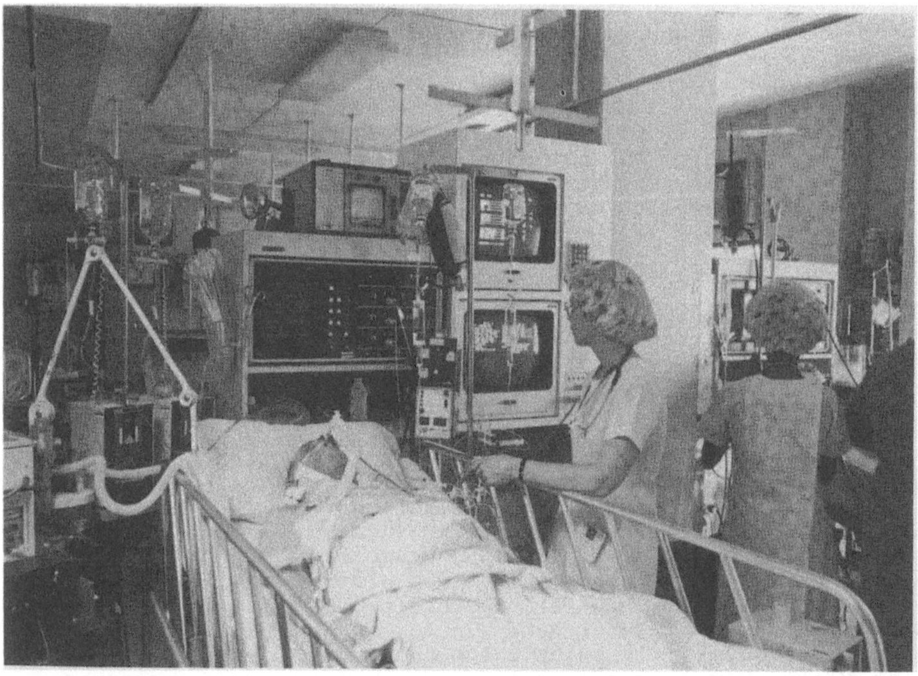

Fig. 1. Computerized intensive system at Charlotte Memorial Hospital and Medical Center. Bedside monitoring equipment and computer digital displays are shown at the patient's head. Computerized pumps are shown at the lower left of photograph

The analog information is displayed on bedside monitoring systems with audio alarms. The digital information is displayed continuously in CRTs located at the bedside (Fig. 4). This information can also be displayed on demand with the proper commands. The accumulated information on patients is stored and can be recalled in either tabular or

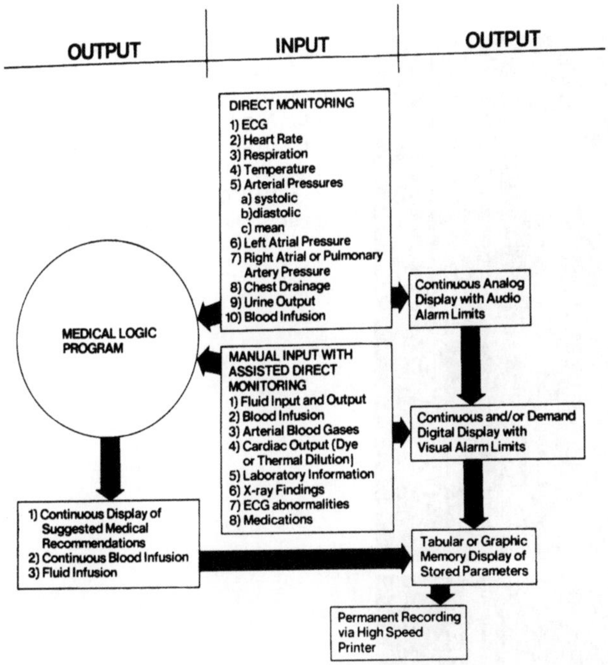

Fig. 2. Diagrammatic representation of the computerized intensive care system with various inputs and outputs relating to different aspects of the system

graphic form (Fig. 5). The patient information is printed out every 4 h and placed in the patient's chart.

The medical recommendation program receives input from both the directly monitored information and the manually entered results. Based on this information, the computer has been programmed to respond with treatment recommendations to alleviate potentially dangerous situations which will or have developed in the patient. The medical recommendations are also displayed continuously on bedside CRTs and are redisplayed automatically every 5 minutes.

The computer system (Series 5000, Roche Medical Electronics, Cranbury, NJ 08512) has been in operation 5 1/2 years. We have monitored approximately 3000 postoperative cardiac surgical patients during this time. The computer-based intensive care system has had very little down-time and nothing major which required more than 12 h to repair. There are presently four computerized beds, all with closed-loop blood infusion. The beneficial aspects of computer-controlled blood infusion suggest a more precise method of administering blood, and as a means of determining this, was the major purpose of the present paper.

One hundred consecutive patients who had undergone only bypass grafting were included in this study. Changes in systolic, diastolic, mean, and left atrial pressures; heart rate; temperature; urine output; chest drainage, and blood infusion were determined for the first 10 h of recovery at hourly intervals.

The blood replacement algorithm is based on an initial replacement of 250 ml of blood per square meter of body surface area as long as the left atrial pressure is below 14-16 mm Hg. After this initial replacement is complete, a blood/drainage ratio is examined. This ratio is calculated from the amount of blood infused divided by the amount of chest drainage. The ratio is normally set at 2 for each patient which indicates that 2 ml of blood is infused for every ml of blood lost. Both the left atrial pressure limit and blood/drainage ratio can be preset in the computer system to correspond to the patient's condition and preoperative values. Therefore, when the blood replacement algorithm is initiated, approximately 500 ml of blood are infused based

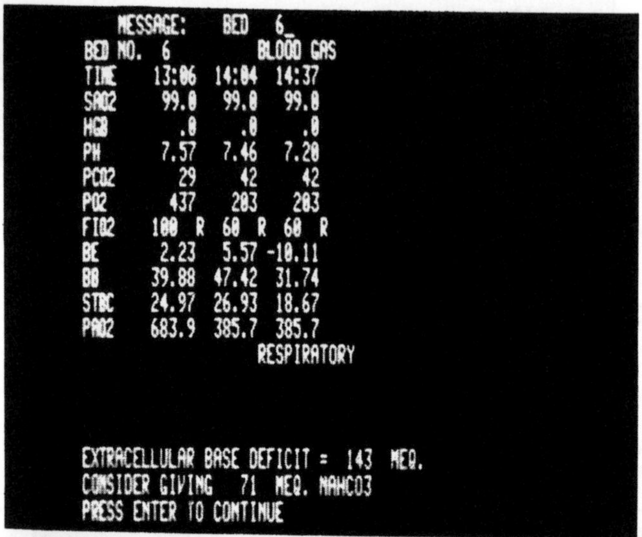

Fig. 3. Display of arterial blood gas information. The parameters are listed on the left. A pH of 7.20 was entered to display the recommendations at the bottom indicating a $NaHCO_3$ requirement to correct the base deficit

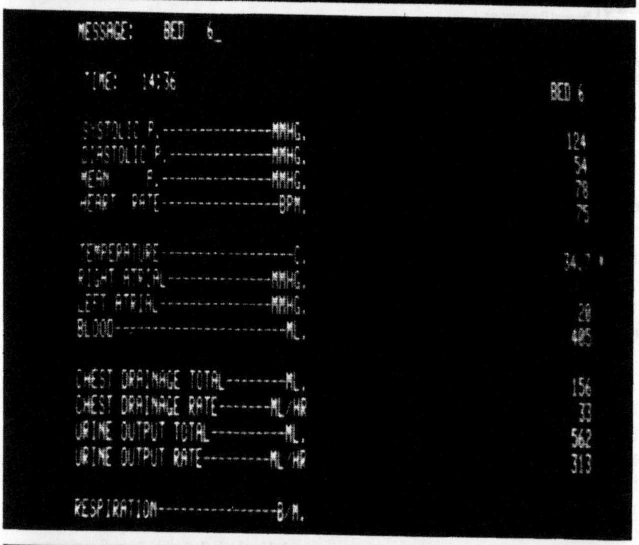

Fig. 4. Digital display of vital signs on bedside CRT. This information is reanalyzed every 2 minutes automatically or manually when required. The asterisk (*) indicates an "out of limit" parameter and indicates a "message" at top of screen

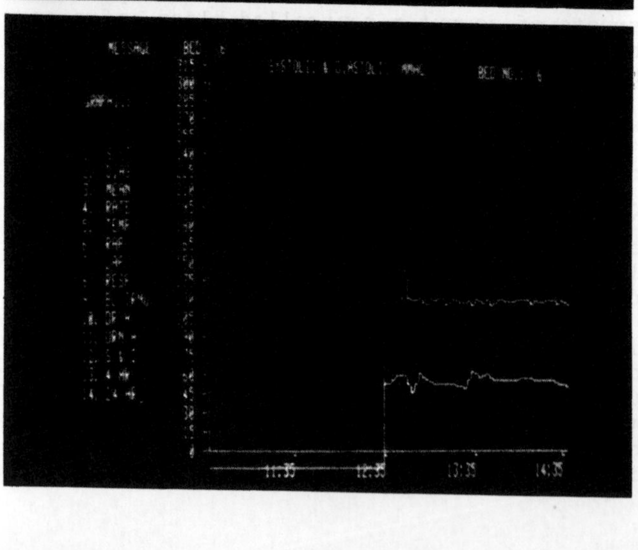

Fig. 5. Graphic display of systolic and diastolic blood pressures of a patient who had been connected to the computer system for 2 h

only on left atrial pressure. Every 2 minutes, the left atrial pressure is examined and if below 14-16 mm Hg, an infusion pump is activated to infuse 20 ml of blood. This continues every 2 minutes until the initial blood requirement has been satisfied, after which both left atrial pressure and blood/drainage ratio must be below the preset limits before blood can be infused. Automatic blood infusion is normally completed within 10-12 h unless a significant bleeding problem develops.

Results

The monitored changes in 100 patients are shown in Table 1. Arterial pressures (SYS, DIA, and MEAN) gradually decreased for the first 6 h and stabilized for the remainder of the observation period. Heart rate was fairly stable throughout the recovery phase with a small but statistically significant decrease after 8 h. Temperature (TEMP) which started at an average of 34.7 ± 0.14°C gradually increased until hour 7 (38.6 ± 0.14°C) and decreased for the remainder of the observation period to 37.9 ± 0.37°C at hour 10.

Chest drainage and urine output decreased throughout the observation period as would be expected. Left atrial pressure did not change significantly throughout the observation period. Since the blood infusion algorithm infuses blood to maintain a predetermined left atrial pressure (LAP, 14-15 mm Hg), the LAP should remain stable.

The observed changes indicate that the initial temperature of patients recovering from cardiac surgery is abnormally low and is a probable cause of vasoconstriction. As the temperature rises, arterial pressure decreases as vasodilation occurs reopening flow channels. Under computer-controlled blood infusion, this vasodilation does not affect the LAP as long as the LAP and the blood infusion/chest drainage ratio is below the preset limits. It was interesting to see that when the LAP was set to be the primary controlling factor on blood infusion, the blood infusion/chest drainage ratio was exceeded only during hours 5 and 6.

The computerized intensive care system in general has been well accepted by our nursing personnel and every aspect of the system is well utilized. The record-keeping aspect is now almost irreplacable from a nursing standpoint as it permits a closer nurse/patient relationship and eliminates the need for constant charting of vital signs, etc. As a result of computer advances in the field of medicine, a humanistic factor has once again returned to nursing applications.

Discussion

The varying methods of myocardial preservation techniques presently employed during cardiac surgery apply profound hypothermia during cardiopulmonary bypass and may result in extreme vasoconstriction with apparently many as yet undefined physiological responses (22). For example, the vasoconstriction is not entirely responsive to vasodilator treatment as found in a study presently being conducted which found the recovery phase of cardiac surgery to not be statistically different from the results reported in the present paper. The slow warming phase is apparently an integral part of the patient's recovery and includes an elevated temperature at approximately hour 7. Once warming has started (hours 2 and 3), larger amounts of blood are administered to compensate for the increasing vascular volume resulting from vaso-

Table 1. Tabulated information on 100 patients recovering from cardiac surgery in a computerized intensive care system with closed-loop blood infusion. The data are for the first 10 h of recovery and include systolic (SYS), diastolic (DIA), and mean (MEAN) pressures; changes in heart rate (RATE); amount of blood automatically infused (BLD); amount of chest drainage (CHEST); amount of urine output (URINE); temperature changes (TEMP); and alterations in left atrial pressure (LAP)

Hour	SYS	DIA	MEAN	RATE	BLD	CHEST	URINE	TEMP	LAP
0	153 ±3	87 ±2	114 ±2	87 ±2	0	0	0	34.7 ±0.14	15.5 ±0.6
1	152 ±2	88 ±2	114 ±2	84 ±2	86.7 ±14.1	152 ±15	616 ±46	34.9 ±0.12	14.0 ±0.6
2	148 ±3	86 ±2	110 ±2	88 ±2	106.8 ±16.1	121 ±12	421 ±33	35.4 ±0.14	13.0 ±0.5
3	139 ±2	81 ±2	110 ±2	88 ±2	118.8 ±20.6	79 ±8	264 ±21	36.0 ±0.13	13.0 ±0.5
4	138 ±2	80 ±2	100 ±2	88 ±2	89.7 ±17.0	64 ±7	171 ±12	36.6 ±0.12	13.0 ±0.5
5	135 ±2	78 ±2	98 ±2	87 ±2	84.4 ±15.3	56 ±7	136 ±13	37.1 ±0.10	13.0 ±0.5
6	134 ±2	75 ±1	95 ±2	87 ±2	95.5 ±15.7	59 ±7	120 ±11	37.5 ±0.80	13.0 ±0.6
7	128 ±2	73 ±2	93 ±2	84 ±1	57.6 ±12.0	68 ±8	99 ±11	38.6 ±0.90	12.0 ±0.5
8	129 ±2	73 ±2	92 ±2	82 ±2	74.4 ±14.0	71 ±9	94 ±8	37.8 ±0.60	12.7 ±0.5
9	129 ±2	72 ±2	92 ±2	83 ±1	35.2 ±10.0	34 ±9	81 ±8	37.9 ±0.47	12.9 ±0.5
10	129 ±2	72 ±2	91 ±2	82 ±1	49.7 ±12.0	35 ±4	62 ±5	37.9 ±0.37	12.6 ±0.5

dilation. Blood requirements can be expected to be the greatest during the hours 2 and 3 with an elevated requirement during hours 4, 5, and 6 with a marked reduction after these periods. The blood infusion algorithm was found to be an effective and more efficient method of infusing blood than could be done manually. The major problem we have had with the program is nursing personnel switching automatic blood infusion to manual control with a preset rate. Many of these patients have been overinfused because the nurse is not able to watch the LAP as closely as the computer can.

The effectiveness of the program is seen by the fact that the LAP in our patients remained generally stable, contrary to infusion of blood where one should expect a greater fluctuation in LAP as well as the remaining monitored parameters. Rises of the temperature coupled with increasing blood loss and urine output usually reduce pressure at a rapid rate which is corrected by increasing blood administration. Large volumes of manually infused blood result in a large increment in blood pressure which could further increase blood loss and urine output. Changes in heart rate and contractility via the sympathetic nervous system would also be expected. These changes could result in large fluctuations of monitored parameters. The computer-assisted infusion of blood eliminated these excusionary changes and resulted in a much smoother recovery for the patient.

Blood utilization per patient since the recovery unit has opened has dropped from 1475 ± 85.8 to 798.8 ± 21.4 ml. This compares to 1600.8 ± 127.5 ml of blood which were required per patient recovering from cardiac surgery without computer-controlled blood infusion (21). There are many factors which might have contributed to these changes: (1) improved surgical techniques, (2) changes in anesthetic procedures, (3) improved nursing care, and (4) smoother recovery due to automatic blood infusion. Whatever the reason, we have observed a highly significant decrease in blood utilization.

Computer algorithm control of blood infusion in patients recovering from cardiac surgery is at present relatively simple. More advanced programs are in use which utilize nitroprusside to maintain blood pressure (20). Undoubtedly in the future more advanced decision-making processes will be utilized. At present, our medical recommendation program only makes suggestions for changes in patient care and requires human inferface to carry out recommended interventions. With additional refinement and better definition and processing of inputted information, computer algorithms will be able to carry out medical interventions rather than making suggestions.

References

1. Acton JC, Sheppard LC, Kouchoukos NJ, Kirklin JW (1974) Automated care systems for critically ill patients following cardiac surgery. National Institutes of Health Conference of Computers in Cardiology, Oct 2-4, 1974, Bethesda, Maryland
2. Afifi AA, Rand WM, Palley NA, Shubin H, Weil MH (1971) A method for evaluating changes in sets of computer monitored physiological variables. Comput Biomed Res 4:329
3. Bleich HL (1971) The computer as a consultant. N Engl J Med 28:141
4. Gerbode F (1973) Computerized monitoring of seriously ill patients. J Thorac Cardiovasc Surg 66:167
5. Glaeser DH, Trost RF (1974) Distributed system for continuous and discrete monitoring for cardiovascular patients. National Institutes of Health Conference of Computers in Cardiology. Oct 2-4, 1974, Bethesda, Maryland
6. Greenburg AG (1974) The role of the computer in patient care. Surg Ann 6:61
7. Greenburg AG, McClure DK, Fink R, Stubbs JA, Peskin GW (1975) Computerization of surgical intensive care unit: Improvement of patient care via education. Surgery 77:799
8. Lewis FJ (1967) Computer techniques in the care of surgical patients. Surgery 62:630
9. Osborn J, Beaumont JO, Raison JCA, Russel J, Gerbode F (1968) Measurement and monitoring of acutely ill patients by digital computer. Surgery 64:1057
10. Osborn JJ, Beaumont JO, Gerbode F (1971) The use of on-line computerized biological data in the management of seriously ill cardio-pulmonary patients. Bull Soc Int Chir
11. Robicsek F, Reichertz PL, Masters TN, Ferrari HA (1975) Computerized intensive care of postoperative cardiac surgical patients. Computers in Cardiology, Rotterdam, Oct 2-4, 1975
12. Sheppard LC, Kouchoukos NT, Kurtis MA, Kirklin JW (1968) Automated treatment of critically ill patients following operation. Ann Surg 168:596
13. Sheppard LC, Kouchoukos NT, Kirklin JW (1973) The digital computer in surgical intensive care automation. Computer 6:29
14. Sheppard LC, Kirklin JW, Kouchoukos NT (1974) Computer controlled interventions for the acutely ill patient. Comput Biomed Res 4:125
15. Vallbona C, Spencer WA, Geddes LA, Blose WF, Canzoneri J III (1966) Experience with on-line monitoring in critical illness. IEEE Spectrum, Sept. 1966, p 136

16. Warner HR, Gardner RM, Toronto AF (1967) Computer-based monitoring of cardio-vascular functions in postoperative patients. Circulation [Suppl 2] 36:263
17. Weil MH, Shubin H, Rand W (1966) Experience with a digital computer for study and improved management of the critically ill. JAMA 198:147
18. Sheppard LC, Kirklin JW, Kouchoukos NT (1974) In: Stacy RW, Waxman BD (eds) Computers in biomedical research. Academic Press, New York, p 135
19. Kouchoukos NT, Kirklin JW, Sheppard LC, Roe PA (1971) Effect of elevation of left atrial pressure by blood infusion on stroke volume early after cardiac operations. Surg Forum 22:126
20. Reves JG, Sheppard LC, Wallach R, Lell WA (1978) Therapeutic uses of sodium nitroprusside and an automated method of administration. Int Anesthesiol Clin 16:51-88
21. Robicsek F, Masters TN (1976) Application of medical logic in computer-based intensive care management of open heart patients. Computers in Cardiology, Oct. 7-9, 139-147
22. Levinsky L, Schimert G, Lajos TZ, Lee AB, Korenyi-Both A, Vladutiu A, Montes M, Siegel JH (1979) The use of steroids as a potentiator of hypothermic myorcardial preservation in man. J Surg Res 26:629-651

Heart Disease in Infancy and Childhood

Chairman: G. Semb, Oslo; Co-Chairman: I. Louhimo, Helsinki

Invited Lecture

The Present State and Future Expectations of Surgery for Tricuspid Atresia

F. Fontan*

*Hôpital Cardiologique du Haut-Leveque, Bordeaux, France

Experience With Palliative Surgery for Tricuspid Atresia

P. A. Sánchez, M. Ferreiros, and F. Alvarez Díaz*

Right atrium-pulmonary artery or right atrium-right ventricle anastomosis has proved to be an excellent technique for the surgical management of different congenital heart defects. Its application in the treatment of tricuspid atresia (11) has been of significant importance. Although long-term results have yet to be carefully evaluated, the follow-up for more than 5 years of several operated children has demonstrated that a certain number of selected patients have benefited greatly from this procedure.

Candidates to Fontan operation have to fulfill predetermined conditions with regard to age, atrial size, pulmonary vascular resistance, left ventricular function, etc. The procedure is usually performed in children over 3 years of age and preferably older. Only few of them, however, reach that age in good condition and many need a previous palliation to survive (10). When dealing with very sick babies and infants, many of them extremely deteriorated, some palliation has to be done, firstly to save their lives and secondly to keep them in the best possible physiological condition until they are fit for the repair. The importance of the palliative procedures is thus clearly understood.

The major aim of palliative procedures, in addition to their effectiveness in the long run, is therefore the maintainance of a good pulmonary vascular bed. What matters is not only to improve the clinical situation by providing an adequate oxygen saturation but to keep the pulmonary arteries normal as well, while avoiding increased pulmonary vascular resistance (24).

In the present report we present our experience in the palliative surgery of tricuspid atresia. It is our intention to outline results and to come to conclusions with regard to surgical indications from now on.

Material and Results

Seventy-two children with tricuspid atresia underwent palliative surgery between 1969 and June 1980. Ages ranged from 2 days to 10 years. A total of 82 procedures were performed, 59 of them (71.9%) within the first year of life. Emergency surgery was indicated in 18% of the cases because of repeated anoxic spells. In the other instances surgical indication was based on severe hypoxemia or cyanosis and heart failure resistant to medical treatment.

In seven cases with increased pulmonary flow, a pulmonary artery banding was performed (Table 1). All but one were operated upon within the first year of life, and in two instances an atrioseptectomy had

*Children Hospital "La Paz" and Centro E. Ramón y Cajal, Madrid, Spain

also to be done due to inadequate atrial drainage with an interatrial gradient above 3 mm Hg.

Table 1. Tricuspid atresia with increased pulmonary flow

	1-3 mo	4-6 mo	7-12 mo	>2 y
PA banding	1 (1)	2	1	1
PA banding + B-H	-	1	1	-

Total seven with one hospital death

In 65 children the first operation was a shunt (Table 2). Overall mortality was 21.5%. Two late deaths of unknown cause occurred in children with a Waterston shunt and atrioseptectomy. As expected, hospital mortaliy was considerably higher in neonates, being steady during the first 6 months of age and decreasing afterwards (Table 3). (One of the deaths among the 11 operated on between 1 and 2 years occurred when reducing the size of the Waterston shunt on the first postoperative day.) In our experience mortality rate was higher in earlier times, having lowered in recent years. Two children were lost due to preoperative renal insufficiency, in another three the cause of death was a postoperative bacterial infection (coli in two cases, meningococcus in one). The other deaths were related to the shunt earlier obstruction or to the large size of it resulting in pulmonary edema and/or right heart failure in the presence of inadequate communication between both atria.

Table 2. Tricuspid atresia – first palliative procedure

Systemic-pulmonary shunts	No.	Hospital mortality
Waterston	26	7
with Blalock-Hanlon	31	6[a]
Blalock-Taussig	1	0
with Blalock-Hanlon	1	0
Glenn	5	0
Ao-P shunt with EPTFE graft	1	0
Total	65	13 (21.5%)

[a]Three with pulmonary atresia

Table 3. Tricuspid atresia — first palliative procedure. Systemic-pulmonary artery shunts

Age	No.	Hospital mortality
Neonates	19	6 (31.6%)
1-3 mo	11	2 (18.2%)
4-6 mo	11	2 (18.2%)
7-12 mo	8	1 (12.5%)
1-2 ys	11	2 (18%)
>2 ys	5	0

Ten of the 52 survivors with systemic to pulmonary shunts required a second operation 1 month to 8 years (average 22.8 months) after the first procedure. Two of these operations were atrial septectomies performed 1 month and 2 years after the initial Waterston shunt. The presence of severe right heart failure with interatrial gradient over 5 mm Hg made the performance of a Blalock-Hanlon septectomy advisable. One of the children died during the postoperative period.

Of the reoperated cases, eight were shunts, seven Blalock-Taussig, and one Potts anastomosis. Hospital mortality was much higher in these children: four Blalock-Taussig and the Potts case were lost in the inmediate postoperative period. Their condition was extremely poor mainly due to severe hypoxemia caused by the obstruction of the previous shunt. Two Waterston shunts performed in babies 10 and 18 days old required a Blalock-Taussig 1 month and 10 months later, respectively. The Potts anastomosis was performed in a 5-month-old infant who had undergone a Waterston and a Blalock-Hanlon as neonate. Three other infants with previous Waterston and atrioseptectomy had a Blalock-Taussig performed 15 months, 2 years, and 4 years later. Two of them survived and are in good clinical condition after 5 years. A right Blalock-Taussig was done in an infant whose left Blalock-Taussig, performed 2 months earlier, had become obstructed. Due to the small size of the subclavian artery, the shunt proved to be insufficient and the infant did not survive. The remaining Blalock-Taussig was performed in a child who had undergone a cavopulmonary anastomosis 8 years earlier. He is in good condition after 2 years.

As already mentioned, in two late deaths the causes remain unknown. At the time of this report, 50 of the 72 children operated on (69.5%) have survived through one or more palliative procedures. Four of them have already undergone surgical repair by means of a Fontan operation. All had a previous Waterston shunt and two an additional Blalock-Hanlon septectomy.

Comments

Long-term results will prove whether right atrium-pulmonary anastomosis can be considered corrective surgery (20) or radical palliative surgery only (19). In any case, only few infants and children will pass through the natural selection up to the age in which they become suitable for the repair. The conditions required to perform a Fontan operation (7) are met by only a small number of those babies born with tricuspid atresia. Natural history of the disease shows that an obstruction to pulmonary blood flow will appear in most infants with normally related great arteries (15). If they are not operated on, very few will survive beyond the first year of life (10). Recent reports have stressed the importance of early palliative procedures (8, 16, 24).

In our opinion the Blalock-Taussig anastomosis is a very useful shunt in tricuspid atresia, being the shunt of choice in many instances. The pericardium does not need to be opened at the operation which makes easier the subsequent repair, and it supplies a controlled pulmonary flow. Hospital mortality is low, too. The results greatly depend, however, on the patient's age at the time when the shunt is performed. In infants under 6 months of age, the size of the subclavian artery is generally too small to give an adequate flow and not infrequently, especially in those infants under 3 months, early obstruction is the result.

In a series of 102 consecutive Blalock-Taussig performed in children with tetralogy of Fallot, the hospital mortaliy has been, in our hands, of 0.9% (4,21). We believe that these excellent results were mainly due to the fact that all shunts but one were performed in infants over 6 months of age when the size of the subclavian artery allows a safer performance of the anastomosis and the chances of kinking at its origin from the aorta are much lower. Although the proximal arterioplasty technique can, in some instances, avoid this latter complication (14), the results in the small infants are not good.

The Waterston anastomosis has shown, in our hands, excellent results in some congenital heart defects, especially in infants under 6 months of age (1 - 3). Hospital mortality in cases of tetralogy of Fallot has remained around 5% in infants less than 3 months old (3, 21), and the usually reported complication of kinking of the right pulmonary artery was only found in 13% of the cases at the time of the complete correction (4). Selective catheterization of the right pulmonary artery also showed absence of pulmonary hypertension (3). Some of the technical details responsible for the results are: 1) small size of the anastomosis, 2) performing it as posteriorly on the ascending aorta as possible, 3) avoiding excessive pulling of the right pulmonary artery during the procedure. The last two can similarly be applied to cases of tricuspid atresia. As for the size, it has to be carefully evaluated to avoid a high flow to the left atrium which increases the pressure and makes the emptying of the right atrium more difficult. Too small an anastomosis, however, may produce early obstruction of the shunt as it occurred in some infants in our series, with the subsequent deleterious result.

It was our policy in babies and small infants with tricuspid atresia to perform a Waterston anastomosis and to assess atrial pressures. If the interatrial gradient was higher than 3 mm Hg, we also performed a Blalock-Hanlon atrioseptectomy. Hospital mortality was then considerably reduced (8). However, we agree that the atrioseptectomy should be avoided, whenever possible, because it prevents to a certain degree the development of right atrial hypertrophy and diminishes the contractile capacity of the atrium, conditions which are required for a successful Fontan operation (6, 11). This pumping capacity of the right atrium has been questioned as the decisive or unique factor to maintain the pulmonary circulation (17, 18). On the other hand, other authors believe that the role played by the left ventricular end-diastolic pressure is more important (13). In our opinion the preservation of the right atrial function is of primary importance with regard to the future repair. Several reported failures of the Fontan operation were attributed to this lack of contractile capacity (6, 12).

In tricuspid atresia, there is usually an atrial septal defect or foramen ovale of appropriate size but in approximately 20% of the children it is too small (9). A balloon atrioseptostomy should be done at the time of hemodynamic study, but this procedure, when a shunt is present, has proved to be inadequate some times later on (22). As mentioned above, two children in our series needed an atrioseptectomy some time after the performance of the Waterston shunt although the previous Rashkind had been very effective. Early occlusion of the shunt occurred in other instances due to the small size of the fistula. A bigger anastomosis prevents the occlusion and in those cases the Blalock-Hanlon can be very useful. Although it decreases the capacity of "ventriculation" of the right atrium and it might be a source of potential arrhythmias, the atrioseptectomy can be in a few cases life-saving by contributing to improve the severe low cardiac output resulting from poor right atrial to left atrial drainage.

On the basis of its good long-term results, the Glenn anastomosis is probably the best shunt used for tricuspid atresia. The actuarial analysis demonstrates that it has the best record for both patient and shunt survival although it shows a remarkable increase in the need for a second shunt 6 to 8 years following the first operation (24). The Glenn anastomosis low surgical mortality and its enlargement with the passing of time provide a good palliation, but unfortunately it cannot be performed in small infants. Only some selected children can benefit from it. When the child outgrows the shunt, a systemic shunt on the left side, as in one of our cases, can provide a good palliation for years, lowering the hematocrit and considerably reducing the hypoxemia.

The combination of a Glenn shunt on the right plus a Blalock-Taussig on the left is a good alternative for children who are not candidates for a Fontan operation (23, 24). When not all the criteria are met to perform a Fontan, the palliative reconstruction of the right ventricular outflow tract, accompanied if necessary by enlargement of the VSD, is also an advisable surgical approach (5). This alternative is certainly a promising one, offering the additional advantage of possibly increasing the size of the pulmonary arteries. That makes feasible a further repair connecting the conduit to the enlarged outlet chamber.

It is too early to know long-term results of systemic-pulmonary shunts done with expanded polytetrafluoroethylene grafts (EPTFE). Although early results seemed encouraging in some congenital heart defects (25), we believe that the grafts are not going to provide better late results than the conventional shunts. At least a 5-6 mm diameter graft has to be used to avoid early thrombosis.

The Fontan operation has certainly presented new and very important horizons to the treatment of tricuspid atresia. The surgical approach as a whole cannot be considered, however, with the exclusive purpose of performing a future conduit repair. The main aim in severely ill infants must be to save their lives. Therefore, surgical management in infancy still is a challenge, and careful anatomic individualization is the first obligatory step. As much remains unkown, especially related to long-term results, the different offered alternatives for palliation still greatly depend on one's own experience (8, 16, 23).

At present, we favour the Blalock-Taussig anastomosis as the palliative procedure of choice in infants and children over 6 months of age with tricuspid atresia and normally related great vessels. A second Blalock-Taussig can be performed on the other side if the child outgrows the shunt and further palliation is considered preferable. In neonates and small infants, we recommend a 3-4 mm Waterston shunt performed with the previously mentioned technical care. An EPTFE graft might also be considered in selected cases. When the balloon atrial septostomy becomes inadequate due to left atrium overflow produced by a shunt, a Blalock-Hanlon septectomy can be useful and life-saving. Although it might make the future conduit repair more difficult, it does not absolutely contraindicate it.

In children over 2 years of age with an inadequate shunt, the Fontan operation is the elective procedure. A Glenn anastomosis has also to be considered depending on patient's age and if not all the criteria for the repair are fulfilled. If the pulmonary arteries are diminutive, the right ventricular outflow tract reconstruction is a very useful alternative.

References

1. Alvarez Díaz F (1976) The treatment of Fallot's tetralogy. In: Dyde JA, Smith RE (eds) Surgery of the heart. Plenum, New York London, pp 119-129
2. Alvarez Díaz F, Brito JM, Cordovilla G, Perez de León J, Sánchez PA, Bordiu C (1973) Ascending aorta-right pulmonary artery anastomosis: Waterston operation. Thorax 28:152
3. Alvarez Díaz F, Sanz E, Sanchez PA, Cordovilla G, Celemin D, Moreno F, Borches D, Gutierrez JR (1978) Fallot's tetralogy-palliation and repair with a previous shunt. In: Anderson RH, Shinebourne EA (eds) Paediatric cardiology 1977. Churchill Livingstone, Edinburgh London New York, pp 273-282
4. Alvarez Díaz F, Sanz E, Cordovilla G, Perez Martinez V, Borches D (1980) Total correction of Fallot's tetralogy with a previous Waterston shunt. World Congress of Paediatric Cardiology, London 1980, Abstract No O33
5. Annecchino FP, Fontan F, Chauve A, Quaegebeur J (1980) Palliative reconstruction of the right ventricular outflow tract in tricuspid atresia: a report of 5 patients. Ann Thorac Surg 29:317
6. Caffarena Raggio JM, Otero Coto E, Gomez-Ullae JM, Peris JJ, Concha M, Ferrer H (1977) La derivación atrio-pulmonar y atrio-ventricular (operación de Fontan) en el tratamiento quirúrgico de la atresia tricúspide. Rev Esp Cardiol 30:375
7. Choussat A, Fontan F. Besse P, Vallot F, Chauve A, Bricaud H (1978) Selection criteria for Fontan's procedure. In: Anderson RH, Shinebourne EA (eds) Paediatric cardiology 1977. Churchill Livingstone, Edinburgh London New York, pp 559-566
8. Cordovilla G, Sanchez PA, Sanz E, Ferreiros M, Borches D, Casanova M, Alvarez Díaz F (1978) Experiencia quirúrgica en 56 casos de atresia tricuspide. Rev Esp Cardiol 31:415
9. Deveral RA, Lincoln JCR, Aberdeen E, Bonhan-Carter RE, Waterston DJ (1969) Surgical treatment of tricuspid atresia. Thorax 24:239
10. Dick M, Fyler DC, Nadas AS (1975) Tricuspid atresia: clinical course in 101 patients. Am J Cardiol 36:327
11. Fontan F, Baudet E (1971) Surgical repair of tricuspid atresia. Thorax 26:240
12. Fontan F, Choussat A, Brom AG, Chauve A, Deville C, Castro-Cels A (1978) Repair of tricuspid atresia: surgical considerations and results. In: Anderson RH, Shinebourne EA (eds) Pediatric cardiology 1977. Churchill Livingstone, Edinburgh London New York, pp 567-580
13. Kreutzer G, Galindez E, Bono M, De Palma C, Laura JP (1973) An operation for the correction of tricuspid atresia. J Thorac Cardiovasc Surg 66:613
14. Laks H, Castaneda AR (1975) Subclavian arterioplasty for the ipsilateral Blalock-Taussig shunt. Ann Thorac Surg 19:319
15. Orlando FG (1970) Progressive obstruction of pulmonary blood flow in tricuspid atresia. J Thorac Cardiovasc Surg 59:447
16. Ostermeyer J, Korfer R, Birks W (1979) Palliative surgery for tricuspid atresia. International Cardiovascular Society, XIV World Congress, San Francisco, Book of Abstracts, p 84
17. Robicsek F, Sanger PW, Golucc V, Daugherty HK (1966) Long-term circulatory exclusion of the right heart. Surgery 59:431
18. Rodbard S, Wager D (1949) Bypassing the right ventricle. Proc Soc Exp Biol Med 71:69
19. Ross DN, Somerville J (1973) Surgical correction of tricuspid atresia. Lancet 1:845
20. Sade RM, Castaneda AR (1975) The dispensable right ventricle. Surgery 77:624
21. Sanchez PA, Cordovilla G, Sanz E, Alvarez Díaz F (1979) Surgical management of Fallot's tetralogy in infants and children. International Cardiovascular Society, XIV World Congress, San Francisco, Book of Abstracts, p 83

22. Santalla A, Sanchez PA, Perez de León J, Gutierrez J, Villagrá F, Gómez R, Dîaz Balda JI, Merino G, Quero M, Brito JM (1980) Role of atrioseptectomy (Blalock-Hanlon) in the surgery of tricuspid atresia in infants. 1st World Congress of Paediatric Cardiology, London
23. Trusler GA, Williams WG (1976) Long-term results of the Glenn procedure for tricuspid atresia. In: Langford Kidd BS, Rowe RD (eds) The child with congenital heart disease after surgery. Futura, Mount Kisco New York, p 79
24. Trusler GA, Williams WG (1980) Long-term results of shunt procedures for tricuspid atresia. Ann Thoracic Surg 29:312
25. Tsunemoto M, Ota Y, Shimada M (1979) Expanded polytetraghoroethylene grafts for construction of systemic-pulmonary shunts. International Cardiovascular Society, XIV World Congress, San Francisco, Book of Abstracts, p 86

Repair of Aortic Coarctation in Neonates

T. K. Kaul, R. R. Chatrath, and D. R. Walker*

Introduction

The infants born with aortic coarctation may frequently have other associated cardiac anomalies (1, 3, 8). These infants commonly present with severe congestive cardiac failure and metabolic acidosis in the early days of life. Mortality at this age group remains considerably high if the surgical treatment is delayed after a fair trial of medical treatment. Although results of the medical treatment have recently improved, surgical treatment is preferred in order to prevent the repeated episodes of congestive cardiac failure and persistance of systemic hypertension. We have studied the operative results in the infants who presented with severe aortic coarctation in the first month of life, during the last 10 years in our unit.

Patients and Methods

Between January 1, 1970, and December 31, 1979, 32 infants (24 males and eight females) underwent repair for aortic coarctation. Mean age at the time of repair was 13.7 days and mean weight 3.7 kg. Sixteen infants were desperately ill at the time of admission and had to be ventilated preoperatively and infused with dopamine (2 to 10 micro gm/kg/minute) to correct the metabolic acidosis, and were operated within a few hours after the admission. All infants had angiocardiography and the diagnosis of coarctation was confirmed preoperatively. Resection of the narrow segment and end-to-end anstomosis or Dacron patch aortoplasty were performed more frequently earlier in the series. Subclavian patch aortoplasty became the surgical procedure of choice in the last 5 years. Postoperatively infants were gradually weaned off the ventilatory or the inotropic support and treated for the residual congenital abnormalities as indicated. The survivors were periodically followed in an out-patient clinic and their drug therapy was reviewed.

*Killingbeck Hospital, Leeds 8, Cardiothoracic Unit, Broadgreen Hospital, Liverpool L14 3 L.B., Great Britain

Results

The aortic coarctation was preductal in 28, juxtaductal in two, and postductal in two infants. The other cardiac anomalies revealed by the angiocardiography are summarised in Table 1.

Table 1. Associated cardiac lesions in 32 infants with aortic coarctation

Patent ductus arteriorus	29
Ventricular septal defect	10
Transposition of great arteries	2
Hypoplastic aortic arch	3
Aortic stenosis	2
Anomalous r. subclavian artery	1
Double outlet r. ventricle and l. superior vena cava	1
AV canal with hypoplastic LV	1

The mortality associated with the definitive surgical procedures is summarised in Table 2. The operative mortality was considerably high in the infants treated with end-to-end anastomosis. There was no early death in uncomplicated cases after subclavian aortoplasty or Dacron patch aortoplasty. An improved survival in these patients could be attributed to pre- and postoperative ventilation, inotropic support, and the correction of the biochemical abnormalities, e.g. plasma glucose and serum calcium. The hypoplastic aortic arch was enlarged in three infants, in two with Dacron patch aortoplasty, and in one with subclavian patch aortoplasty; unfortunately none of these infants survived in the postoperative period.

The correction of the associated cardiac anomalies at the time of surgery or at a later date may also contribute to the poor survival in these infants. One late death was associated with the banding of the pulmonary artery, and two infants have died after the correction of the transposition of the great vessels. The 21 survivors have been followed for a mean follow-up period of 43.4 months. Recoarctation occurred in two infants after the end-to-end anastomosis and in one infant after subclavian aortoplasty which was subsequently repaired with a Gor-Tex patch.

Systemic hypertension persisted in two infants after subclavian aortoplasty (in one infant with recoarctation and in one without recoarctation) and cold arm with no pulse but a normally functional limb was noticed in one child.

Discussions

An early surgical intervention after an initial resuscitation has considerably improved the survival of the infants born with severe aortic coarctation (1, 3). An almost complete regression of systemic hypertension may occur when the repair of aortic coarctation is undertaken early in infancy; however, the residual hypertension even in the absence of

Table 2. Surgical correction of aortic coarctation in 32 infants

Operation	No.	Hospital deaths
Subclavian patch aortoplasty	22	Nil
Dacron patch aortoplasty	2	Nil
End-to-end anastomosis	5	3
Additional surgical procedures		
Ligation of PDA	29	Nil
PA banding	4	Nil
Enlargement of hypoplastic segment:		
Dacron patch	2	2
Subclavian patch	1	1

recoarctation may persist. The reason for it remains obscure. In view of a high mortality for the additional surgical procedures, we no longer band the pulmonary artery at the initial operation. The repair of ventricular septal defect should be done subsequently if the cardiac failure persists.

The end-to-end anastomosis is usually associated with a higher early mortality due to the technical difficulties in the mobilisation of a long coarctation segment, tension at the anastomosis, or an incomplete relief of the coarctation. These factors and the failure of the anastomosis to grow may contribute to a high incidence of recoarctation seen after an end-to-end anastomosis (2, 4, 6, 8). The growth potential is likely to be retained in the posterior wall of the aorta after Dacron patch aortoplasty and a satisfactory long-term survival without recoarctation has been reported (3). However, the possibility of infection of the patch and the complications associated with it have limited its use (5, 7). Subclavian patch aortoplasty was first introduced in 1966 (9). Technically it is an easier procedure in which the growth potentials are well preserved, and is also free from the complications associated with a prosthetic material. The ligation of subclavian artery is unlikely to cause a major disability. In view of a satisfactory record of a long-term survival without recoarctation, subclavian patch aortoplasty is now accepted as a surgical procedure of choice for the repair of aortic coarctation in neonates (1, 3).

Acknowledgement. The authors are thankful to Miss J.G. Luxton for her secretarial help in preparation of this manuscript.

References

1. Hamilton DI, Eusanio GD, Sandra Sagra FA, Donnelley RJ (1978) Early and late results of aortoplasty with a left subclavian flap for coarctation of the aorta in infancy. J Thorac Cardiovasc Surg 75:699-704
2. Hartmann AF, Goldring D, Hernandez A, Behrer MR, Schad N, Ferguson T, Burford T (1970) Recurrent coarctation of the aorta after successful repair in infancy. Am J Cardiol 25:405
3. Herrmann VM, Laks H, Fagan L, Terschluse D, Willman VL (1978) Repair of aortic coarctation in the first year of life. Ann Thorac Surg 25:57-63
4. Ibarra-Perez C, Castaneda AR, Varco RL, Lillehei CW (1969) Recoarctation of aorta. Nineteen year clinical experience. Am J Cardiol 23:778
5. Moor GF, Ionescu MI, Ross DN (1970) Surgical repair of coarctation by patch grafting. Ann Thorac Surg 14:626-630
6. Pelletier C, Davignon A, Ethier MF, Stanley P (1969) Coarctation of the aorta in infancy: Postoperative follow-up. J Thorac Cardiovasc Surg 57:171-179
7. Reul GL, Kabbani SS, Sandiford FM, Wukash DC, Cooley DA (1974) Repair of coarctation of the thoracic aorta by patch graft aortoplasty. J Thorac Cardiovasc Surg 68:696-704
8. Shinebourne EA, Tam A, Elseed AM, Paneth M, Lennox SC, Cleland WP, Lincoln C, Joseph MC, Anderson RH (1976) Coarctation of the aorta in infancy and childhood. Br Heart J 38:375-380
9. Waldhansen JA, Nahrwold DL (1966) Repair of the coarctation of the aorta with a subclavian flap. J Thorac Cardiovasc Surg 51:532-533

Pacemaker Implantation in Children

W. Ruschewski, B. Heisig, K. Hellberg, W. Krebs, and R. de Vivie*

Introduction

Total AV block after surgery of congenital heart lesions in infancy and childhood is a severe complication. Before introduction of permanent cardiac pacemaker therapy in children in 1962, the mortality rate was high. Since the number of open-heart procedures in early infancy and childhood has rapidly increased, pacemaker implantation in children has become more and more important. In comparison, the number of patients with congenital heart block who need permanent cardiac pacemaker therapy is relatively low.

In the adult the technique of implantation is well established and much experience has been gained in the last 20 years. But there are only a few follow-up studies on permanent cardiac pacing in children. The particular problems in children are their smaller size, lack of muscular and subcutaneous tissue, extensive growth, greater physical activity, and long life expectancy. To minimize psychological stress, complications and hospitalization frequency must be kept low, and a good cosmetic result is important.

Patients

Between August 1964 and June 1980, 41 children ranging in age from 3 months to 13 years underwent implantation of a permanent cardiac pacemaker at our hospital. The average age was 7.5 years. The patients ranged in weight from 4.8 to 34 kg (average 19.3 kg), in height from 50 to 143 cm (average 113 cm). The indication for pacemaker implantation was surgically induced heart block in 34 patients, congenital heart block in seven. The different heart lesions and surgical procedures leading to total AV block are listed in Table 1. During the nearly 16-year follow-up period, 3868 pediatric open-heart operations have been performed at our hospital. That means that our rate of pacemaker-dependent patients with postoperative heart block has been 0.88%.

*Klinik für Thorax-Herz-Gefäßchirurgie, Klinikum der Universität, Robert-Koch-Str. 40, D-3400 Göttingen

Table 1. Permanent pacemaker implantation in children with surgical and congenital total AV block

Congenital heart lesion		Surgery
Tetralogy of Fallot	10	Total repair
VSD type 2	9	Patch closure
TGA	2	Mustard's operation
Corrected TGA + VSD	1	Patch closure
Incomplete AV canal	3	Patch closure + suture of cleft
Complete AV canal	1	Total repair
Mitral valve defect	4	MVR
LVOTO	2	Aortoventriculoplasty
Aortic stenosis	1	AVR
Fibrous subaortic stenosis	1	Excision
Congenital total AV block	5	
Romano-Ward syndrome	1	
Sick-Sinus syndrome	1	
Total	41	

Indication

The indication for permanent pacemaker implantation was seen when the following criteria were present: 1) Adams-Stokes attacks or 2) congestive heart failure, and 3) a ventricular rate less than 50 bpm without adequate increase during exercise. All children with congenital heart block received a permanent pacemaker because of Adams-Stokes attacks. Surgically induced heart block was primarily treated by temporary myocardial stimulation for 2-4 weeks. After this period, the recurrence of sinus rhythm was rare. We saw late restitution only in five cases (14.7%) 6 weeks to 5 years after surgery.

During the first years of the follow-up period, we tried treatment by medication of orciprenaline in four cases without permanent success. One child developed congestive heart failure after malabsorption because of diarrhea 3 months after surgery; the other three experienced Adams-Stokes attacks 3 years after surgery though orciprenaline was taken regularly.

Operative Technique

In 37 patients (90%) epicardial pacemaker electrodes were implanted initially. One or two leads were attached to the anterolateral wall of the left ventricle through a left anterior thoracotomy. The pulse generator was implanted in the submuscular tissue beneath the rectus and external or internal oblique muscles. We did not perform subcutaneous or subfascial insertion because a higher rate in skin erosion and infection has been observed. In one case an intrapleural application was used in a 10-year-old very small boy in 1972. Unfortunately we lost this patient from observation after a period of 3.5 years without complications. The intrapleural, subdiaphragmatic, and intrapelvic application was not performed because it requires invasion of major body cavities and offers bad possibilities for fixation and programming. The retroperitoneal position has not been used because downward migration into the pelvis has been reported.

The disadvantages of the epicardial technique are a higher rate of wire breakage because of frequent and extensive movement between the anterior abdominal wall and the chest and the frequent increase of stimulation threshold with exit block due to epicardial scarring. Therefore, in 15 patients transvenous pacemaker leads were inserted via the right cephalic vein or the external and internal jugular vein. In these cases the generator was placed beneath the pectoralis major muscle. The transvenous technique was chosen secondarily in 11 patients because of multiple complications with the epicardial lead, such as infection (five), wire breakage near the heart (five), and extensive increase of stimulation threshold (one). In four patients the transvenous technique was performed initially, as subpectoral battery application was anatomically possible.

Pacemaker Systems

During the 16-year follow-up period, we implanted 86 devices of 19 different types: Biotronik (IP 44, IRP 44, IDP 44, and IDP 54), Chardack-Greatbach 5859, Devices Demand 3821 F, Stanium AM Baby, Edwards (8114 and 8116), Siemens-Elema Baby, Pacesetter UD 102, Arco Li 2 D, Cordis (Ventricor, Ectocor, Omni-Stanicor, and Omni-Stanicor Lambda), and Intermedics (Interlith 223, Thinlith II 227, and Cyberlith 253-01) with different electrodes. The last 39 devices have been lithium pacemakers and the last 32 programmable systems with the advantage to change rate, output, and other data if necessary. With these systems the rate can be adjusted to hemodynamic requirements and the output raised with increasing threshold. A rechargeable system was used only once by request of the patient's parents.

Results

During a cumulative follow-up period of 1744 months, we performed 100 reoperations because of generator depletion or complications. The overall mean lifetime of a complete pacemaker system was only 17.4 months (ranging from 1 to 49 months). Eight programmable lithium systems are still doing well after initial implantation for a cumulative follow-up period of 173 months (mean lifetime until now 21.6 months). We observed 53 complications in 25 children (61%), mostly wire breakage, increased stimulation threshold, and infection (Table 2). There was one death because of increased stimulation threshold with exit block. Four patients (10%) had four or more complications (50%). Cumulatively there was one complication every 36 months.

Comparison of the epicardial and the transvenous techniques shows a much higher frequency of complications with the epicardial. With epicardial leads we had one complication every 33 months, with transvenous only every 89 months, although there was only a small difference in average age (transvenous 9 years, ranging from 2 to 13 years; epicardial 7.7 years, ranging from 3 months to 13 years).

Table 2. Complications during a cumulative follow-up period of 1744 months

Wire breakage	19
Increase of threshold	15
Infection	11
Insulation defect	2
Lead dislocation (transvenous)	2
Stimulation of muscles	1
Battery leakage	1
Parasystole (fixed rate)	1
Death (battery failure)	1
	53
Battery change	47

Discussion

The results of this follow-up study show that lifetime of pacemaker systems in children has been markedly improved after introduction of programmable lithium devices. The complication rate is, however, still much higher than in adults. The main reason seems to be the preference for epicardial electrodes with the tendency of stimulation threshold increase because of epicardial scarring and frequent wire breakage because of the thoracoabdominal course of the lead. Therefore, now we try to implant a transvenous pacemaker system with a subpectoral battery application whenever it is anatomically possible. With the new small-sized lithium generators there are now rarely space problems. The youngest patient has been 2 years of age. By the use of highly flexible screw-in electrodes a long redundant loop can be inserted into the cavity of the superior vena cava and the heart without dislocation to avoid wire breakage and lead dislocation because of growth. Regular medical check-up every 3 months is absolutely necessary. Further development will be needed in the design of longer-lived electrodes. The implantation of rechargeable and nuclear power sources and atrial programmed pacemakers in children at the present time does not seem recommendable because the frequency of complications is too high and the expected lifetime of the new lithium devices is adequate for a pacemaker system.

Summary

Between 1964 and 1980, 41 children, 3 months to 13 years of age, underwent implantation of a permanent cardiac pacemaker (PM) for total AV block after cardiac surgery (34), congenital AV block (five), and other bradyarrhythmias (two). Until 1975, only epicardial electrodes had been used. Preferred pocket location was preperitoneal beneath the rectus and external or internal oblique muscles. Since our experience showed much higher frequency in PM malfunction because of increased pacing threshold and wire breakage for the thoracoabdominal systems, now we prefer transvenous electrodes and subpectoral pocket location whenever it is anatomically possible with reduced complication rate. For the new small-sized lithium devices, there are rarely space problems even in small children. The last 32 generators have been programmable ones. During our cumulative follow-up period of 1744 months, PM malfunction has occurred 100 times, including generator depletion (47), wire breakage (19), increase of threshold (15), and infection (11). There was one case of death because of battery failure. The overall mean lifetime of a complete pacemaker system was 17.4 months. There was one complication every 33 months with the epicardial systems, with the transvenous systems only every 89 months. Therefore, the implantation of transvenous electrodes should be preferred.

References

1. Amato JJ, Payne DD, Rheinlander HF, Cleveland RJ (1977) Intermuscular abdominal implantation of permanent pacemakers in infants and children. Ann Thorac Surg 25:243-247
2. Benrey J, Gillette PC, Nasrallah AT, Hallman GL (1976) Permanent pacemaker implantation in infants, children, and adolescents. Long-term follow-up. Circulation 53:245-248
3. Daicoff GR, Aslami A, Tobias JA, Miller BL (1974) Management of postoperative complete heart block in infants and children. Chest 66:639-641
4. Donahoo JS, Haller JA, Zonnebelt S, Neill C, Gott VL, Brawley RK (1976) Permanent cardiac pacemakers in children: Technical considerations. Ann Thorac Surg 22: 584-587
5. Idriss FS, Otto R, Nikaidoh H, Newfeld E, Paul MH (1973) Implantation of permanent pacemaker in the first month of life for congenital complete heart block. J Thorac Cardiovasc Surg 65:851-855
6. Mulch J, Wüsten B, Georgi M, Hehrlein FW (1980) Verbesserte Möglichkeiten der transvenösen Schrittmacherbehandlung durch Anwendung von aktiv verankerbaren Endocardelektroden. Herz/Kreislauf 12:212-219
7. Smyth NPD (1979) Cardiac pacing. Ann Thorac Surg 27:270-283

Aortic Valve Replacement in Children With Rheumatic Heart Disease

A. Appelbaum, M.S. Gotsman, A. Simcha, and J.B. Borman*

Between 1968-1978, 20 children, aged 7-16, were operated on for severe rheumatic disease of the aortic valve. There were 14 males and six females. Eleven patients were in F.C. grade III and nine in grade IV (NYHA). The dominant pathology was AI in 19 and aortic stenosis in one. In addition to aortic valve disease, four patients had mitral incompetence (MI), three had MI + tricuspid insufficiency, and one had MI + MS, TI + TS. Nineteen patients were in sinus rhythm and one in atrial fibrillation at the time of surgery. Three patients were operated on during acute rheumatic activity including two children with MI + AI who required emergency double valve replacement because of severe CHF and pulmonary edema. The child with the triple valvular disease had had previous closed mitral commissurotomy. All 20 patients had aortic valve replacement (AVR), five patients had AVR + MVR, one had AVR + MVR + TVR, and one had AVR + MVR + tricuspid De-Vega annuloplasty. The prostheses used were changed during the years. One had Hufnagel valve, seven had Starr-Edwards ball valves, ten had Björk-Shiley disc valves, and two had Ionescu-Shiley biological valves. In one patient, the No. 8A S-E valve had to be replaced 4 years later as a result of severe stenosis.

There were no operative deaths: 16 patients (80%) improved significantly during a follow-up period of 1-12 years. There were four late deaths (20%), 2 months to 7 years after surgery. The cause of death was unknown in one patient, stuck valve in one, S.B.E. in one, and residual mitral incompetence in one. Three patients had recurrent episodes of rheumatic activity.

We conclude that rheumatic aortic valvular damage is a life-threatening condition in the young. Aortic valve replacement may be carried out with low mortality. Rheumatic activity is not a contraindication for surgery if the child's condition deteriorates. There is a marked clinical improvement with an acceptable incidence of late complications.

*Hadassah University Hospital

The Preserved Dura Mater for Repair of Congential Cardiac Anomalies

B. A. Koroljev, A. V. Koroljev, V. A. Yjaznicov, and V. V. Sokolov*

Today the majority of patients with congenital cardiac anomalies should have reconstructive operations with the necessary use of different plastic materials. Synthetic materials are not always available for correction of ventricular septal defects, the tetralogy of Fallot, and other anomalies.

The dura mater as a plastic material has been used at Gorky Medical Training Institute. It has been demonstrated that a sufficiently high elasticity of the dura mater is combined with a high tensile strength – the dura mater is able to sustain dynamic loadings of greater than 6 atm for 24 h or longer in experiments with both constant and impulse pressure loading without any appreciable stretching. The structural features of the dura mater are thought to explain this. Collagenous fibers, constituting the main mass of the dura mater, make up bundles which lie in criss-cross directions; the elastic fibers are known not only to join the isolated collagenous fibers, but also to penetrate through adjacent layers so forming the strong three-dimensional structure. The cellular elements, predominantly fibroblasts, constitute a relatively small part of the dura mater general mass. This is the cause of its extremely low antigenicity.

In order to test the value of the dura mater as a plastic material, experimental studies were performed on ten mongrel dogs. Artificially created defects of the lateral aortic wall were repaired by dura mater grafts. The results were obtained at follow-up from 1 month to 1 year.

Neither macro- nor microscopic studies of the grafts revealed any severe inflammatory reactions in the neighbouring tissues. In all cases the elasticity remained, the grafts pulsated, and were capable of withstanding the systemic pressure. Gradually increasing dystrophic changes of the graft and substitution of it by the connective tissue of the host resulted in the following observations. Within 5 to 6 postoperative months, the graft tissues did not differ in macro- and micropreparations from adjacent areas of the aorta. Occasionally solitary regions of fibrous interruption were observed within the friable connective tissue and many cellular elements could be seen. At 1 year, the graft as a whole was indistinguishable practicably from the aortic wall. Full endothelialisation took place. Taking into account these findings, one can reasonably suggest that it is possible to use dura mater for reconstructive operations in cardiovascular surgery in the clinical field.

We have used human dura mater taken after death from trauma. Tissues were taken during the initial 8 to 16 hours after death only from cadavers which had been stored in a refrigerator at +2°C to +4°C. Both lophilized and xenogenic dura mater grafts have been used. The most convenient and simple method is the technique of tissue preservation in 0.75% formalin with subsequent cooling to +2°C to +4°C. This method provides sterile material after 10 to 12 days of storage at +4°C even if the cadaver tissues had been taken in a non-sterile state. The dura

*Gorky Medical Institute, 8a - 3, Zhdanov Embankment, Gorky, USSR, 603005

mater so preserved retains its fibrous and cellular structure for 6 months. Moreover, at the end of this period, the tensile strength of the graft is unchanged. To January 1, 1980, in Gorky Cardiovascular Center 174 clinical operations have been performed for correction of congenital cardiac anomalies using dura mater as a plastic material. The distribution of patients according to their anomalies is given in Table 1. Table 2 shows the character of operations performed using dura mater homografts.

The late follow-up revealed varying degrees of residual ventricular septal defect in 7.3% of cases. In four patients late septic endocarditis was the cause of this complication; two of these patients were reoperated upon successfully. In conclusion we would like to emphasize that the dura mater is a good plastic material. It possesses durability, elasticity, and a low antigenicity. Our results from the clinical use of preserved dura mater make it possible for us to recommend dura mater for use as a plastic material in cardiovascular surgery.

Table 1. Distribution of patients according to the types of congenital cardiac anomalies

Anomaly	Number
Tetralogy of Fallot	83
Ventricular septal defect	78
Atrial septal defect	7
Miscellaneous	6
Total	174

Table 2. Character of repair with the dura mater homografts

Character of repair	Number
Repair of ventricular septal defect	136
Repair of ventricular septal defect plus right ventricular outflow tract	24
Repair of ventricular septal defect plus the main pulmonary artery	4
Repair of atrial septal defect	7
Repair of anomalous pulmonary venous drainage	1
Indirect isthmoplasty of supravalvular aortic stenosis	1
Total	174

Clinical Experience With Aortoventriculoplasty for Different Types of Left Ventricular Outflow Tract Obstruction (LVOTO)

R. de Vivie, J. Koncz, G. Rupprath, and A. Beuren*

Introduction

Left ventricular outflow tract stenoses can be divided into isolated or combined forms of supravalvular, valvular, or subvalvular aortic stenoses. Isolated obstructions are observed all three levels. Valvular forms are dysplastic, often bicuspid aortic valves combined with a narrow valvular ring. Subvalvular forms are 1) diaphragma, 2) diffuse (fibromuscular), either localised or tunnellike, 3) dynamic forms, known as HOCM or IHSS. Common are combinations and overlapping of all forms at different levels multiple level stenosis. The "Shone complex" is one example.

The results of conventional operative methods for different types of congenital left ventricular outflow tract obstructions (LVOTO) are up to now still unsatisfactory. This is valid particularly for tunnel type and multilevel stenoses. Especially in the case of congenital valvular aortic stenosis with narrow annulus and dysplastic valves commissurotomy can only be regarded as a palliative operation.

Introducing a new surgical procedure to enlarge the stenotic left ventricular outflow tract solved in our opinion a surgical-technical problem. The so-called aortoventriculoplasty (AVP) has been developed by Rastan and Koncz (8, 9) and applied in Göttingen as a routine since 1974. Independently Konno et al. (7) employed a similar operative procedure in 1975 which was used by Symbas (11) in 1976. In the following years, there were additional methods of treatment for left ventricular outflow tract stenoses in the literature. Cooley performed a left ventricular to abdominal aorta conduit to relieve the obstruction. Bernhard et al. (1, 2) also published clinical results with this method. Ross and Sommerville (10) reported in 1980 their experience concerning total aortic valve and root replacement with aortic homograft and reimplantation of coronary arteries for diffuse left ventricular outflow tract obstruction.

Operative Technique

Infusion cardioplegia according to Bretschneider et al. (4) is used for myocardial protection. After cardiac arrest, a longitudinal aortotomy is made between right and left coronary ostia (Fig. 1a). In the course of aortotomy care must be taken to be far enough to the left from the ostium of the right coronary artery. Then the right ventricular outflow tract is opened by a transverse incision just beneath

*Klinik für Thorax-Herz-Gefäßchirurgie, Klinikum Göttingen, Robert-Koch-Str. 40, D-3400 Göttingen

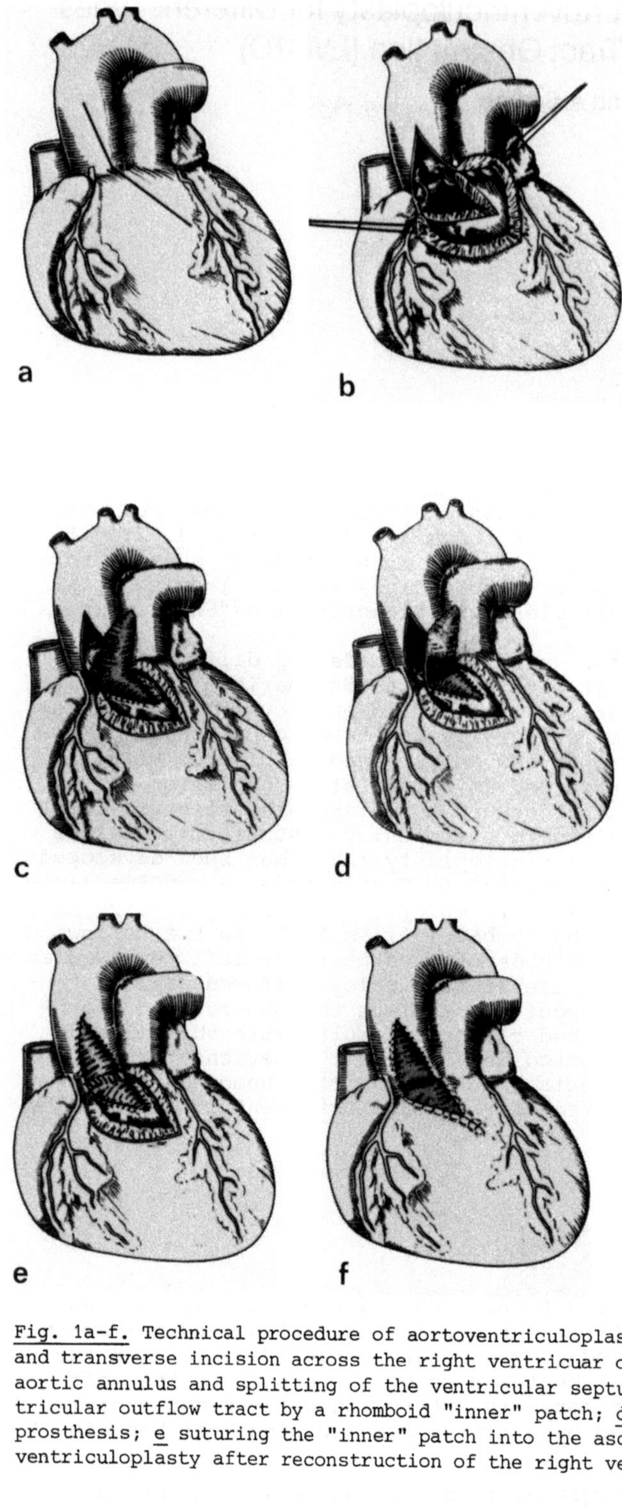

Fig. 1a-f. Technical procedure of aortoventriculoplasty. a Longitudinal aortotomy and transverse incision across the right ventricuar outflow tract; b dividing of the aortic annulus and splitting of the ventricular septum; c roofing of the left ventricular outflow tract by a rhomboid "inner" patch; d implantation of a valvular prosthesis; e suturing the "inner" patch into the ascending aorta; f completed aortoventriculoplasty after reconstruction of the right ventricular outflow tract the pulmonary valve. The aortic and right ventricular incisions are joined after dividing the infundibulo-ventricular fold and the aortic annulus. Now the septum is incised with scalpel exactly in the commissure between left and right cusp as far as possible. The length of the incision depends on the desired size to which the annulus has to be expanded and the thickness of the ventricular septum (Fig. 1b). The aortic valve and – if necessary – subaortic fibrous tissue are excised. The reconstruction of the left ventricular outflow tract is started with a rhomboid "inner" patch (Dacron) inserted in the V-shaped septal defect (Fig. 1c). The running suture beginning in the angle is directed from the right side through the septum to the left side and then through the patch. In this manner, the patch roofs the septal defect on the right side thus allowing the widest possible exit of the left ventricular outflow tract. An adequate prosthesis, fitting the enlarged annulus, is now sewn to the posterior (natural) annulus, whereas the anterior position of the sewing ring is fixed to the outflow patch with an outer running suture (Fig. 1d). We implanted the following prostheses: two Starr-Edwards (sizes 9 and 12) in the first patients, 37 Björk-Shiley (sizes 21 to 29), and nine St. Jude Medical (SJM, sizes 23 to 29).

The right ventricle is reconstructed by a second triangular "outer" patch (Dacron), suturing the upper edge of the patch directly to the "inner" patch. Care must be taken to remold adequately the roof of the ventricle to avoid narrowing of the right outflow (Figs. 1f and 2a,b).

Patients

From 1961 to 1980, 1089 children with various types of congenital aortic stenoses were diagnosed at Göttingen University Hospital. Four hundred and thirty-eight out of these patients were operated on by conventional methods. Patient material is divided into three groups:

1) Valvular aortic stenosis	246
2) Supravalvular aortic stenosis	51
3) Subvalvular aortic stenosis	141
Diaphragma	42
Diffuse (fibrous)	85
Tunnellike	14

Since 1974, we operated in Göttingen on 47 patients with aortoventriculoplasty. Patients age ranged from 4 to 35 years; most of the operations have been performed at ages between 8 and 15 years. There were 32 male patients and 16 females. It is noteworthy that for only 12 patients was the aortoventriculoplasty the first operation. Twenty-seven patients had one and eight patients had two unsuccessful previous attempts to relieve the outflow tract stenosis (Fig. 3).

Among a total of 47 patients, 23 had diffuse subaortic stenoses, eight had valvular stenosis with a narrow annulus, and nine had a subaortic tunnel, four of them associated with a Shone complex. In three cases a small aortic prosthesis implanted in childhood was changed with enlargement of the valvular ring. Four patients had hypertrophic obstructive cardiomyopathy (HOCM) (Table 1). The mean time of ischemic cardiac arrest was 71 ± 14 minutes and ranged from 48 to 155 minutes. The first nine patients were operated on with intermittent coronary perfusion. In this group, we had three deaths. The following 38 patients have been protected by infusion cardioplegia.

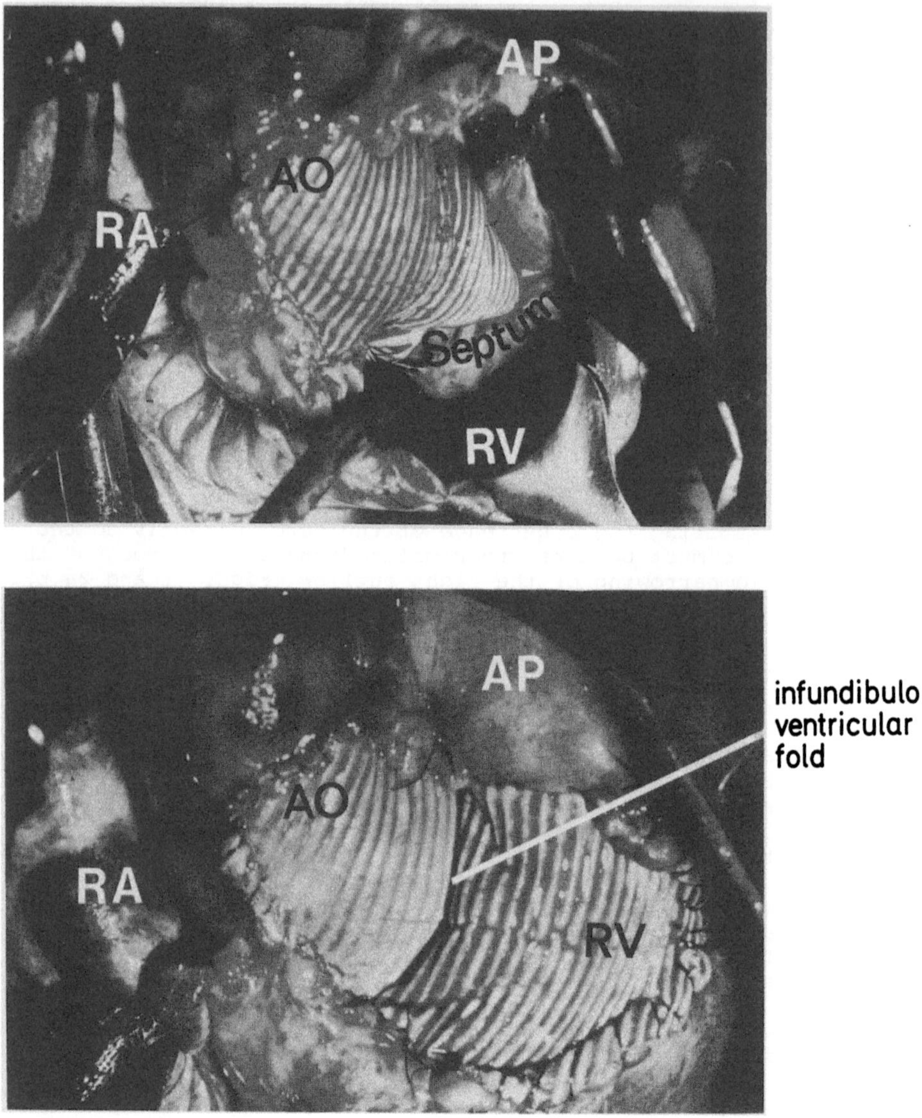

a

b

Fig. 2a,b. Aortoventriculoplasty. a Intraoperative view into the right ventricle, "inner" patch after aortic valve replacement; b completed. *RA* right atrium; *AO* aorta; *AP* pulmonary artery; *RV* right ventricle

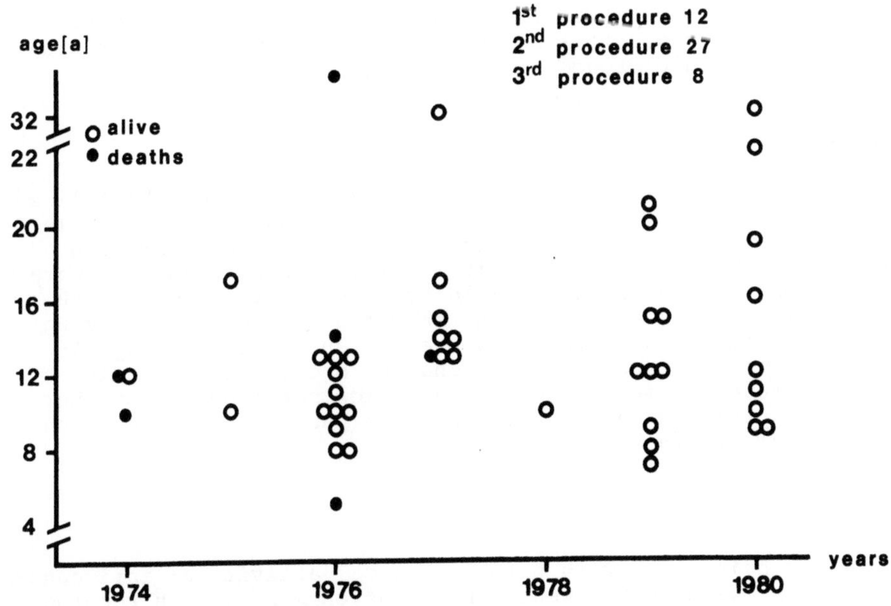

Fig. 3. Aortoventriculoplasty

Table 1. Aortoventriculoplasty (AVP) for left ventricular outflow tract obstruction (LVOTO)

Diagnosis	Patients	Mortality
Diffuse subaortic stenosis, multilevel stenosis	23	3
Narrow aortic annulus	8	0
Tunnel subaortic stenosis (4 x Shone complex)	9	2
Outgrown prosthesis	3	0
HOCM	4	1
Total	47	6 (12.7%)

Results

Mortality

Out of 47 patients, six died at operation or 1 to 12 days postoperatively. The total mortality rate was 12.7%. There was no late death. The causes of death were as follows: In the first 12-year-old patient who had two previous operations, it was impossible of come off bypass; furthermore, we had bleeding disorders. One child had an ischemic lesion according to an anomaly of the right coronary artery, and two patients myocardial failure. One patient suffered renal failure caused by an underestimated coarctation of aorta. One patient died of cerebral damage, apparently due to a perfusion disorder; we used retrograde arterial cannulation in presence of a coarctation.

Complications

The follow-up examinations of all surviving patients showed the following complications: Two patients with Shone complex had mild mitral insufficiency, two patients had small fistulas to the right ventricle. In one patient, there was a mild aortic insufficiency caused by a paravalvular leak, one patient showed a mild outflow tract stenosis with a gradient of 37 mm Hg, another patient showed a gradient of 60 mm Hg between left ventricle and aorta. Only one patient developed a postoperative hepatitis. Postoperative ECG changes showed right bundle branch block in seven patients and left anterior hemiblock in another three cases. Two patients needed a transvenous pacemaker implantation due to a permanent AV block.

Restudies

All patients are doing well with normal physical activities; anticoagulation therapy is obligatory. Twenty-three patients have been recatheterised between 1 month and 3 years after operation. The mean gradients between left ventricle and aorta has been lowered from 98 to 14 mm Hg. Even after provocation with isoproterenol, no gradient increased more than 15 mm Hg, except one patient with a gradient of 60 mm Hg over the aortic valve prosthesis. This patient had been operated in the first series and the implanted Björk-Shiley prosthesis of 21 mm was too small. Left ventricular end-diastolic pressure did not increase significantly after operation. The gradients between the right ventricle and the pulmonary artery did not change significantly; they were in the normal range. In two patients, we measurd small ventricular defects which do not require reoperation.

Conclusions

Reviewing our operative experience, we suggest some technical aspects:
1. Due to the long time of cardiac ischemic arrest, an optimal myocardial protection is necessary. We use the infusion cardioplegia according to Bretschneider et al. (4).
2. Preclotting with fibrin glue of the Dacron-velour patch material is a safe prevention against postoperative bleeding.
3. In case of hypertrophic septum, the patch material is inserted using a special large atraumatic needle (CTX needle, Ethicon).

According to our clinical results, the following indications for aortoventriculoplasty are concluded:
1. We see the main application of AVP *for all forms* of *diffuse SAS* from collarlike to tunnellike obstruction.
2. Another indication is the narrow aortic annulus. The associated lesions are to be duly observed.
3. Because of the tendency of recurrence in some cases of HOCM, AVP can be considered as a second intervention.
4. In multilevel obstructive lesions of the so-called Shone complex, the AVP opens a promising way for corrective surgery, provided that a significant coarctation has been removed previously. In addition, the method may be applied in some cases of diffuse supravalvular stenosis.

5. Finally, AVP in our opinion is the method of choice in cases of "outgrown" aortic prosthesis in a growing child. The diameter of the aortic annulus can be doubled if necessary. This operation gives the child the chance to reach adult life without exchange of the prosthesis.

Summary

Since the first clinical application of the aortoventriculoplasty for tunnel subaortic stenosis in 1974, the indication for this method was extended to other types of left ventricular outflow tract stenoses. The operation technique consists in enlarging both the left and right ventricle outflow tract and inserting an aortic prosthetic valve.

Forty-five operations have been performed in patients with various types of LVOTO: Seven narrow annulus, 22 diffuse subaortic stenosis (multiple level stenosis), nine complex forms of tunnel subaortic stenosis (Shone complex), three outgrown prosthesis, four obstructive idiopathic hypertrophic subaortic stenosis. Patient age ranged from 4 to 35 years. Overall mortality was 13%, no late deaths; in the last 34 patients no death. In 25 patients, there were one and in 13 patients two previous procedures. As a result of the operation, nine patients developed complete right bundle branch block or left anterior hemiblock, in two patients total AV block was observed with the need of permanent pacemaker implantation. Twenty-five patients had catheterization postoperatively. Mean gradient across the left ventricular outflow tract was significantly reduced from 91.5 ± 21 mm Hg to 13.1 ± 15 mm Hg. According to our experience, aortoventriculoplasty can be used routinely in all forms of diffuse subaortic stenosis, narrow aortic annulus, reoperation in HOCM, multiple level stenosis, and outgrown aortic prosthesis.

References

1. Bernhard WF, Keane JF, Fellows KE, Litwin SB, Gross RE (1973) Progress and problems in the surgical management of congenital aortic stenosis. J Thorac Cardiovasc Surg 66:404
2. Bernhard WF, Poirier V, La Farge CG (1975) Relief of congenital obstruction to left ventricular outflow with a ventricular aortic prosthesis. J Thorac Cardiovasc Surg 69:223
3. Björnstad PG, Rastan H, Keutel J, Beuren AJ, Koncz J (1979) Aortoventriculoplasty for tunnel subaortic stenosis and other obstructions of the left ventricular outflow tract. Circulation 60:59
4. Bretschneider HJ, Gebhard MM, Preuße CJ (1980) Optimalisation of myocardial protection. In: Advances in clinical cardiology, vol I. Witzstrock, New York
5. Cooley DA, Norman JC, Mullius CE, Grace RR (1975) Left ventricle to abdominal aorta conduits for relief of aortic stenosis. Cardiovasc Dis Bull Texas Heart Inst 2:376
6. Hatcher CR (1976) Aortic valve replacement: The problem of the small aortic annulus (Editorial). J Thorac Cardiovasc Surg 71:400
7. Konno S, Imai Y, Iida Y, Nakajima M, Tetsuno K (1975) A new method for prosthetic valve replacement in congenital aortic stenosis associated with hypoplasia of the aortic valve ring. J Thorac Cardiovasc Surg 70:909
8. Rastan H, Koncz J (1975) Plastische Erweiterung der linken Ausflußbahn — Eine neue Operationsmethode. Thoraxchirurgie 23:169

9. Rastan H, Koncz J (1976) Aortoventriculoplasty, a new technique for the treatment of left ventricular outflow tract obstructions. J Thorac Cardiovasc Surg 71:920
10. Ross D, Sommerville J (1980) Total aortic valve and root replacement with aortic homograft and reimplantation of the coronary arteries for diffuse left ventricular outflow tract obstruction. First World Congress of Pediatric Cardiology, London, Abstract 313
11. Symbas PN, Ware RE, Hatcher CR, Temesy-Armos PN (1976) An operation for relief of severe left ventricular outflow tract obstruction. J Thorac Cardiovasc Surg 71:245

Session XI Vascular Surgery

Vascular Forum III

Chairman: K.V. Hall, Oslo; Co-Chairman: R.C. de Sobregrau, Barcelona

Hemodilution in Arterial Reconstructive Surgery

Z. M. Daciewicz, and T. Orlowski*

Intraoperative hemodilution is a method which allowed us to obtain a certain amount of the patient's own blood. This blood used during or after the operation eliminates the need for stored homogenous blood transfusions. The advantages of this method are well known and therefore hemodilution has been widely introduced in different types of operation. However, in arterial reconstructive surgery, there are some fears of coagulopathy due to dilution leading to a leaking anastomosis and affecting graft clotting.

Experimental

Material and Method

The experiment was carried out on 19 mongrel dogs of mean body weight 17 kg. Under general anesthesia, excision and then reconstruction of the lower abdominal aorta was performed using woven or knitted Dacron grafts. After completion of proximal anastomosis grafts were preclotted in the animals' own blood. Heparin was not used.

The animals were divided into three groups. Group A (six animals) was regarded as a control. In group B (six animals) 20% of circulating blood volume was drawn just prior to the operation with simultaneous volume replacement using multielectrolyte solution and 5% glucose. In group C (seven animals) 40% of circulating blood volume was drawn with similar volume replacement. The drawn blood was reinfused after the end of surgery.

Samples of blood for morphology, biochemistry, and coagulological examinations were taken before the operation, at the end of surgery, and on the 1st, 5th, and 10th postoperative days. The animals were killed between the 10th and 37th postoperative days and pathomorphological examination was performed with special consideration of the reconstructed part of the aorta.

Results

1. Clinical observations. In the majority of cases the postoperative course was uneventful. On the 5th postoperative day, full recovery was noted. In two animals of group A, paresis of the hind limbs occurred and groin pulses were absent. This complication occurred in one animal in group B and in one in group C.

*Centre of Postgraduate Education M.M.A., Institute of Surgery, ul. Szasevów 128, Warsaw - 60, Poland

2. Results of laboratory studies. Mean laboratory values are shown in Tables 1 and 2.

3. Pathomorphology. During postmortem examination, only various degrees of passive hyperemia of internal organs were observed in all the animals. In group A, the graft was thrombosed in two cases. This was found in one animal in group B and in one in group C. In two cases in group C, a hematoma was found around the graft.

Table 1. Mean results of some laboratory studies. *I*, before operation; *II*, end of the operation; *III*, 1st day after operation; *IV*, 5th day after operation; *V*, 10th day after operation

Type of laboratory study	Group	Time of investigation				
		I	II	III	IV	V
HCT vol%	A	37.7	40.5	46.3	30	43.0
	B	39.7	36.8	44.2	38.2	41.8
	C	42.6	31.0	40.0	36.4	39.0
Platelets x $10^3/mm^3$	A	163	108	128	173	170
	B	161	135	156	174	181
	C	163	130	180	175	168
Ca^{++} mg%	A	9.9	8.9	9.6	9.6	9.8
	B	9.5	7.9	9.4	9.7	9.9
	C	9.7	7.1	8.9	9.7	9.7
Fibrinogen level mg/ml	A	2.9	2.6	6.4	5.2	4.0
	B	2.9	2.6	5.3	4.6	3.3
	C	3.1	1.7	5.2	4.6	3.4

Clinical

Material

During recent months, we have performed 79 arterial reconstructive operations; 32 of them (40.5%) were done using hemodilution. Inclusion criteria for hemodilution were: age under 65, hematocrit value not lower than 40%, and hemoglobin level at least 13 g/dl.

Table 3 depicts types of operations with and without hemodilution and the amount of stored blood transfused in both groups. Moderate hemodilution was done in the theatre and on an average 800 ml of blood was drawn with simultaneous volume replacement using electrolyte and glucose isotonic solutions.

Grafts were preclotted using Souvage method. Samples of blood for laborabory evaluations were taken before and at the end of operation, and on the 1st, 5th, and 10th postoperative days.

In some cases, especially with a forefoot necrosis, sisomicin was given prophylactically. There were no serious infection complications.

Table 2. Some mean results of the coagulation study. *I*, before operation; *II*, end of the operation; *III*, 1st day after operation; *IV*, 5th day after operation; *V*, 10th day after operation

Type of study	Group	Time of study I	II	III	IV	V
Recalcination time (s)	A	63	35	48	64	63
	B	63	86	62	60	61
	C	62	108	89	74	61
Prothrombin time (s)	A	6.5	5.8	7.5	5.9	6.6
	B	6.6	9.2	6.9	7.2	6.8
	C	6.4	7.6	6.6	6.3	6.3
Thrombin time (s)	A	11.5	11.8	10.0	13.4	11.2
	B	12.0	18.3	10.0	14.4	12.8
	C	11.5	13.6	9.9	11.7	12.8
Euglobulin lysis time (min)	A	26	25	92	48	39
	B	21	26	56	36	24
	C	23	20	49	35	23

Table 3. Type of operation and amount of donor blood which was transfused

	Type of operation	Hemodilution			No hemodilution		
		No. of cases	Trans- fusion	Blood amount (ml)	No. of cases	Cases with transf.	Blood amount (ml)
Bypass operations	Fem-pop (vein)	12	1	1000	6	4	6000
	Fem-pop (prosthesis)	5	1	500	13	9	8250
	Aorto-fem bifurcated (Leriche syndrome)	3	2	1500	10	9	11250
	Aorto-fem bifurcated (aorta aneurysm)	-	-	-	4	4	8750
	Ilio-fem	8	2	1000	3	1	500
Others		4	1	1000	11	9	8500
Total		32	7	5000	47	36	43250

Results

1. Results of surgery. During surgery, there were no significant differences between patients operated on with or without hemodilution. Grafts and arterial anastomoses were tight after preclotting. The postoperative course was similar in both groups as well as late clinical results.

Intraoperative hemodilution allowed us to obtain 62 units of the patients' own blood which was reinfused during or just after surgery. Only in seven cases (21.9%) in the group with hemodilution, there was a need for transfusion of donor blood. The total amount of blood transfused in this group was 5000 ml. In three cases surgery with hemodilution was repeated two or three times without any donor blood. In the group operated on without hemodilution, 36 patients (76.6%) required blood transfusions in the total amount of 43 250 ml.

2. Results of laboratory studies. Selected mean laboratory values are presented in Table 4.

Table 4. Some mean results after operations with hemodilution. *I*, before operation; *II*, end of the operation; *III*, 1st day after operation; *IV*, 5th day after operation; *V*, 10th day after operation

Type of investigation	Time of study				
	I	II	III	IV	V
HCT vol%	46	35	39	36	39
Platelets x $10^3/mm^3$	193	123	194	207	269
Fibrinogen mg/ml	5.72	4.05	5.92	6.92	6.45
Ca^{++} mg%	9.72	8.10	9.13	9.04	9.33
Thrombin time (s)	12.9	13.3	12.6	13.0	13.2
Prothrombin time (s)	13.4	15.2	14.0	-	-
Euglobulin lysis time (min)	155	170	212	209	188
FSP μg	3.7	4.9	5.4	4.0	3.9

Discussion

In the experiment it was found that intraoperative hemodilution decreases the number of morphotic elements, protein complexes, and enzymes. These changes seem to be proportional to the degree of hemodilution. Even profound hemodilution (40% of circulating blood volume) does not significantly impair basic functions of blood such as gas exchange and hemostasis mechanisms.

Clotting tests have shown in the control group (without hemodilution) there was a tendency to a hypercoagulability state especially at the end of surgery and on the 1st postoperative day. This phenomenon did not occur in animals operated on in hemodilution. In group B (moderate hemodilution), hemostasis was not impaired and did not differ from normal values. In group C (profound hemodilution), a tendency to hypocoagulability was seen but not to a pathological degree. Moderate hemodilution would therefore appear to be an optimal method for application in normal clinical practice.

Thirty-two reconstructive vascular operations in human patients were performed using intraoperative moderate hemodilution. No coagulation and fibrinolysis disorders were observed. Intraoperative hemodilution in vascular surgery decreases the risk of early thrombosis of the graft and the possibility of embolic complications. Hemodilution also decreases the amount of stored homogenous blood transfused. This kind of treatment protects the patient from infections and immunological complications which can occur in case of massive and frequent transfusions.

Conclusions

1. Intraoperative hemodilution is a safe method of supplying blood for patients undergoing operations.
2. Intraoperative hemodilution can be used in arterial surgery.
3. A moderate intraoperative hemodilution (about 20% of circulating blood volume) seems to be optimal in arterial surgery.
4. This method lessens the risk of early graft thrombosis and incidence of infections and immunological complications.
5. A profound intraoperative hemodilution (about 40% of circulating blood volume) can lead to a hypocoagulability impairing proper graft healing due to hematoma.

Increased Calf Blood Flow and Haemoglobin Delivery Following Haemodilution in Patients With Intermittent Claudication

C. Yates, A. Berent, M. Bailey, and J. Dormany*

Experimental work in animals and a few clinical trials suggest that, in patients with coronary artery disease and peripheral vascular disease, haemodilution from haematocrits in the upper range of normal is of clinical benefit. However, there has been no quantitative measurement of the changes in calf blood flow patients with intermittent claudication.

We performed limited normovolaemic haemodilution in 15 patients with stable intermittent claudication in whom surgery was not indicated at that time. Calf resting and reactive hyperaemic blood flow was measured using strain gauge plethysmography. 500 ml of blood were withdrawn at weekly intervals and replaced with 500 ml of Dextran 70 in normal saline. All measurements were repeated within one week of completion of haemodilution.

Results: For a mean 20% reduction in the haematocrit, there was a mean increase of 170% in the peak blood flow ($p < 002$) and a 110% increase in peak haemoglobin delivery ($p < 0.02$).

Eleven out of the 15 patients reported subjective improvement in their walking distance.

Patients have been followed for up to 18 months and the variable rise in the haematocrit and the accompanying changes in the blood flow and haemoglobin delivery were noted.

---

*St. James' Hospital, London, Great Britain

Thermal Entrainment of Peripheral Blood Flow

A. J. Mearns and J. B. Harness*

Thermal entrainment of peripheral blood flow is a new non-invasive approach to the assessment of cardiovascular function. This paper describes an instrument to generate a square wave thermal signal which will entrain the following cardiovascular parameters: peripheral blood flow, heart rate variability, blood pressure, and intra-cranial pressure. Comments will be restricted to the measurements of peripheral blood flow.

Introduction

Frequency analysis techniques (4) show that within the cardiovascular system there are well-recognised frequencies occurring at less than heart rate; these frequencies are generated by normal body functions. The most readily recognised identifiable parameter is the regular rhythm of respiration. Under normal circumstances in a healthy individual at rest, the breathing pattern is 15 times per minute; this will generate a frequency of 0.25 Hz. The effect of breathing upon the impedence of the pulmonary vasculature alters the rate of right-to-left transfer of blood across the lungs. There is a change in the left ventricular filling and thus a change in the left ventricular output; this respiratory variation can be demonstrated in the blood pressure signal. The presence of this respiratory component within the blood pressure signal is described as entrainment. The power of this entrainment frequency will depend on the depth of the respiration, that is how much change in intra-thoracic impedence to blood flow has occurred. The Traube-Hering-Mayer frequency was first described by Traube (9) when he identified the slow waves occurring in the outer envelope of the blood pressure in curarised animals. Hering (5) studied these waves but suggested they were respiratory in origin. However, Mayer (8) described these waves in the presence of normal respiration and suggested that they were separate from respiration as Traube had initially thought. Today the evidence is that the Traube-Hering-Mayer wave (10) as it now tends to be called, has its origin in the coordinated contraction of the smooth muscle of the arterial tree. This frequency seems to be coordinated centrally by the vasomotor centre and appears to be directly related to the activity of the baro-receptors. For any increase in baroreceptor response, for instance, when a prone patient stands up, there is an increase in the power of the Traube-Hering-Mayer frequency.

The third frequency that occurs is the thermo-regulatory wave and it was first identified by Burton (2). Burton and Taylor (3) performed

*Bradford Royal Infirmary and Schools of Chemical and Control Engineering, University of Bradford, Bradford BD7 1DP, Great Britain

a sophisticated series of experiments which demonstrated that the wave form was an essential thermo-regulatory frequency that varied between once every 30 s and once every 90 s depending on the necessary rate of heat loss. They showed that as the need to lose heat increased so the frequency decreased and as the patient cooled down and had less need to lose body heat the frequency of thermo-regulatory wave increased. Kitney (7) has demonstrated that thermal entrainment of this peripheral thermo-regulatory frequency was possible by alternately immersing the hand in water at 18 and 46°C at a regular frequency. He was able to detect the entrainment of this frequency in peripheral blood flow and heart rate variability. It is very difficult to control the frequency accurately when the patient has to move his hand from one reservoir of water to the other; this difficulty is most apparent when the patient is obliged to move quickly from one reservoir to the other. In order to bring this principle to a wider range of patients some of whom may not be able to cooperate at all, we have developed an instrument which is able to deliver an alternating flow of air through a plastic sleeve, over a limb at the temperatures of 18 and 46°C. With this instrument we are able to strictly control the frequency and deliver the set temperatures at will (6).

Instrument: The Thermal Entrainment Device

An industrial hot air blower (Fig. 1), somewhat similar to a hair dryer, is used to deliver a constant flow of air through a plastic sleeve over either the arm or the leg. With the blower on continuously air heating is provided by switching on the heating element at a pre-set frequency; the temperature of the cool air is maintained by controlling the temperature of the air delivered to the blower. The hot air temperature is controlled by a thermistor immediately proximal to the delivery point at the limb so that the air temperature is controlled by a feedback mechanism during the heating phase; thus overheating is not possible. The air passes over the limb within its plastic sleeve and is allowed to escape from the top to atmosphere. The hot air temperature is 46°C and the cool air temperature is preferably at 18°C but may be allowed to rise to 24°C. Timing of the heating period is controlled using a constant frequency oscillator which is divided down until the last bi-stable circuit in the chain is running at the required period. Variable time is achieved by changing the frequency of the oscillators, so with this equipment we are able to deliver a hot-cold square wave signal to the limb which may be varied.

Physiology

When the square wave hot-cold signal is delivered over the limb, the temperature change is detected by the cutaneous receptors in the skin. Essentially under these circumstances the hot receptors are stimulated directly and the cold receptors are stimulated paradoxically because they are raised initially to the temperature of 46°C and then the cool air comes at 18°C; although this is higher than the normal triggering of their response, they respond to a rate of change of fall in temperature. A temperature difference of greater than 20°C should stimulate the cold receptors paradoxically if the higher temperature is slightly greater than normal body temperature. Under these circumstances an alternating hot and cold recpetor impulse passes up the lateral columns

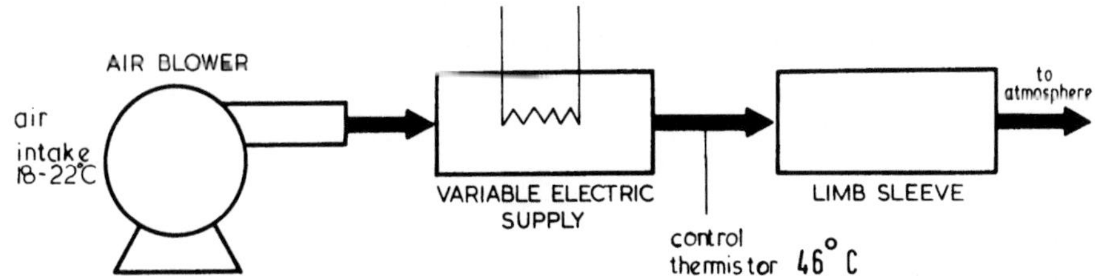

Fig. 1. Flow sheet for providing hot or cold air periodically to the limb sleeve

in the spinal cord to the hind brain and in some way which is not understood, this frequency of oscillation entrains the vasomotor centre. The vasomotor output is conducted both down the vagus nerve to the sinus node and back down the lateral columns to feed into the sympathetic chain. These frequencies now register within the vascular system. This input signal manifests itself in heart rate variability, peripheral blood flow, and within the blood pressure; it can also be detected within the intra-cranial pressure if there is some slight increase of the stiffness of the brain (1).

A series of experiments (6) on fit adults and children have demonstrated the normal behaviour pattern. Twenty patients at rest received the hot/cold square wave signal from the thermal entrainment device to a limb. Their peripheral blood flow was detected with an infra-red plethysmograph and the signal analysed by fast Fourier transform (4). Spectra were produced as in Figure 2. The experiments showed that for period times from 8 to 80 s the body of a healthy adult would follow this periodic temperature variation (Fig. 3) and this defined the period of entrainment. In all the subjects studied, the greatest entrainment occurred with a period time of approximately 30 s and no entrainment occurred with a period time greater than 80 s or less than 8 s. At rest in an ambient temperature, when the patient was neither cold nor had a heat load, the normal temperature control mechanism oscillated 0.03 Hz and therefore we felt it not surprising that the best entrainment occurred close to this frequency. This pattern of entrainment was clearly shown in heart rate variability, peripheral blood flow, and blood pressure. Figure 3 demonstrates the powers generated in a patient; it showed a pattern with two maxima and one minimum. This was a constant finding in all patients but the younger fitter patients tended to have quite a marked minimum between the primary and subsidiary maxima, but with older subjects or less fit subjects this minimum may only show as a point of inflection.

Clinical Aspects

If vasodilators such as sodium nitroprusside (Nipride) or phenoxybenzamine are used, the thermo-regulatory wave form disappears from the peripheral blood flow and blood pressure signals. The thermal entrainment device does not produce its signal in the peripheral flow or blood pressure but it does occur in heart rate variability.

The coordination of the thermo-regularity wave is within the sympathetic nervous system and the oscillation occurs simultaneously throughout the body (3). If the sympathetic chain is blocked locally by local anaesthetic or surgical intervention, central control into the local blood flow is lost and thermal entrainment will not be present in the other limbs. It is very difficult to demonstrate these oscillations if the peripheral temperature is less than 32°C (3).

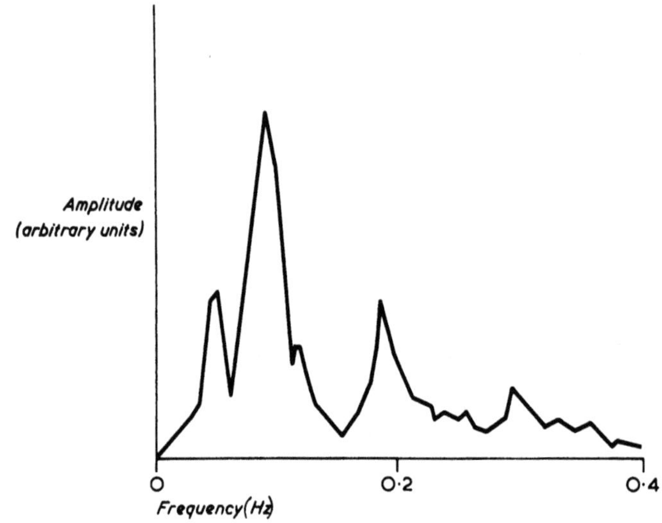

Fig. 2. A typical Fourier transform of the frequency content less than 1 Hz. The lowest peak 0.03 Hz is the thermo-regulatory frequency. The second peak is the Traube-Hering-Mayer wave at 0.1 Hz and the first and second harmonics of respiration are at 01.8 and 0.36 Hz

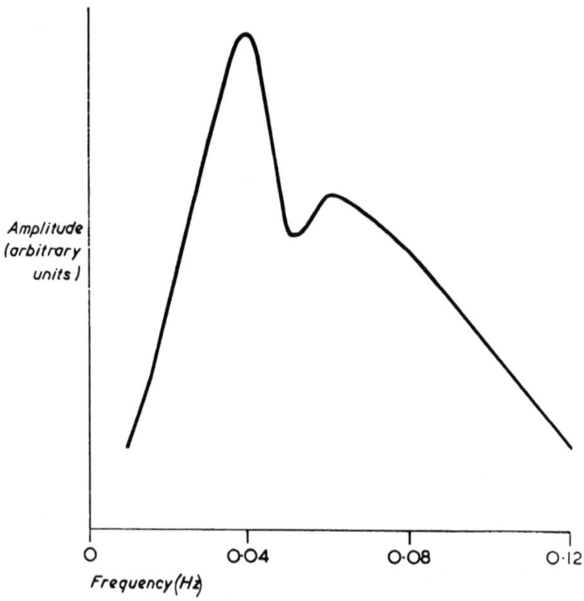

Fig. 3. This demonstrates the entrainment limits for the thermal entrainment device between 0.0125 and 0.125 Hz. The maximum power is at 0.033 Hz. There is a minimum at 0.05 Hz and a secondary maxima at 0.6 Hz

References

1. Ahmed AD, Harness JB, Mason J, Mearns AJ (to be published) Relationships between blood pressure and intra-cranial pressure wave forms.
2. Burton AC (1939) The range and variability of the blood flow in the human fingers and the vasomotor regulation of body temperature. Am J Physiol 127:437-452
3. Burton AC, Taylor RM (1940) A study of the adjustment of peripheral vascular tone to the requirements of the regulation of body temperature. Am J Physiol 129:565-577
4. Cooley JW, Tukey JW (1965) Math Comput 19:297-301
5. Hering E (1869) Über den Einfluß der Atmung auf den Kreislauf. Ver Akad Wiss Wien 60:829
6. Hitchen M, Harness JB, Mearns AJ (to be published) A thermal entrainment device for cardiovascular investigation. J Med Eng Technol
7. Kitney RI (1975) The analysis of and simulation of the human thermoregulatory control system. Med Biol Eng 12:57-64
8. Mayer S (1876) Über spontane Blutdruckschwankungen. Ver Akad Wiss Wien 74:281
9. Traube L (1865) Über periodische Tätigkeitsänderungen des vasomotorischen und Hemmungs-Nervenzentrums. Cgl Med Wiss 56:880
10. Wagner R (1954) Probleme und Beispiele biologischer Regelung. Thieme, Stuttgart

Significance of Red Cell Deformability

J. Dormandy, P. Matthews, M. Boyd, E. Ernst, and D. Bennett*

Although for centuries we have realised that the red cells have to deform in order to negotiate the microcirculation, it is only very recently that the possible pathological significance of abnormalities in red cell deformability has begun to be considered. This has partly been due to the difficulty of assessing red cell deformability (RCD) in the clinical context. A number of techniques such as cinemicrophotography and suction into a micropipette are clearly not applicable clinically. Currently the most widely used method involves the filtration of red cells through small pores. The technique used in the studies reported here involved the filtration of red cells resuspended at a 5% concentration in their own plasma (after elimination of the white cells and platelets) and filtered under the force of gravity through cylindrical pores measuring 5 μ in diameter (1). The possible clinical significance of such measurements in various types of ischaemia is illustrated in three groups of patients.

RCD was measured in 52 patients with ischaemic disease in the legs of varying severity. The results are summarised in Figure 1 which shows that the patients as a whole had a significantly lower RCD than an age- and sex-matched group of normal controls, that is their red cells were more rigid ($p < 0.01$). The prognostic significance of the degree of abnormality became apparent when the patients were followed clinically; patients with more rigid red cells had a worse prognosis than patients with more flexible cells. In Figure 1 only the results in relation to hard criteria of clinical ischaemia are shown. Patients who went on to have reconstructive vascular surgery tended to have lower RCD while the patients who required a major amputation during the subsequent 2 years after the measurement of RCD had significantly more rigid red cells initially than patients with ischaemic legs who did not require amputation ($p < 0.01$).

The second group of patients studied underwent a variety of operations including arterial reconstructions, varicose vein surgery, hernia repairs, and cystoscopies. The general pattern of change in RCD seemed to be independent of the magnitude of the operation; in all cases there was a decrease of RCD, usually reaching a minimum on the second postoperative day and returning to the preoperative level in the subsequent 5 to 10 days. The change in RCD was unrelated to the type of anaesthesia, transfusion of blood during operation, or other intravenous infusions. Nor could the pattern of RCD change be correlated with the postoperative changes in whole blood viscosity (at low or high shear rates) or the changes in plasma fibrinogen.

Further experiments were carried out to try and identify the possible cause for these changes in RCD. Figure 2 summarises the results of these studies in patients having hernia repairs. There was no dif-

*St. James' and St. George's Hospitals, Departments of Surgery, London, Great Britain

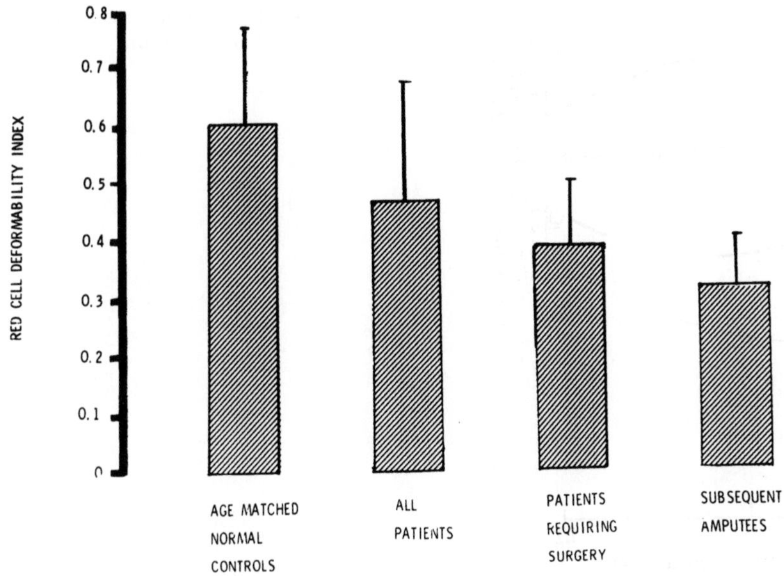

Fig. 1. Red cell deformability in patients with leg ischaemia and its prognostic value

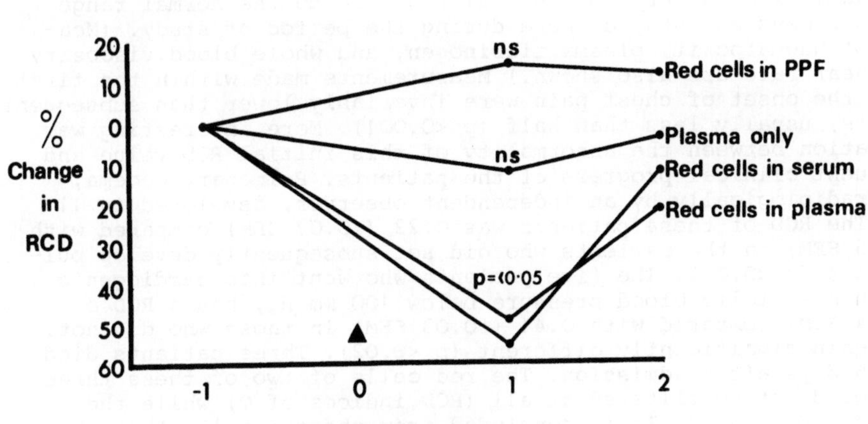

Fig. 2. Five patients having hernia repair

ference in the RCD change, whether the red cells were suspended in their own plasma or serum, confirming that plasma fibrinogen does not affect RCD. Red cells resuspended in purified protein fraction did not alter their filterability following surgery. It would therefore seem that the changes in RCD following operation are due to a plasma factor affecting the red cells. (Plasma alone, without any cells, filtered at an unchanged rate.) The last type of patient studied consisted of 43 cases admitted to hospital as an emergency with acute myocardial infarction. (Patients in whom the clinical diagnosis was not confirmed by electro-

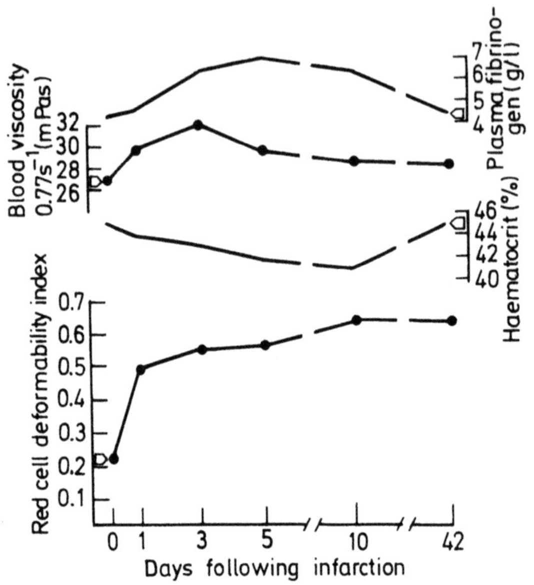

Fig. 3. Haemorrheological changes after myocardial infarction

cardiography and cardiac enzyme studies had been eliminated.) Figure 3 shows the pattern of changes in various haemorrheological measurements following admission. A very low initial RCD rose to the normal range within 1 to 2 days and stayed there during the period of study. (Measurements of haematocrit, plasma fibrinogen, and whole blood viscosity at a low shear rate are also shown.) Measurements made within the first 24 h after the onset of chest pain were invariably lower than subsequent measurements, usually less than half ($p < 0.001$). More interesting was the correlation between the abnormality of this initial RCD value and the subsequent clinical progress of the patients. Pulmonary oedema, diagnosed radiologically by an independent observer, developed in 11 patients. The RCD of these patients was 0.22 (±0.07 SEM) compared with 0.47 (±0.05 SEM) in the patients who did not subsequently develop pulmonary oedema ($p < 0.01$). The five patients who went into cardiogenic shock, with a systolic blood pressure below 100 mm Hg, had a RCD of 0.11 (±0.04 SEM) compared with 0.44 (±0.03 SEM) in those who did not. This was again significantly different ($p < 0.02$). Three patients died 1, 3, and 5 days after admission. The red cells of two of these three patients could not be filtered at all (RCD indices of 0) while the third had a RCD of 0.22. It is concluded from these results that not only are the red cells of patients with recent myocardial infarction much more rigid than normal, at least for the first 24 to 48 h, but also that the degree of abnormality has a prognostic significance in relation to their subsequent clinical course.

The findings in these three studies suggest that there are certain reproducible and constant changes in the deformability of red cells which may have a pathological and clinical significance. The results in patients with chronic ischaemia of the legs and acute ischaemia of the myocardium suggest a correlation between the severity of the ischaemia and the abnormality of the RCD. It is not, however, known which is the cause and which the effect. Possibly a reciprocal interaction may exist, setting up a vicious cycle where some product of ischaemic tissue renders the red cells more rigid and this in turn decreases the perfusion to the area of marginal ischaemia. In both these types of patients the degree of abnormality in RCD appears to be a significant predictor of clinical progress. The study on postoperative patients is mostly of interest as it suggests that changes in RCD, at least following surgery, are not due primarily to a change in the red cell itself, but rather to a plasma factor affecting the red cells secondarily.

The whole field of red cell deformability is clearly still in its infancy. Much further work will be necessary before we can define its exact role in the pathophysiology of circulatory disease and decide the importance of aiming our therapy at this new aspect of haemorrheology. The present report merely suggests that such further work may be profitable.

References

1. Dodds AJ, O'Reilly MJG, Yates CJP, Cotton LT, Flute PT, Dormandy JA (1979) Haemorrheological response to plasma exchange in Raynaud's syndrome. Br Med J 2:1186-1191

Extensive Vascular Surgery on Combined Aorto-iliac and Femoro-popliteal Diseases. Indications and Results

J. A. Gutiérres-Sánchez, J. I. Gallo-Mezo, and J. L. Vega-Fernandez*

Introduction

Significant arteriosclerotic lesions of aortoiliac and femoropopliteal arteries are frequently found. Complete revascularization would seem to be the ideal anatomic and physiological result to relieve the occlusive disease involving the lower extremities. The importance of the profunda femoris artery was emphasized by Morris et al. (12). Since then, many authors have cited the importance of this artery as a collateral vessel for revascularizing ischemic limbs with combined segmental occlusive disease (5, 6, 10, 11, 15). In some patients, proximal revascularization alone will not improve symptoms. In others, an initial good result from proximal revascularization may be followed by sudden or gradual deterioration. Hemodynamic tests have been proved to evaluate or distinguish between aortoiliac and femoropopliteal disease, but no one can demonstrate with certainty which of the patients will need a distal revascularization. Most of the authors have advocated and done staged revascularization (2, 4, 7), and bypass of multiple lesions by one-stage aortofemoropopliteal reconstruction has not been widely practiced, mainly because it was a longer and more formidable procedure with higher mortality and graft failure rates (2, 11). Continued improvements in the care of the patients and the surgical procedures for revascularization has allowed performance of extensive vascular surgery when revascularization of the profunda femoris is not sufficient (8, 14).

We will limit our discussion to our experience in extensive vascular surgery realized on patients with significative unilateral or bilateral aortoiliac and femoropopliteal diseases.

Material and Methods

During the period from January 1975 to January 1980, 70 patients underwent one-stage extensive vascular reconstructions which represents 13.4% of our patients with combined aortofemoropopliteal lesions. All patients were male and ages ranged from 39 to 79 years (average 60.5 years).

Risk factors and associated diseases are recorded in Table 1. Virtually all patients smoked. Hypertension was found in 18.5% of patients; 12.8% had peptic ulcer whereas 18% had evidence of coronary artery disease; 10% of patients had diabetes.

Severe intermittent claudication in 83% of patients and ischemic rest pain or tissue necrosis in 16% were the primary indications for

*Centro Médico Nacional "Marquès de Valdecilla", Servicio de Cirugía Cardiovascular, Santander, Spain

Table 1. Extensive vascular surgery on combined aortofemoropopliteal diseases (N = 70)

Risk factors	No. patients	%
Smoking history	63/70	90
Hypertension	13/70	18.5
Hyperlipidemia	4/70	5.7
Concomitant diseases	**No. patients**	**%**
Coronary artery disease	13/70	18.5
Peptic ulcer	9/70	12.8
Pulmonary syndrome	5/70	7.1
Diabetes	7/70	10.0
Renal disease	4/70	5.7
Cerebrovascular disease	3/70	4.2

Table 2. Clinical and arteriographic findings

Arteriographic findings	Claudication				Rest pain or necrotic lesions	
	100-200 m		20-100 m			
	No.	%	No.	%	No.	%
Unilateral significative lesions (group I)	12/31	38	14/31	45	5/31	16.1
Bilateral significative lesions (group II)	4/39	10	18/39	46	17/39	43.5

operation in 31 patients with unilateral significative lesions of both aortoiliac and femoropopliteal segment (group I). In contrast, rest pain or ischemic necrosis in 43.5% patients and severe intermittent claudication in 56% were the indications for operation in 39 patients with bilateral significative lesions (group II) as shown in Table 2. One-stage aortoiliac and femoropopliteal revascularization procedure was performed on the basis of preoperative angiograms and operative findings if a collateral circulation through profunda femoris artery and distal vascular bed had not sufficient runoff to ensure patency.

Operations performed in each group are shown in Figure 1. In group I, 15 patients were treated by iliac endarterectomy and associated femoropopliteal graft. Another 16 patients were operated by either iliac or aortofemoral graft and concurrent femoropopliteal bypass. In group II, all patients were treated by aortofemoral bifurcation graft. Unilateral femoropopliteal bypass was associated in 74% of patients and 23% of them suffered a bilateral femoropopliteal bypass. All proximal grafts were done with knitted Dacron. An autogenous greater saphenous vein

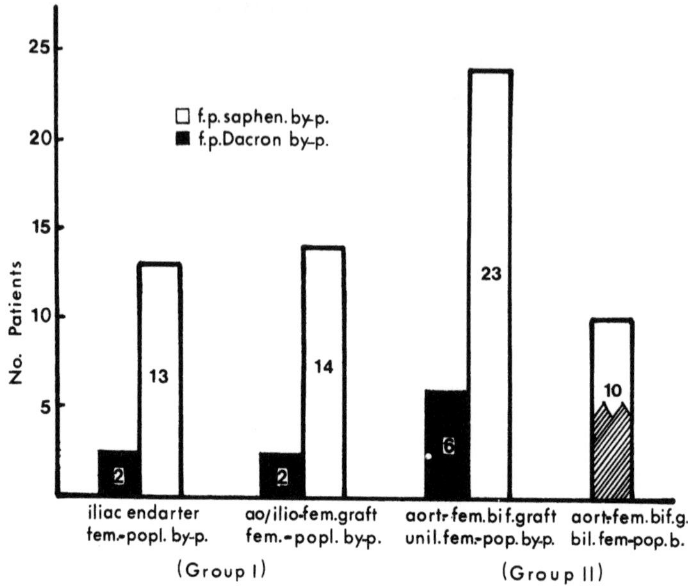

Fig. 1. Operative procedures. Group I, unilateral and group II, bilateral reconstructions

was most commonly used for distal revascularization. Concurrent profundoplasty was performed in 27% of patients and lumbar sympatectomy in 23%. Abdominal aortic aneurysm was resected in six patients. In bilateral extensive reconstructions, two surgical teams were present and the time of operation was reduced.

Results

Average follow-up was 33 months (range 3 to 60 months). There were one early and two late deaths. Mortality causes are shown in Table 3. Comparison of cumulative survival rates for both groups is recorded in Figure 2. Overall survival rate was of 83% at 5 years (heavy line).

Table 3. Operative mortality rate: Causes

	Group I	Group II
Early		
Myocardial infarction (1 mo. postop.)	1	
Late		
Sepsis post-reoperation for graft infection (46 mo. postop.)	-	1
Mesenteric infarction (52 mo. postop.)	-	1

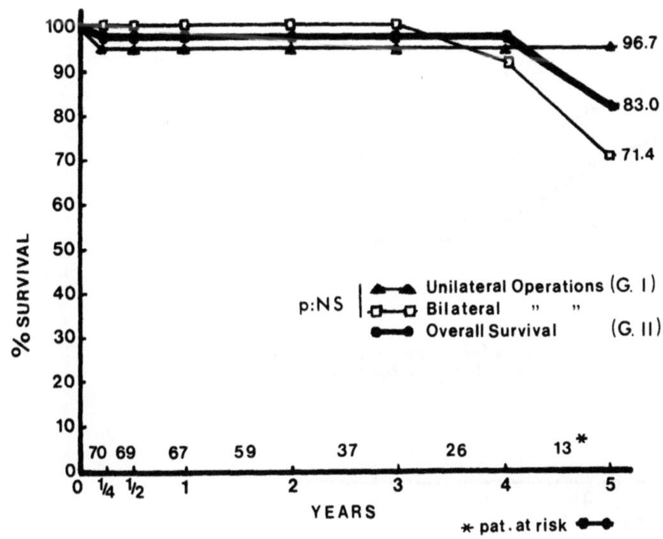

Fig. 2. Cumulative survival rates

Table 4. Cumulative patency rates of unilateral reconstructions (group I)

Interval (mo.)	Limbs at risk	Limbs failing	Cumulative patency (%)
Ilio/femoral endarterectomy + femoropopliteal bypass			
0- 3	15	0	100
3- 6	14	0	100
6-12	14	1	93
12-24	13	0	93
24-36	10	1	84
36-48	6	1	70
48-60	1	0	70
Aorto/iliofemoral graft + femoropopliteal bypass			
0- 3	16	2	88
3- 6	14	0	88
6-12	13	1	81
12-24	7	2	58
24-36	2	0	58
36-48	1	0	58

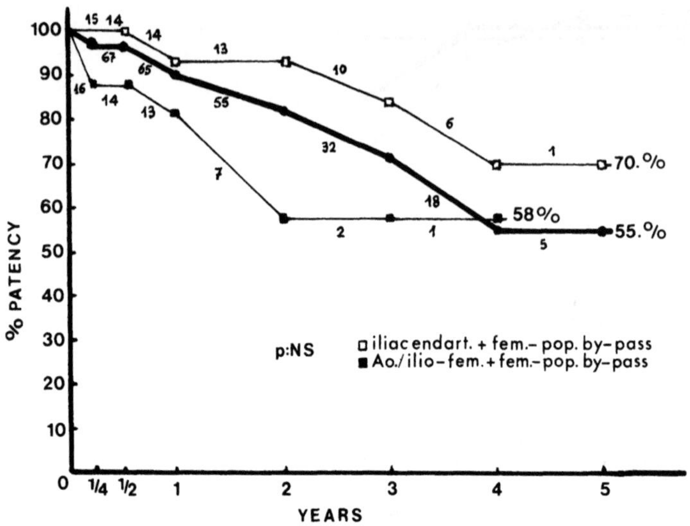

Fig. 3. Cumulative patency rates of unilateral vascular procedures (group I)

Comparison of cumulative patency rates of alternative procedures in group I is shown in Table 4 and Figure 3. Aorto/iliofemoral graft and iliac endarterectomy have an important incidence of failure with time, although both procedures have highly satisfactory long-term patency rates. Superiority of iliac endarterectomy was not statistically significant.

Late patency rates of group II, as determined by life-table analysis, are shown in Figure 4 and Table 5. When compared to other procedures, aortofemoral bifurcation graft with associated unilateral femoropopliteal vein graft demonstrated a superior patency rate at 5 years. Average patency rate of both groups was 55% at 5 years (heavy line).

Eleven patients needed a limb amputation. A comparison of cumulative patency rates and cumulative limb salvage rates in both groups is represented graphically in Figures 5 and 6. Patients with a femoropopliteal Dacron graft had a higher incidence of limb amputation.

Two graft infections occurred and ten patients with femoropopliteal graft thrombosis were reoperated; six of them with initial success needed amputation several months later. The limbs of five patients without possibilities of reoperation were amputated, and five other patients who refused a new reconstruction complain of claudication at present. A total of 67% of patients had excellent or good results.

Discussion

The occurrence of combined arteriosclerotic occlusive disease in both the aortoiliac and superficial femoropopliteal segments is a common clinical entity. Previous series have placed the incidence of occlusion of femoral artery between 45% and 63% (13). Morris et al. (12) drew attention to the value of reconstruction of the profunda femoris artery as a means of salvaging limbs with such advanced arterial disease. Under these circumstances, proximal revascularization and profundoplasty will be successful in most patients (1, 3, 5, 6, 10, 11, 15).

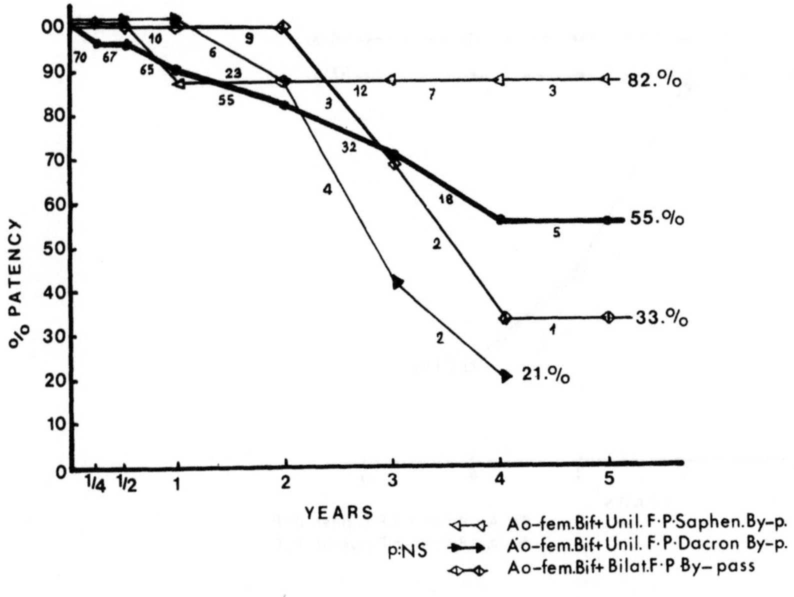

Fig. 4. Cumulative patency rates of bilateral operations (group II)

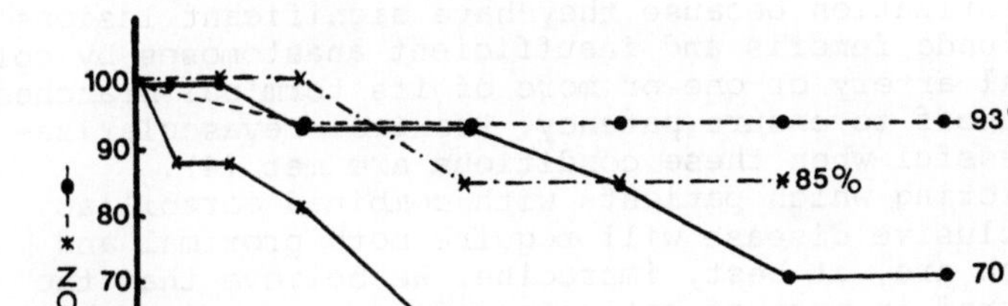

Fig. 5. Comparison between cumulative patency and cumulative limb salvage rates in unilateral vascular operations (group I)

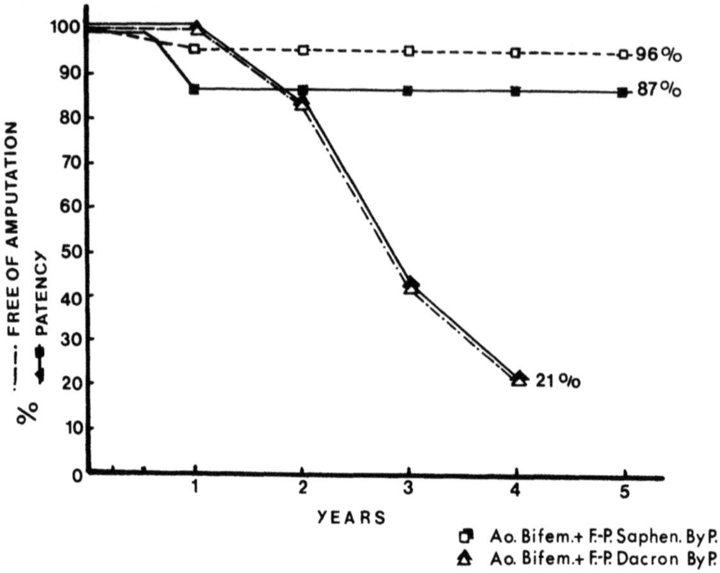

Fig. 6. Comparison between cumulative patency and cumulative limb salvage rates in bilateral vascular reconstructions (group II)

But some patients may have not improvement of lower extremity ischemia after proximal revascularization because they have significant lesions of the branches of profunda femoris and insufficient anastomoses by collateral to the popliteal artery or one or more of its terminal branches that have sufficient runoff to ensure patency. Proximal revascularization will be less successful when these conditions are met (4).

Techniques for predicting which patients with combined aortoiliac and femoropopliteal occlusive disease will require both proximal and distal revascularization are, at best, imprecise. We believe that the staged method is preferred in most of patients and we agree with the experience previously cited by different authors (3, 4, 7, 8, 14). But if preoperative arteriograms and operative findings demonstrate significative lesions of profunda femoris branches and technical difficulties to repair it, we prefer to perform a total aortofemoropopliteal reconstruction in one stage.

Continued improvements of vascular surgery, anesthesic procedures, and postoperative care of patients can reduce the mortality and morbidity rates to acceptable levels, as we have illustrated. Meticulous attention to sterile techniques and the use of prophylactic antibiotics, and reduction of time of operation will reduce possibilities of postoperative infection (9). We believe when one-stage procedure is performed, complications due to reoperation can be avoided.

Our experience in extensive vascular surgery indicates a better long-term result when femoropopliteal vein bypass is associated. Control of risk factors is important in lessening the progression of the basic atherosclerotic process and thereby ensuring the continuation of the good results obtainable by surgical reconstructions.

Table 5. Cumulative patency rates of bilateral reconstructions (group II)

Interval (mo.)	Limbs at risk	Limbs failing	Cumulative patency (%)
Aortofemoral bifurcation graft + unilateral femoropopliteal vein graft			
0- 3	23	0	100
3- 6	23	0	100
6-12	23	3	87
12-24	20	0	87
24-36	12	0	87
36-48	7	0	87
48-60	3	0	87
Aortofemoral bifurcation graft + unilateral femoropopliteal Dacron graft			
0- 3	6	0	100
3- 6	6	0	100
6-12	6	0	100
12-24	6	0	100
24-36	4	2	83
36-48	2	1	21
Aortofemoral bifurcation graft + bilateral femoropopliteal bypass			
0- 3	10	0	100
3- 6	10	0	100
6-12	9	0	100
12-24	9	0	100
24-36	3	1	67
36-48	2	1	33
48-60	1	0	33

References

1. Baird RJ, Feldman P, Miles JT, Madras PM, Gurry J (1977) Subsequent downstream repair, after aortoiliac and aortofemoral bypass operations. Surgery 82:785-793
2. Benson JR, Whelen TJ, Cohen A, Spencer FC (1966) Combined aortoiliac and femoro-popliteal occlusive disease. Limitations of total aortofemoropopliteal bypass. Ann Surg 163:121-130
3. Brewster DC, Darling C (1978) Optimal methods of aortoiliac reconstruction. Surgery 84:739-748
4. Collins GJ, Rich MM, Andersen CA, McDonald PT (1978) Staged aortofemoropopliteal revascularization. Arch Surg 113:149-153

5. Cormier JM, Janneau D (1979) Revascularization associeé des artères fémorales superficielle et profonde par greffe veineuse. Nouv Presse Med 8:1753-1755
6. David TF, Drezner AD (1978) Extended profundoplasty for limb salvage. Surgery 84:758-762
7. De Bakey ME, Crawford ES, Cooley DA, Morris GC (1958) Surgical considerations of occlusive disease of the abdominal aorta and iliac, and femoral arteries: An analysis of 803 cases. Ann Surg 148:308
8. Edwards HW, Wright RR (1974) A technique for combined aortofemoralpopliteal arterial reconstruction. Ann Surg 179:572-579
9. Ehrenfeld WK, Wilson BG, Olcot CN, Stoney TF (1979) Autogenous tissue reconstruction in the management of infected prosthetic grafts. Surgery 85:82-100
10. Hill DA, Jamieson CW (1977) The results of arterial reconstruction utilizing the profunda femoris artery in the treatment of rest pain and pregangrene. Br J Surg 64:359-361
11. Hill DA, McGrath MA, Lord RSA, Tracy GD (1980) The effect of superficial femoral artery occlusion on the outcome of aortofemoral bypass for intermittent claudication. Surgery 87:133-136
12. Morris GC, Edwards W, Cooley DA (1961) Surgical importance of profunda femoris artery. Arch Surg 82:32-37
13. Royster TS, Lynn R, Mulcare RJ (1976) Combined aortoiliac and femoropopliteal occlusive disease. Surg Gynecol Obstet 143:949-952
14. Viver E, Callejas JM, Rodriguez-Mori A, Sobregrau RC (1979) Reconstrucción simultánea de las lesiones obliterantes de los sectores aortoilíaco y fémoropoplíteo. Angiología 31:163-171
15. Ward AS, Morris-Jones W (1978) The role of the profunda femoris in aortoiliac surgery. Br J Surg 65:308-312

Intraoperative Monitoring, Preoperative and Intraoperative Investigation With the Aid of the Ophthalmodynamogram

F. Klinke, H. Dittrich, R. Achatzy, V. Jelesijević, and E. Anyanwu*

The most dangerous complication during operation on the supraaortic arteries is cerebral ischemia which is caused by the temporary interruption of blood flow, with resultant hypoperfusion of the brain.

Several measures are being employed to protect the brain from injury, especially during operations on the carotids. These measures include back flow pressure measurement, EEG monitoring, intraoperative Doppler sonography, determination of the venous oxygen saturation in the jugular vein, operations in hypercapnia, hyperbaria, hypothermia, or in local anaesthesia.

The surest and the simplest way to protect the brain has proved to be the installation of an intraluminal shunt. Despite the high degree of safety which the shunt method offers, we feel that an additional monitoring of the cerebral perfusion is necessary; hence we give preference to the ophthalmodynamography as a method of synchronised measurement on both sides.

With the ophthalmodynamography as described by Hager (2), largely the volume pulse of the ophthalmic artery is measured which as the first large intracranial branch of the internal carotid artery representatively reflects the blood pressure of this artery up to the point of measurements. The analysis of the registered pulse curve allows an assessment of the haemodynamic effectiveness of a stenosis. Furthermore, an assessment of the collateral circulation, the necessity for the use of a shunt, and the recognition of an interruption of blood flow intraoperatively, e.g. through kinking of the shunt or overt exteriorization of the vessel, are made possible. We are able to judge the immediate postoperative success (1, 3, 5, 6).

Material and Methods

Since 5 years, we have performed well over a hundred operations on the supraaortic arteries under ODG monitoring because we reckoned with interference in the cerebral perfusion. We made use of the Infraton Ophthalmodynamograph of Hager-Otte, Boucke Model 350. Having modified this apparatus further, we employ it during the intraoperative monitoring.

The following examples demonstrate not only the procedure, but also the reliability of the preoperatively and intraoperatively recorded ophthalmodynamogrammes. A preoperative ODG investigation on anaesthetised patients who were referred with the diagnosis of a one-sided occlusion of the carotid, can eventually demonstrate on the contralateral side stenosis which was not obvious at the initial examination.

*Chirurgische Universitätsklinik, Abt. Thorax-, Herz- und Gefäßchirurgie, D-4400 Münster

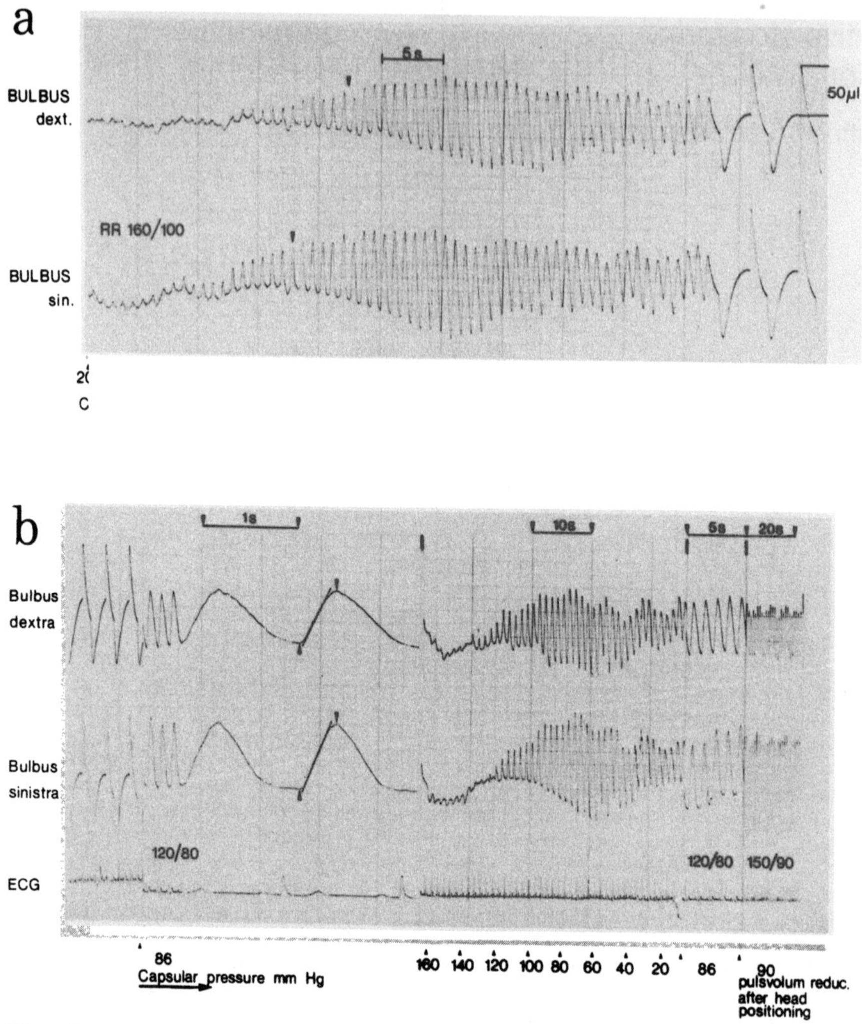

Fig. 1. a Preoperative ophthalmodynamogram in case of subclavian steal syndrome. b Intraoperative ophthalmodynamogram before correction of the left subclavian steal syndrome

A 58-year-old man with a left subclavian steal syndrome, presented in dynamic ODG (Fig. 1a), recorded just before the operation a delayed pulsation and a significant reduction of the amplitude on the right side, thus indicating the presence of a stenosis. The presence of such a stenosis in the area of the origin of the internal carotid was suggested by the angiogram. The ODG from the same patient intraoperatively showed insufficiency of the circulus arteriosus of Willis, thus demonstrating the exigency of the operation of this stenosis at a later date.

A 64-year-old woman, likewise with a subclavian steal syndrome, showed in a preoperative recording (Fig. 1b) only a little reduction of the amplitude both under diastolic capsular pressure and in the dynamic ODG. The form of the curve is otherwise normal. The positioning of the head for the operation led to a significantly higher reduction in the blood perfusion.

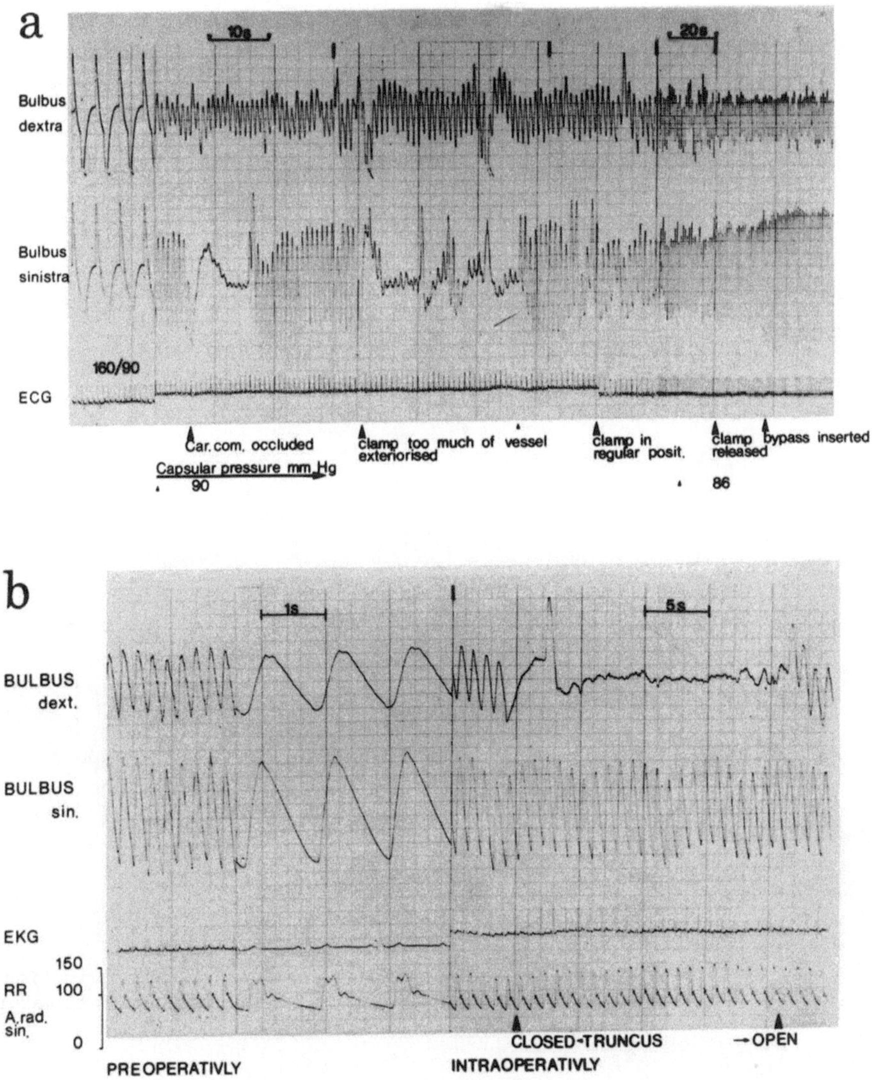

Fig. 2. a Intraoperative ophthalmodynamogram during correction of left subclavian steal syndrome. b Stenosis of the brachiocephalic trunk. Ophthalmodynamogram

Figure 2a shows that clamping of the left common carotid artery leads to cessation of the blood flow. We concluded that the circulus arteriosus of Willis is insufficient. The sequential recordings show that the clamping manoeuvres have to be guarded because extensive exteriorization occludes the vessel and the position of the clamp has to be corrected.

In stenosis of the brachiocephalic trunk, it is important to know if cerebral perfusion is compromised when the vessel is cross-clamped. The recording in a 50-year-old patient (Fig. 2b) demonstrates that the perfusion is interrupted when the trunk is cross-clamped because the circulus arteriosus is insufficient. The clamping would have led to severe cerebral damage in the absence of an adequate vascular compensation.

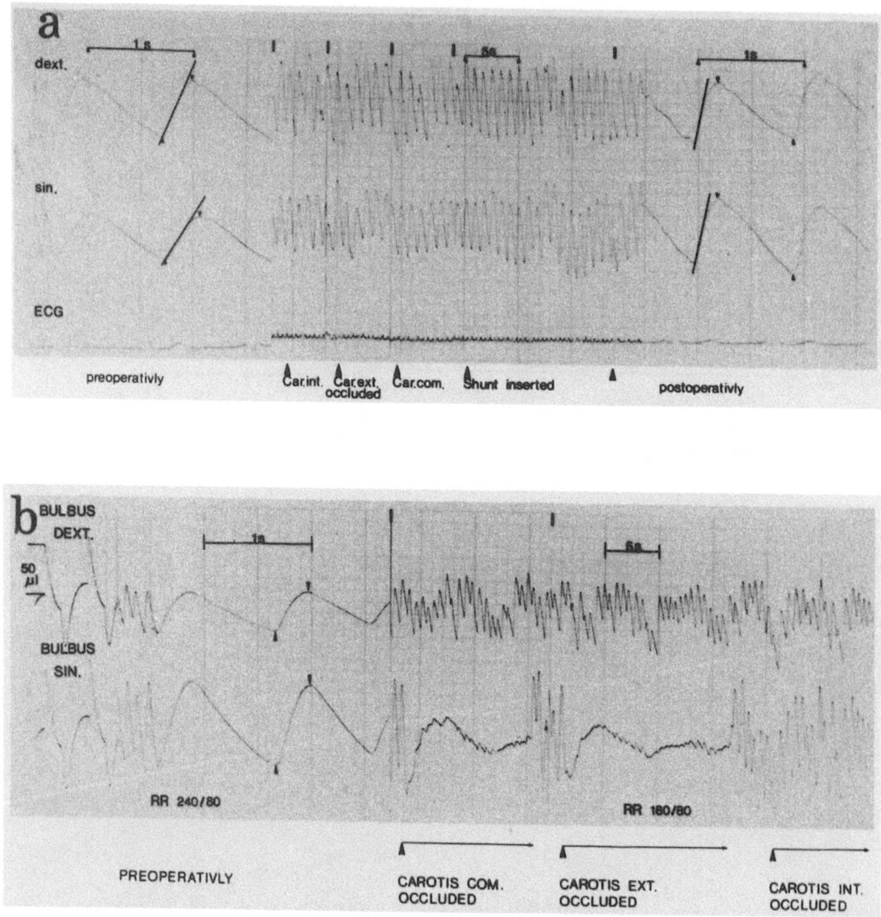

Fig. 3. a Stenosis of left common carotid. Ophthalmodynamogram during correction. b Intraoperative ophthalmodynamogram during correction of the left internal carotid stenosis

A 51-year-old man with the stenosis of the left common carotid has – as judged from the immediately preoperative ODG recording (Fig. 3a) – a good collateral circulation. Following the cross-clamping of both the internal and external carotids, a good collateral circulation is displayed via the circulus arteriosus – as would be expected from the previous recording. We recognise a flat anacrotic angle and a delay of the summit time. Here, too, the operation was carried out employing a shunt.

The recording from a 60-year-old woman (Fig. 3b) shows a good collateralization. She had a subtotal occlusion of the left internal carotid and obvious stenosis on the right side. A trial cross-clamping of both the internal carotid and the external carotid demonstrates that perfusion on the left side does not come from the contralateral vessels via the circulus arteriosus, but exclusively from the external carotid. Clamping of the external carotid would have caused severe cerebral damage. The operation was carried out under the use of a shunt from the common carotid to the external carotid.

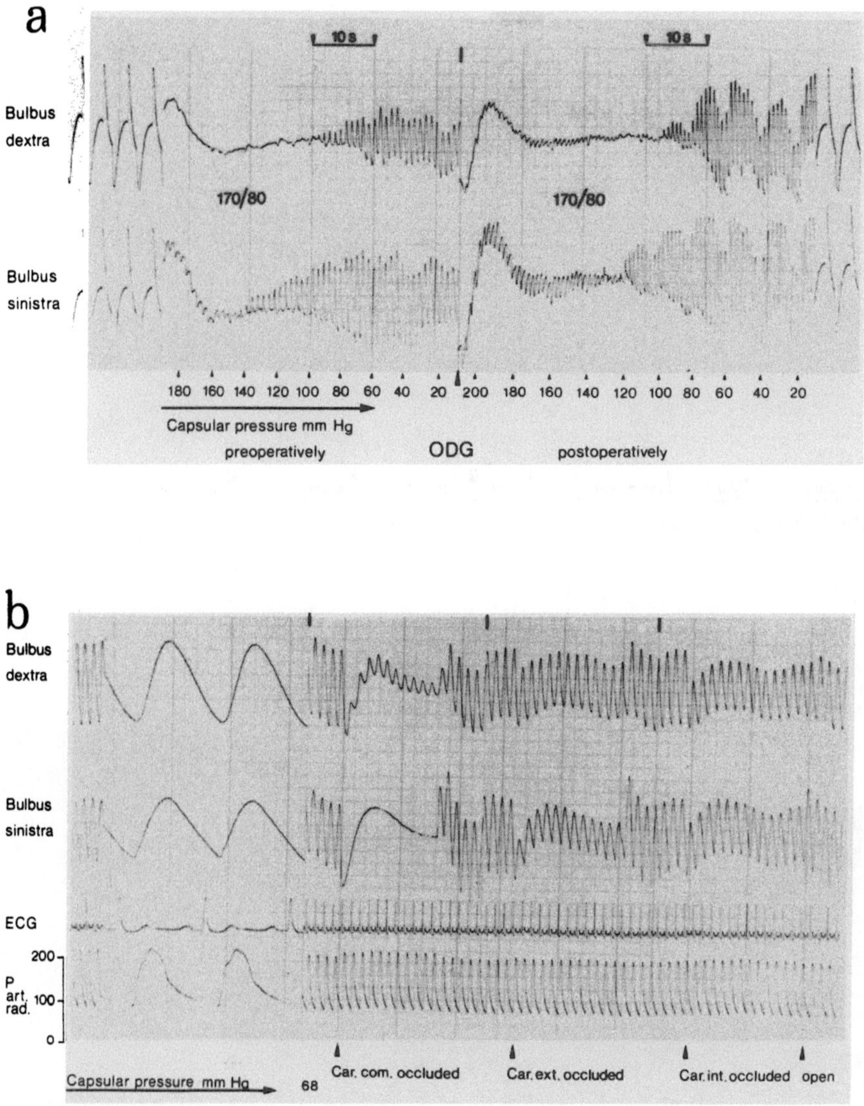

Fig. 4. a Right common and internal carotid obliteration, left internal carotid stenosis. b Intraoperative ophthalmodynamogram during correction of the left internal carotid stenosis

A 66-year-old woman presented with a complete obliteration of the right common carotid and the internal carotid. An explorative dissection revealed an obliterated cord and a stenosis at the origin of the left common carotid. In the dynamic preoperative ODG, a delayed pulse could be recorded (Fig. 4a) on the left side, and on the right, only a collateral pulsation.

c

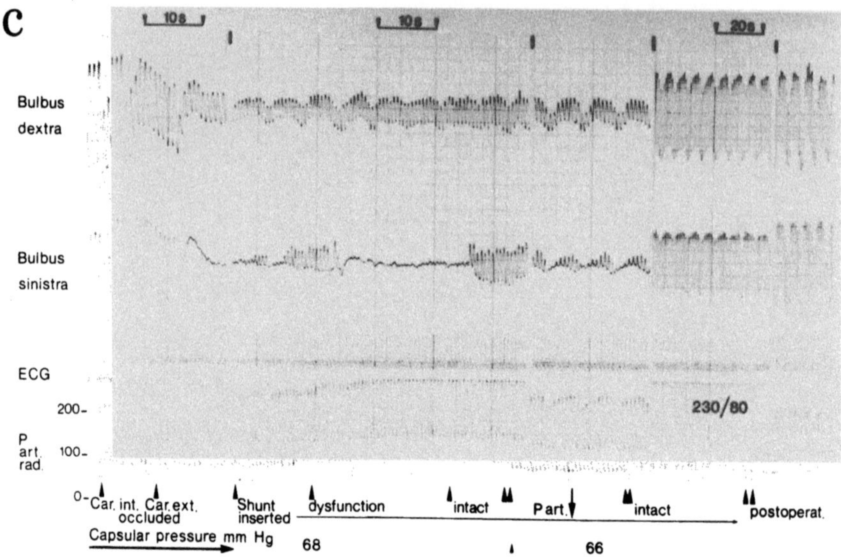

d

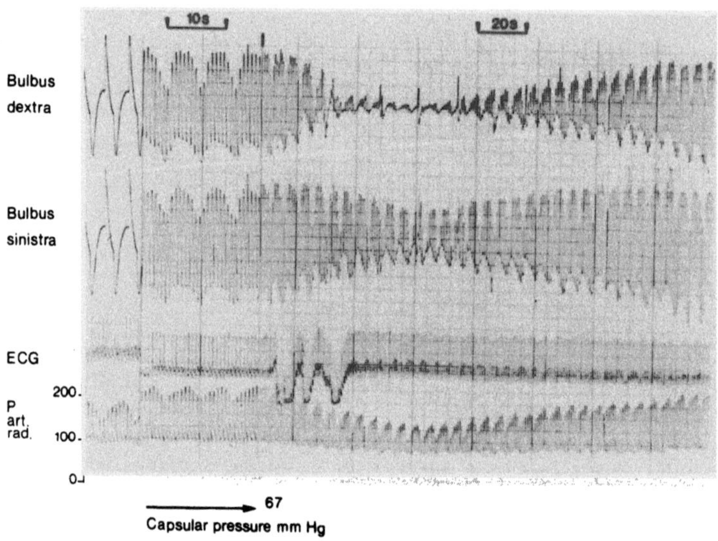

Fig. 4. c Intraoperative ophthalmodynamogram during correction of the left internal carotid stenosis. d Postoperative ophthalmodynamogram after correction of the left internal carotid stenosis

We recorded a little pulsation on the right side, and on the left side we registered a complete interruption of the blood flow on application of the clamp (Fig. 4b). Following the introduction of a shunt between the common carotid and the internal carotid, a reduced blood flow was registered which was very much dependent on the blood pressure. With a fall in pressure, the blood flow was totally interrupted. Raising the systemic pressure allowed a good shunt function (Fig. 4c). Following a patch plastic, good perfusion could be demonstrated on both sides, even with a drop in pressure. This could be documented postoperatively, too (Fig. 4a). The same female patient who, by the way, is hypertensive, had postoperatively a pharmacologically induced drop in blood pressure, the result of which is demonstrated in Figure 4d.

A systolic pressure of 130 mm Hg allows the failure of the collateral perfusion on the right side, while on the left side the perfusion is considerably reduced. This demonstrates the risk of drastically reducing the blood pressure in such a patient.

Summary

In the absence of the obliteration of the ophthalmic artery, the ODG is well suited for the pre-, intra-, and postoperative diagnosis because of its high reliability as a result of a synchronous measurement on both sides, and as a routine monitoring method during all operations on the carotids and when danger to cerebral perfusion arises. The device is not unwieldy; The method is simple, too. The surgeon is not hindered and he can at all stages of the operation get information as to the state of cerebral perfusion. The hemodynamic changes resulting from abnormal convolusions can, in our opinion, be best shown by this method (4). Since we use the ODG as an intraoperative monitoring device, we have not observed any postoperative neurological complications.

References

1. Derka H (1973) Ophthalmodynamographische Überwachung während gefäßchirurgischer Eingriffe an den Halsschlagadern. Vasa 2:233
2. Hager H (1963) Die Bedeutung des Bulbus-Orbitapulses (Ophthalmodynamographie) für die Diagnose der Verschlüsse im Bereich der Carotiden und des Aortenbogens. Verh Dtsch Ges Kreislaufforsch 29:212
3. Hermanns B, Dittrich H, Heger R (1976) Intraoperatives Monitoring der Gehirndurchblutung bei rekonstruktiven Eingriffen an den Karotiden (Abstract). Thoraxchirurgie [Suppl] 1:59
4. Hermanns B, Dittrich H, Jelesijevic V, Knoll D, Storm G (1980) Ophthalmodynamic studies in kinking of the internal carotid artery. Surgical implications. Thorac Cardiovasc Surg 28:61
5. Klinke F, Hermanns B, Storm G, Dittrich H (1980) Monitorische Registrierung der Hirndurchblutung bei chirurgischen Eingriffen an den extrakraniellen Arterien (Abstract). Zentralbl Chir 105:347
6. Strik F (1974) Graphische Analyse der ODG-Pulsationen. In: Frinke J (ed) Ophthalmodynamographie. Schattauer, Stuttgart New York

The intra-arterial Permanent Perfusion With Prostaglandin E_1 for Limb Salvage in Cases With Severe Inoperable Occlusive Diseage in Stage IV

J.D.Gruß, D.Bartels, C.Karadedos, and T.Ohta*

Introduction

Since January 1978, we have been using prostaglandin (Pg) E_1 in our department as a last attempt in advanced inoperable arterial occlusive disease in stage IV. We were able to report about first encouraging results with this substance at the 27th International Congress of Cardiovascular Surgery in June 1978 in Lyon, at the annual meeting of the German Society of Angiology in September 1978 in Heidelberg, as well as at the 11th Congress of the Austrian Society of Vascular Surgery in October 1979 in Graz. We have learned the latter described technique from Shionoya in Nagoya who has been successfully employing this substance in Buerger's disease since 1976 (5, 6). Apart from one report by Carlson and Erikson (1) from 1973, there are – as far as we know – no publications about the administration of Pg E_1 in vascular diseases in the European and Anglo-American literature. Only recently have there been first reports about treatments with Pg E_1, e.g. Sethi (4).

Material and Methods

From January 1, 1978, to December 31, 1979, we found an indication for the intra-arterial perfusion with Pg E_1 in 34 patients. During this period, 1305 reconstructive procedures on the arterial system were carried out. From the numerical proportion you can assume that our indication for this treatment is extremely severe, and this also shows that the choice of patients is an absolutely negative one. All patients were in an advanced inoperable stage IV. Every surgical possibility and all conservative methods had been exhausted. All together, in our 34 patients 67 operations including lumbar sympathectomy were carried out. In each case the amputation of the lower limb would have been the obligatory next step in the treatment schedule.

Twenty-three of our 34 patients were male, 11 female. The average age is 67 years, the youngest patient was 30, the oldest one was 88 years old. The Doppler index of all patients whose gangrenous changes allowed this examination was below 0.2. The local inoperability was, in every case, proved angiographically. Eighteen patients suffered from a severe diabetes requiring insulin; four other diabetic patients were treated with diet or tablets. Ten patients suffered from atheriosclerosis. In six cases, our diagnosis was an endangiitis obliterans regarding the age and the country of origin of the patients as well as the peripheral localization of the occlusions.

*Kurhessisches Diakonissenhaus, Department of Vascular Surgery, D-3500 Kassel

Technique

The femoral bifurcation is exposed from a short inguinal incision under local or general anaesthetic. After inspection and palpation of the vessels, the percutaneous puncture of the common femoral artery is done under direct vision. In order to surely avoid a dissection of the intima, it can sometimes even become necessary to make a short arteriotomy. A thin plastic catheter with an inner diameter of 0.5 mm is inserted through the canula as far as possible, either into the superficial or the deep femoral artery, depending on the angiographic condition. Sometimes, the catheter can only be pushed forward for a few centimeters, in other cases we succeeded in advancing it up to the ankle area. The catheter localization can be controlled by intraoperative angiography. The satisfactory position can be taken from the retrograde blood filling of the catheter. In order to avoid a catheter thrombosis, there must be an instantaneous perfusion with heparin after these manipulations, respectively the intra-arterial infusion has to start at once. The catheter is attached with two 6-0 sutures at the adventitia of the common femoral artery as well as with two 4-0 sutures at the abdominal skin. After this, the plastic tube is fixed with a broad adhesive tape on the lower abdomen. The continuous perfusion is carried out by a portable roller pump produced by the Sharp company (Pip MP-21). The pump is operated by a clock mechanism and disposes of a reservoir with a capacity of 25 ml. In a period of 24 h, 5 ml are continuously perfused. The perfusion liquid contains 0.1 to 0.2 ng of Pg E_1 per kg body weight per min, furthermore 8000 units of heparin/day in a physiological NaCl solution. Our average perfusion period is 33.9 days, the shortest treatment period was 2 days, the longest one was 59 days.

Results

In 11 of 34 cases, a large limb amputation was not avoidable. Four patients died, one of them after an above-knee amputation and one patient after a below-knee amputation; two patients died in the course of the therapy before the fate of the extremity had been decided. Nevertheless, in 21 cases a lower extremity could be kept in function and thus a supply with prostheses or wheel chair could be avoided. In 13 of these patients, however, more or less extensive amputations of toes or forefeet were necessary. In eight cases, large and deep necroses on foot and lower leg healed completely within an amazingly short period of time. The rest pain disappeared. Another partition of our patients is of high interest: Among the 18 diabetic patients needing insulin treatment, 11 had to bear an extensive limb amputation, i.e. all 11 large limb amputations were to be found in the group of severe diabetics. In the group of endangiitis (six patients), only one toe amputation was necessary. Therefore, the results of this treatment may be considered as most successful in this group. The group of uncomplicated atherosclerotics consisting of ten patients is placed, in its results, between patients with diabetes and endangiitis. It is astonishing that the good results once achieved, obviously remain constant for a longer time. During the observation period of 2 years, no later amputations were necessary. After leaving the hospital, all patients received a combined medical treatment with aspirin and dipyridamol which is known under the name Asasantin in West Germany. In those cases without contraindications, the patients were anticoagulated with dicumarol in addition.

Complications

Three times an operative revision, once due to an acute arterial thrombosis, twice because of bleeding after removing the catheter, was necessary. In a third patient, bleeding could be stopped by means of compression and conservative management. A local infection at the point of insertion of the catheter healed without complications after removing the catheter. Local pains with a swelling and red colouring in the area of the catheter tip have been observed in seven cases. After reduction of the Pg E_1 dose or withdrawing the catheter, these complications could be controlled in every case. Once we saw an allergic dermatitis. All other secondary effects of Pg E_1 described in the literature such as generalised formation of oedemas, increasing temperature, tachycardia, hypotonia, lack of appetite, diarrhoea, leucocytosis, increased transaminases, anaemia, and agranulocytosis could not be observed.

Discussion

The above results have two weak points: 1) this is not a randomized study, and 2) the number of patients is far too small. However, as 21 of 34 extremities which actually required an amputation could be saved and kept in a good stage of function, a randomization seems at least critical from the ethic point of view. We do not have any long-term results yet. Contrary to our procedure, Sethi et al. (4) apply Pg E_1 in a dose of 10 ng/kg body weight/h for 72 h. They introduce their perfusion catheter without direct vision, i.e. according to the Seldinger technique which has not shown any disadvantage. With this method, the authors were able to avoid an extensive limb amputation in nine of 25 cases.

The pharmacological mechanism of Pg E_1 has not been fully cleared up until now. In case of the intra-arterial application, the substance has the effect of a strong vasodilator. The vascular dilatation concerns both muscle and skin vessels. The effect of vasodilatation could be angiographically proved by Carlson (1-3). In these obervations, Carlson et al. (3) also describe an opening and increasing diameter of the collateral arteries. It is presumed that Pg E_1 also has a positive effect on the rheological properties of the blood. Moreover, Pg E_1 is an aggregation inhibitor. And furthermore, the substance influences the cell metabolism itself and increases, among others, the permeability of the capillaries. It is not proved to what extent the effects on the cell metabolism as well as the inhibition of the lipolysis represent characteristics which have an essential influence on the peripheral tissue supply. An analgetic effect is being discussed. Pg E_1 is practically fully metabolised on the first lung passage. A smaller portion is also eliminated by kidney function.

Our favourable results considering the desperate condition of the patients in question encourage us to continue the described concept. The patients treated so far will be further followed-up which will enable us, in the future, to present long-term results.

References

1. Carlson LA, Erikson I (1973) Femoral-artery infusion of prostaglandin E_1 in severe peripheral vascular disease. Lancet 1:155
2. Carlson LA, Olsson AG (1976) Intravenous prostaglandin E_1 in severe peripheral vascular disease. Lancet 1:810
3. Carlson LA, Ericsson M, Erikson U (1972) Prostaglandin E_1 (PGE_1) in peripheral arteriographies. Acta Radiol [Diagn] (Stockh) 14:583
4. Sethi GK, Scott SM, Takaro T (1980) Effect of intra-arterial infusion of PGE_1 in patients with severe ischemia of lower extremity. J Cardiovasc Surg 21:185
5. Shionoya S (1978) Continuous intra-arterial infusion therapy of Prostaglandin E_2 for ischemic ulcer of the extremities. XIth International Congress of Angiology, Prague
6. Shionoya S, Matsubara J, Hirai M, Kawai S (1976) Intra-arterielle Dauerperfusion mit Prostaglandin E_1 bei peripheren arteriellen Verschlußkrankheiten. Gekachiryo 213:34
7. Gruß JD, Kawai S, Bartels D, Karadedos C, Tsafandakis E (1979) Indikation, Technik und Ergebnisse der intraarteriellen Dauerperfusion mit Prostaglandin E_1 bei der fortgeschrittenen inoperablen Verschlußkrankheit im Stadium IV. 11. Jahrestagung der Österreichischen Gesellschaft für Gefäßchirurgie, 18-20 Oct 1979, Graz
8. Gruß JD, Kawai S, Karadedos C (1978) Preliminary results with intra-arterial long-term perfusion with prostaglandin E_1 in advanced peripheral arterial occlusive disease in stage IV. 27th International Congress of the European Society of Cardiovascular Surgery, Lyon
9. Gruß JD, Kawai S, Karadedos C, Bartels D (1978) Erste Erfahrungen mit der intraarteriellen Langzeitperfusion von Prostaglandin E_1 bei fortgeschrittener arterieller Verschlußkrankheit der unteren Extremitäten im Stadium IV. Dtsch Med Wochenschr 41:1624
10. Kawai S, Gruß JD, Karadedos C (1978) Erste Erfahrungen mit der intra-arteriellen Dauerperfusion mit Prostaglandin E_1 bei fortgeschrittener arterieller Verschlußkrankheit im Stadium IV. Jahrestagung der Deutschen Gesellschaft für Angiologie, Heidelberg

Preliminary Experience With Prostaglandins E_1 and I_2 in Peripheral Vascular Disease

B. J. Pardy, J. D. Lewis, and H. H. G. Eastcott*

Severe extremity ischemia frequently cannot be relieved by surgical means and failure of current drug therapy results in prolonged disability or amputation. Prostaglandins E_1 (PGE_1) and I_2 (prostacyclin, PGI_2) are potent vasodilators and inhibitors of platelet and leukocyte aggregation, and have been reported to be of value in peripheral ischemia (1, 2).

Twenty patients with severe extremity ischemia have been treated by intravascular infusion of PGE_1 or PGI_2 over 3-4 days. Diagnoses included Buerger's disease, arteriosclerosis, Raynaud's phenomenon, "trash foot", and vasculitic ulceration.

In patients with patent proximal axial arteries, pain was relieved for prolonged periods, tissue healing was excellent, and foot temperature increased by $4.9^{\circ} \pm 3.1^{\circ}C$. In contrast, occlusion of the proximal axial artery was associated with a brief or absent clinical response, and the increase in foot temperature was $0.6^{\circ} \pm 1.7^{\circ}C$. High dose intravenous infusion of PGE_1 was as effective as intra-arterial infusion despite 86% pulmonary inactivation. Side effects of intravenous treatment were not serious and were more prominent with PGI_2.

We conclude that when surgical measures are inappropriate, intravenous infusion of PGE_1 or PGI_2 is the treatment of choice in severe distal arteriopathy.

1. Carlson LA, Eriksson I (1973) Femoral artery infusion of prostaglandin E_1 in severe peripheral vascular disease. Lancet 1:155-156
2. Szczeklik A, Nizankowski R, Skawinski S, et al. (1979) Successful therapy of advanced arteriosclerosis obliterans with prostacyclin. Lancet 1:1111-1114

*St. Mary's Hospital, London and Northwick Park Hospital, Harrow, Great Britain

Vascular Forum IV

Chairman: P. Balas, Athens; Co-Chairman: J. van der Stricht, Brussels

Aortofemoropopliteal Reconstruction in One and Two Acts

B. Vujadinović, S. Anojčić, P. Petrović, M. Djordervić, V. Arsov, and S. Lotina*

The authors have presented their experience in the revascularization of the aortofemoropopliteal region in 88 patients.

Reconstructions have been performed in one or two stages. Reconstructions in one stage (58 patients) have been applied in patients with diffuse lesions of the AFP region, particularly in advanced ischemic lesions of the foot. Reconstructions in two stages were performed:
a) In 10 patients in whom the femoropopliteal reconstruction had already been performed previously but in whom proximal reconstruction has been subsequently performed due to the development of atherosclerotic lesions in the aortoiliac segment.
b) In 20 patients in whom the reconstruction of the aortoiliac segment necessitated the revision of the ostium of artery femoralis profundus in the first stage and in whom subsequent femoropopliteal reconstruction had to be performed due to the development of occlusive processes.

Patients with AFP reconstruction by applying closed desobstruction form a separate group. Due to unfavorable long-term results that type of revascularization has been abandoned.

After one year we performed control examination in 52 patients or 59% of operatively treated.

We found that 86% of aortofemoral grafts were patent, 84% of femoropopliteal grafts above the knee were also patent, 68% of femoropopliteal grafts below the knee revealed patency on control examinations.

*Second Surgical Clinic, University of Belgrade, Yugoslavia

Preventing and Detecting Problems With Femoro-popliteal Grafts

W. T. Davies*

Introduction

Femoropopliteal bypass with autogenous saphenous vein is effective in saving the limbs of patients threatened by ischaemia, with major amputation, even though we are dealing with elderly, and often unfit, patient population. In this personal series, one-third were diabetic, more than one-half had significant cardiac disease and all the non-diabetics were cigarette smokers. On life-table analysis (Fig. 1) it appears that at 5 years approximately 60% will be alive with their own limbs. This is reassuring, but as with many statistical statements, it conveniently omits those patients with ischaemia who were denied the procedure in the first place. For example, in 100 consecutive cases referred to me, of severe limb ischaemia due to clinically diagnosed femoropopliteal disease, only 68 were submitted to arteriography and of these only 39 had femoropopliteal bypass grafting. In other words, case selection can distort results and compensate for surgical errors – if examined in terms of graft patency only.

Femoropopliteal surgery is usually quite straightforward but, as we all know, problems can arise which challenge the surgeon. In the limited time available, I wish to concentrate on four, as listed:

1) Improper placement of the graft.
2) Alternatives to an unsuitable vein.
3) Problems with the outflow tract.
4) Verification of graft patency during follow-up.

Twisting of the Graft

If a vein graft inadvertently becomes twisted during placement in the thigh, this may not be detected at the time of surgery, but will almost certainly lead to early failure.

Marking the vein with an indelible marker or thread along the adventitia, before it is harvested from the thigh, can be misleading, since the in situ vein already has a twist which has occurred during limb development. There are many ways of tackling this problem. For several years, I have relied on this simple instrument (Fig. 2). It consists of two flexible segments of stainless steel which telescope one into the other. It is designed to stabilise the graft during its preparation and to make twisting impossible during subsequent insertion into the thigh.

*University Department of Surgery, Welsh National School of Medicine, Heath Park, Cardiff, CF4 4XN, South Wales, Great Britain

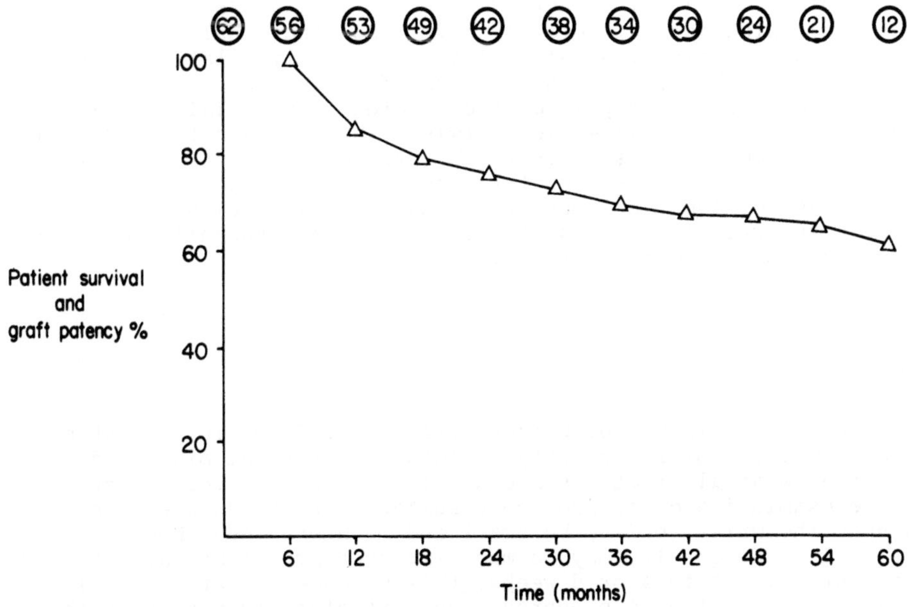

Fig. 1. Cumulative graft patency and patient survival in patients submitted to femoropopliteal bypass surgery using autogenous saphenous vein

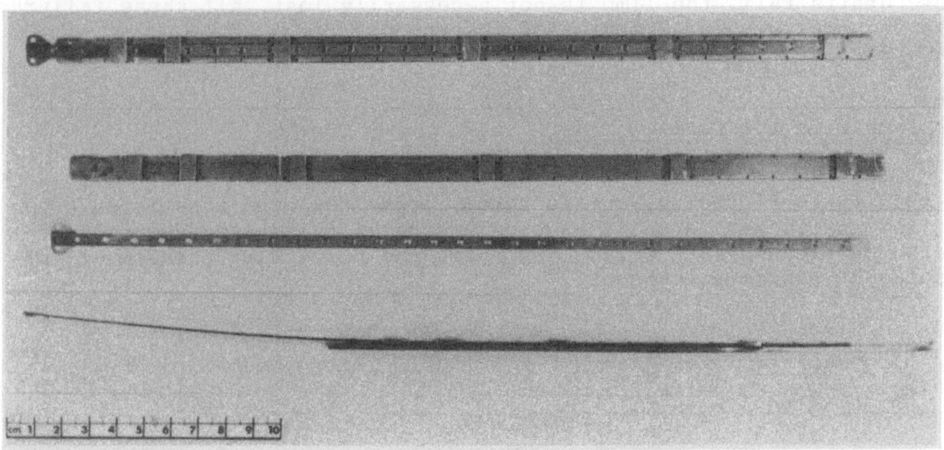

Fig. 2. Photograph of stainless steel vein holder, designed for femoropopliteal surgery

The removed vein is first sewn to the tip of the instrument with two sutures (which are deliberately left long) and a bulldog clip is placed across the vein. The vein can then be gently dilated, so that side branches may be ligated and adherent fat removed.

When preparation is completed, the dilated vein is laid out along the holder. The gentle distension untwists the vein and further rotation is prevented by two sutures to the stem of the instrument (which is adjusted to the required length). The holder and vein can then easily be passed down the lumen of a tunnelling instrument. After picking up the sutures with haemostats, the holder and tunneller are removed using long alligator forceps.

Alternatives to Saphenous Vein

If the saphenous vein has been previously removed (or is present but unsuitable because of its quality, length, or critical minimum diameter), then what alternatives are available? The arm veins should always be examined and may produce a suitable graft. However, the veins near the wrist tend to be small and much branched. Where time is available, the quality may be much improved by a temporary arteriovenous fistula. Within 4 or 5 weeks, this produces a very suitable arterialised vein. I have prepared eight satisfactory grafts in this way. If one does not have time to arterialise the vein, then the human umbilical vein graft may be suitable although, as yet, I can describe no personal experience.

In 18 cases, using synthetic grafts alone or as composite grafts, I have been rather disappointed (Table 1). The figures are small and not worthy of any statistical analysis, but they do show that when these grafts fail, the limb is not necessarily lost. All these failures have occurred within 18 months of insertion.

Problems with the Outflow Tract

In this type of surgery, one is rarely presented with a satisfactory outflow tract. Many authors have demonstrated that this adversely affects the prognosis. I would here raise the particular problem of the "isolated" popliteal segment.

Table 1. Results of femoropopliteal bypass grafting using synthetic or composite (synthetic and vein) grafts

	No.	Failed	Amputations
Dacron	5	4	3
Dacron/vein	6	2	2
Gore-Tex	4	4	3
Gore-Tex/vein	3	0	0

By this I mean the surgical dilemma of whether one should place one's graft into a blind popliteal segment (with the vessels of the trifurcation occluded), or bypass both occlusions into the tibial vessels. I examined this problem with Professor Mannick in Boston, in 60 or so cases, where either procedure was feasible on the preoperative arteriogram. The study showed that with autogenous vein, better early and late patency was obtained by grafting into the popliteal segment. This study (2) was performed a few years ago, but remains my personal conviction.

Verification of Graft Patency

Where one wishes to be objective and critical of one's own performance, careful follow-up is necessary. In the majority it is not difficult using clinical methods to detect whether a graft is patent or not. In a minority it is almost impossible – particularly during the critical period when the graft is near to failure, with a markedly diminished blood flow through it. Most of us would regard arteriography at this stage as too invasive to be acceptable.

In the vascular laboratory I have attempted to measure limb and muscle blood flow, before and after surgery, using a system where the limb under examination is supported in a cradle and able to perform a standard exercise, so as to stress the circulation. A strain gauge around the calf enables plethysmography to be performed in the resting and recovering phases, whilst isotope removal from muscle may be performed during resting, exercise, and recovery periods. In this way, reproducible data are obtained for each subject (1). In a normal limb there is a marked increase in muscle blood flow during the exercise.

In the ischaemic limb, isotope removal may stop completely during exercise. Successful bypass grafting returns this pattern to that of a normal limb. Such laboratory methods are time consuming, expensive, and cumbersome for routine follow-up.

Recently, we have been using a technique of in vivo labelling to study these grafts. This is surprisingly easy and safe. It involves an intravenous injection of stannous methylene diphosphonate (this is allowed to mix in the circulation before the small dose of isotope technetium is introduced into the arm vein). The stannous ion coats the red cells and efficiently binds the isotope to the erythrocytes and avoids the problems of in vitro labelling. Imaging is performed using a conventional gamma camera system with data analysis. Dynamic and static studies can be performed for at least 60 min after injection and the technique is applicable to a variety of vascular studies. It is particularly useful for femoropopliteal grafts and we are now evaluating its semiquantitative application. In six patients, this method has been invaluable in prolonging the patency of a graft about to fail. When this situation was detected, further limited procedures to prolong the patency could be performed.

In summary, therefore, I believe that autogenous vein has "stood the test of time". Alternative grafts produce less satisfactory results but if carefully monitored by clinical and non-invasive physical methods, may still offer an acceptable rate of limb salvage.

References

1. Davies WT (1980) Blood flow measurement in patients with intermittent claudication. Angiology 31:164-175
2. Davis RC et al. (1975) Bypass vein grafts in patients with distal popliteal artery occlusion. Am J Surg 29:421-425

The Haemodynamics of the Side-to-end A-V Fistula in the Wrist

M. Hashmonaai, O. Adler, A. Eithan, A. Rosenberger, and A. Schramek*

Introduction

The consequences of the opening of an AV fistula are changes in the haemodynamics of the systemic and the limb circulation, pressure alterations resulting in regional flow pattern changes near the fistula, and changes in the wall of the vessels between which the fistula was created. Several studies deal with these alterations (1-4, 6, 7, 9-14, 16), the fistula being in the majority of the side-to-side and in a few of the end-to-side types. None of these investigated the haemodynamics of the side-to-end type of AV fistulae. The present study deals with the changes in the regional flow pattern of the side-to-end radiocephalic fistula near the wrist and with the clinical significance of these alterations.

Material and Methods

During the period 1971-1979, 200 side-to-end AV fistulae between the radial artery and the cephalic vein near the wrist were created in 182 patients with terminal renal failure (Table 1). The proximal part of the transected cephalic vein, cut at 45°, was bent and anastomosed to the side of the radial artery by a 6/0 continuous Tevdek suture, creating a stoma of 8 mm and a branching angle of 135° (Fig. 1). There were 17 early occlusions, the remaining fistulae functioning for a period varying from a few months and up to 9 1/2 years.

Table 1. The series

200	fistulae		
182	patients		
		17	early occlusions
		12	low output fistulae
		2	ischaemia of hand
		3	limb swelling

*Departments of Surgery B and Diagnostic Radiology, Rambam Medical Centre, Haifa, Israel

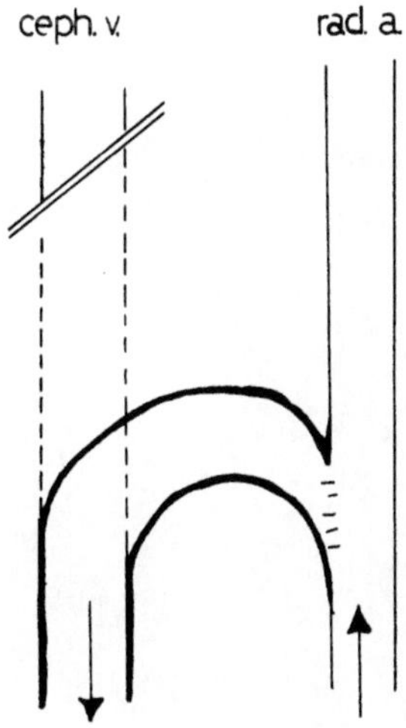

Fig. 1. Diagrammatic representation of the fistula

The flow pattern of the fistula was studied by means of a serial brachial angiography. A 20 gauge needle was inserted into the brachial artery and 20 cc of meglumine diatrizoate and sodium diatrizoate (Urografin 60%, Schering AG) were injected with maximal manual pressure. Four exposures of the forearm and hand were taken with 1 to 1 1/2 s intervals, starting immediately at the end of injection of the contrast material.

In the majority of cases, angiography was performed only in order to assess the haemodynamics of a normally functioning fistula. In 17 patients, the purpose was to study flow disturbances.

Results

In all cases with normally functioning fistulae, the following angiographic pattern was recorded: The blood flow through the radial artery was more rapid and the contrast material filled the fistula while the ulnar artery was still visualized at this stage only up to the middle of the forearm (Fig. 2a). All the proximal radial flow was diverted into the fistula. The flow in the ulnar artery advanced into the hand and all fingers. However, part of it entered the palmar artery arches, backwards into the distal radial artery, and finally the fistula, at a stage in which all contrast material had already disappeared from the proximal part of the radial artery (Fig. 2b). In all long functioning fistulae, the radial and – to a lesser degree – the ulnar arteries were dilated. In most of the cases, there was no retrograde filling of the veins in the hand.

In 12 patients, small outflow of the fistula impaired its utilisation for haemodialysis. Angiography in all these cases demonstrated a stenotic obstacle to the venous outflow of the fistula and no reverse flow in the radial artery distal to the fistula (Fig. 3).

Painful ischaemia of the hand was noticed in two patients. In both, the distal part of the ulnar artery had been ligated during previous shunt operations. Angiography visualized the radial artery up to the fistula only and, even in late pictures, no filling of the arteries of the hand, via either the radial or the ulnar artery. The venous outflow limb of the fistula was very wide in both cases. Clinically,

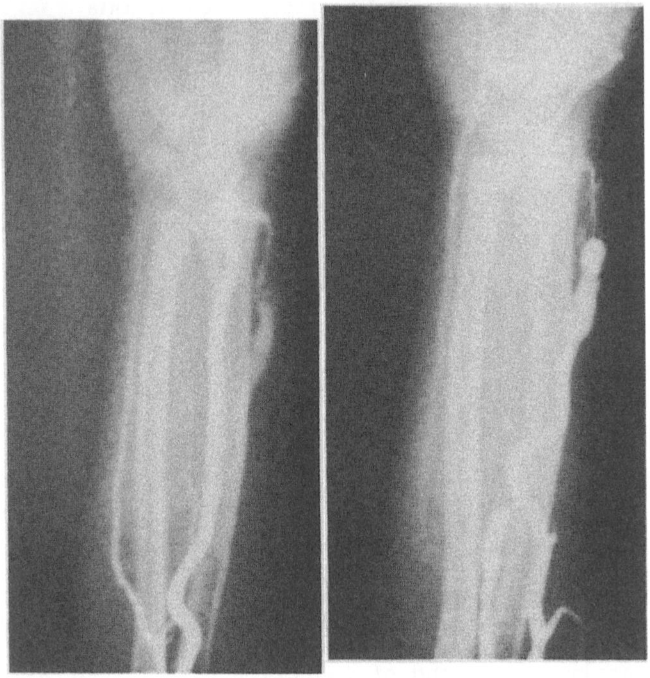

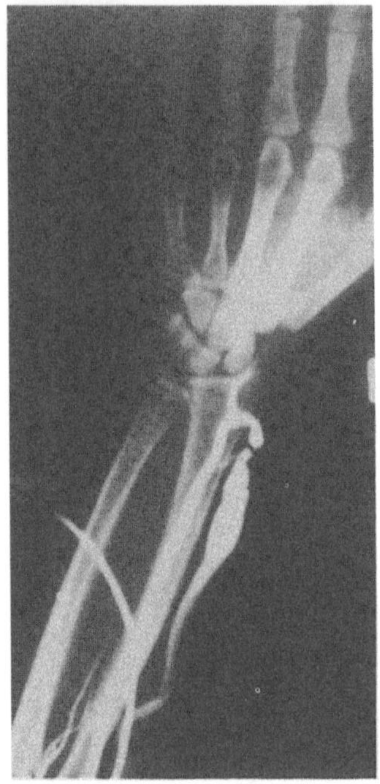

Fig. 2a b Fig. 3

Fig. 2a,b. Angiography of a normally functioning fistula. a Early phase; b late phase

Fig. 3. Angiography of a malfunctioning fistula: early phase

ischaemia was overcome by band narrowing of the fistula in one case, but necessitated complete ligation of the fistula in the second patient.

Extreme swelling of the hand occurred only in three patients accompanied in the first case by severe pain in the hand. Angiography showed in all three cases that most of the contrast material was diverted into the fistula. In all the cephalic vein was occluded and the flow entered the mid-metacarpal vein in a retrograde direction filling an enlarged venous network in the hand. A very poor visualization of the arteries of the hand was obtained, particularly in the patient suffering from pain. Ligation of the fistula in two and of the mid-metacarpal vein in one resulted in complete regression of the swelling in all three patients as well as of the pain in the first case.

Discussion

The direction of flow in the artery distal to an AV fistula depends on the presence of an arterial collateral circulation and on resistance to the outflow in the venous limbs of the fistula. In the femoral region, the anatomical collateral circulation is not always well developed. Thus, reversed flow in the artery distal to the fistula is variable (4, 6, 7, 13, 16). In the radial region, the palmar artery arches are an excellent collateral pathway. Therefore, flow in the radial artery distal to the fistula, as shown in the present and other studies (1, 3, 8, 9, 14), is apparently always reversed. However, if outflow in the venous limb of the fistula is impaired, as in 12 patients of our series, the flow direction in the distal radial artery remains normal.

Despite radiological "steal", clinical ischaemia of the fingers is very rare. Ischaemic symptoms are apparently enhanced by a) an occluded ulnar artery, as in two of our cases, or an occluded proximal radial artery (14), and b) a large stoma and very well-developed venous outflow. Ligation of the distal limb of the radial artery or an end-artery type fistula has been suggested to prevent ischaemia (1, 3). However, flow is diminished in the end-artery type of fistulae (4). Therefore, the authors are of the opinion that rather than making this type of fistula, an accurate evaluation of the arterial circulation of the forearm and hand prior to using a limb for creating an AV fistula should be done.

Swelling of the limb seems to be connected with a reverse flow, dilatation, incompetence of valves, and finally, increased venous pressure in the distal part of the limb (17). Experimental data (6) have shown that in side-to-side fistulae, the pressure in the distal venous limb was significantly elevated as compared with normal values, resulting in oedema. In the published clinical material, this complication occurred mainly in side-vein type fistulae or, as in our series, when the runoff vein flow is impaired (17). As elevated pressures in the runoff channel have been measured (5, 6), it may appear surprising that swelling of the hand occurs so rarely. The answer to this question may be in negative pressures which have been recorded at some levels of the runoff vein (7, 10, 11, 16). The Venturi phenomenon may explain these negative values (7) and may also be the mechanism which prevents venous congestion and swelling in the majority of cases.

The angle at which the vein branches off the artery is important in determining the regional haemodynamics on an AV fistula. In the side-to-side type, the angle of major outflow is a very sharp one. In the end-vein type, many degrees of angulation are feasible. In the present series, an angle of 135° has been used. This was considered to be an intermediate between the 90° angle which, based on mathematical computer model, is supposed to obtain maximum efficiency of flow (12), and the 180° angle (straight line) which gives the least helical pattern of flow and applies the smallest shear stresses on the vessels' walls beyong the fistula (6). These may cause aneurysmal dilatation at the site of the fistula. An obtuse angulation results as well in the minimal intimal changes of the wall of the vein (2, 12). Another advantage of the 135° angle is that it allows the creation of a mild bend, thus overcoming the problem of reversing the direction of flow from the proximal artery into the cardiad vein. The follow-up of the present series (up to 9 1/2 years) has shown that, indeed, no aneurysms developed at the site of the fistula, while those occasionally found in a more cardiad location were always connected with trauma due to repeated punctures in the same segment of the vein.

Conclusions

Based on angiographic studies in the present series of 182 patients with 200 fistulae, we have reached the following conclusions:

1. The radiocephalic fistulae near the wrist result in an anatomical "steal" of blood from the hand.
2. Functional, clinical "steal" develops only when a) the ulnar or proximal radial flow is impaired and b) a large arteriovenous stoma with a very wide cardiad venous limb of the fistula exists.

3. When flow through the cardiad venous limb is impaired, no "steal" is found.
4. Extreme swelling of the hand is connected with massive congestion of the veins of the hand, by reversed flow into these veins.
5. An angle of 135° between the proximal artery and runoff vein of the fistula bears no danger of aneurysm formation at the site of the fistula.

Summary

The haemodynamics of the side-to-end radiocephalic fistula in the wrist have been studied by serial brachial angiographies. Whenever an unimpaired venous outflow existed, a reverse flow in the distal part of the radial artery was observed. Despite this "steal" phenomenon, no ischaemia of the hand was noticed except in two cases in which the ulnar artery had been ligated in previous operations. When the venous runoff of the fistula was impaired by stenosis or segmental occlusion of the major venous channel, the flow in the radial artery distal to the fistula was not reversed. Swelling of the hand in three patients was connected with reverse flow and congestion of the veins of the hand. In the authors' series of 200 side-to-end AV fistulae in the wrist, a 135° angle between the proximal artery and the runoff vein has produced no aneurysms.

References

1. Abbott JA, Campbell M, Bussell JA, Lim RC (1973) Blood flow in end-to-side arteriovenous fistulae and saphenous vein grafts. Kidney Int 3:342-344
2. Bond MG, Hostetler JR, Karayannacos PE, Geer JC, Vasco JS (1976) Intimal changes in arteriovenous bypass grafts. Effects of varying the angle of implantation at the proximal anastomosis and of producing stenosis in the distal runoff artery. J Thorac Cardiovasc Surg 71:907-916
3. Bussell JA, Abbott JA, Lim RC (1971) A radial steal syndrome with arteriovenous fistula for hemodialysis. Ann Intern Med 75:387-394
4. Dawkins HG Jr, Vargish T, James PM (1975) Comparative hemodynamics of surgical arteriovenous fistulae in dogs. J Surg Res 18:169-175
5. Hobson RW II, Wright CB (1973) Peripheral side-to-side arteriovenous fistula. Hemodynamics and application in venous reconstruction. Am J Surg 126:411-414
6. Hobson RW II, Croom RD III, Swan KG (1973) Hemodynamics of the distal arteriovenous fistula in venous reconstruction. J Surg Res 14:483-489
7. Holman E, Taylor G (1952) Problems in the dynamics of blood flow. II. Pressure relations at site of an arteriovenous fistula. Angiology 3:415-430
8. Hurwich BJ (1968) Brachial arteriography of the surgically created radial arteriovenous fistula in patients undergoing chronic intermittent hemodialysis by venipuncture technique. AJR 104:394-402
9. Johnson G Jr, Blythe WB (1970) Hemodynamic effects of arteriovenous shunts used for hemodialysis. Ann Surg 171:715-723
10. Johnson G Jr, Dart CH Jr, Peters RM, Steele F (1966) The importance of venous circulation in arteriovenous fistula. Surg Gynecol Obstet 123:995-1000
11. Johnson G Jr, Peters RM, Dart CH Jr (1967) A study of cardiad vein negative pressure in arteriovenous fistula. Surg Gynecol Obstet 124:82-86
12. Kennedy JH, Wieting DW, Hwang NHC, Anderson MS, Bayardo RJ, Howell JF, De Bakey ME (1974) Hydraulic and morphologic study of fibrous intimal hyperplasia in autogenous saphenous vein bypass grafts. J Thorac Cardiovasc Surg 67:805-813

13. Lavigne JE, Brown CS, Fewel J, Swan KG (1975) Hemodynamics within a canine femoral arteriovenous fistula. Surgery 77:439-443
14. Medical Staff Conference, University of California, San Francisco (1972) Hemodynamic consequences of an arteriovenous fistula. Calif Med 117:38-43
15. Patel DJ, Vaishnav RN, Gow BS, Kot PA (1974) Hemodynamics. Annu Rev Physiol 36:125-154
16. Schenk WG Jr, Martin JW, Leslie MB, Portin BA (1960) The regional hemodynamics of chronic experimental arteriovenous fistulas. Surg Gynecol Obstet 111:44-50
17. Storey BG, George CRP, Stewart JH, Tiller DJ, May J, Sheil AGR (1969) Embolic and ischemic complications after anastomosis of radial artery to cephalic vein. Surgery 66:325-327

Late Results of Femoropopliteal and Femorotibial Bypasses Examined by Transvenous Xeroarteriography

J. Roder*, P. C. Maurer*, M. Reiser**, S. Feuerbach**, and B. Kraman**

Up to now, our experiences with transvenous xeroarteriography (in the following abbreviated TVXA) were concerned mostly with traumatic vessel lesions or localized vascular alterations. The method has proved to be most useful for postoperative control after reconstructive vascular surgery in trauma. In the study presented here, we adopted for the first time TVXA in a series of patients with comparable lesions and operations.

Patients and Methods

In a follow-up study of femoropopliteal and femorotibial bypasses performed in our department, we used TVXA 18 times to clear uncertain findings. Fifteen males and 3 females underwent this procedure. The youngest patient was 58 years old, the oldest was 78. Preoperatively three patients had mild claudication corresponding to Fontaine's stage II a, four patients suffered from severe claudication, i.e., stage II b, four patients had rest pain (stage III), seven patients showed gangrene corresponding to stage IV. Today we agree with most other vascular surgeons that there is no indication for surgery at stage II a.

All bypasses were anastomosed proximally end-to-side to the femoral artery. In four cases, the distal anastomosis was carried out above, in 11 cases below the knee joint. Three patients underwent femorotibial surgery with distal anastomoses to the tibial artery. In 12 cases, we used the saphenous vein, in five cases a Gore-Tex^R graft, to bypass the occluded vessel. One patient received a composite graft consisting of vein and lyophilized bovine carotid artery. This bypass was implanted in 1974.

All patients have been examined periodically. In addition to clinical examination, these patients underwent a treadmill test. We determined the systolic ankle pressure index (in the following abbreviated SAPI) by ultrasound Doppler pressures.

Supplementary to this, we used TVXA in cases with uncertain results. For this examination, we modified a cassette changer for Xerox cassettes. The device has a frame speed of one exposure per second for eight Xerox cassettes. For maximum resolution, the extremity being examined is laid directly on the cover plate of the cassette changer which is equipped with an adjustable support, so that it can be positioned at

*Abteilung für Gefäßchirurgie, Klinikum Rechts der Isar der Technischen Universität München, Ismaninger Straße 22, D-8000 München 80
**Institut für Röntgendiagnostik, Klinikum Rechts der Isar der Technischen Universität München, Ismaninger Straße 22, D-8000 München 80

the level of the table on which the patient lies. The popliteal region and the foot are positioned in lateral view to avoid osseous structures.

In principle, any high concentrated contrast medium can be used. Because of minimal side effects, we prefer Telebrix 380®, a product of ByK Gulden. The usual dose is 1 cc/kg body weight. However, the maximum dose does not exceed 65 cc even if the patient's weight exceeds 65 kg. After warming, the contrast medium is injected into a cubital vein, preferably with the arm raised. The injection is performed manually and usually takes 7 to 10 s. After finishing the injection, we started the cassette changer with an extended interval between the exposures of 2 s.

We did not see serious side effects except a clear flush due to the fast injection of contrast medium. In two cases transient nausea was observed. The study was done on out-patients only. Ten of them were on anticoagulative drugs. All of them left the hospital after a recovery period of 30 min without any problems.

Results

The time between surgery and the study amounted to a maximum of 8 years and a minimum of 2 years. We found seven patients at Fontaine's stage I, eight patients at stage II a, two patients at stage II b. In both patients with stage II b, we had to stop treadmill ergometer test due to cardiac·insufficiency (one case) and arthrosis of the hip (one case).

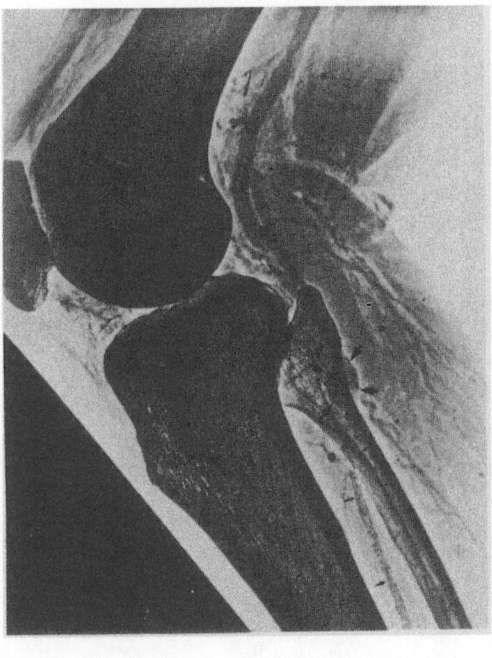

Fig. 1

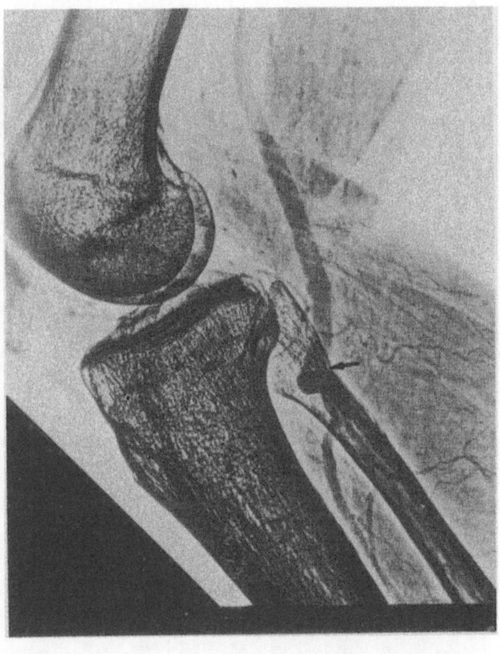

Fig. 2

Fig. 1. Femoropopliteal vein bypass implanted in 1972. Aneurysm of the distal anastomosis. Calcifications along the peripheral vessel

Fig. 2. Patent femoropopliteal vein bypass implanted in 1973

In detail, eight patients with an occluded graft presented sufficient collateralization. In all these cases, we could estimate the runoff. In cases with a SAPI below 1 and occluded graft, we could show good correlation of the extent of collateral circulation and the degree of SAPI. Values in the range of 0.7 and 0.9 correlated with an excellent collateral circulation. Furthermore, we were able to detect an aneurysm of the distal anastomosis (Fig. 1). In another case, we found a stenosis of the saphenous vein bypass close to the distal anastomosis. The bovine composite graft showed ectatic dilatations. Finally in ten patients the graft was patent (Figs. 2 and 3).

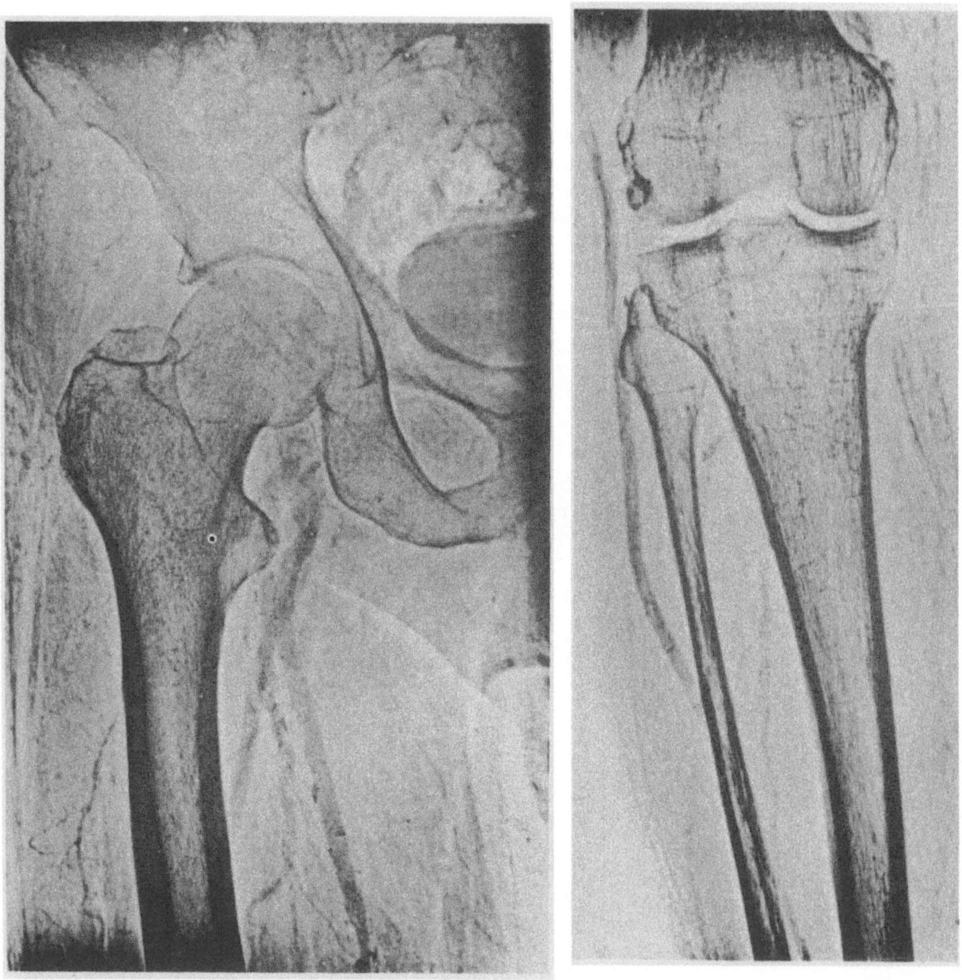

Fig. 3. Extraanatomical femorotibial Gore-Tex® graft implanted in 1977. Patent proximal and distal anastomosis

In comparison to conventional arteriography, there are some disadvantageous facts. The uniform size of cassettes allows examination of localized arterial segments only. In addition, there is a higher radiation exposure. The phenomenon of extinction by overlapping osseous structures creates problems which cannot always be solved by exact position of the extremity.

In conclusion, we may state that the noninvasive transvenous xeroarteriography which can be performed on out-patients by a simple intravenous injection, is a valuable supplementary method to the clinical angiological examination. Avoiding additional injury to an already alterated artery, a definitive statement is possible about the bypass functions even in patients on anticoagulative drugs.

References

1. Kramann B (1979) Transvenous xeroarteriography: Noninvasive method for demonstration peripheral arteries. AJR 133:245-250
2. Maurer PC, Kramann B, Lange J (1978) Erfahrungen mit der transvenösen Xero-Arteriographie in der Gefäßchirurgie. Thoraxchirurgie 26:140-143

Our Experiences With Surgical Treatment of the Asymptomatic Lesions of the Extracranial Cerebral Blood Vessels

P. Petrović, S. Avramov, and J. Pfau*

Indications for surgery, operative risks, and values of prophylactic treatment are now among the main interests in asymptomatic lesions of extracranial segments of the cerebral blood vessels. On earlier investigations it was found that approximately 40% of asymptomatic lesions underwent acute evolutions without previous neurological symptoms. Possibilities of surgical treatment and rehabilitation after acute or chronic neurological lesions are very limited.

We operated 51 cases of the asymptomatic lesions, mainly stenosis on the carotid bifurcation. Comparing results of the operative treatment in the stage of the acute or chronic neurological deficits with those in asymptomatic period, earlier active surgery of the asymptomatic stenosis is highly justified.

Follow-up of our patients varied between 3 months and 7 years. Permanent complications (1.95%) had been found mainly in the first ten operated cases, without immediate postoperative mortality.

Serious prognosis of the natural evolution of the cerebral vessel disease and good results with acceptable operative risk justify prophylactic surgical treatment. In every case of subtotal stenosis, ulcerative atheromas and contralateral lesions as indications for the operation are strictly proposed.

Introduction

Evolution of the asymptomatic lesions of the extracranial cerebral blood vessels is well known and prognosis very serious. The beginning of the disease cannot be predicted and it is sudden, without previous prodromal symptoms, and becomes manifested with acute plaegia. In our previous investigations (6), these developments of the asymptomatic atheromas had been found in over 40% of cases.

Possibilities of the treatment of neurological sequelas and rehabilitation of these patients are very limited. Preventive surgery in the transitory and especially in the asymptomatic stage of the disease are justified only if the risks of the operation are less than risks of the natural evolution of the disease.

*Medical Faculty Novi Sad, Department of Vascular Surgery, Novi Sad, Yugoslavia

Material and Methods

Operative treatment in 51 patients with asymptomatic lesions of the extracranial cerebral blood vessels were analysed. The period of the postoperative evaluation of the results varied between 3 months and 7 years. All patients were operated by standard techniques. Neuroleptanalgesia used for these operations allowed permanent and highly effective neurological control of the brain tissue tolerance on interruption of the cerebral circulation. In every case of inadequate tolerance, Javid intraluminal shunts were used (in approximately 25% of cases on this material).

Typical localization of atheroma on the carotid bifurcation was found in 50 cases. In one patient, central thrombosis of the left subclavian artery was found (Fig. 1), but expected vertebrovertebral steal did not develop because of the anatomic variety of the left vertebral artery originating directly from the aortic arch. In the literature, this variety had been found in 6% of cases (5).

On the arteriography, steal between external carotid and subclavian artery was evident (Fig. 2), but had been asymptomatic. The case was solved by carotid-subclavian bypass, performed from two separate incisions that can be seen on the control arteriography (Fig. 3).

Results

Immediate postoperative results of the prophylactic surgery in the stage of asymptomatic and transitory neurological lesions are presented in Table 1. All intraoperative and early complications were found in the first ten operated patients. Respiratory arrest, thrombosis after successful endarterectomy, and paresis of the recurrens nerve had been transitory, but homolateral plaegia in one patient with later stabilization were permanent complications in this group of asymptomatic patients.

In the patients with TIA, one transitory complication, paresis of the recurrens nerve, and one permanent contralateral plaegia, as results of technical imperfection, were found. We had no mortality in this series of patients. Long-term results of the prophylactic surgery are shown in Table 2.

Table 1. Operative results in prophylactic surgery of CVI

Clinical category	Without any complic. (%)	Transient complic. (%)	Permanent complic. (%)	Op. mort. (%)	Total (%)
Asymptom.	47 (92.17)	3 (5.88)	1 (1.95)	0 (0.0)	51 (100)
TIA	70 (97.22)	1 (1.39)	1 (1.39)	0 (0.0)	72 (100)

One case of worsening after desobstruction of the asymptomatic carotid stenosis was due to malignant hypertension, and another died 8 months after operation from chronic leucemia.

Late mortality in the TIA stage belongs in all cases to the extracranial origin: cardiac insufficiency or infarction (four), acute thrombosis of the abdominal aorta (one), and acute thrombosis of the mesen-

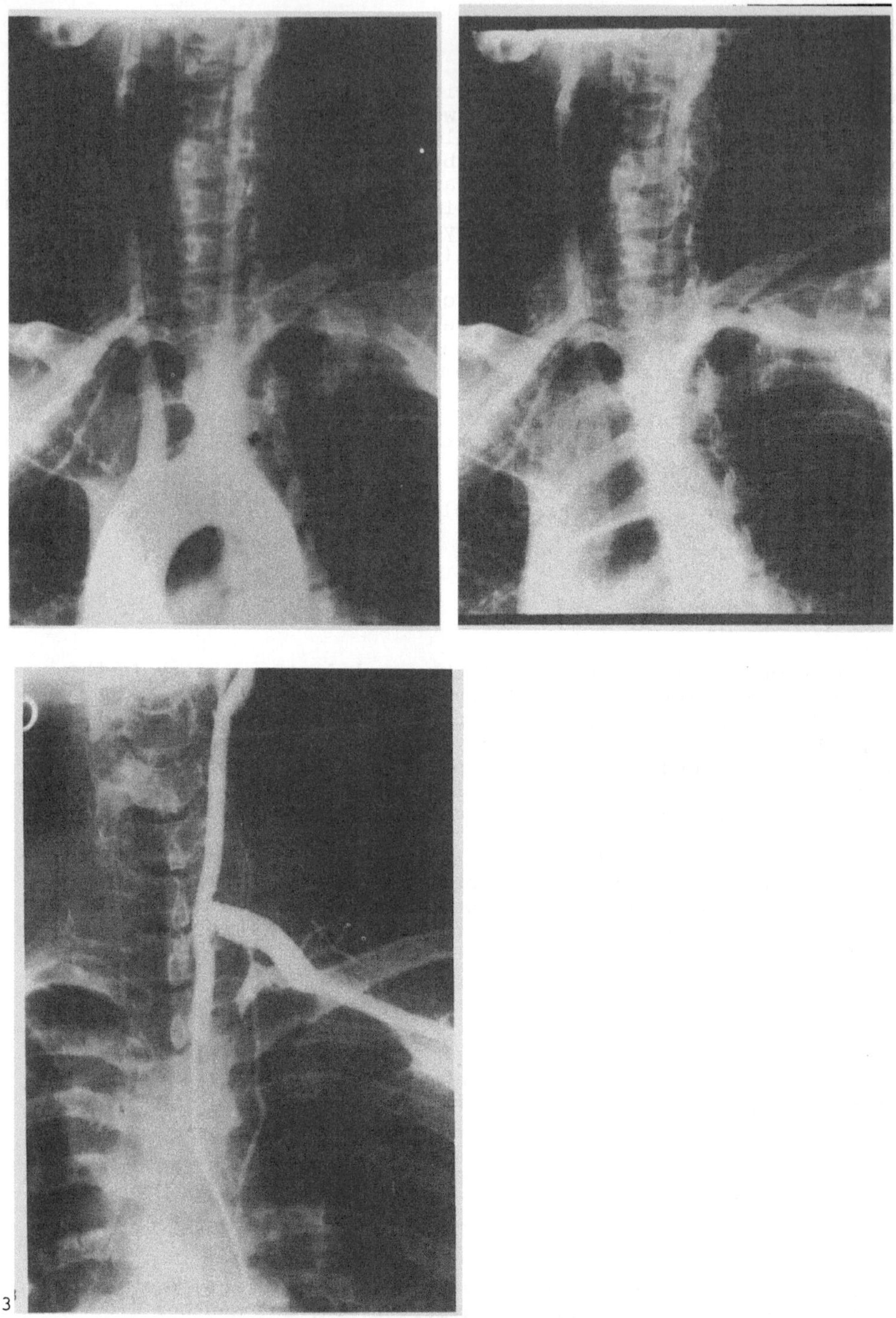

1 2 3

Fig. 1-3. For explanation see text

teric artery (one). Late results of surgery in the stage of chronic or acute neurologic deficits are presented in Table 3.

Results of the surgery in chronic neurologial lesions are average and mortality quite high. In the acute stage of cerebral infarction, however, mortality is enormously high, even when only cases of the successful desobstruction are taken into account. Results of the prophylactic surgery are significantly better than those in the stage of the chronic or acute neurological lesions, both immediately postoperative and later.

Table 2. Late results and mortality in prophylactic surgery of CVI

Clinical category	Good (%)	Worse (%)	Late mortality (%)	Total (%)
Asymptom.	49 (96.08)	1 (1.96)	1 (1.96)	51 (100)
TIA	60 (83.33)	6 (8.33)	6 (8.33)	72 (100)

Table 3. Late results and operative mortality in surgical treatment of chronic and acute CVI

Clinical category	Good (%)	Unchanged (%)	Op. mortal. (%)	Total (%)
Chronic CVI	37 (78.72)	8 (17.02)	2 (4.26)	47 (100)
Acute CVI	16 (53.33)	8 (26.66)	6 (20.00)	30 (100)

Discussion

Operations performed in the neroleptanalgesia permitted good neurological control during test of cerebral blood flow interruption as well as later during operations which are performed in full comfort for both the patients and the surgeon. In case of positive neurological tests, we used a Javid intraluminal shunt. Using this approach with correct operative techniques, the percentage of permanent or fatal complications in the asymptomatic stage of the disease was lowered to a level such that risks of operation are less than that of the natural development of the disease (2, 3). Javid et al. (4) on 208 operations had had 0.5% and Thompson (7) on 94 operations 1.06% permanent complications. In the same category of the patients in our series (51 cases), we had 1.95% permanent complications.

Problems of detection of asymptomatic lesions of extracranial blood vessels must be solved with use of both modern noninvasive and angiographic diagnostic procedures (8).

Subtotal asymptomatic stenosis, ulcerated atheromas of the carotid bifurcation, and contralateral occlusion are strict indications for surgical treatment. Sometimes, urgent surgery after short diagnostic evaluations is necessary in these cases.

Conclusion

Natural evolution of asymptomatic extracranial cerebral blood vessel lesions is well known, serious neurological sequelas probable, and beginning of the clinical presentation could not be predicted. Intra-operative protection of the brain tissue, during temporary interruption of the cerebral blood flow with use of Javid shunts, when indicated by positive neurological tests, as well as good surgical techniques greatly lowered operative risks. Successful operative results and stable effects of surgery in the asymptomatic stage of the disease justify indications for the prophylactic operations.

References

1. Fields WS (1979) Selection of patients with ischaemic cerebrovascular disease for arterial surgery. World J Surg 3:147-154
2. Hejhal L, Firt P (1970) Chirurgicka prevence a liecba mozgove ishemie. Avicenum, Praha
3. Javid H, Ostermiller WE, Hengech JW, Dye ES, Hunter JA, Najafi H, Julian OC (1970) Natural history of carotid bifurcation atheroma. Surgery 67:80
4. Javid H, Julian OC, Dye WS, Hunter JA, Najafi H, Goldin MD, Serry C, De Laria GA (1979) Seventeen year experience with routine shunting in carotid artery surgery. World J Surg 3:167-177
5. Lie TA (1968) Congenital anomalies of the carotid arteries. Excerpta Medica, Amsterdam New York London Paris
6. Orovcanec K, Petrovič P, Zikič M, Ičurup M, Ristič S (1976) Karotidne lezije. Klinicka slika i tretman. Zbornik V Kongresa Neurologa i Psihijatara Jugoslavije, Ljubljana
7. Thompson JE (1979) Complications of carotid endarterectomy and their prevention. World J Surg 3:155-165
8. Thompson JE (1978) Cerebrovascular disorders: A clinical and research classification. In: Goldstein M, Bolis C (eds) WHO Publication No 43, Geneva

Resting and Effort E.C.G. Findings in Patients With Peripheral Vascular Disease

R. J. Vecht, E. Brandao, K. Daskalakis, and A. N. Nicolaides*

Fifty patients with PVD had resting and treadmill ECG (leads I, II, III, AVR, AVL, AVF, V5). Recordings were made at 1-min intervals during exercise, up to 5 min or when limited by symptoms. Postexercise ECG was recorded at 1-min intervals for 5 min.

Results

The mean resting heart rate was 72.5 beats/min rising to a mean of 105 beats/min after exercise ($p < 0.001$). All patients were in sinus rhythm except five with atrial fibrillation. Thirty-seven patients were able to do 5 min exercise, the others were limited by symptoms. Five patients developed ventricular extrasystoles during exercise (one multifocal; one bigeminy).

Twenty-seven patients (54%) had abnormal ECG at rest: eight patients had inferior infarction, one anteroseptal infarction, and 20 ST/T wave changes. Five patients had LAD and two RAD.

Twelve patients (24%) had positive effort ECG; of these eight had abnormal resting ECG.

Summary

More than 50% of patients with PVD had abnormal resting ECG (18% had evidence of previous myocardial infarction); 24% had positive effort tests. More patients would probably have developed positive effort ECG, had they not been limited by symptoms.

Patients with PVD need careful cardiac investigation and monitoring during treadmill exercise in order to identify those at high risk.

*Clinical Cardiovascular Laboratory, Academic Surgical Unit, St. Mary's Hospital, London W.2., Great Britain

Angiography, Ultrasound and the Vascular Surgeon

M. Thick and F. Ellis*

We would like to present our experience with Doppler shifted ultrasound used to extract diagnostic information about diseased arteries. This is offered as the practical viewpoint of a surgeon required to make decisions by the bedside. We are not physicists.

We are fortunate because we have in our hospital an enthusiastic and energetic group investigating the uses to which ultrasound may be applied in the diagnosis of peripheral vascular disease. We have been able to submit our vascular cases to a routine ultrasonic diagnostic assessment and we receive a detailed report on the state of many of the vessels, and their circulation. It occurred to us to consider whether these reports may contain enough detailed information to be sufficient in themselves, and thus make angiography unnecessary in some circumstances. This would certainly be an advantage, because unlike arteriography, ultrasound is entirely non-invasive, has no apparent complications, and is cheaply and simply performed by trained personnel. We have a limited experience with upper limb and carotid disease and therefore confine our remarks to the investigation and diagnosis of lower limb vascular pathology.

Material and Methods

We examined the last 50 consecutive patients who have had both ultrasonic and angiographic investigation. All our results are therefore retrospective. Angiography was usually performed by the translumbar approach, or occasionally transfemorally. Monoplanar views were produced, except when lesions of the profunda femoris were suspected, and then some oblique views were taken. Diagnostic ultrasound was performed using the technique devised by Woodcock and Gosling, and developed by Gosling and his group at our hospital.

Information is extracted by comparing simultaneous velocity profiles of the arterial pulsation at the input and output of an arterial segment. Wave forms are taken from the aorta, the iliofemoral junction, the popliteal artery, and the three ankle vessels. These profiles are displayed as a sonagram where the Doppler shifted signal is plotted as change of frequency on the y axis, and time is plotted on the x axis. The actual density of the plot is a measure of the amplitude of the returned signal.

Three parameters are used to establish normality or disease. The first is pulsatility index which is the ratio of the peak-to-peak height divided by the mean height. The second factor is called the damping factor which is the ratio of the pulsatility indices at the

*Guy's Hospital, Department of Vascular Surgery, London, Great Britain

input and output of the arterial segment examined. The final factor is the transit time which is the time delay between the start of the sonagram at the input of the segment and the start at the output. It represents the delay induced as the pulse passes down the vessel, and is expressed in milliseconds. These parameters have been collected from a large series of both normal and abnormal arteries.

By plotting damping factor on the y axis and transit time on the x, a scattergram is produced. It is found that patients with particular types of lesions fall onto different areas of the scattergram, and therefore it may be used as a diagnostic map by plotting the co-ordinates of the patient upon it.

The actual written reports have been presented to the clinician in a variety of formats. At first we were presented with the wave forms themselves drawn out, but this proved too complex for routine clinical use. At present we receive a typewritten report describing each segment investigated, or a line drawing diagrammatic explanation.

Results

Our comparison of the ultrasound reports with the angiograms show a 26% false negative rate and a 34% false positive rate, using the angiogram as the diagnostic baseline.

Examples of false positive include: 1) Blocks or stenoses reported on ultrasound, but not visible on angiography; 2) ectasia diagnosed as stenosis on ultrasound; 3) poor run-off seen to be good on X-ray. False negative include: 1) Aneurysm or atheroma easily seen on X-ray; 2) segments said to be normal, but the angiogram shows either a block or significant stenosis; 3) run-off said to be good, but seen to be poor on angiography.

The figures given were calculated by scoring each patient report as entirely correct or as containing a false positive or negative statement. It must be stressed that the ultrasound report contains many detailed statements and so, while it is not often completely right, it is very rarely entirely wrong. Of our series of 100 limbs, significant pathology was detected in 96, even though the exact details may have been incorrect.

Conclusions

The ultrasound reports were compared with monoplane X-rays which may have concealed pathology and would therefore count as a false positive ultrasound score. The diagnostic ultrasound reports are limited by the technique. Information can only be offered on the whole segment of vessel lying between the probes whose sites are fixed. No comment can be made about the actual site and length of blocks or stenosis, or of the calibre of the normal vessel. Further, it cannot comment on other relevant pathology or anomaly, for example, a low aberrant renal artery, a blocked internal iliac or profunda femoris artery. This last is particularly important for attempting surgical salvage of limbs of doubtful viability. The particular advantage of ultrasound is that it may be used as a screening investigation for those with symptoms of uncertain origin, and as a monitor of those patients on whom surgery is either not yet required or has already been performed.

We therefore conclude that ultrasonic diagnosis based on pulsality index cannot yet replace angiography in the diagnosis of vascular disease of the lower limbs. However, even now this method significantly narrows the indications for angiography, and it cannot be long before wave form analysis and imaging techniques are sufficiently reliable to relegate angiography to a minor role.

Ultrasonic Doppler Scanning and B Mode Imaging of the Carotic Artery

R. J. Lusby, M. Horrocks, W. D. Jeans, P. C. Clifford, D. T. Hope, R. Skidmore, J. Woodcock, and R. N. Baird*

Cerebral ischaemic attacks may be due to carotid bifurcation disease (3, 4, 6, 10) from emboli arising from atheromatous ulcers or haemodynamically significant stenosis or occlusion of the internal carotid artery (ICA). The need to determine the presence and nature of carotid lesions has been increased with the success of carotid endarterectomy in preventing stroke (8). While preoperative evaluation requires angiography for full assessment of extra- and intracranial vessels, it is not suitable to screen all patients with suspected cervical carotid vessel disease, due to the associated risks (7).

Ultrasound systems have been developed to image the carotid bifurcation directly; they may be Doppler pulsed or continuous wave systems, or real time B-mode scanners. For the past 2 years, we have used the pulsed Doppler system MAVIS (GEC Medical) to image the common femoral bifurcation (1) and the carotid artery (9). Recently, we acquired the real time duplex B mode ATL scanner and now report the results of a prospective trial evaluating the use of these systems in detecting carotid artery disease.

Materials and Methods

Forty-six carotid arteries in 23 patients (17 men and six women, aged between 40 and 63 years) undergoing investigation for attacks of transient cerebral ischaemia were assessed prospectively. Each patient underwent non-invasive testing using techniques: 1) pulsed Doppler imaging using MAVIS, 2) Duplex scanning using the Advanced Technology Laboratory system. All underwent contrast angiography. Each investigation was carried out independently and reported in the absence of any knowledge of the other findings.

Pulsed Doppler Imaging System

MAVIS is a directional 30-channel range-gated pulsed Doppler flowmeter with a focused ultrasound transducer mounted on a position-sensing gantry. The system was developed by Fish (5) for GEC Medical and has a transducer which emits pulsed ultrasounds at 5 MHz. The 30 gates can be adjusted to a suitable depth and the movement of blood is detected by the Doppler shift principle in any or all of the gates.

By moving the probe manually across the skin, an image of the moving column of blood is built up on a storage oscilloscope; a permanent record is obtained by means of a polaroid photograph. Images in antero-

*Department of Surgery, Bristol Royal Infirmary, Bristol BS2 8HW, Great Britain

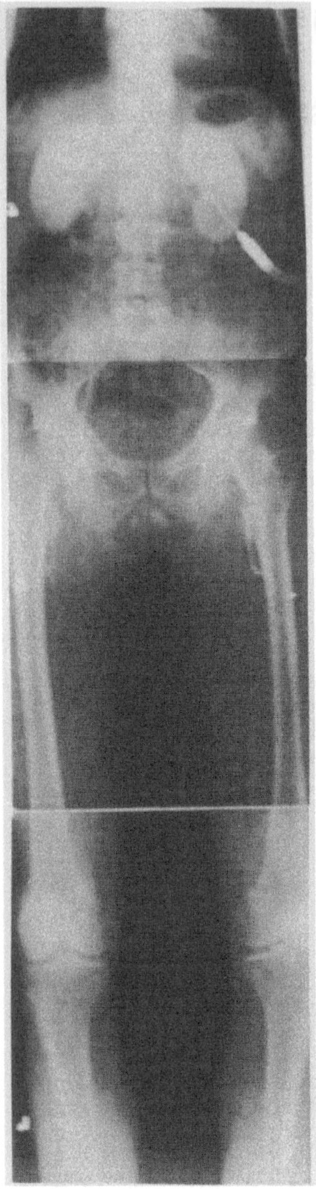

Fig. 1

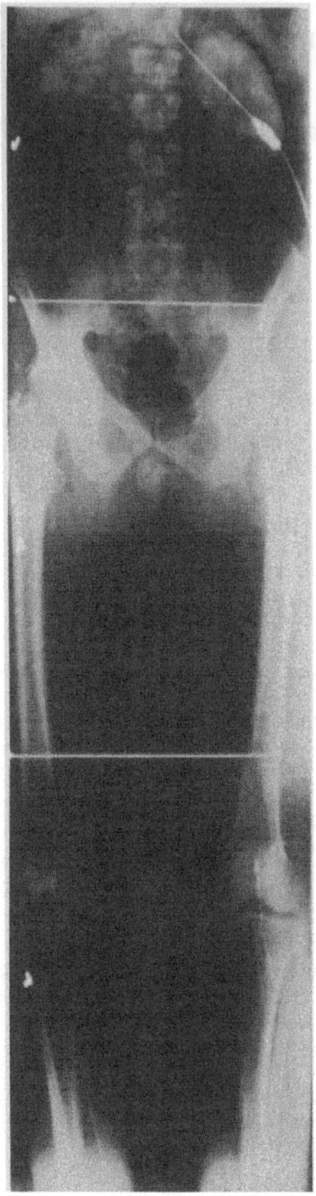

Fig. 2

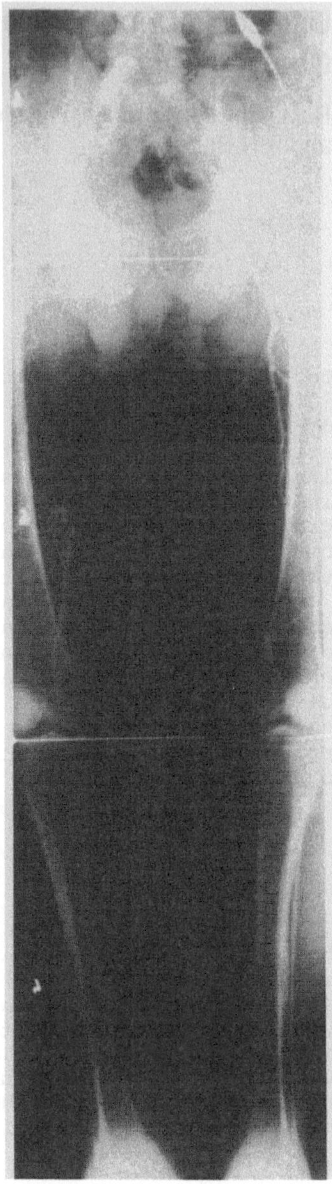

Fig. 3

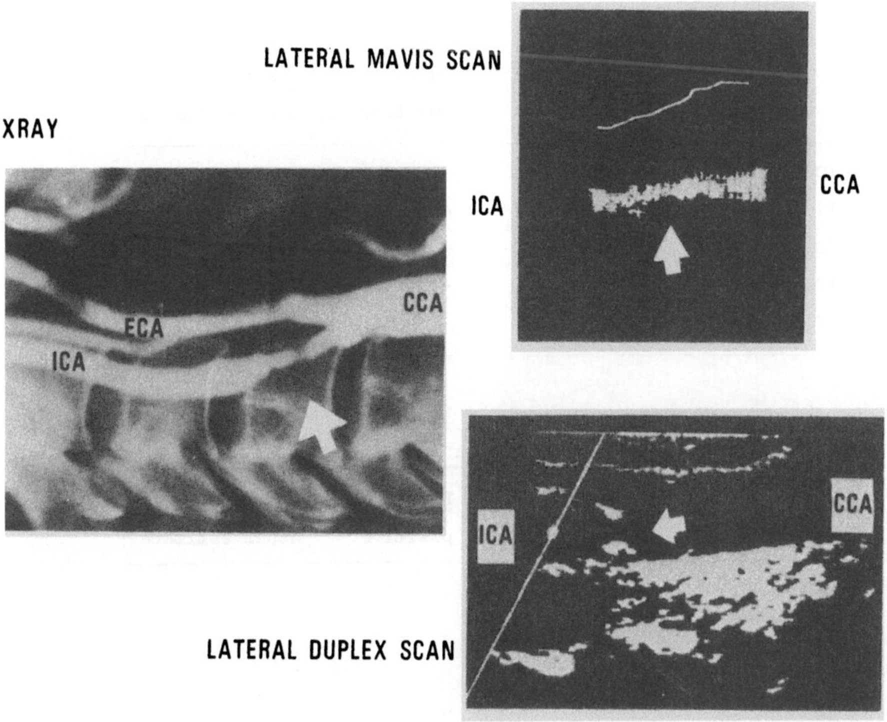

Fig. 1. Arteriogram, lateral MAVIS pulsed Doppler image and lateral duplex scan. The MAVIS scan shows narrowing, arrowed, at the origin of the ICA. The duplex scan shows plaque pushed into the lumen of the same site. Confirmation of the lesion is seen on arteriography

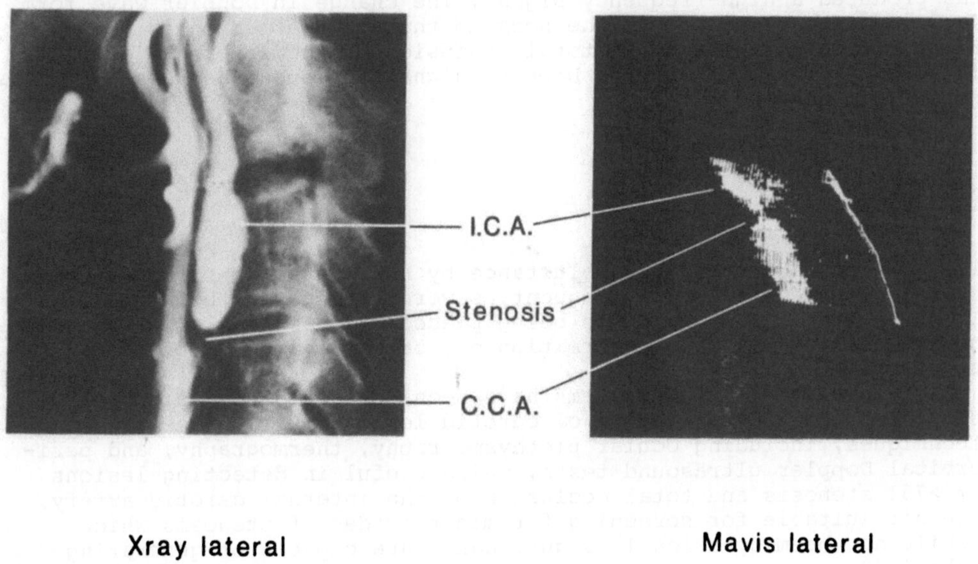

Fig. 2. Lateral MAVIS scan and arteriogram. Note the tight stenosis clearly demonstrated with the pulsed Doppler system

Table 1. MAVIS pulsed Doppler

	No. of vessels	Agreement No.	Agreement %	False positive	Positive other estimate
Normal	10	10	100	-	-
0%-25%	14	10	71	4	-
26%-50%	10	9	90	-	1
51%-99%	10	70	10	-	3
100%	2	2	100	-	-

Table 2. Duplex B mode

	No. of vessels	Agreement No.	Agreement %	False positive	Positive other estimate
Normal	9	9	90	1	1
0%-25%	12	12	85	-	1
26%-50%	9	9	90	-	1
51%-99%	8	8	80	-	1
100%	1	1	50	1	-

In high-grade stenotic lesions, turbulence can be noted on the pulsed Doppler signal and this is seen in Figure 3 where the stenosis has produced a high-frequency signal. The change in Doppler wave form from common carotid low in the neck to that in the lesion is marked. Further towards the head, a total occlusion of the internal carotid is noted by the absence of a Doppler signal although the vessel appears potent on scanning.

Discussion

There is an understandable reluctance by many physicians to perform angiology unless TIAs are frequent, severe, and of textbook quality. This results in many patients being placed on antiplatelet or anticoagulant therapy without confirmation of, or estimation of, arterial stenosis.

Non-invasive imaging systems have been developed to assist in the screening and identification of carotid lesions. Early non-invasive techniques, including ocular plethysmography, thermography, and periorbital Doppler ultrasound tests, while useful in detecting lesions of >75% stenosis and total occlusion of the internal carotid artery, are not suitable for screening for minor grades of stenosis which (while not haemodynamically significant) are capable of generating emboli (2).

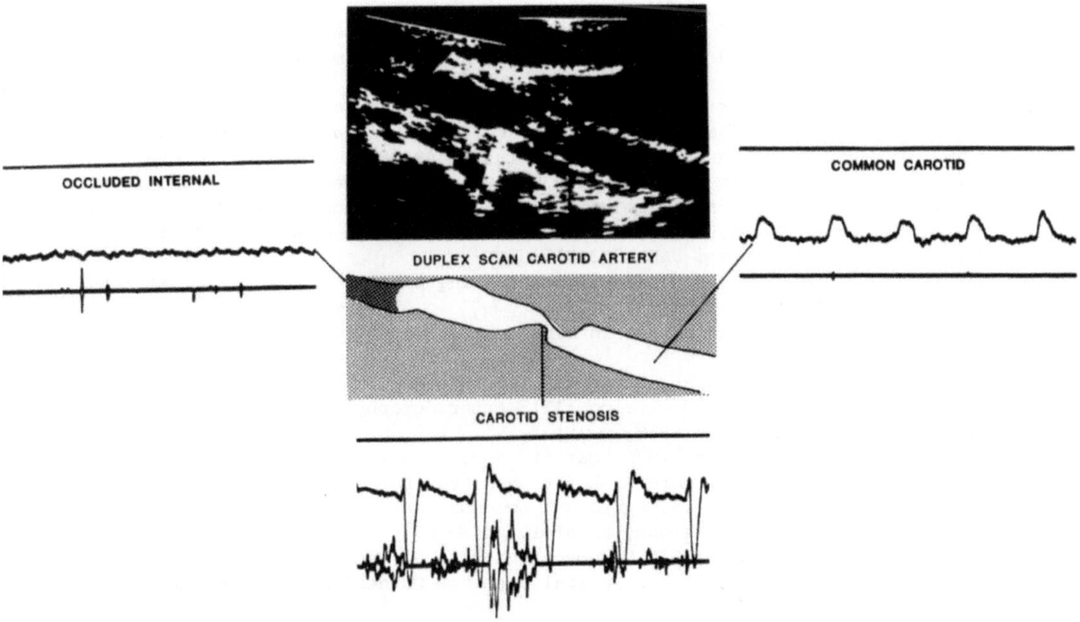

Fig. 3. Composite duplex scan with Doppler wave forms. Note the change in wave form shape in passing from the lower CCA to the stenosis. Occlusion of the ICA is demonstrated by absence of pulsatile flow although the scan shows an apparently patent vessel. Soft thrombus is not detected with B mode imaging

This study suggests that screening for all grades of stenosis may be possible using direct imaging of the bifurcation. Ultrasound systems are most suitable in the assessment of vessels near the surface such as the carotid and femoral arteries (1).

Limitations in their use are those related to heavy calcification at the bifurcation. With the ATL duplex, an umbria or ultrasound lucient area appears under the plaque which, if in the anterior wall, may limit the assessment of the posterior wall. With the MAVIS system this problem also exists but both systems have the advantage of providing multiple views which help overcome the difficulty.

Although our experience is limited, we feel that both systems are able to detect lesions of clinical significance in >90% of instances; in particular they detect the low grade as well as high-grade stenoses. Both are non-invasive and with experience take about 1/2 h to conduct a study.

In practice, we have found physicians now referring patients for ultrasound screening prior to angiography. In addition, the system offers a means of following the results of therapy whether surgical or medical and the progression of disease.

References

1. Baird RN, Lusby RJ, Bird DR, Giddings AEB, Skidmore R, Woodcock JP, Horton RE, Peacock JH (1979) Pulsed Doppler angiography in lower limb arterial ischaemia. Surgery 86:818-825
2. Barnes RW (1978) Doppler ultrasonic arteriography and flow velocity analysis in carotid artery disease. In: Bernstein EF (ed) Non-invasive diagnostic techniques in vascular disease. Mosby, St Louis, pp 40-48
3. Chiari H (1905) Über das Verhalten des Teilungswinkels der Carotid Communis bei der Endarteritis chronica deformans. Verh Dtsch Ges Pathol 9:326-330
4. Fields WS, North RR, Hass WK (1968) Joint study of extra cranial arterial occlusion as a cause of stroke. JAMA 203:955-960
5. Fish PJ (1974) Multi channel direction-resolving Doppler angiography. Excerpta Med Congr Ser 363:153-159
6. Fisher M (1951) Occlusion of the internal carotid artery. Arch Neurol Psychiatr 65:346-377
7. Hass WK, Fields NS, North RR, Kricheff II, Chase NE, Bauer RB (1968) Joint study of extra cranial arterial occlusion (II): Arteriography, techniques sites, and complications. JAMA 203:961-968
8. Thompson JE, Talkington CM (1976) Carotid endarterectomy. Ann Surg 184:1-15
9. Woodcock JP, Hope DT, Skidmore R, Lusby RJ (1980) Doppler scanning of the extra cranial carotid arteries. In: Baird RN, Woodcock JP (eds) Diagnosis and monitoring in arterial surgery. Wright, Bristol, pp 63-68
10. Yates PO, Hutchinson EC (1961) Cerebral infarction. The role of stenosis of the extracranial cerebral arteries. Medical Research Council Special Report Series No 300. HMSO, London

Film Session Cardiovascular Surgery

Chairman: H. Dalichau, Cologne; Co-Chairman: J. Chr. Reidemeister, Essen

Anatomy and Surgical Correction of Total Anomalous Pulmonary Venous Drainage (TAPVD), Supracardiac Type

G. A. Tolis, G. Papas, and C. Stathatos*

1) Anatomy and surgical correction of total anomalous pulmonary venous drainage (TAPVD), supracardiac type (12')

2) Resection of large left atrial myxoma (12')

*"Evangelismos" Hospital, Athens, Greece

Truncus Arteriosus (Rastelli-McGoon Operation)

C. Lolas, H. Karapistolis, M. Iakovidou, V. Hatzigiannakis, and K. Tountas*

This 16 mm *color movie* of 7 min duration is about a female child, 3 years old, who on 20th January 1977, at the age of 7 months, had left pulmonary artery banding for congestive heart failure due to Truncus Arteriosus, type II. Since then, she has improved and she was electively readmitted to our unit. On 24th May 1979, at the age of 3, she had the Rastelli-McGoon corrective procedure.

Technique

1. Cannulations were made to ECC, placing the aortic cannula more distal than usual to permit clamping of the aorta above the level of the pulmonary artery.
2. Hypothermia at 28°C.
3. Transection of the aorta for better access to pulmonary orifices.
4. The conduit containing a porcine heterograft valve was sutured to the open pulmonary trunk with a continuous suture of 5-0 prolene.
5. Restoration of the aortic continuity with continuous suture of 5-0 prolene.
6. The VSD was closed through the right ventriculotomy with a patch of Dacron material, using interrupted sutures of 4-0 silk.
7. The widely beveled proximal end of the conduit was anastomosed to the right ventricle, using a continuous suture of 3-0 prolene. The old "banding" was left in place, not compromising significantly the left pulmonary artery lumen. The "bypass" time was 2 h and 15 min.

The patient survived the main procedure and her arterial blood gases and the hemodynamics were restored to the physiologic level.

*University of Athens, 2nd Surgical Department, Cardiac Division, Athens, Greece

Left Atrial Tumor Simulating Mitral Stenosis Combined With Rheumatic Mitral Insufficiency – Removal of the Tumor and Heart Valve Replacement With the St. Jude Medical Prosthesis

F. W. Hehrlein, J. Mulch, P. Walter, and H. Scheld*

In a 55-year-old patient with mitral insufficiency (stad. II-III NYHA), additional atypical syncopal attacks are registered. The echocardiogram shows multiple signals of a tumor behind the anterior leaflet during systole of the atrium. In the cine-angiogram, a pediculate tumor moving toward the valve orifice can be detected. Resection of the tumor and mitral valve replacement using the new bileaflet St. Jude Medical Prosthesis is demonstrated. Histopathologic examination of the tumor shows a hamartoma. Normal hemodynamic parameters are ascertained by recatheterization 6 months postoperatively.

16 mm magnet-sound, Duration 13 min.

*Klinik für Herz- und Gefäßchirurgie, Justus-Liebig-Universität, D-6300 Giessen

Flow Dynamics xof the Deep Femoral Artery

J. Lange, D. Liepsch, and P. C. Maurer*

Introduction

As early as 1972, Caro (1) expressed the opinion that depositions of cholesterol in the vessel wall occur preferentially in the vessel wall region with flow disturbance, such as we find at vessel branchings and junctions. After Caro postulated that these are a prestage of the arteriosclerotic plaque, Stein and Sabbah (16) measured turbulences for the first time in animal experiments in 1974 and detected a linear relation between the degree of turbulence and deposition of thrombin In detailed investigations, Sandmann et al. (11-14) were able to measure volume, flow, rate of flow, profiles, and turbulences with the pulsed Doppler ultrasound technique reconstructed vessel regions. On the basis of the investigations, we investigated the flow behavior at stenoses at the point of origin of the deep femoral artery or after profunda grafting together with the group of flow engineers.

Statement of the Problem

Up to a certain degree, the arterial system can be treated according to principles of pure hydrodynamics, especially in the region of the large vessels. Under physiological conditions, laminar flow prevails in straight sections of the arterial system. This means that all fluid particles move in parallel with the axis of the vessel at a maximum velocity in the middle of the longitudinal axis and no flow at the wall. A parabolic flow profile results. The limiting value of this laminar flow is expressed by the critical Reynolds number, the value of which is 2000-2300 in a straight tube. If this value is exceeded, disturbed, unstable flow appears which may increase to completely turbulent flow. Transverse movements in all directions then occur besides the main movement in the longitudinal axis of the flowing fluid. This turbulence leads to a reduction of the flow rate in the middle of the tube, to a movement of particles in the direction of the wall and thus to a raised concentration of corpuscular constituents which are retained in the field of turbulence. If these particles now collide with the wall, they may be damaged (especially the thrombocytes) and agglutinate on the vessel wall. In order to show the significance of hydrodynamic disturbances, we have attempted to simulate the flow conditions in stenosed deep femoral artery or after profunda grafting in scale models of the original vessels and to make them visible by various methods.

*Department for Vascular Surgery, Klinikum Rechts der Isar, Technical University of Munich, Ismaningerstr. 22, D-8000 München 80

Methods and Experimental Arrangement

In order to be able to compare an arteriosclerotically altered deep femoral artery with a deep femoral artery widened by patch grafting, we removed the femoral bifurcation with its branching into the superficial femoral artery and the deep femoral artery from cadavers with generalized chronic occlusive arterial disease. In half of the cases, a PTFE extension patch was sewn on previously. Scale models of these preparations were made from transparent elastic silicon rubber. We used the following procedure to make the flow visible:

1. *Flow-Diffractive Fluid*

For qualitative observation of the flow process in the models, various flow-diffractive fluids (vanadium pentoxide and alphanol true yellow) are run through the models. The processes are observed with a photoelastic apparatus with stationary and pulsating flow.

The processes are recorded with a 60 mm camera. In this way, one obtains a complete picture of the flow course. The sites at which all disturbances and turbulences occur can be localized. Information is obtained as to the vessel section in which flow is disturbed. However, these pictures can be evaluated only qualitatively, since with three-dimensional flow an integral effect over the entire transverse section is shown in the pictures. Nevertheless, a certain quantitative interpretation is possible, since the black line shows the current maximum in laminar flow and the colored lines with the same main current difference are different. The sites at which especially high strain occur can thus be shown.

2. *Staining of Flow Threads*

Here one obtains information on the entire flow field, in contrast to the first method. A single flow thread is stained in each case with different high-contrast dye solutions. It is possible in this way to follow the flow course of this flow thread. Thus various processes observed with the flow-diffractive solution can be explained in more detail. This procedure is suitable only for stationary flow conditions. The adjusted flow rates correspond to the physiological rate of blood flow.

Results

Both techniques were now applied to a healthy femoral bifurcation, in a stenosis at the point of origin of the deep femoral artery, and after profunda grafting. The following results were found: From a certain volume flow ratio of the bifurcating vessel flow to the total flow, such as exists in a stenosis at the profunda artery and its point of origin, there are severe turbulences and secondary flow at the origin. A pronounced zone of disturbance opposite to the origin of the superficial femoral artery as well as before and after the origin of the deep femoral artery is found in the region of the stenosis. A laminar flow is no longer present and lines of equal shear are no longer recognizable poststenotically. The dye threads which still arrive bundled together in the common femoral artery are pulled apart at the stenosis and directly after it. Poststenotically, there is a turbulence over the entire cross section of the deep femoral artery (Fig. 1). These flow lines begin to become parallel again very much farther in the

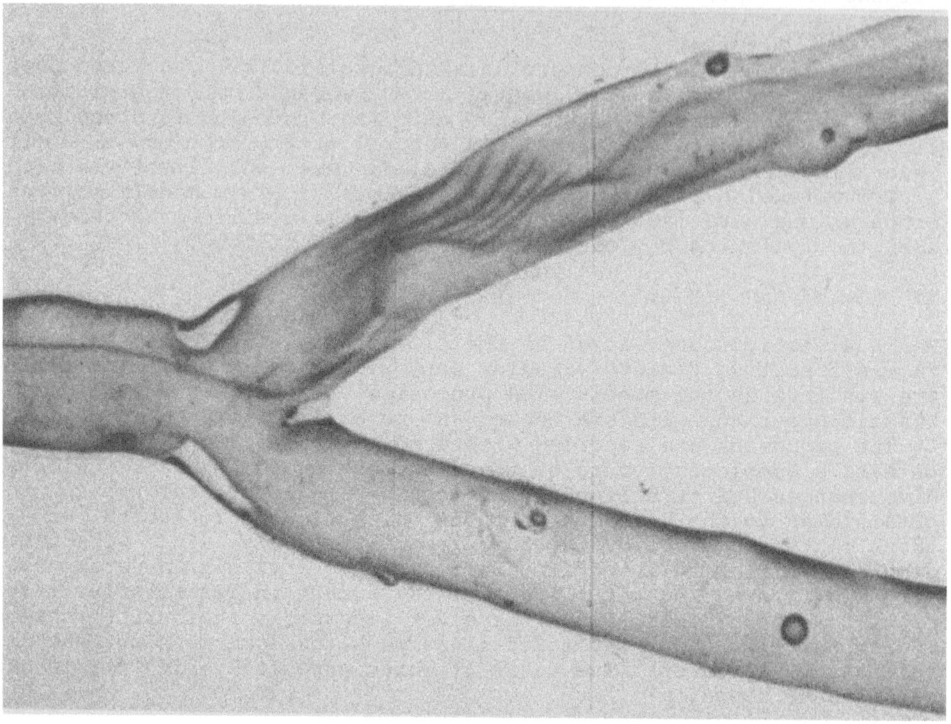

a

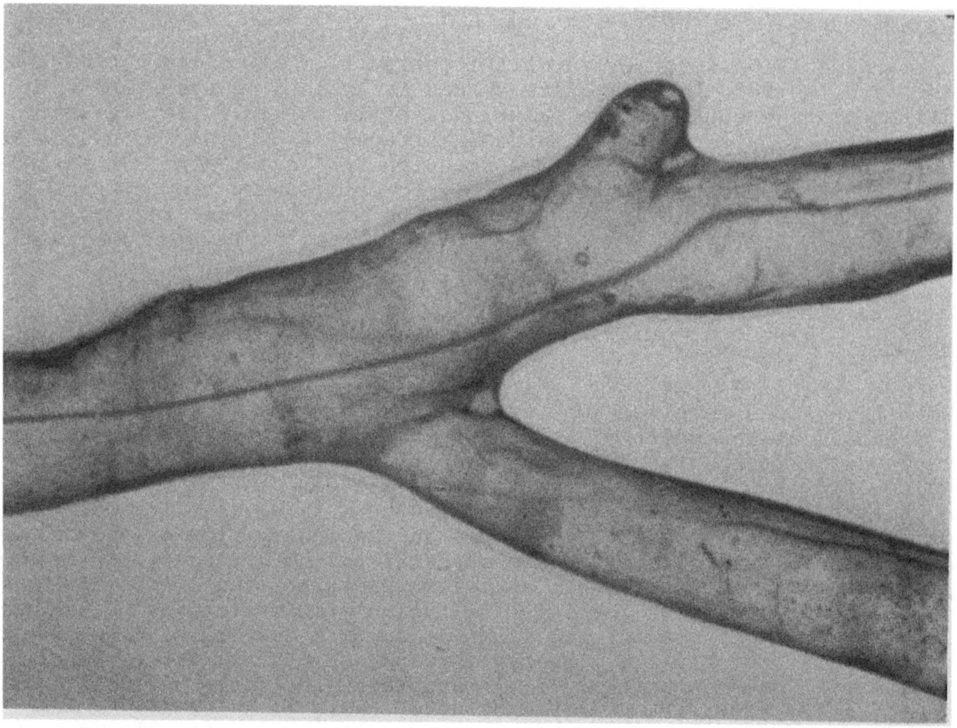

b

Fig. 1a,b. For explanation see text

distal direction, but there are still marked wall detachments even in this region.

If one now corrects the profunda stenosis with an extension patch, a completely different flow behavior results. Turbulences decline and a laminar nondisturbed flow develops again. The fluid particles move parallel to the longitudinal axis of the vessel in the direction of the main flow lines. Only slight wall disturbances which no longer affect the flow course are still found at the edge (Fig. 2). The extension patch thus leads to a marked calming of the flow and to an abolition of the turbulences.

On the basis of these studies, we believe that profunda grafting leads to an appreciable improvement of the flow dynamics in the stenotically altered deep femoral artery. It is to be concluded from this that an ateriosclerotically altered deep femoral artery with stenosis of the profunda artery and its origin, which induces a disturbance of peripheral arterial blood flow, should be widened with a patch graft.

References

1. Caro CG (1971) Atheroma and arterial wall shear; observations, correlations, and proposal of a shear-dependent mass transfer mechanism for atherogenesis. Proc R Soc London 177:109-159
2. Föppl L, Möch E (1972) Praktische Spannungsoptik. Springer, Berlin Heidelberg New York
3. Hagmüller GW (1977) Diskussionsbemerkungen zur IX. Jahrestagung der Österreichischen Gesellschaft für Gefäßchirurgie. Vienna 1976. In: Denck H., Hagmüller GW (eds) Das Therapiekonzept beim chronischen femoro-poplitealen Arterienverschluß. Egermann, Vienna
4. Hagmüller GW, Hold M, Russe OJ (1977) Hämodynamik verschiedener anastomosen Formen beim femoropoplitealen Venenbypass. In: Denck H., Hagmüller GW (eds) Das Therapiekonzept beim chronischen femoropoplitealen Arterienverschluß. Egermann, Vienna
5. Lange J, Maurer PC, Lipesch D (1979) Strömungsdynamik der Arteria profunda femoris: Experimental-physikalische Untersuchungen am naturgetreuen Modell vor und nach Profundoplastik. In: Wagner O, Kibiena K (eds) Der Rezidivverschluß nach Gefäßrekonstruktion an der unteren Extremität. Egermann, Vienna
6. Liepsch D (1975) Strömungsdoppelbrechung. Ein einfaches Verfahren zur Beobachtung von Strömungsvorgängen. Chem Prod 1/2:6
7. Liepsch D (1975) Untersuchungen der Strömungsvorgänge in Verzweigungsmodellen der Herzkranzgefäße mit einer Laser-Doppler-Sonde. Chemie Ingenieur Technik 47:347
8. Linke H (1970) Strömungsfaktoren als Grundlage von Arterienverschlüssen. In: Rotter W., Kief E., Gross D.(eds) Lokalisierende Faktoren für Arterien- und Venenverschlüsse. Schattauer, Stuttgart
9. Malan E, Noseda G, Longo T (1969) Approach to fluid dynamic problems in reconstructive vascular surgery. Surgery 66:994
10. Maurer PC, Lange J, Liepsch D (1979) Experimentelle Untersuchungen zur Strömungsdynamik im femoro-poplitealen Bypass und in der A. profunda femoris (vor und nach Profundaplastik). In: Maurer PC, Fischer M, Scholze H, Thisinger W, Pfohl G (eds) Behandlungsgrundsätze der Chirurgie. Schattauer, Stuttgart
11. Sandmann W (1978) Blutige und unblutige Flußmessung zur Qualitätskontrolle in der Arterienchirurgie. Jahrestagung der Deutschen Gesellschaft für Angiologie. Heidelberg, Sept 21-23, 1978, pp 11-13
12. Sandmann W, Peronneau P, Ulrich B, Bornat CP, Exhaard M, Gisbertz KH (1976) Die Messung von Turbulenz mit Ultraschall-Doppler-Verfahrungen am Strömungsmodell, am Hund und am Menschen. In: Zeitler E (ed) Hypertonie — Risikofaktor in der Angiologie. Witzstrock, Baden-Baden

13. Sandmann W, Peronneau P, Gisbertz G, Bournat JP, Ulrich B, Exhaard M (1976) Untersuchungen zur Turbulenz im normalen und stenotischen Gefäß. Langenbecks Arch Chir [Suppl Chir Forum] 157
14. Sandmann W, Peronneau P, Schweins G, Bournat JP, Hinglais J (1978) Turbulenzmessung mit dem Doppler-Ultraschall-Verfahren: Eine neue Methode der Qualitätskontrolle in der Arterienchirurgie. In: Kriesmann A., Bollinger A. (eds) Ultraschall-Doppler-Diagnostik in der Angiologie. Thieme, Stuttgart
15. Schlicht L (1966) Hydraulic aspects of arteriosclerosis and arterial repair. Prog Surg 5:123-161
16. Stein PD, Sabbah HN (1974) Measured turbulence and its effect on thrombus formation. Circ Res 36:608
17. Wegener K, Goettler K (1970) Die Strömung als Lokalisationsfaktor von Gefäßverschlüssen. In: Rotter W., Kief E., Gross D.(eds) Lokalisierende Faktoren für Arterien- und Venenverschlüsse. Schattauer, Stuttgart

Cardiac Valve Replacement Using Omniscience Pivoting Disc Prosthesis

A. Thevenet*

The new generation of Omniscience valves, an improved version of the Lillehei-Kaster prosthesis, introduces hydrodynamically advantageous specific changes:

1. A radiopaque concave-convex pivoting disc;
2. replacement of the struts by two rounded elevations and reduction of the height of the housing;
3. increase in size of the smaller orifice and larger effective orifice area relative to the tissue annulus diameter.

These design refinements permit maximum unobstructed flow and produce minimal pressure gradients with enhanced flow.

Two cases of valve replacement (calcified aortic disease and mitral, and aortic insufficiency) are described with demonstration of technical steps, as well as myocardial protection, using hypothermic cardioplegia.

Valve function is shown by cinefluoroscopic study and echocardiogram. Long-term effective anticoagulation is recommended. At the present time and for want of ideal valvular substitute, Omniscience valve constitutes a reasonable alternative in the choice of a prosthetic cardiac valve.

Length of film 14 min
Color
Sound = optical
16 mm film

*Hôpital Aiguelongue, C.H.U. Montpellier, France

Mitral Valve Replacement

J. V. Garcia*

This 16-mm color-sound, 30-min duration film shows the operation of a mitral valve replacement in a 12-year-old child who had severe mitral regurgitation secondary to rheumatic endocarditis, frequently observed in the younger population of the Venezuelan Andes.

The film illustrates the usual surgical method employed with this condition at the cardiovascular surgery service of the Andes University.

*Cardiovascular Surgery Service. Medicine School, Andes University, Venezuela

Subject Index

Medical and Surgical Management of Tachyarrhythmias

Editors: W. Bircks, F. Loogen, H. D. Schulte, L. Seipel

1980. 95 figures, 12 tables. VIII, 185 pages
ISBN 3-540-09929-8

Contents: Introduction. – Electrophysiology of Reentrant Ventricular Arrhythmias in the Late Myocardial Infarction Period. – Surgical Therapy of Ventricular Tachyarrhythmias: Experimental Models and Cardiac Activation Mapping Techniques. – Effect of Various Interventions on Myocardial Activation During Ischemia. – Management of Patients with Malignant Arrhythmias. – Pacemaker Therapy in Ventricular Arrhythmias. – Implantable Pacemakers for Management of Supraventricular Tachyarrhythmias: Current Status. – The Automatic Implantable Defibrillator: A New Avenue. – Anatomic Substrates of Ventricular Preexcitation. – Preoperative Localization of Bypass Tract(s) in the Wolff-Parkinson-White Syndrome. – Electrophysiologic Observations During Cardiac Surgery of Patients with the Wolff-Parkinson Syndrome. – Intraoperative Localization and Division of Accessory Pathways Associated with the Wolff-Parkinson-White Syndrome. – Correlations Between Latest Delayed Potentials in Sinus Rhythm and Earliest Activation During Chronic Ventricular Tachycardia. – Is the Reentry Concept a Guide to the Surgical Treatment of Chronic Ventricular Tachycardia? – Intraoperative Delineation of the Conduction System in Corrective Surgery for Congenital Heart Disease. – Surgical Therapy of Ventricular Tachyarrhythmias in Ischemic Heart Disease Using Conventional Techniques. – Subject Index.

1979 marked the 30th anniversary of the Düsseldorf Heart Center. Since its founding, the successful cooperation between the cardiologic and the surgical working groups has produced a number of noteworthy advances, among them the introduction of open heart surgery by means of surface-cooling hypothermia, cardiac catheterization and surgery in patients with acquired and congenital heart disease, and the diagnosis and treatment of arrhythmias.
In recent years, interest at the Düsseldorf Heart Center has turned increasingly to the tachyarrhythmias. New pacing techniques for treating these conditions have been devised, surgical interventions developed to eliminate the "focus" of intractable arrhythmias, and intraoperative electrophysiologic studies (endocardial and epicardial mapping) applied to enhance the success of the surgical procedures. This volume contains the contributions to a special symposium convened in honor of the Düsseldorf Heart Center's 30th anniversary. The papers review past achievements while seeking to stimulate further activities, particularly in the medical and surgical therapy of tachyarrhythmias.

Springer-Verlag
Berlin
Heidelberg
New York

MIX
Papier aus verantwortungsvollen Quellen
Paper from responsible sources
FSC® C105338

If you have any concerns about our products,
you can contact us on
ProductSafety@springernature.com

In case Publisher is established outside the EU,
the EU authorized representative is:
Springer Nature Customer Service Center GmbH
Europaplatz 3, 69115 Heidelberg, Germany

Printed by Libri Plureos GmbH
in Hamburg, Germany